A Dictionary of

Dentistry

ROBERT IRELAND

D0865574

( ) SEE WEB LINKS

Many entries in this dictionary have entry-level web
links. When you see the above symbol at the end of an
entry go to the dictionary's web page at www.oup.com/
uk/reference/resources/dentistry, click on **Web links**
in the Resources section and locate the entry in the
alphabetical list, then click straight through to the
relevant websites.

Over 100 illustrations are also available on the
dictionary's web page. When you see this symbol at
the end of an entry, go to the web page (details
above), click on **Illustrations** in the Resources section
and locate the entry in the alphabetical list.

Robert Ireland was formerly Professor of Primary
Dental Care and Director of the Dental Therapy School
at the University of Liverpool. He is currently Associate
Clinical Professor at the Postgraduate Dental
Education Unit at The University of Warwick Medical
School and is also a presiding examiner for the
National Examination Board for Dental Nurses.

OXFORD
UNIVERSITY PRESS

Great Clarendon Street, Oxford OX2 6DP

Oxford University Press is a department of the University of Oxford.
It furthers the University's objective of excellence in research, scholarship,
and education by publishing worldwide in

Oxford New York

Auckland Cape Town Dar es Salaam Hong Kong Karachi
Kuala Lumpur Madrid Melbourne Mexico City Nairobi
New Delhi Shanghai Taipei Toronto

With offices in

Argentina Austria Brazil Chile Czech Republic France Greece
Guatemala Hungary Italy Japan Poland Portugal Singapore
South Korea Switzerland Thailand Turkey Ukraine Vietnam

Oxford is a registered trade mark of Oxford University Press
in the UK and in certain other countries

Published in the United States
by Oxford University Press Inc., New York

British Library Cataloguing in Publication Data

Data available

Library of Congress Cataloging in Publication Data

Control number: 2010920516

Typeset by SPI Publisher Services, Pondicherry, India
Printed in Great Britain
on acid-free paper by
Clays Ltd., St Ives plc

ISBN 978-0-19-953301-5

1 3 5 7 9 10 8 6 4 2

Preface

This first edition of *A Dictionary of Dentistry* provides full coverage of all the important terms and concepts used in dentistry today. Contributions have been made by a team of distinguished practising dental specialists and dental authors. It is intended primarily as a handy guide for dental practitioners and dental students, but it should prove invaluable as a reference source for all members of the dental team, medical practitioners, lawyers involved with the dental profession, or members of the public. Each entry contains a basic definition followed, where appropriate, by a more detailed explanation or description. Entries are written in clear and concise English without the use of unnecessary dental or medical jargon.

The dictionary defines terms in a broad range of dental specialist areas including primary care, anatomy and comparative anatomy, physiology, biochemistry, radiography, radiology, orthodontics, periodontology, restorative dentistry, dental public health, paediatric dentistry, oral surgery, embryology, homeopathy, pharmacology, sedation, histology, implantology, ethics, and oral medicine. For completeness, some drugs, techniques, or instruments of historical interest have been included. A limited number of biographies of those who are considered to have made a highly significant contribution to dentistry are also described. The frontiers of dentistry are continually expanding with new terms and definitions being defined; where there is a significant level of consensus these new terms have been included.

Entries for dental drugs are given under their recommended international non-proprietary names; where these differ from the names commonly used in Britain, the latter are included both as synonyms and as cross-reference entries. Entries of trade names of drugs or materials have been avoided as much as possible but they are included where they are in either wide or long-term usage.

Derivative words (e.g. adjectival forms of nouns that are defined) are listed at the end of the definitions of the words from which they are derived. A number of entries are supplemented by clear and fully labelled line drawings, where it is considered that their addition complements the written description. An asterisk against a word used in a definition indicates that this term has its own entry in the dictionary and that additional information can be found there. Cross-reference entries simply refer the reader to another entry, indicating that they are synonyms or abbreviations or that they, together with their related terms, are most conveniently explained in one of the dictionary's longer articles. Synonyms and abbreviations are shown in brackets after the defined term. Where within an entry an associated term is described which does not have its own entry elsewhere in the dictionary, the term is written in bold type. A number of feature entries focus on an aspect of dentistry considered to merit a more extensive and detailed description. Many entries could have been expanded had space permitted; in such cases the reader is directed to 'further reading' which provides a reference to articles or research papers which are considered to provide additional relevant and more extensive information.

To avoid cluttering the entry list with a large number of names of anatomical structures, the principal muscles, nerves, arteries, veins, foramina, and sinuses of the head and neck, together with illustrations, are grouped together in the appendices; also included is a list of common symbols and abbreviations used in both the UK and America.

Disclaimer

Oxford University Press makes no representation, express or implied, that any drug dosages in this book are correct. Readers must therefore always check the product information, clinical procedures, and clinical guidelines with the most up-to-date product information and data sheets provided by the manufacturers, and the most recent codes of conduct and safety regulations. The authors and publishers do not accept responsibility or legal liability for any errors in the text or for the misuse or misapplication of material in this work.

List of Contributors

Editor

Professor Robert Ireland BDS, MPhil, MFGDP(UK). University of Warwick.

Contributors

Dr Colette Balmer BSc, BChD, FDSRCS(Edin.), DipCE, PGCertEd. University of Liverpool.
Dr Carole Boyle, BDS, FDSRCS(Eng.), MMedSci, MFGDP(UK), MSNDRCS(Ed.). King's College, London.
Professor David Coleman BA (Mod.), PhD, FTCD, FRC.Path. Trinity College, Dublin.
Dr David Craig, BA, BDS, MMedSci, MFGDP. King's College, London.
Professor Richard Cure BDS, MDSRCS(Eng.), FDSRCS(Edin.), FFGDP(UK), MOrthRCS(Edin.). University of Warwick.
Dr Sarah Ellison BDS, FDSRCS(Eng.). University of Bristol.
Professor Paula Farthing BSc, BDS, PhD, FDSRCS, FRCPath, ILT. University of Sheffield.
Dr Stephen Fayle BDS, MDsc, FDSRCS(Eng.), FRCD(Canada). Leeds Dental Institute.
Dr Andrew Ginty BSc, PGCE, PGLTHE, PhD, FHEA, CBiol. MIBiol. University of Central Lancashire.
Professor William A Gregory DDS. University of Michigan.
Dr Bryan D Harvey BDS, DGDP. Dental Defence Union.
Dr Anna Ireland BDS, MFGDP(UK), MPH. Buckinghamshire Priority Dental Service.
Dr Jane Luker BDS, LDSRCS, PhD, DDR RCR, FDSRCS(Edin.). University of Bristol.
Dr Denise MacCarthy BDS NUI, MA, MDentSc, FDS RCS (Edin.). Trinity College, Dublin.
Mr Joseph McIntyre CGLI Advanced (Orthodontics), LCGI, TQFE (Jordanhill College, Science and Applied Science). NHS Education for Scotland.
Dr N.O. Palmer BDS, PhD. University of Liverpool.
Dr Anthony J. Preston BDS, PhD, FDS, FDSRCS(Eng.), ILTHE. University of Liverpool.
Dr Paul Sutcliffe BSc, DPhil. University of Warwick.
Dr Philip Wander BDS, MGDSRCS, DDFHom. General dental practitioner.
Dr Michael D. Wilkinson BDS. General dental practitioner.

Contents

a- (an-) Prefix denoting absence of, lacking, without; e.g. **atoxic** (not poisonous), **abacterial** (without bacteria).

abapical *adj.* Opposite to or directly away from the *apex.

abarticulation *n.* The displacement or *dislocation of a bone from its normal position (e.g. the *temporomandibular joint).

Abbé–Estlander operation (also known as a **cross-flap**) [R. Abbé (1851–1928), American surgeon; J. A. Estlander (1831–81), Finnish surgeon] A full thickness flap of tissue taken from the middle portion of usually the lower lip and transferred to the upper lip below the nose in order to correct inadequate lip length and fullness caused by surgical excision or growth deficiency. The flap is attached by means of a pedicle to maintain the blood supply. *See also* GRAFT.

ABCDE approach The method of assessment of critically ill patients and those suffering from cardiorespiratory arrest. A = Airway, B = Breathing, C = Circulation, D = Disability, E = Exposure. It provides an aide-memoire for providing assessment in an appropriate chronological sequence.

⊕ SEE WEB LINKS

• The Resuscitation Council (UK): Medical emergencies and resuscitation.

abdomen *n.* (*adj.* **abdominal**) That part of the body cavity below the chest and separated from it by the diaphragm. It contains a number of organs including the stomach, liver, kidneys, spleen, pancreas, and intestines.

abdominal thrust *See* HEIMLICH MANOEUVRE.

abduction *n.* Movement away from the midline; e.g. the lateral rectus muscle is an abductor of the eye.

aberrant *adj.* Deviating from the normal. Usually applied to a blood vessel or nerve that fails to follow its normal course.

abfraction *n.* The loss of tooth structure in the *cervical region of the *crown of a tooth. Some research studies suggest that this is owing to flexural forces applying an excessive biomechanical loading to one or more *cusps of the tooth, resulting in stress concentration. 🔘

Further Reading: Bartlett D. W., Shah P. A critical review of non-carious cervical (wear) lesions and the role of abfraction, erosion, and abrasion. *J Dent Res* 2006;85:306–12.
Rees J. S. The biomechanics of abfraction. *J of Engineering in Medicine* 2006;220:69–80.

ablation *n.* The removal or excision of a piece of tissue, usually by surgery. Surface ablation of the skin may be carried out by chemicals or *laser.

abrasion *n.* 1. The non-bacterial loss of tooth tissue due to frictional wear by extrinsic agents. Common causes are *toothbrushing, particularly with abrasive pastes, pipe smoking, and pencil chewing. The lesions produced by toothbrush abrasion are typically wedge-shaped and are most commonly associated with the labial and buccal surfaces of the premolars, canines, and incisors of the permanent dentition. Similar causes can result in **gingival abrasion** with loss or damage to the gingival tissues. 2. A minor wound in which the surface of the skin or mucous membrane is worn away by frictional trauma. *See also* TOOTH WEAR. 🔘

Further Reading: Bartlett D. W., Shah P. A critical review of non-carious cervical (wear) lesions and the role of abfraction, erosion, and abrasion. *J Dent Res* 2006;85:306–12.

abrasive *n.* A material used to smooth or roughen a softer material by mechanical wear. It may be delivered in a high pressure stream of air (*air abrasion) or by adhesion to strips, discs, wheels, or points. An **abrasive strip (finishing strip)** consists of a piece of linen, acetate, or thin metal of varying width coated on one or both sides with abrasive grit of differing textures. It is used for smoothing and contouring the proximal surfaces of restorations.

abscess *n.* A localized accumulation of *pus in a cavity caused by tissue breakdown as a result of infection or foreign materials. It is a tissue defence reaction to prevent the spread of infection to other parts of the body. An abscess may be

The ABCDE approach: the method of assessing critically ill patients

		Assessment	Action
A	**Airway**	Look for: • signs of airway obstruction • abnormal chest and abdominal movements (see-saw respiration) • use of accessory neck muscles • blue lips and tongue • gurgling noise • snoring • or no breathing.	• Call for help. • Head tilt/chin lift or *jaw thrust. • Remove any foreign bodies. • Consider inserting airway adjunct. • Give oxygen (10–15 litres per minute).
B	**Breathing**	• Look, listen, and feel for signs of respiratory distress. • Count the respiratory rate (normally 10–15 breaths per minute in adults and up to 20–30 in children). • Check for bilateral chest expansion and tracheal deviation. • Undertake *auscultation and *percussion of the chest if trained to do so.	• Use bag and mask (if trained) or pocket mask. • Ventilate with supplemental oxygen. • Attach a *pulse oximeter to measure oxygen saturation if available.
C	**Circulation**	• Check colour of skin (is it blue, pink, pale, or mottled?). • Assess limb temperature e.g. are hands cool or warm? • Check for *pulse rate and measure blood pressure. • Measure capillary refill time: apply thumb pressure to the sternum at heart level (or just above) for 5 seconds, with enough pressure to cause blanching. Time how long it takes for the skin to return to the colour of the surrounding skin after releasing the pressure; the normal refill time is less than 2 seconds.	• Lay patient flat. • Gain intravenous (IV) access and consider giving an intravenous fluid challenge and emergency drugs as appropriate.

D	**Disability**	• Assess patient's conscious level using either the *Glasgow Coma Scale or more easily using the AVPU scale.
		  • A = Alert
		  • V = Responds to voice
		  • P = Responds to pain
		  • U = Unresponsive
		  • Examine the pupils (size, equality, and reaction to light).
		• Check patient's drug record.
			• Check blood glucose level and give glucose if less than 3mmol/l.

E	**Exposure**	Remove patient's clothing and check the whole body for signs of trauma or blood loss, while maintaining patient's dignity and minimizing heat loss.	

described as **acute** when there has been a rapid onset frequently associated with pain, or **chronic** when it has developed over a longer period of time and is usually painless. A **gingival abscess (gumboil)** is associated with the free gingival margin (*see* GINGIVA) of a tooth. These are frequently caused by foreign bodies, or food impaction: they may be associated with a non-vital primary tooth and be asymptomatic. A **periapical abscess** is associated with the root apex of a tooth and the surrounding bone and is a sequel of pulpal infection. A lateral **periodontal abscess** involves the *periodontal attachment tissues and usually arises from an established *periodontal pocket. It may occur because of an increase in virulent organisms, a compromised immune response, or reduced drainage from the periodontal pocket. The last may occur following root debridement with superficial tissue healing and residual infection in the periodontal pocket. A **pericoronal abscess** is related to the flap of gum (*operculum) overlying a partially erupted tooth, most commonly the third molar. Treatment is by establishing drainage and addressing the cause.

absolute risk reduction (ARR) *See* RISK DIFFERENCE.

absorbable gelatin(e) sponge *n.* A material applied topically to aid *haemostasis, usually following a dental extraction. It provides a structure for clot formation.

absorbent *adj.* Describing a material capable of taking up other substances by suction e.g. an absorbent paper point.

absorption *n.* The passage of one substance to another by penetration or solution. For example, the passage of liquids into the mucosa, skin, or dental materials.

absorption layer *n.* An amorphous zone on the dentine surface into which adhesive agents can flow. *See also* HYBRID LAYER.

abuse *v.* and *n.* Inappropriate use or treatment of materials, techniques, persons, programmes, or language. *See also* CHILD ABUSE.

abut *v.* To touch or border upon. To have a common boundary.

abutment *n.* A tooth, tooth root, or implant used to support a fixed or removable *prosthesis (bridge or partial denture). It may provide either the terminal support for a prosthesis or additional intermediate support (**pier abutment**). In implant dentistry, **healing abutments** are designed to allow peri-implant soft tissues to heal; they may be screwed into the implant at the time of implant insertion or several months later; they are

usually made of titanium. **Restorative implant abutments** are designed to attach the restoration to the implant and can compensate for soft tissue contour or implant position, angle, or depth.

acanthion *n.* The tip of the anterior *nasal spine of the maxillary bone.

acantholysis *n.* The breakdown of epidermal or epithelial cells due to a loss of intercellular substance. It is often seen in conditions such as *pemphigus vulgaris, where it is caused by autoantibodies, but may also occur in other conditions.

acanthosis *n.* (*adj.* **acanthotic**) An increase in the number of cells within the prickle cell layer (the middle part) of the *epithelium.

accelerator *n.* A substance that speeds up a chemical reaction, such as the addition of *plaster of Paris to *mineral trioxide aggregate. Heat may also act as an accelerator in speeding up the setting reaction of an impression or restorative material. *See also* CATALYST.

access *n.* An approach or pathway, either natural or prepared, to view, instrument, or treat an area of interest. An **access cavity** is prepared in a tooth to identify root canal entrances in the pulp chamber or to enable the instrumentation and removal of carious tissue.

accessory *adj.* Additional, supplementary, subsidiary to the main thing. An **accessory root canal** is a branch of the principal root canal frequently occurring in the apical third of the root.

Access to Health Records Act 1990 (in Britain) A British act of parliament that established legislation for controlling a patient's access to their written clinical health records. This act has largely been replaced by the *Data Protection Act 1998.

accidental extraction *n. See* TOOTH EXTRACTION.

accident book A book used to record all accidents to staff, patients, and visitors in a dental practice or clinic. Entries should include the time, date, and nature of the accident, where it took place, who was involved, and what action was taken. The accident record does not have to be in book format, and may for example be stored as a file, written log, or electronic record.

(⊕) SEE WEB LINKS
• Health and Safety Executive guidance details.

accreditation *n.* A process of formal recognition by a professional external body whereby an educational establishment or programme meets certain agreed quality standards.

accredited prior learning (APL) *n.* Credit given for previously gained skills or knowledge.

accretion *n.* An accumulation of material such as *calculus, *plaque, or dental cement on tooth surfaces.

accretion lines *n.* Lines visible in microscopic sections of *enamel marking successive layers of added material.

acellular *n.* Describing any tissue or part of a tissue that does not contain cells.

acesulfame-potassium (ace-K, acesulfame-K) *n.* A calorie-free artificial sweetener known in Europe under the additive code **E950**. It is 150–200 times sweeter than *sucrose. It is used in many foods, including cakes and low-calorie drinks. It is not metabolized or stored in the body and after ingestion is rapidly excreted unchanged.

acetate strip *n.* A clear plastic strip of celluloid acetate used as a *matrix band for tooth-coloured restorations in anterior teeth, to restore the contour of the proximal surface.

acetone *n.* A colourless liquid ketone used as a solvent in some dental restorative *primer materials. Primers with high acetone content can cause significant erosion of calcium hydroxide lining materials.

acetylsalicylic acid *n. See* ASPIRIN.

ache *n.* A dull persistent pain.

acheilia *n.* Congenital absence of the lips.

achlorhydria *n.* An absence of hydrochloric acid in the stomach. It may not be associated with disease.

achondroplasia *n.* A genetic disorder in which the bones of the arms and legs fail to grow to normal size, due to a defect in both cartilage and bone, resulting in dwarfism. It can result in delayed exfoliation of the primary teeth.

aciclovir (acyclovir) *n.* An antiviral drug that acts by inhibiting DNA synthesis in cells infected with the *herpes virus. It can be applied to the lips as a cream in the treatment of herpes labialis (cold sores), or can be used systemically for severe infections or in the immunocompromised patient. Trade name: **Zovirax**.

acid *n.* Any chemical compound which when dissolved in water produces a solution with a *pH of less than 7. An **acid bath** is an acid (usually

hydrochloric or sulphuric) solution used to remove the oxide layer of a metal, a process known as *pickling. **acidic** *adj. Compare* ALKALINE.

acid-etch technique *n.* A technique for bonding resin-based materials to enamel or dentine. An acid, usually phosphoric acid, is applied in either gel or liquid form to the previously dried and isolated tooth surface for about 30 seconds. The dissolution of the mineral element of the tooth creates micro-porosities into which the subsequently applied unfilled resin can flow and provide a mechanical lock by means of resin tags. It is used to bond *fissure sealants, restorative materials, orthodontic *bands, and adhesive *bridges (prostheses).

acidogenic *adj.* Describing the ability to produce acid.

acidogenic theory A theory describing the cause of dental caries, first postulated by Willoughby D. Miller in 1890, which stated that non-specific bacteria in the plaque fermented refined carbohydrates to produce acid that demineralized tooth enamel.

acidosis *n.* A condition in which the acid–base balance in the body is characterized by an excess of acid or a deficiency of alkali. In health this is regulated by the respiratory and renal systems. *Compare* ALKALOSIS.

acidulated phosphate fluoride gel (APF) *n. See* FLUORIDE GEL.

aciduric *adj.* Describing the ability to tolerate exposure to pH environments lower than 7.

acinic cell tumour *n.* A malignant tumour of the salivary glands in which the cells typically resemble salivary acini. It is now classified by the *World Health Organization (WHO) as **acinic cell carcinoma**. It is most commonly seen in the *parotid gland and may produce symptoms of pain and tenderness. Tumours arising from non-epithelial tissue of the salivary glands (*sarcomas) are very rare.

acinus *n.* (*pl.* **acini;** *adj.* **acinous) 1.** A small sac-like dilatation surrounded by excretory cells in a compound gland such as the salivary glands. **2.** (in the lung) The tissue supplied with air by one terminal bronchiole.

aclusion (disclusion) *n.* The condition of not having the teeth in contact with each other.

acne (acne vulgaris) *n.* A common skin condition occurring particularly during adolescence that affects the hair follicles and sebaceous glands in the skin. In puberty, acne occurs because of changes to hormone levels. These cause the sebaceous glands to produce increased amounts of sebum which, together with dead skin, block the hair follicles. Acne is characterized by the presence of spots ranging from blackheads and whiteheads to painful red nodules usually occuring on the face, hands, and neck. Acne during puberty normally corrects itself in time without treatment. **Acne rosacea** *see* ROSACEA.

aconite *n.* An alkaloid from the dried roots of the herbaceous plant *Aconitum napellus* used in the homeopathic treatment of dental fear or acute anxiety. It was formerly used as a *tincture for toothache. Its use is controversial in view of its low safety margin and evidence of its being a cardiotoxin.

acquired immunodeficiency syndrome (AIDS) *n. See* AIDS.

acrodont *adj.* Having tooth attachment in which the teeth are fused (*ankylosed) to the jaw bone, rather than being located in sockets within the bone. It is common in reptiles and fish.

acrodynia (pink disease) A rare severe illness of children of teething age, possibly leading to the early loss of the primary teeth and permanent tooth germs. It is characterized by pink cold clammy hands and feet, rapid pulse, raised blood pressure, stomatitis, periodontitis, and premature loss of teeth. It is thought to be caused by an allergy to mercury, which used to be a constituent of teething ointments, lotions, and powders. Since mercury-containing paediatric preparations have been banned, the disease has virtually disappeared.

acromegaly *n.* A chronic metabolic disorder caused by the presence of excess growth hormone. It results in gradual enlargement of body tissues, including the bones of the face (*frontal bossing), jaw, hands, feet, and skull.

acrosclerosis *n.* A skin disease thought to be a type of generalized *scleroderma mainly affecting the hands, face, and feet.

acrylic (polymethylmethacrylate) resin *n.* A thermoplastic vinyl polymer made by free radical vinyl polymerization from methyl methacrylate monomer. It was first developed in 1928 and eventually replaced *vulcanite as a material in the construction of acrylic resin complete and partial dentures. It is also used for the construction of temporary resin crowns and bridges and in the manufacture of resin teeth and removable orthodontic appliances. The material is supplied as a polymethylmethacrylate powder and a liquid monomer. To construct a denture

base, the powder and liquid are mixed together to form a dough, which is packed into an appropriate mould and subjected to prolonged heat to produce the final rigid product. Acrylic resin may be polymerized at room temperature by including a chemical initiator, such as a tertiary amine, in the liquid monomer: these resins are known as **self-curing** or **auto-curing** resins. The impact strength of acrylic resin may be increased by grafting a rubber-like butadiene-styrene polymer to the acrylic molecules. Acrylic resin can produce an allergic contact reaction with the soft tissues and in such cases may then be substituted with a *polyamide resin.

Actinobacillus actinomycetem comitans A carbon dioxide-requiring (capnophilic), microaerophilic, *Gram-negative rod-shaped bacterium associated with chronic periodontitis. Toxins released by these bacteria produce an inflammatory response in the gingival tissues with a consequent increase in gingival crevicular fluid flow. Virulence factors include collagenese, endotoxin, IgA proteases making it capable of evading normal host response and destroying connective tissue and bone.

Actinomyces *n.* A genus of non-spore forming Gram-positive bacteria that can be *anaerobic or facultatively anaerobic. Individual bacterial cells tend to be rod-shaped, whereas bacteria in colonies form branched networks of hyphae-like fungi. Several *Actinomyces* species are opportunistic pathogens of humans, especially in the oral cavity, and can be isolated from plaque. *See also* ACTINOMYCOSIS.

actinomycosis *n.* An uncommon bacterial disease of humans generally caused by *A. israelii* and *A. gerencseriae* and species of propionibacteria. The disease is characterized by painful abscesses in the oral cavity, lungs, or digestive tract. Treatment is by antibiotic therapy.

action potential *n.* The electrical signal that rapidly propagates along the *axon of nerve cells as well as over the surface of some muscle and glandular cells. It is due to a change in membrane electrical potential caused by a change in flow of ions across the membrane, in turn due to voltage-activated ion channels.

actisite *n.* A trade name for a polyvinyl acetate fibre impregnated with *tetracycline used as a form of *chemotherapy to provide a *topical antibiotic for the treatment of periodontal disease. The impregnated fibres are packed into the gingival pocket and retained for about 10 days by means of a *cyanoacrylate adhesive.

activator *n.* 1. A substance used to initiate the *polymerization reaction of an *impression material. 2. A removable myofunctional orthodontic appliance used to guide jaw growth and development. *See* FUNCTIONAL APPLIANCE. 3. An alkali (sodium carbonate), forming a component of photographic developing solution that softens and swells the gelatin of the film emulsion and provides the required alkaline medium for the developing agents to react with the sensitized silver halide crystals.

active *adj.* (*v.* **activate**) Describing an orthodontic appliance which has been adjusted to provide an effective force on a tooth, teeth, or jaw. *Compare* PASSIVE.

active metabolite *n.* An agent produced following metabolism of a drug, which has its own therapeutic effect (e.g. salicylate from aspirin).

acupressure *n.* The pressure applied by hands, elbows, or fingers to acupuncture points on various parts of the body as an alternative to using needles (*acupuncture).

acupuncture *n.* The insertion of a solid needle into any part of the human body for the purpose of disease prevention, therapy, or maintenance of health. It is a form of traditional Chinese medicine used by some dental practitioners to relieve symptoms of pain, nausea, dental anxiety, and the gag reflex. It is based on the theory of energy pathways that run through the body (the *meridian system). Needles are used to stimulate the nerves in skin or muscle to increase the release of endorphin and serotonin (neuro-endocrine theory). **Electro-acupuncture** uses a device to pass a small electrical current across acupuncture points. 📷

Further Reading: Thayer M. L. T. The use of acupuncture in dentistry. *Dent Update* 2007;34:244–50.

🌐 **SEE WEB LINKS**
• The British Medical Acupuncture Society website.

acute *adj.* 1. Describing a condition of rapid onset, severe symptoms, and brief duration, e.g. acute pulpitis. *Compare* CHRONIC. 2. Describing any intense symptom such as acute toothache or acute inflammation.

acute ulcerative gingivitis *n. See* GINGIVITIS, NECROTIZING.

Adams crib *n. See* CRIB.

Adams pliers *n. See* PLIERS.

adaptation *n.* 1. The close approximation of a prosthetic appliance to the oral tissues. 2. The adjustment of a band or restorative material to

closely approximate against a tooth surface. 3. The process by which a sense organ shows a progressively diminishing response to continuous or repetitive stimulation. 4. The alteration that an organism gradually undergoes to adjust to a changing environment.

Adcortyl in orabase *See* TRIAMCINOLONE ACETONIDE.

addiction *n.* Psychological and bodily dependence, on a substance or practice, which is beyond voluntary control. Treatment is aimed at gradual withdrawal of the substance or behaviour and eventually complete abstention.

Addison's disease [Thomas Addison (1793–1860), English physician] Hypo-secretion of the adrenal glands characterized by symptoms of tiredness, weakness, weight loss, and thirst. An early oral sign is blue-black pigmentation usually of the gingivae or mucous membrane of the cheek but may involve other parts of the mouth and face. An acute infection or severe adrenal hypofunction can precipitate an **Addisonian crisis** manifested by low blood pressure and collapse. Treatment is by replacement hormone therapy.

addition curing *See* POLYMERIZATION.

adduction *n.* The movement towards the midline of the body.

adenitis *n.* Inflammation of a gland or lymph node.

adenocarcinoma *n. See* CARCINOMA.

adenofibroma *n.* A tumour consisting of fibrous tissue and containing glandular structures.

adenoid *n.* Lymphatic tissue covered by ciliated epithelium situated on the posterior wall of the *nasopharynx (pharyngeal tonsils). They function as part of the body's immune system and form part of the ring of lymphatic tissue known as *Waldeyer's ring.

adenoid cystic carcinoma *n.* A *malignant salivary gland *neoplasm which is more common in the minor glands than the major. It has a characteristic 'Swiss cheese' pattern arrangement of the epithelial cells and spreads widely along nerves. Patients present with slow growing swelling with pain and ulceration. Treatment is wide local excision.

adenolymphoma *n.* (**Warthin's tumour**) [A. S. Warthin (1866–1931), American pathologist] A benign cystic tumour that occurs exclusively in the *parotid gland. It contains epithelial and lymphoid tissue and accounts for about 5% of all parotid tumours. It is frequently bilateral (affects both glands). *See also* ADENOMA.

adenoma *n.* A benign epithelial tumour of glandular origin. A **pleomorphic adenoma** is a benign tumour of *salivary glands and is the most common tumour of the *parotid gland. It has a variable histological appearance in terms of the proportions and arrangements of epithelial cells and connective tissue stroma and is usually enveloped by a fibrous capsule. It may grow to a large size and treatment is by surgical excision. Recurrence is rare. Longstanding tumours may become malignant. Other types of adenoma arising in the salivary glands are **basal cell adenoma** and **canalicular adenoma**.

adenomatoid odontogenic tumour *n.* A benign *odontogenic tumour that is often associated with the crown of an unerupted tooth, particularly the upper canines. It is composed of odontogenic epithelium and mesenchyme and characterized by *ameloblast-like cells that form ducts and tubules. Calcification is common. It is treated by excision and does not usually recur.

adenosine triphosphate (ATP) *n.* A nucleotide which provides the energy to drive sodium (sodium pump) out of the nerve cell as part of the repolarization phase following nerve stimulation. It stores energy in muscles which is released on hydrolysis to **adenosine diphosphate (ADP)**.

adhesion *n.* 1. The sticking of two surfaces together (e.g. an orthodontic *bracket to tooth enamel, or a denture to the roof of the mouth). Adhesive systems in restorative dentistry permit the bonding to dentine and enamel using an *acid-etch technique. 2. The tissue that provides the pathological joining of two normally separate surfaces. 3. The healing process by which the edges of a wound are united. This may be **primary** with minimal *granulation tissue or **secondary** when the edges are joined by granulation tissue. *See also* WOUND.

adipose *adj.* Fatty or pertaining to fat. Adipose tissue is connective tissue with a predominance of fat cells which serves as an insulating layer and an energy store.

adipsia *n.* The inability to drink or the avoidance of drinking. It is the extreme form of an abnormally diminished thirst (**hypodipsia**) and is usually caused by damage to the thirst centre in the anterior hypothalamus.

adjudication *n.* (US) A part of a dental peer review process in which a peer review committee expresses a non-binding opinion of a dispute brought before it.

adjuvant *n.* A pharmacological or immunological agent which is added to modify the effectiveness of the main ingredient (e.g. an adjuvant drug used to enhance the pain relief provided by another drug). **Adjuvant therapy** is additional treatment supporting primary treatment such as radiation therapy following surgery for the removal of a malignant lesion.

adnexa *pl. n.* Accessory or adjoining anatomical parts or appendages to an organ.

adolescence *n.* The stage of development from *puberty to adulthood. Puberty in girls starts usually at the age of 10 years and in boys at about 12 years. The behaviour and identity of an adult usually starts at about the age of 19 years.

adrenal crisis Acute adrenocortical insufficiency characterized by headache, nausea, vomiting, rapid weak *pulse, circulatory collapse, and coma. It may occur in response to the additional stress of dental treatment in patients with adrenal suppression or who are being treated with cortisone therapy. Treatment is by intravenous or intramuscular *hydrocortisone and *oxygen.

adrenal glands The two *endocrine glands situated above each kidney. The outer part (**adrenal cortex**) produces corticosteroid hormones e.g. cortisone and hydrocortisone and the inner part (**adrenal medulla**) produces epinephrine (*adrenaline) and norepinephrine (*noradrenaline).

adrenaline (epinephrine) *n.* A hormone secreted by the medulla of the adrenal gland. It is a directly acting sympathetomimetic amine with both alpha and beta adrenergic activity and stimulates the heart, blood vessels, and respiratory system. Adrenaline may be injected in the treatment of *cardiac arrest (intravenously) or *anaphylactic shock (intramuscularly). In the dose used in cardiopulmonary resuscitation (CPR), it stimulates alpha 1 and alpha 2 receptors, causing vasoconstriction, and thereby increasing systemic vascular resistance during CPR and causing a relative increase in cerebral and coronary *perfusion. In the beating heart, adrenaline acts on beta 1 receptors to increase the heart rate and force of myocardial contraction. It is added as a *vasoconstrictor in dental local analgesic solutions to prolong the action of the analgesic.

adrenal shock *n. See* ADDISON'S DISEASE.

adrenocorticotrophic hormone (ACTH) *n.* A hormone produced by the pituitary gland which stimulates the *adrenal glands to produce cortisone. Large amounts are produced in response to stress.

adsorption *n.* The adhesion of a gas, liquid or dissolved substance onto the surface of a solid material or body.

adult dental health survey A review carried out in the UK and many EU states and countries worldwide every ten years since 1968, to provide information on the current state of adults' teeth and oral health in the four countries of the UK and to measure changes in oral health since the previous survey. The specific aims of the survey are to establish the condition of the natural teeth and supporting tissues; to investigate dental experiences, attitudes, and knowledge; dental care and oral hygiene; to establish the state and use made of dentures worn in conjunction with natural teeth; to identify those people who have lost all of their natural teeth and investigate their use of dentures; and to monitor the extent to which oral health targets set by government are being met. *See also* CHILDREN'S DENTAL HEALTH SURVEY.

(⊕) SEE WEB LINKS

• Summary of the 1998 survey on the government's Office of National Statistics site.

adumbration *n.* Sketchy or lack of sharp-edge definition of an image on a radiographic film.

advanced life support (ALS) Medical care provided by trained personnel to assess a patient's condition, administer drugs, defibrillate, and provide advanced airway management prior to transfer to a hospital. *See also* BASIC LIFE SUPPORT.

(⊕) SEE WEB LINKS

• The Resuscitation Council (UK) information on advanced life support.

adventitia (tunica adventitia) *n.* 1. The outer coat of the wall of an artery or vein. 2. The outer covering of various organs.

adventitious *adj.* Describing something occurring in an unexpected location.

adverse effect An abnormal or harmful event for which the causal relation between the drug or intervention and the event is at least a reasonable possibility. It can be applied to all interventions, unlike an **adverse drug reaction** which is applied only to drugs. Adverse effects are indicated usually by pathological changes, illness, or even death.

aerobic *adj.* 1. Living or occurring only in the presence of oxygen. 2. Cellular respiration by which carbohydrates are completely oxidized by atmospheric oxygen to achieve maximum energy production.

aerodontalgia *n. See* BARODONTALGIA.

aerodontia *n.* The science of the effect of either increased or reduced atmospheric pressure on the teeth.

aerosol *n.* A suspension of very small solid or liquid particles that range in size up to 50μm diameter in air or gas: they may be suspended in passive air for several days. Aerosol sprays are used for the delivery of some drugs (e.g. Ventolin for the treatment of asthma). Aerosols are a possible hazard when using high speed turbines and ultrasonic scalers because of the potential spread of infected material.

Further Reading: Day C. J., Sandy J. R., Ireland A. J. Aerosols and splatter in dentistry—A neglected menace. *Dent Update* 2006;33:601–6.

aetiology (*US* **etiology)** *n.* 1. The study of the causes of disease. 2. The cause of a disease.

afferent *adj.* 1. Conducting information inwards. 2. Designating the part of the peripheral nervous system which transmits impulses from organs or tissues to the central nervous system, i.e. any sensory nerve or neurone. 3. Describing blood vessels that feed a capilliary network. 4. Designating lymphatic vessels that enter a lymph node. *Compare* EFFERENT.

agar (agar-agar) *n.* A vegetable polysaccharide gel made from seaweed extract (*Gelidium cartilagineum, Gracilaria confervoides,* and related red algae) and used as a sterile, solid, bacterial culture medium (**agar plate**) contained in a *Petri dish. Agar is the principal ingredient of reversible *hydrocolloid impression material.

agate *n.* A hard gemstone used in the construction of spatula blades. They are used for mixing tooth-coloured materials because of their resistance to abrasion and their ability not to cause discoloration of the material, unlike some metallic spatulas.

age change An alteration in the form or function of a tissue or organ over a period of time. Age changes which take place in the oral soft tissues include a decrease in the thickness of the mucosa, a reduction in taste bud function, and an increase in the number of *sebaceous glands; there is an increase in the incidence of mucosal disease such as *oral cancer, *lichen planus, and *candida. The dental hard tissue changes include a reduced permeability of the enamel, a reduced rate of secondary dentine formation, and a progressive occlusion of the dentinal tubules with calcified material. *See also* GERODONTOLOGY.

ageusia *n.* Total loss of the ability to taste sweet, sour, salty, or bitter substances. It has many causes including neurological damage particularly affecting the lingual and hypoglossal nerves. The loss of taste may only be partial (*hypogeusia).

agglutination *n.* Clumping together often as a result of infection, antibodies, or inflammation (e.g. red blood cells or bacteria).

aggressive periodontitis *n.* See PERIODONTITIS, AGGRESSIVE.

aglossia *n.* The congenital absence of the tongue.

agnathia *n.* The total failure of development of the mandible or maxilla.

agomphious *adj.* The condition of being toothless (*edentulous). *See also* ANODONTIA.

agonist *n.* 1. A muscle whose contraction causes movement of part of the body at the same time as another muscle (*antagonist) relaxes. 2. A drug that acts at a cell receptor site and mimics the action of the body's natural *neurotransmitters.

agranulocytosis *n.* An acute blood disorder in which there is a severe deficiency in *granulocytes. It can be caused by drugs, chemicals, or *neoplasia. Oral signs are necrotic ulcers of the gingivae, tongue, and buccal mucosa.

AIDS (acquired immunodeficiency syndrome) *n.* A disease caused by the human immunodeficiency virus (*HIV). The syndrome was first identified in Los Angeles in 1981. AIDS is essentially a sexually transmitted disease although transmission can also be via infected blood, blood products, or breast milk. The virus may also be present in saliva. The virus can only survive for a few minutes outside the body and must enter the bloodstream to cause infection. High standards of clinical practice are required by all clinical dental health workers in order to avoid inadvertent infection via blood or body fluids from HIV positive people. *See also* KAPOSI'S SARCOMA.

air abrasion A method of delivering an abrasive material, usually aluminium oxide, under high pressure. The average particle size is 27.5 microns and the nozzle tip exit pressure commonly employed ranges between 60 and 120 pounds per square inch. It is a non-rotary technique used to cut small cavities in enamel, dentine or to remove surface accretions or stain. The nozzle tip is usually placed less than 1mm from the tooth surface to minimize the cone-shaped particle scatter. It is an alternative in some situations to using the *air turbine for cavity preparation.

Further Reading: Banerjee A., Watson T. F. Air abrasion: Its uses and abuse. *Dent Update* 2002;29:340–46.

⊕ SEE WEB LINKS
• WebMD page providing an overview of restorative dentistry using air abrasion.

air block *n.* A material, such as petroleum jelly, applied to the surface of a resin composite restoration prior to curing. It acts as a barrier to oxygen which is a polymerization inhibitor. *See also* OXYGEN INHIBITION LAYER.

air embolism *n.* A bubble of air present in the tissues. It may occur in an artery, vein, or tissue space as a result of surgery, injury, or injection.

air syringe *n.* An instrument for delivering compressed air to a given location for the purpose of removing fluids or loose particles.

air turbine handpiece *n.* A handpiece with a turbine powered by compressed air. Used with diamond or tungsten carbide burs and a water coolant spray to dissipate the heat produced when removing enamel, dentine, or other hard materials. *See also* HANDPIECE.

airway *n.* 1. The passageway allowing air to pass into and out of the lungs. 2. A device to facilitate free passage of air to the lungs when the patient is unconscious. **Oropharyngeal airways** are made in a range of sizes from newborn to large adult. The airways are rigid curved plastic tubes with a reinforced flange. They are inserted in the mouth in the inverted position and rotated 180° as the tip passes into the *oropharynx. **Nasopharyngeal airways** are an alternative if the patient is not deeply unconscious and should be inserted via the nostril, following lubrication, with a twisting action into the oropharynx. 📷

airway obstruction *See* CHOKING.

akinesia *n.* An inability to move or a difficulty in beginning or maintaining a body motion. It is a symptom of *Parkinson's disease.

ala *n.* (*pl.* **alae**) A wing-like structure such as the ala of the crista galli, part of the projection from the cribriform plate of the ethmoid bone, the ala of the vomer, and the alar part of the nasalis muscle. The **alar cartilage** is the U-shaped structure on the lateral aspect of the external naris (nostril) which forms the tip of the nose.

ala-tragal line A line from the lower border of the ala of the nose to the upper border of the *tragus of the ear. It is used as a reference line in orthodontics, radiography, and the construction of complete dentures. Also known as **Camper's line** [P. Camper (1722–89), Dutch anatomist].

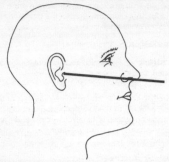

Ala-tragal line

Albers–Schönberg disease *See*
OSTEOPETROSIS.

Albright syndrome *See* DYSPLASIA.

alcohol *n.* Compounds with a hydroxyl (OH) group attached to a carbon atom. Alcoholic beverages contain ethyl alcohol (ethanol) which has the formula C_2H_5OH. It has a depressant effect on the central nervous system. Ethyl alcohol potentiates the effects of carcinogens (e.g. cigarette smoke), by increasing the permeability of the oral mucosa and it is therefore a risk factor for oral carcinoma. Excessive alcohol consumption over a short period of time (**binge drinking**) can lead to acetaldehyde accumulation in the oral mucosa which is thought to be a carcinogenic factor. Alcohol consumption during pregnancy can have a detrimental effect on foetal development. A frequent high intake of alcohol can lead to physical deterioration and mental impairment (**alcohol abuse**). Prolonged alcohol consumption can lead to cirrhosis of the liver, enteritis, and heart damage. A mental or physical desire to consume alcohol can lead to **alcohol dependence** (**alcoholism**), which is characterized by a strong craving, anxiety, and tremor, and a reliance on the intake of alcohol despite adverse physical,

mental, and social consequences. Support groups are available, such as **Alcoholics Anonymous** for sufferers from alcoholism and **Al-Anon** for friends and families of alcoholics.

(((●))) SEE WEB LINKS
• Alcoholics Anonymous website.
• Al-Anon website.

-algia Suffix denoting pain e.g. **neuralgia** (pain in a nerve).

alginate *n.* Any salt of alginic acid (e.g. sodium alginate, calcium alginate). **Alginate impression material** is a mixture of sodium, potassium, and triethanolamine alginate, calcium sulphate (gypsum), and a filler (65–75%) such as diatomaceous earth which, when mixed with water, forms calcium alginate, an irreversible hydrocolloid. Trisodium phosphate is added (1–3%) to control the setting time. Alginate is used for primary impressions for complete and partial dentures and for the construction of study casts. Because of its dimensional instability it is not a suitable material for crown or bridge preparations.

align *v.* 1. To set prosthetic teeth up in the line of the dental arch. 2. To orthodontically bring teeth into the normal arch position. This is usually achieved by the use of flexible nickel or stainless steel *archwires attached to a *fixed appliance.

alignment (of tooth) *n.* The location of the tooth relative to the supporting alveolar *bone and adjacent and opposing teeth.

alimentary tract *n.* The digestive passage extending from the mouth to the anus. Each region is specialized to undertake mechanical breakdown (in the mouth), chemical digestion and absorption (in the stomach and small intestine), and faeces formation and water absorption (in the colon and rectum).

alkaline *adj.* Describes any chemical compound which, when dissolved in water, produces a solution having a pH greater than 7. *See also* ACID.

alkalosis *n.* A condition in which the acid-base balance in the body is characterized by an excess of alkali or a deficiency of acid. In health this is regulated by the respiratory and renal systems. *Compare* ACIDOSIS.

allergen *n.* (*adj.* **allergenic**) A substance capable of inducing hypersensitivity or an allergic reaction e.g. *latex.

allergy *n.* A condition in which the body has an exaggerated response to a substance (e.g. material, food, or drugs). Latex allergy is particularly significant in healthcare workers. In dentistry, allergy to metals such as nickel, copper, and chromium has been reported; the recent popularity of *oral piercing has placed susceptible patients at greater risk of developing allergies to metals. Dental resins such as di- and mono-methacrylate resins present in restorative materials and bonding agents, eugenol-containing products, and polyether impression materials can induce an allergic *hypersensitivity reaction. An allergic reaction can be immediate or delayed. An **immediate reaction** (Type I) affects multiple body systems and is characterized by itching of the skin or mucosa, reddening, and swelling (oedema), hay fever-type symptoms, asthma, and, more rarely, *anaphylaxis. A **delayed reaction** (Type IV) is characterized by a red itchy rash usually localized to the area of contact.

allodynia *n.* Pain due to a stimulus that does not normally provoke pain. This is exemplified by non-painful stimulation such as touch, gentle pressure, cold, or gentle joint movement producing symptoms of pain. *Compare* HYPERALGESIA.

allograft *n. See* GRAFT.

allopathy *n.* Treatment of disease by the use of medicines or drugs that oppose the presenting symptoms.

alloplasty *n.* (*adj.* **alloplastic**) A surgical procedure utilizing a synthetic material, i.e. a material not from the human body.

alloy *n.* A mixture, either in solution or compound, of two or more metals. *Gold, *palladium, *titanium, *nickel-chrome, and nickel metal–ceramic alloys may be used in the construction of bridges and crown restorations. Copper is added to gold to reduce the density and melting point and increase the strength and hardness; however, the corrosion resistance is reduced. The addition of silver to gold increases the hardness and strength but also increases porosity and the degree of tarnish. Zinc or indium are added as scavengers to prevent the oxidation of other metals during melting and casting. A **eutectic alloy** has a melting point which is lower than that of any of the individual metals of which it is constituted. *See also* AMALGAM.

Further Reading: Brown D. Alloys for metal-ceramic restorations. *Dent Update* 2005;32:583–6.

alumina *n.* Aluminium oxide (SiO_2), a component of dental *porcelain. Also used as an abrasive material.

aluminium *n.* A silvery white metallic element. It is used as a filter in x-ray machines to block x-rays over a certain wavelength. It is also added to some dental waxes to modify the hardening properties. **Aluminium chloride hexahydrate** is a powerful antiperspirant used in the treatment of excessive sweating.

alveolalgia *n. See* ALVEOLITIS.

alveolar *adj.* Pertaining to an alveolus.

alveolar bone *n. See* BONE.

alveolar crest *n.* The most coronal part of the alveolar *bone. In the healthy periodontium, the distance between the alveolar crest and the cement–enamel junction is 1–2mm, as measured on a radiograph.

alveolar mucosa *See* MUCOSA.

alveolar osteitis *See* ALVEOLITIS.

alveolar process *n.* That part of the *mandible or *maxilla that forms a U-shaped dental arch housing the teeth.

alveolar ridge *n.* The bony ridge of the *mandible or *maxilla which contains the tooth sockets and the teeth.

alveolectomy *n.* The removal of part or all of the *alveolar process, often associated with the removal of teeth or to achieve surgical correction of a deformity.

alveolitis (dental) *n.* Inflammation of the alveolus also known as **dry socket**, **alveolar osteitis**, or **alveolalgia**, caused by premature loss or the destruction of the blood clot formed in the socket following a tooth extraction. The acute condition is characterized clinically by pain 1–3 days post-operatively with surrounding mucosal inflammation. There may be exposed bone or food debris in the socket. Predisposing factors are a traumatic extraction, pre-existing periapical infection, reduced blood supply (notably in the mandible rather than the maxilla), smoking, premature mouth rinsing, and premature clot removal by the patient. It is more common in the permanent than the primary dentition. Management is by irrigation with warm saline to remove food debris and covering the exposed bone with either a resorbable or non-resorbable antiseptic dressing. Analgesics are normally required, e.g. non-steroidal anti-inflammatory drugs. Prescription of an antibiotic is only advisable if there is associated evidence of systemic infection. Healing normally takes place in 10–14 days. There is evidence to suggest that the incidence of alveolar osteitis can be reduced by rinsing pre-operatively with a *chlorhexidine mouthwash.

alveoloplasty *n.* The surgical modification of the alveolar bone, such as a tooth socket following the extraction of a tooth, or prior to the insertion of a prosthesis. It is usually undertaken to produce a smoother bony contour.

alveoloschisis *n.* A cleft of the *alveolar process.

alveoloscopy *n.* The examination of the *alveolus following tooth extraction by means of an *endoscope. It may be used to identify the presence of root fragments as well as to determine alveolar defects during augmentative surgery.

alveolus *n.* **1.** A bony socket in the alveolar ridge of the jaw bones which holds a tooth or tooth root. **2.** An air sac in the lungs involved in gas exchange situated distal to the terminal *bronchioles.

Alvogyl *n.* The trade name for a resorbable dressing containing butamben, eugenol, and iodoform used in the treatment of *alveolitis (dry socket). It is contraindicated in patients allergic to procaine or iodine compounds.

Alzheimer's disease [A. Alzheimer (1864–1915), German physician] A disease caused by a degeneration of nerve fibres in the brain. It is a cause of dementia that results in a decline in intellectual capacity. The symptoms include short-term memory loss, confusion, incontinence, speech difficulty, and personality changes. Medication may result in *xerostomia, potentially leading to a high *caries incidence.

amalgam

n. An alloy of *mercury with one or more other metals. **Dental amalgam alloy** typically contains approximately 60% silver, 27% tin, 13% copper and 0–2% zinc. *Zinc, included as an oxygen scavenger, can be omitted if the alloy is manufactured in an oxygen-free environment. The alloy particles can either be **spherical** in shape, irregular (**lathe-cut**) or **admixed**, consisting of a mixture of spherical and lathe-cut particles. Spherical alloys are more easily condensed and therefore require a lower mercury content, which can lead to superior physical properties. Amalgam is transferred to the tooth using an *amalgam carrier, and is packed into the cavity using an amalgam *condenser. During the setting reaction, the silver/tin phase (Ag_3Sn or γ phase) of the powdered alloy reacts with the mercury to form a solid material according to the formula:

$$Ag3Sn(\gamma) + Hg$$
$$\rightarrow Ag_3Sn(\gamma) + Ag_2Hg_3(\gamma1) + Sn_7Hg(\gamma_2)$$

The hardened material consists of unchanged particle cores surrounded by a matrix of γ_1 and γ_2. The γ_2 is associated with increased corrosion and lower strength and is kept to a minimum in modern alloys by the inclusion of high amounts of copper. Amalgam is strong, hard-wearing, and has low abrasivity but doesn't bond to tooth substance so requires a mechanically retentive cavity when used as a restorative material; however, **amalgam bonding** can be achieved using adhesive resins which reduce pulpal sensitivity and the need for mechanical cavity retentive features. Because of its durability and poor aesthetics amalgam is used mainly to restore posterior teeth. Amalgam *corrosion at the margins of a restoration over a period of time can result in *ditching. The potential health risk from **amalgam toxicity** because of its mercury content is the subject of ongoing research. Sweden, Denmark, and Germany have proposed restrictions on dental amalgam use to diminish both human exposure to, and environmental release of, mercury, and not because of any documented health effects associated with exposure to dental amalgam.

Further Reading: A review of the future of amalgam as a restorative material: Osborne J. W. Amalgam: dead or alive? *Dent Update* 2006;33(2):94–8.
McCullough M. J., Tyas M. J. Can patients be allergic to amalgam? *International Dental Journal* 2008;58:3–9.

amalgamation *n.* The mixing together of a metal or alloy and mercury to form an amalgam. The alloy and mercury are normally contained within an *amalgam capsule. *See also* TRITURATION.

amalgamator *n.* A machine for mixing amalgam alloy and mercury. *See also* TRITURATION.

amalgam capsule *n.* A round-ended hollow plastic cylinder containing amalgam alloy, mercury, and a mixing pestle. It is mechanically activated to bring the mercury into contact with the alloy and then vibrated in an *amalgamator.

The capsules are visually coded to designate different quantities (**spills**) of alloy and mercury.

amalgam carrier *n.* An instrument used to transfer amalgam alloy to a tooth cavity. It has a hollow working end at an angle to the long axis of the instrument through which amalgam is expelled by a plunger mechanism. It may be made of metal or plastic; the inside of the working tip may be coated with a material to prevent adhesion of the plastic amalgam.

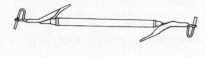

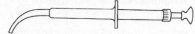

Types of amalgam carrier

amalgam condenser *n. See* CONDENSER.

amalgam tattoo An *iatrogenic lesion caused by traumatic implantation of dental amalgam into soft tissue. It is characterized by a blue-grey discoloration, usually located on the gingiva or alveolar mucosa. As the amalgam corrodes, macrophages take up the amalgam particles and collagen fibres become darkly stained by the silver component. Treatment by excision is usually unnecessary, except for cosmetic reasons or to exclude the diagnosis of a melanotic lesion. 📷

amalgam waste Excess amalgam following the completion of a dental procedure. It may be either excess amalgam mix which has not come into contact with the patient (**non-contact amalgam waste**) or amalgam contaminated by a patient's bodily fluids (**contact amalgam waste**). It may be present in chairside traps, vacuum pump filters, extracted restorations or teeth, amalgam separators, or discarded amalgam capsules. Amalgam waste is classed as hazardous in the European Waste Catalogue and is subject in England to the Hazardous Waste (England and Wales) Regulations (SI2005/894). Amalgam waste should be stored separately in an airtight and clearly labelled container distant from any heat source prior to disposal according to national guidelines or legislation. Commercially supplied storage containers usually contain a mercury vapour suppressant such as activated charcoal or an oxidizing agent used to convert the mercury to a less hazardous form.

(( )) SEE WEB LINKS

- Department of the Environment and Rural Affairs guidance document on waste disposal.
- Proposed American National standard/American Dental Association Specification No.109: Procedures for storing dental amalgam waste and requirements for amalgam waste storage containers.

ameloblast *n.* A cell from which enamel forms. Cells lining the inner surface of the *enamel organ (the inner enamel epithelium) differentiate into ameloblasts. They secrete the enamel proteins *enamelin and *amelogenin, which later mineralize to form enamel. The cells are columnar in shape and have a pyramidal extension at the secretory end called the *Tomes' process.

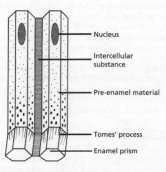

Ameloblast

ameloblastic carcinoma *n.* A malignant *ameloblastoma.

ameloblastic fibrodentinoma *n.* An ameloblastic *fibroma which contains dentine. Some were previously classified as dentinoma.

ameloblastic fibroma *n. See* FIBROMA.

ameloblastic fibro-odontome *n.* An ameloblastic *fibroma associated with an odontome.

ameloblastic odontosarcoma *n.* A very rare *neoplasm containing primitive enamel and dentine.

ameloblastoma *n.* A *benign but locally aggressive *neoplasm of the jaw of unknown cause, derived from *odontogenic epithelium. It is characterized histologically by columnar cells resembling preameloblasts and the stellate reticulum of the developing tooth germ arranged in islands or strands. It may be cystic. It affects young adults and is most common in the fourth decade of life. Radiographically it has a radiolucent multilocular 'soap bubble' appearance and is most common at the angle of the mandible where it may cause expansion. Treatment is by surgical excision with a margin.

amelo-cemental junction *n.* See CEMENTO-ENAMEL JUNCTION.

amelodentinal junction *n.* The point at which the enamel and dentine meet. Microscopically it has a scalloped appearance.

amelogenesis *n.* See ENAMEL.

amelogenesis imperfecta *n.* A group of hereditary defects of either the matrix or the mineralization of enamel. The clinical features depend on which gene is defective. The enamel may be *hypoplastic and appear thin or pitted; *hypocalcified and appear opaque white-, honey-, or brown-coloured; or hypomatured and appear mottled or frosty-white, sometimes confined to the incisal third of the tooth (**snow-capped teeth**). Where there is hypocalcification, the enamel is soft and subject to excessive tooth wear. There may be symptoms of thermal sensitivity. Treatment is usually by restorative intervention. *See also* DENTINOGENESIS IMPERFECTA. 📷

amelogenin *n.* A low-molecular weight extracellular protein secreted by *ameloblasts associated with the formation of enamel. It is thought to be associated with the initiation and growth of *hydroxyapatite crystals.

Ametop (amethocaine) gel *n.* The trade name for a topical analgesic with 4% tetracaine (amethocaine) as the active ingredient. It is used on the skin prior to venepuncture or venous cannulation, especially in children and anxious patients. It needs to be left in situ for approximately 30 minutes prior to venepuncture and 45 minutes prior to cannulation. *See also* TETRACAINE.

amide local analgesic *n.* See ANALGESIC.

amino acid An organic compound containing both an amino group (NH₂) and a carboxylic acid group (COOH). They are synthesized by living systems to form peptides, *polypeptides, and proteins. Amino acids which the body cannot synthesize or store are known as **essential amino acids**. Those generally regarded as essential for humans are histidine, isoleucine, leucine, lysine, methionine, phenylalanine, threonine, tryptophan, and valine.

amiodarone *n.* A drug used in *advanced life support (ALS) for shock resistant ventricular fibrillation (VF) and pulseless ventricular tachycardia (VT). It acts as a membrane stabilizing anti-arrhythmic drug. It slows the *action potential and *refractory period of the *myocardium. It should be given where possible via a central line or, if used peripherally, should be given with a large flush. It is used as a 300mg bolus diluted with 5% *dextrose to 20ml and administered just prior to the fourth shock in cardiopulmonary resuscitation (CPR) (*see* BASIC LIFE SUPPORT).

amnesia *n.* Partial or total loss of memory.

amorphous *adj.* Having no definite shape or form.

amorphous calcium phosphate (ACP) *n.* See CASEIN PHOSPHOPEPTIDE-AMORPHOUS CALCIUM PHOSPHATE.

amoxicillin *n.* A broad spectrum antibiotic effective against both Gram-positive and Gram-negative bacteria, but ineffective against beta-lactamase-producing bacteria. It is a form of *chemotherapy given orally in tablet form or as a suspension and is well absorbed. Side-effects may include nausea, vomiting, diarrhoea, maculopapular rashes, and *angioedema. It should not be prescribed for patients allergic to penicillin. Trade name: **Amoxil**.

amphotericin *n.* A polyene antifungal drug. It is usually administered by intravenous infusion but may be administered by mouth for the treatment of oral *candidiasis (thrush). Side-effects include headache, fever, muscle pains, and diarrhoea. Trade names: **Abelcet, AmBisome, Amphocil, Fungilin, Fungizone**.

ampoule (ampule) *n.* A sealed sterile glass phial or bottle containing a solution for injection.

amputation *n.* The surgical removal of part of the body (e.g. pulp or the root or part of the root of a tooth).

amylase *n.* See PTYALIN.

amyl nitrite A potent *vasodilator and heart stimulant used as an inhalant in the treatment of *angina and cyanide poisoning.

amyloid *n.* A protein substance deposited in extracellular sites in various tissues and organs. It may be idiopathic (unknown cause) or associated with chronic inflammatory diseases or malignancy. It is also found in the brains of individuals with *Alzheimer's disease. The tongue may become enlarged.

amyxorrhoea *n.* An absence of the normal secretion of *mucus.

anabolism *n.* The biological process by which living organisms synthesize simple substances (e.g. sugars and amino acids), into more complex compounds. It is the opposite to *catabolism.

anachoresis *n.* The attraction of micro-organisms to a local tissue lesion.

anaemia (*US* anemia) *n.* A shortage of the oxygen-carrying pigment, *haemoglobin, in the blood, reducing its ability to carry oxygen around the body. **Aplastic anaemia** is a condition where the bone marrow fails to produce any or sufficient red blood cells (*erythrocytes). **Haemolytic anaemia** results from the increased destruction of red blood cells and is seen in congenital conditions such as *sickle-cell trait/disease. This condition is a potential problem during general anaesthesia, owing to the low blood oxygen level. Anaemias can be classified according to the size and shape of the red blood cells. They may be larger than normal (**macrocytic**), smaller (**microcytic**), or normal (**normocytic**) in size. Macrocytic anaemia is due to a deficiency of vitamin B12 and folate, and is treated by replacement therapy. Normocytic anaemia has many causes including acute blood loss, rheumatoid arthritis, tuberculosis, and leukaemia. Microcytic anaemia is due to faulty haemoglobin production, usually because of iron deficiency.

anaerobe *n.* An organism that does not require oxygen for growth and reproduction and may even die in its presence. An **obligate anaerobe** will die in the presence of atmospheric levels of oxygen. A **facultative anaerobe** (e.g. staphylococci and *Escherichia coli*) is an organism, usually a bacterium, that can grow in the presence of oxygen and makes *adenosine triphosphate (ATP) by aerobic respiration if oxygen is present but is also capable of switching to fermentation.

anaerobic *adj.* Describing a biological process which occurs in the absence of oxygen. **Anaerobic respiration** refers to the production of energy by the oxidation of molecules in the absence of oxygen, in contrast to aerobic respiration which does use oxygen.

anaesthesia (*US* anesthesia) *n.* A loss of feeling or sensation in part or all of the body. It may occur as a result of disease, injury, the administration of drugs, or by alternative medical therapies such as *hypnosis or *acupuncture. **General anaesthesia** occurs when there is total loss of consciousness, usually induced by the administration of drugs by inhalation or injection. Risk factors for general anaesthesia include age, smoking, alcohol, drug abuse, and *sickle-cell trait. **Local anaesthesia** (more correctly described as local *analgesia) is achieved by administering a drug to a very localized part of the body (e.g. the oral mucosa). **Regional or block anaesthesia** occurs when one or more nerves are anaesthetized, resulting in loss of sensation to the area of supply (e.g. inferior dental nerve block).

anaesthetic (*US* anesthetic) 1. *n.* An agent that reduces or removes sensation. It can affect the whole body (**general anaesthetic**) or a defined area or region (**local anaesthetic**). General anaesthetics depress the activity of the central nervous system producing loss of consciousness. Local anaesthetics inhibit the conduction of impulses in sensory nerves in the region where they are applied or injected. 2. *adj.* reducing or eliminating sensation.

analgesia

n. Insensibility to pain without loss of consciousness. It is usually produced by the administration of a drug, although it may occur as a result of injury or disease. When drug-induced, an analgesic works by blocking the passage of sodium ions into the nerve cell, thereby interrupting the passage of a nerve stimulus. **Topical analgesia** is used in dentistry to reduce the sensation of *needle penetration prior to a local analgesic. It may be applied as an aerosol spray, ointment, gel, lozenge, tablet, paste, powder, solution, or patch. It can also be delivered as a jet in powder or liquid form. Effective topical analgesics are *lignocaine and *benzocaine. **Infiltration (local) analgesia** is achieved by injecting a local analgesic agent beneath the epithelium of the oral mucosa but above the periosteum. In adults, infiltration analgesia is more effective in the *maxilla than the *mandible because of the comparatively thinner layer of cortical *bone. Mandibular infiltration analgesia may be indicated in children since the mandibular cortical bone is less well developed. **Intraosseous analgesia** is achieved by using a 6mm 27 gauge needle to deliver a small quantity of solution directly into the cancellous bone in the vicinity of the operative area. It may be used where infiltration analgesia has been unsuccessful but it is contraindicated where there is *periodontal disease, limited attached gingival, or minimal *interradicular bone. **Intrapulpal analgesia** is achieved by injecting directly into the pulpal tissue under pressure. **Regional (block) analgesia** is obtained by injecting an analgesic solution close to a nerve trunk (e.g. inferior dental nerve), at some distance from the operating field. This achieves an area of analgesia related to the distribution of the nerve distal to the site of injection. Complications can include haematoma or nerve injury. **Subepithelial analgesia** is accomplished by placing the analgesic agent immediately beneath the epithelial layer of the gingival tissues. Injection into the periodontal ligament achieves **intraligamentary analgesia** which is specific to the tooth concerned and does not extend to the surrounding tissues; it requires a specially designed *syringe which will deliver the analgesic under pressure and provide approximately 15 minutes of pulpal analgesia. **Intrapapillary analgesia** may be indicated for gingival surgery and is achieved by injecting a very small amount of solution into the interdental papilla.

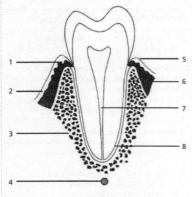

1. Intrapapillary
2. Subepithelial
3. Intraosseous
4. Nerve block
5. Topical
6. Infiltration
7. Intrapulpal
8. Intraligamentary

Analgesia: methods of delivering local analgesic

Failure to achieve analgesia may be due to patient anxiety, inflammation at the site of injection, or anatomical variation. Complications of analgesia include fainting, trauma, allergy (rare), toxicity, *methaemoglobinaemia, and drug interactions. The use of an aspirating *syringe reduces the risk of intravascular injection, particularly when giving regional block injections.

analgesic 1. *n*. An agent that alleviates pain without loss of consciousness. There are many different types of analgesics including non-steroidal anti-inflammatory drugs (e.g. *aspirin, *ibuprofen); para-aminophenols (e.g. *paracetamol); opioid analgesics (e.g. morphine); combined analgesics (e.g. co-codamol); topical analgesics (e.g. *benzydamine hydrochloride); topical and local anaesthetics; anticonvulsants and antidepressants. There are two classes of local anaesthetic agents (more correctly described as local analgesic agents). **Amide local anaesthetic** agents have a tertiary amine base delivered as a water-soluble hydrochloride. Within this group *lignocaine (lidocaine), *prilocaine, *mepivacaine, *articaine, *bupivacaine, levobupivacaine, and *ropivacaine are used in dentistry. These amides are mainly metabolized by the liver. **Ester local anaesthetic** agents are rapidly metabolized in plasma by pseudocholinesterases. Those that are used in dentistry are *procaine, *benzocaine, and amethocaine (*see* AMETOP® GEL). *Cocaine, which is also an ester, is no longer used because of its highly addictive properties and its potential for misuse. The half-life of the esters is very much shorter (only a few minutes) than the amides. 2. *adj*. relieving pain. *See also* ANALGESIA.

Further reading: Ramacciato J. C., Meechan J. G. Recent advances in local anaesthesia. *Dent Update* 2005;32:8–14.

(⊕) SEE WEB LINKS
● World Anaesthesia online. It provides details of the pharmacology of local anaesthetic agents.

analysis of covariance (ANCOVA) A statistical procedure that uses the *F-ratio to investigate the overall fit of a linear model by controlling for the effect that one or more *covariates have on the outcome *variable.

analysis of variance (ANOVA) A statistical test to determine whether there is a significant difference between the means of a number of treatment groups.

anamnesis *n*. The past medical or dental history of a patient based on information recalled by the patient at the time the history is taken.

anaphylaxis *n*. (*adj*. anaphylactic) An immediate and severe life-threatening reaction to a substance. It is characterized by itching, nausea, vomiting, swelling of the mouth and airway, and a fall in blood pressure (*hypotension). Patients may exhibit a rash and show significant peripheral *oedema (swelling). In its acute form it presents as **anaphylactic shock** which can occur within minutes of contact with an *allergen (e.g. penicillin, latex, bee stings, eggs, peanuts). The condition is characterized by severe hypotension, laryngeal swelling, an asthma-like wheeze, and difficulty in breathing due to the restricted airway. Treatment is by injection of *adrenaline, airway maintenance, and administration of oxygen. *See also* SHOCK.

anaplasia *n.* (*adj.* **anaplastic**) A loss of normal cell differentiation or characteristics. It is a characteristic of rapidly growing malignant tumours.

anastomosis *n.* The joining of two structures, organs, or spaces (e.g. two blood vessels), to provide a direct connection between them.

anatomist *n.* A person who studies the structure of the parts of the body.

anatomy *n.* (*adj.* **anatomical**) 1. The science of the dissection or the taking apart of parts of the body. 2. The study of the structure of the parts of the body of an animal or plant.

ANCA-associated granulomatous vasculitis (Wegeners granulomatosis)
A progressive, occasionally fatal disorder affecting the respiratory tract and sometimes the oral cavity. There is marked destruction, and lesions typically affect the gingivae, which appear red and raised. The aetiology is unknown but antibodies against neutrophils (c-ANCA antibodies) are characteristic. It is treated with steroids and cytotoxic drugs.

anchorage *n.* 1. A structure or structures used to provide support or resistance to unwanted tooth movement for an orthodontic appliance. **Absolute anchorage** describes the use of an *implant or *onplant as a specific aid to achieve anchorage during orthodontic treatment. **Extra-oral anchorage** is obtained from outside the mouth (e.g. by linking the appliance by means of hooks and elastics to a head cap). **Intra-oral anchorage** is obtained from within the mouth and may be **simple**, where there is active movement of one tooth versus several anchor teeth, **compound**, where teeth of greater resistance to movement are used as anchorage for the movement of teeth which have less resistance to movement, or **reciprocal**, where two groups of teeth are pitted against each other resulting in equal reciprocal movement of both groups of teeth. Intra-oral anchorage may also be described as **intra-maxillary** (anchorage obtained from teeth in the same jaw) or **inter-maxillary** (anchorage obtained from teeth in the opposing jaw). **Mini-plate anchorage** is obtained by securing small titanium plates with screws to the cortical bone of either jaw: they do not *osseointegrate and therefore do not need to be exposed and can be loaded immediately

after placement. **Micro-screw anchorage** is achieved by using titanium or surgical steel screws approximately 1–2mm in diameter and 4–9mm in length placed in alveolar bone; they are less invasive than *implants, *onplants, or mini-plates. Since they do not osseointegrate they can be loaded immediately after placement and can be removed by simply unscrewing. 2. The means of retention of a restoration. 3. The means of retention of a crown or bridge.

Further Reading: A review of research papers on orthodontic anchorage: Feldmann I., Bondemark L. Orthodontic anchorage: a systematic review. *Angle Orthod* 2006;76 (3):493–501.

ancillary 1. *adj.* Subordinate, subsidiary, or supplementary. 2. *n.* An early term used to describe a dental assistant or nurse.

Andresen appliance [V. Andresen (1870–1950) Norwegian orthodontist] A functional orthodontic appliance used to correct Class II *malocclusions. It is made in one block of acrylic resin and is designed to hold the mandible forwards and increase the distance between the maxilla and mandible. *See also* ORTHODONTIC APPLIANCE.

Andrews' six keys to occlusion A definition of the optimal *occlusion in the permanent dentition as defined by Lawrence F. Andrews in 1972.

Andrews' six keys to occlusion
1   Molar relationship: the distal surface of the disto-buccal cusp of the upper first permanent molar occludes with the mesial surface of the mesio-buccal cusp of the lower second molar.
2   Crown angulation (mesio-distal tip): the gingival part of the long axis of the crown is distal to the incisal part of the axis. The extent of angulation varies according to tooth type.
3   • Crown inclination (labio-lingual, bucco-lingual): the incisors are at a sufficient angulation to prevent overeruption. • Upper posterior teeth: the lingual tip is constant and similar from canine to second premolar and increased in the molars. • Lower posterior teeth: the lingual tip increases progressively from the canines to the molar.
4   Rotations are not present.
5   There are no interdental spaces.
6   There is a flat plane of occlusion.

They have significant clinical implications for routine orthodontic therapy.

Further Reading: Andrews L. F. The six keys to normal occlusion. *Am J Orthod* 1972;62:296-309.

anencephaly *n.* A neural tube defect involving severe structural defects of the brain and skull.

anesthesiology *n.* (US specialty) The branch of medicine that deals with the administration of pain relief during clinical procedures.

aneurysm *n.* (*adj.* **aneurysmal**) A balloon-like swelling or dilatation in the wall of an artery due to *atheroma, infection, or inflammation. A **berry aneurysm** is a small sacular aneurysm that occurs in the *circle of Willis. An atheromatous aneurysm is most common in the abdominal aorta.

aneurysmal bone cyst *See* CYST.

anexate *n.* *See* FLUMAZENIL.

angina *n.* A choking sensation or pain or feeling of strangulation. *See also* ANGINA PECTORIS.

angina bullosa haemorrhagica Large blood-filled blisters, usually seen unilaterally on the soft palate and generally in the elderly. The blisters occur rapidly and spontaneously burst, leaving an area of ulceration. The aetiology is unknown.

angina, Ludwig's *n.* *See* LUDWIG'S ANGINA.

angina pectoris *n.* Chest pain caused by a reduced blood flow to the heart, when the demand for blood by the heart exceeds the supply as during exercise, stress (such as stress induced by a dental visit), or vascular constriction. The pain may spread to the neck, jaws, or arms and there may be additional symptoms of nausea, sweating, or shortness of breath. The most common cause is coronary artery *atheroma. Angina is treated or prevented by sublingual *glyceryl trinitrate tablets or spray and *propranolol. Long-term treatment may be by coronary *angioplasty or a coronary artery bypass.

angina, Vincent's *See* GINGIVITIS, NECROTIZING.

angioedema *n.* Swelling beneath the skin instead of on the surface. Angioedema is characterized by deep swelling around the eyes and lips and sometimes of the hands and feet. If it proceeds rapidly, it can lead to airway obstruction and suffocation, and it should therefore be treated as a medical emergency. It can be hereditary but more commonly occurs as an *allergic response or as a side-effect of some medications such as *angiotensin converting enzyme (ACE) inhibitors.

angiofibroma *n.* A benign tumour composed of blood vessels and fibrous tissue.

angioma *n.* A benign tumour composed of lymph or blood vessels.

angio-oedema (angioneurotic oedema) *n.* *See* URTICARIA.

angioplasty *n.* A surgical procedure in which a narrowed or diseased artery is widened by the insertion of a thin tube (catheter) which is inflated so as to dilate the lumen of the artery and improve the blood flow.

angiosarcoma *n.* A rare but highly malignant *neoplasm arising from vascular endothelial cells.

angiotensin converting enzyme (ACE) inhibitors A group of drugs (e.g. **lisinopril, captopril**) used in the treatment of *hypertension and congestive cardiac failure. Side-effects include dry mouth (*xerostomia), *glossitis, dry cough, *angioedema, and *lichenoid-type reactions. Captopril is associated with depression of the bone marrow and can lead to anaemia and spontaneous bruising or bleeding.

Further reading: Wakefield Y. S., Theaker E. D., Pemberton M. N. Angiotensin converting enzyme inhibitors and delayed onset, recurrent angioedema of the head and neck. *Br Dent J* 2008;205:553-6.

angle *n.* The space between two meeting lines or surfaces. An **angle board** is a device used for positioning the patient's head in relation to the x-ray beam and x-ray film when taking extra-oral radiographs. The **cavosurface angle** in a prepared cavity is formed by the junction of the cavity wall with the surface of the tooth. The **cusp angle** is made by the slope of the cusp of a tooth with a perpendicular line bisecting the cusp. A **line angle** is formed at the junction of two tooth surfaces or two cavity walls; it is designated by the names of the walls forming the angle e.g. disto-buccal line angle. The **angle of the** *mandible** is formed by the junction of the ramus and the body. The **angle of the mouth** forms the junction of the upper and lower lips.

Angle, Edward Hartley (1855–1930) An American dentist regarded as the father of orthodontics. He graduated from the Pennsylvania College of Dentistry in 1876 after 18 months of study. In 1885 he was appointed professor of orthodontics at the University of Minnesota and was subsequently appointed professor at Northwestern University, the Marion Simms College of Medicine, and the Washington University Medical Department. In 1900 he established the Angle School of Orthodontia in St Louis, Missouri. In 1922 the Edward H. Angle

Society of Orthodontia was established by some of Angle's graduates and survived until 1928; it was replaced in 1930 by a new organization, the Angle Orthodontist. Angle classified abnormalities of occlusion (*see* MOLAR RELATIONSHIP) and designed appliances for their treatment; he also devised a number of surgical techniques.

Angle's classification of malocclusion *n. See* MOLAR RELATIONSHIP.

angular cheilitis (perlèche, cheilosis) A condition characterized by redness, soreness, and cracking of the corners of the lips. It is frequently caused by infection with *Candida species but, where there is crusting, secondary infection with *Staphylococcus aureus should be considered. It is associated with *overclosure due to worn dentures, or excessive *tooth wear, and nutritional deficiencies such as vitamin B12, folate, or iron. Treatment is by the application of topical antimicrobial cream and, depending on the cause, restoration of the vertical height, or prescription of nutritional supplements.

angulation *n.* The direction of the primary beam of radiation in relation to the teeth and the radiographic film.

anhidrosis *n.* The failure to sweat in response to an appropriate stimulus such as physical exertion or heat. It is a characteristic of anhidrotic ectodermal *dysplasia.

anhidrotic 1. *n.* A drug that inhibits sweating. 2. *adj.* Inhibiting sweating.

anhidrotic ectodermal dysplasia (hypohidrotic ectodermal dysplasia) *See* DYSPLASIA.

anhydrous *adj.* Without water. Anhydrous forms of dental cements are initiated by the presence of water.

anisodont *adj.* Describing the condition of having unequal or irregular teeth as typified by insectivores and carnivores. *Compare* ISODONT.

anisognathous *adj.* Describing a condition in which the maxillary and mandibular arches or jaws are of unequal size, with the upper jaw being of greater width than the lower jaw.

ankylocheilia *n.* The adhesion of the lips to each other.

ankyloglossia *n.* A congenital abnormality in which a short lingual *fraenum limits the movement of the tongue (**tongue-tie**). It may affect breast-feeding, speech, or the self-cleansing mechanism of the mouth. Surgical intervention is usually unnecessary but if advocated is usually delayed until late childhood.

(⊕) SEE WEB LINKS

• Bandolier website section that provides evidence-based information on ankyloglossia.

ankylosis *n.* (*adj.* **ankylotic**) 1. The pathological fusion of bones across a joint space. Fusion across the temporomandibular joint may occur as a result of trauma, mastoid infection, or juvenile chronic arthritis. Treatment may be by replacement with a prosthetic joint or by a graft if the facial development is incomplete. 2. The fusion of a tooth directly to bone with no intervening *periodontal ligament. This may occur as a result of trauma, most frequently to the upper incisor teeth or spontaneously (e.g. primary molars). Ankylosed teeth can become submerged (infra-occluded), which may necessitate restoration or extraction.

Further reading: An overview of the management of ankylosed teeth: Kurol J. Impacted and ankylosed teeth: why, when, and how to intervene. *Am J Orthod Dentofacial Orthop* 2006;129: S86–90.

ankylotomy *n. See* FRAENOTOMY.

anneal *v.* The heating and cooling of metals or glass to alter their physical characteristics such as hardness or brittleness. *Gold foil is annealed immediately prior to condensation, solely to drive off any volatile impurities.

anodontia *n.* A congenital absence of teeth. When all teeth are missing it is described as **total anodontia**; when only some teeth are missing it is described as **partial anodontia** or *hypodontia.

anodontism *n.* Congenital absence of tooth bud development.

anodyne *n.* Any treatment or drug that relieves or soothes pain.

anomalad *n.* A pattern of anomalies arising from one structural defect.

anorexia nervosa An eating disorder characterized by low body weight, disturbed body image, and a pathological fear of weight gain. It is most common among female adolescents. Physiological signs include electrolyte disturbances from the excessive use of laxatives, depression, impaired nutrition, and cardiac dysrhythmias. Low oestrogen levels contribute to significant losses in bone density. In addition, individuals with anorexia often produce excessive amounts of the adrenal hormone *cortisol, which is known to trigger bone loss. Low bone mass (osteopenia) is not uncommon in anorexics and occurs early on in the course of the disease. Girls with anorexia are less likely to reach their peak bone density and therefore may be at increased risk of osteoporosis and bone fracture throughout life. Self-induced vomiting causes marked acid *erosion of the teeth, particularly affecting the palatal and occlusal surfaces. A tendency towards fanatical oral hygiene can lead to tooth *abrasion and significant *gingival recession. Treatment is by psychotherapy, family therapy, nutritional guidance, and antidepressants for prevention of relapse. *See also* BULIMIA NERVOSA.

Further Reading: Ashcroft A., Milosevic A. The eating disorders: 1 current scientific understanding and dental implications. *Dent Update* 2007;34:544–54.

(((⊕))) **SEE WEB LINKS**

• Medicine.net page that provides information on the symptoms, treatment and causes of anorexia nervosa.

anosmia *n.* Absence of the sense of smell. It can be temporary, as with the common cold, or permanent, such as following certain viral infections. Partial loss of the sense of smell is called **hyposmia**.

ANOVA *See* ANALYSIS OF VARIANCE.

ansa cervicalis A loop of nerves derived from the cervical plexus which supplies the sternothyroid, sternohyoid, and omohyoid muscles. A superior root (C1) joins the inferior root (C2, C3) to form the handle or **ansa anterior** to the common carotid arteries.

antagonist *n.* (*n.* **antagonism**) 1. A tooth in one jaw that occludes with a tooth in the opposing jaw. 2. A muscle that acts against or in opposition to another muscle. 3. A drug which counteracts or blocks the action of another drug; for example, flumazenil is the antagonist for benzodiazepines; naloxone is the antagonist to opioid drugs.

ante- Prefix denoting before. Examples: **antenatal** (before birth), **anteprandial** (before meals).

antealveolism *n.* A condition in which the *alveolar process is normal in height and width but is positioned anteriorly on the respective jaw base. *Compare* RETROALVEOLISM.

antegenia *n.* A condition in which the chin prominence is too far forward in relation to the rest of the facial skeleton. *Compare* RETROGENIA.

antemaxillism *n.* A condition in which the base of the maxilla is normal in length and width, but is positioned too far anteriorly. *Compare* RETROMAXILLISM.

anterior open bite (AOB) *n. See* BITE.

anterior triangle The anterior cervical region of the neck whose borders are formed posteriorly by the anterior border of sternocleidomastoid muscle, superiorly by the lower border of the body of the mandible and a line extending from the angle of the mandible to the mastoid process, and anteriorly by the midline of the neck. *See also* POSTERIOR TRIANGLE.

Ante's law First postulated by Irwin H. Ante, a Canadian dentist, in 1926. It states that the combined pericemental area of all abutment teeth supporting a fixed dental prosthesis should be equal to or greater in pericemental area than the tooth or teeth to be replaced. Ante's law is generally considered to be a guide rather than a law.

anthropoid space *See* PRIMATE SPACE.

antibiotic *n.* A substance produced by or derived from a micro-organism which has the capacity, in low concentration, to inhibit the growth of or kill other micro-organisms. They are used to treat antibiotic-sensitive infections. Antibiotics active against a wide variety of organisms (**broad-spectrum antibiotics**) may cause the proliferation of resistant organisms. **Systemic antibiotics** may be appropriate for oral or dental conditions where there are systemic signs of illness (e.g. *pyrexia, gross facial swelling, significant *lymphadenopathy, and *trismus). **Topical antibiotic** delivery systems can deliver a high dosage in a closely defined area (e.g. *tetracycline and *minocycline inserted into a gingival pocket), and may be used in conjunction with other localized treatment. Adverse oral reactions to antibiotics are *glossitis, *angular cheilitis, and *hairy tongue due to *allergy, sensitivity, or a proliferation of resistant organisms. **Antibiotic prophylaxis** involves the use of an antibiotic to protect the individual from an anticipated bacterial invasion. It is particularly useful for certain medically compromised patients; however, antibiotic resistance can occur as a result of inappropriate or excessive use. Any benefits from prophylaxis need to be weighed against the risks of adverse effects for the patient and of antibiotic resistance developing. As a result, the National Institute for Health and Clinical Excellence (NICE) recommends in guideline 64 that antibiotic prophylaxis should no longer be offered routinely for defined interventional procedures.

(((⊕))) **SEE WEB LINKS**

• Access to the National Institute for Health and Clinical Excellence (NICE) guidance.

antibody *n.* A specialized protein produced by the white blood cells (plasma cells) of the immune system in response to a foreign substance (*antigen). It acts specifically on the foreign substance and destroys it. Antibodies form an important part of the body's natural defence mechanism and they are classified according to their structure and function.

anticoagulant *n.* A substance that prevents or retards the clotting of blood. Anticoagulants may be natural (e.g. *heparin) or synthetic (e.g. *Warfarin). Anticoagulant therapy is a potential haemorrhage risk factor for patients undergoing dental treatment.

anticonvulsant *n.* A drug used to prevent or relieve seizures or convulsions. Anticonvulsants are frequently used in the treatment of *epilepsy but are also used in the management of chronic pain and *trigeminal neuralgia e.g. *carbamazepine, gabapentin, lamotrigine, and *phenytoin. *See also* BENZODIAZEPINE.

antidote *n.* A substance that counteracts injurious or unwanted effects. Antidotes may be used for the treatment of drug overdose or the ingestion of poisons or toxins. For example, naloxone is the antidote for morphine overdose.

antiemetic *n.* A drug that reduces or prevents vomiting or nausea.

antiflux *n.* A coating placed on metal to prevent the flow of applied solder (e.g. graphite). *See also* FLUX.

antigen *n.* Any substance that is capable of stimulating the production of antibodies.

antihistamine *n.* A chemical that blocks the effect of *histamine produced during an allergic reaction. Antihistamines have a drying effect on the nasal mucosa.

antioxidant *n.* A substance capable of reducing damage due to oxygen such as that caused by free radicals produced by various disease processes, radiation, smoking, poisons, and other agencies. Antioxidants occur naturally in the body, may be ingested as supplements, or are added to certain foods to prolong their shelf-life.

antiplaque *adj.* Describing substances, such as *chlorhexidine gluconate and *triclosan, used to control the formation of dental *plaque.

antipyretic *n.* An agent that lowers the body temperature thus reducing fever. Some analgesic drugs (e.g. *paracetamol) have antipyretic activity.

anti-rotation *n. See* RETENTION.

antisepsis *n.* The process of using an antimicrobial substance or agent to inhibit the growth of micro-organisms while in contact with them.

antiseptic *n.* A substance that destroys (*bactericidal) or inhibits (*bacteriostatic) the growth of bacteria or other micro-organisms. A *bisguanide antiseptic such as *chlorhexidine may be applied to wounds of the oral mucosa or used as a mouthwash. Natural herbal antiseptics such as sanquinarine have been used in both toothpastes and mouthwashes.

antisialogogue *n.* A drug, such as atropine, that diminishes the flow of saliva.

antitoxin *n.* An antibody produced by the body with the ability to neutralize a specific toxin produced by invading bacteria, other micro-organisms, or from any other source.

antitrismus *n.* A condition of tonic muscular spasm that prevents closing of the mouth.

antitussive *n.* A drug that suppresses coughing.

antrocele *n.* An accumulation of fluid in the *maxillary sinus.

antrolith *n.* A calcified mass in the *maxillary sinus (antrum). It is usually asymptomatic and is formed by calcification of a *nidus such as a bone chip, root fragment, or foreign object. It may be associated with *sinusitis.

antrostomy (antrotomy) *n.* A surgical procedure to produce a permanent or semipermanent artificial opening in the maxillary antrum in order to secure drainage for any fluid.

antrum *n.* A cavity in a bone. *See also* MAXILLARY SINUS.

ANUG *n. See* GINGIVITIS, NECROTIZING.

anxiety *n.* A feeling of apprehension characterized by fear, tension, nervousness, or restlessness, and associated with increased activity of the *sympathetic nervous system. In the dental context it can be measured using the *dental anxiety scale or the *modified dental anxiety scale. An **anxiety state** is a condition in which anxiety dominates the patient's life. **Anxiety control** is important in improving patient comfort and dental attendance. It can be achieved using a variety of methods including behavioural techniques, distraction, control strategies, relaxation techniques, positive reinforcement, local analgesia, and *anxiolytic drugs (e.g.

*benzodiazepines). Management may be aided by the use of *hypnosis, and inhalation, intravenous, oral, or intranasal *sedation.

Further Reading: Mellor A. Management of the anxious patient: what treatments are available. *Dent Update* 2007;34:108–14.

anxiolytic *adj.* Describing a drug that reduces or treats acute or chronic anxiety.

apertognathia *n.* A type of malocclusion in which either the anterior or posterior teeth of the mandible do not occlude with those of the maxilla. Possible causes include fracture of the mandible, dislocation of the temporomandibular joint, or deformity of either the mandible or maxilla. *See also* BITE.

Apert syndrome (acrocephalosyndactyly) [E. Apert (1868–1940), French physician] A congenital disorder characterized by fusion of the fingers and toes (**syndactyly**) and cranial malformations. Oral manifestations include mandibular *prognathism, a narrow high arched palate, and crowded teeth.

apex *n.* The tip of a tooth root. The **anatomic apex** is usually defined as the apical constriction in the root canal at the cemento-dentinal junction. **Apex locators** are instruments used to determine the position of the apical foramen in endodontic therapy by measuring electrical resistance; recent electronic apex locators (EALs) have multiple frequencies which are claimed to reduce the clinical inaccuracies caused by the presence of blood or irrigants in the root canal.

Further Reading: Khaled A. B. Modern electronic apex locators are reliable for determining root canal working length. *Evid based Dentistry* 2006;7:31–2.

apexification *n.* Treatment to induce the closure of an open root apex containing a necrotic pulp. *Necrotic tissue is removed with the intention of promoting the formation of a calcified barrier across the open apex of the tooth so that obturation with a root canal filling material may be achieved.

apexigraph *n.* A device used to measure the size and position of the root *apex of a tooth.

apexogenesis *n.* Treatment for a tooth with an open apex designed to preserve apical pulp tissue to encourage the completion of the formation of the root apex.

aphagia *n.* The loss of the ability to swallow. It is often used to refer specifically to an inability to eat. Aphagia can be due to lesions in the hypothalamus of the brain, damage to the cranial nerves, or to a blockage or constriction of the *oesophagus.

aphasia (dysphasia) *n.* A neurological disorder affecting the generation and content of speech and its understanding. It is commonly associated with reading or writing difficulties.

aphthous ulcer A discrete white or red ulcerated spot occurring on the mucous membrane. They are relatively common particularly in younger individuals and are of unknown aetiology. Predisposing factors include stress, trauma, hormonal changes such as menstruation and puberty, and haematological disorders such as vitamin B_{12} and iron deficiency anaemia. There is a hereditary disposition in about 45% of patients. **Herpetiform aphthous ulcers** are small-sized ulcers which occur in crops. **Minor aphthous ulcers** are characteristically very painful ulcers 2–5mm in diameter covered by a grey slough, located on non-keratinized mucosa; they last for 10–14 days and have a variable time interval for recurrence; the surrounding mucosa may be reddened (erythematous). **Major aphthous ulcers** are usually 6–10mm in diameter, often multiple, and affecting both the keratinized and non-keratinized mucosa. They are commonly located on the lips, cheeks, or soft palate. They are painful, last for 4–6 weeks, and may heal with residual scarring. Treatment of aphthous ulcers is symptomatic once the predisposing factors have been excluded. The application of topical hyaluronic acid may be of transient benefit in providing a protective barrier to stimuli produced within the mouth. *See also* ORAL ULCERATION. 📷

apical *adj.* Relating to the apex of the tooth root.

apical abscess *n. See* ABSCESS.

apical granuloma An accumulation of granulation tissue (fibroblasts and endothelial cells) and inflammatory cells at the apex of a non-vital tooth. The bone and periodontal ligament is destroyed by infection from the non-vital tooth and appears as a radiolucency (dark area) on a radiograph.

apicectomy (apicoectomy) *n.* (Also known as peri-radicular surgery, apical surgery or surgical endodontics.) The surgical removal of the apex or apical portion of a tooth. The procedure involves the raising of a mucoperiosteal flap to expose the alveolar bone, buccal bone removal over the area of the root apex, the removal of at least 3mm of the root apex, the preparation of a small cavity in the root apex into which a biocompatible filling material such as *mineral trioxide aggregate or glass ionomer *cement is placed (retrograde *root filling), and finally the closure of the soft tissue wound using suture material. An apicectomy may be indicated in situations where there is a failure of conventional endodontics such as a sclerosed root canal, inaccessible lateral canals, apical root fracture, a fractured root canal instrument that cannot otherwise be removed, a symptomatic apically extruded root filling, an open apex that cannot be sealed using a conventional root filling, an apical cyst needing to be removed, or when an apical *biopsy is indicated.

apicoectomy *n. See* APICECTOMY.

apicoscopy *n.* The application of *odontoscopy to endodontic surgery.

apicotomy *n.* Incision into an apical structure.

aplasia *n.* Total or partial failure of development of an organ or tissue.

aponeurosis *n.* A fibrous or membranous sheet histologically similar to a tendon which connects a muscle to the part it moves.

apoptosis *n.* The body's normal process of terminating the life cycle of a damaged, malfunctioning, unwanted, or dead cell through cellular self-destruction involving the fragmentation of cell membranes which are then *phagocytosed by neighbouring cellular activity.

apoxemena *n.* An obsolete term used to describe the material removed from a periodontal pocket.

apoxesis *n.* An archaic expression used to describe the *debridement of the root surfaces.

appliance *n.* A device used to improve function or to provide therapeutic benefit. An *orthodontic appliance is used to move teeth or to stabilize their position.

appraisal *n.* The act or process of estimating value. **Performance appraisal** is a periodic evaluation of an individual's assigned duties and responsibilities; it may be applied to all members of the dental team. The basis for performance appraisal is the performance which may be expected after a reasonable or defined period of training of an individual. **Practice appraisal** is a method of assessing the quality of care delivered in a primary care setting, together with providing advice and guidance on any necessary or desirable changes that need to be made. Practice appraisal may also include a valuation of the practice to establish its asset value.

approximal (proximal) *adj.* Near to or adjacent. Approximal surfaces are those surfaces of the teeth that adjoin each other in the same dental arch. *See also* TOOTH SURFACE.

apron spring *n. See* SPRING.

apyrexia *n.* The absence of fever. *Compare* PYREXIA.

arch *n.* A curved or bow-shaped structure. The **alveolar arch** is the bow-shaped alveolar process of either the maxilla or mandible. The first **branchial arch** is located between the stomodeum and the first pharyngeal groove and develops into the mandibular and maxillary processes. The **palatine arch** (pillars of the fauces) consists of the two curved folds of mucous membrane enclosing the muscles at the sides of the mouth at the entrance to the *pharynx. The **zygomatic arch** is formed by the *zygomatic bone and the zygomatic process of the *maxilla and the *temporal bone.

archaea *pl. n.* A group of *prokaryotic micro-organisms originally called archaebacteria. Archaea were originally described in extreme environments and were known as **extremophiles** but have since been found to be ubiquitous. Unlike bacteria, archaea are not known to cause disease in humans or animals. Archaea and bacteria are similar in that they are both prokaryotic, but they have evolved differently. *See also* PROKARYOTES.

archwire *n.* That part of an *orthodontic appliance that is placed into the bracket slots and applies the force through the brackets to the teeth to guide tooth movement. It may be passive or active in applying a force to one or more teeth. In cross-section, the archwire may be either round, which in a rectangular slot will produce a tipping force around the fulcrum of the tooth in response to a buccolingual force, or it may be rectangular, which in a rectangular slot can produce buccolingual apical movement. The wire used is usually stainless steel, variations of nickel titanium, or tungsten molybdenum alloy (TMA) based. A **pre-posted archwire** has hooks already attached; these hooks are fixed in a set position on the wire. A **sectional archwire** occupies less than the complete arch; it engages only a few teeth (e.g. only the four incisors or only a posterior dental segment), through crown attachments.

areca nut *n. See* BETEL QUID.

areola *n.* (*pl.* **areolae**; *adj.* **areolar**) A small space in a tissue. Also used to describe small circular areas such as the inflamed region around a pimple.

argyria *n.* A rare condition resulting in a permanent blue-grey discoloration of the skin or mucous membrane due to the ingestion of silver, usually in the form of ointments or silver containing drugs. It may be generalized or localized.

Arkansas stone A fine grained abrasive quartz rock (**novaculite**) used for sharpening non-disposable surgical and dental instruments; it is found in the Ouachita mountains of Arkansas and Oklahoma. The grain of the silica crystals that form novaculite are approximately the same size (3–5µ), whether the stone is classified as soft Arkansas or hard Arkansas. After use the stone should be cleaned using a solvent.

armamentarium *n.* The materials and equipment of a dental or medical practitioner.

arnica montana *n.* A topical remedy used in *homeopathic dentistry for the management of trauma and bleeding. It has been known to cause contact dermatitis. It is derived from the rhizomatous arnica genus of plants. Current research evidence for the efficacy of arnica is lacking.

Further Reading: Ernst E., Pittler M. H. Efficacy of homeopathic arnica: A systematic review of placebo-controlled clinical trials. *Arch Surg* 1998;133:1187–90.

aromatherapy *n.* The use of smells derived from natural herbs as therapeutic agents such as to aid relaxation and reduce stress. The herbs are usually diluted in carrier oils. The evidence base for their effective use in the dental environment is currently lacking.

ART *See* ATRAUMATIC RESTORATIVE TREATMENT.

arteriosclerosis *n.* A generic name for a group of degenerative diseases characterized by the constriction of the lumen of an artery due to a thickening of the wall resulting in a reduced blood supply (*ischaemia) to the area of supply. *See also* ATHEROSCLEROSIS.

arteritis *n.* An inflammatory disease of the muscular walls of the arteries. **Temporal arteritis** occurs in the elderly and most commonly affects the arteries of the scalp.

artery *n.* (*adj.* **arterial**) A blood vessel carrying blood away from the heart. All arteries except the pulmonary artery carry oxygenated blood. The walls of an artery consist of three layers: an inner layer (**tunica intima**), a middle smooth muscle and elastic tissue layer (**tunica media**), and an outer fibrous layer (**tunica adventitia, tunica externa**). *See* Appendix C for the main arteries of the head and neck.

arthritis *n.* (*adj.* **arthritic**) The inflammation of one or more joints. It may be acute (sudden onset) and characterized by swelling, pain,

redness, warmth, and reduced function. Chronic forms result in progressive destruction of the joint and are commonly due to wear and tear (*osteoarthritis) or autoimmune disease such as *rheumatoid arthritis.

arthrocentesis *n.* The irrigation of joint spaces using saline under pressure. It is used in the treatment of inflammatory conditions of the *temporomandibular joint.

arthrogram *n.* A radiographic imaging technique involving the injection of radiopaque dye into a joint, such as the temporomandibular joint, to demonstrate the position of soft tissues within it. It has now been superseded by *magnetic resonance imaging (MRI).

arthroplasty *n.* The surgical remodelling of a joint or joint abnormality. Temporomandibular arthroplasty may be indicated in conditions of intractable pain during normal function (chewing, opening, yawning, and talking).

arthroscopy *n.* The direct visual examination of a joint cavity using a rigid telescope fitted with a lens system and fibreoptic illumination (**arthroscope**). The instrument also has interchangeable ends which can allow for some minimal surgical procedures to be carried out such as the division of joint adhesions and minor re-modelling of the articular surfaces.

articaine (carticaine) *n.* An amide local *anaesthesia agent used in dentistry currently available as a 4% solution. When used with a *vasoconstrictor, usually *adrenaline, the efficacy is similar or better than *lignocaine with adrenaline; common findings include greater success in producing anaesthesia, more profound anaesthesia, and faster onset of action. It has a shorter half-life than lignocaine with adrenaline. Swelling and persistent *paraesthesia of the oral tissues (e.g. the lips) have been reported after inferior dental block injections. Trade names: Septocaine, Septanest*.

Further Reading: Wells J. P., Beckett H. Articaine hydrochloride: a safe alternative to lignocaine? *Dent Update* 2008;35:253–6.

articular disc *n.* A fibrocartilaginous plate or ring separating the articular surfaces of the bones of a joint.

articulating paper *n.* A thin non-adhesive paper strip coated in coloured or fluorescent ink or dye-containing wax. It is used for marking occlusal contacts or interferences.

articulation *n.* 1. The jointed movement of the upper and lower teeth when they come into contact. 2. The arrangement of artificial teeth to simulate the natural dentition. **3.** The process of producing or shaping the sounds of speech.

articulator *n.* A device that artificially attempts to reproduce the movement of the jaws. A **hinge articulator** only permits movement on a vertical hinge axis. **Plane line** and **average value articulators** allow limited lateral and protrusive movement. The average value articulator is usually set at 25–30° for condylar guidance angle, 15° for incisal guidance, and 110mm for intercondylar distance. The **semi-adjustable articulator** allows the recording of multiple positions of the mandible and the recording of these positions in relation to the maxilla. It requires the use of a facebow and interocclusal records. There are two types: the **arcon** (**ar**ticulator-**con**dyle) type has an adjustable condylar fossa mechanism that sits on a fixed condylar sphere; it has features of the joint mechanism that are anatomically similar to the arrangement in a natural temporomandibular joint; the **non-arcon** type is the reverse of the arcon type in that it has a moving condylar sphere set in a non-removable track. **Fully adjustable articulators** provide for more adjustments and greater accuracy; border movements of the mandible can be duplicated with a high degree of accuracy. They usually require *pantographic tracings to set the adjustments. A **maxillofacial articulator** is used for model planning prior to the surgical correction of dentofacial and craniofacial deformities.

Further Reading: Milosevic A. Occlusion: 3. Articulators and related instruments. *Dent Update.* 2003;30(9):511–15.

artifact (artefact) *n.* (in radiography) An artificial blemish appearing on an image suggesting a defective technique or image receptor as opposed to the true appearance of the patient: an artifact indicates something that is not really there.

asbestos *n.* A group of minerals with long fibrous crystals formerly used as a lining material in laboratory casting procedures. Its use has been discontinued because of the highly toxic nature of the material. Inhalation of asbestos dust can result in serious long-term lung disease such as **asbestosis** and *malignant tumours of the lungs.

asepsis *n.* (*adj.* **aseptic**) The practice to reduce or eliminate microbial contaminants (including bacteria, fungi, viruses, and other micro-organisms) from the operative field in surgery (including dentistry) to prevent or minimize infection.

aseptic technique A procedure that is free from contamination by any bacteria, fungi, virus, or other micro-organism.

Asperger's syndrome [H. Asperger (1906–80), Austrian paediatrician] *n.* A

psychiatric disorder of childhood. It is a variant of autism spectrum disorder. Features of dental significance are *bruxism, prolonged retention of food in the mouth increasing the prevalence of caries, and possible gingival overgrowth due to medication with *phenytoin.

asphyxia *n.* Suffocation; a life-threatening condition in which there is insufficient or no oxygen reaching the tissues due to obstruction or damage to a part of the respiratory system. Brain cells cannot normally live for more than about 4 minutes without oxygen.

aspiration *n.* **1.** The inhalation of a foreign body into the respiratory system. **2.** The removal of gases, liquids, or solids from the body or a body cavity by means of vacuum suction. It is achieved using equipment called an **aspirator**. This may consist of a needle used to draw up fluid into a syringe or cartridge (e.g. blood aspiration prior to block analgesia); *see* SYRINGE. Intra-orally, aspiration of fluids is achieved with either low-level aspiration using the vacuum created by running water (saliva *ejector) or by high-speed suction capable of additionally removing solid debris (e.g. tooth and restoration fragments).

aspirin (acetylsalicylic acid) *n.* A non-steroidal anti-inflammatory drug that reduces fever and inflammation; it is taken orally, alone or in combination with other analgesics, for the relief of pain such as headache, toothache, neuralgias, and the pain of rheumatoid *arthritis. Aspirin inhibits both cyclo-oxygenase 1 and 2 irreversibly, thus preventing binding of arachidonic acid to the active sites of the enzymes and thereby inhibiting prostaglandin synthesis. It also has anti-platelet activity leading to an increase in bleeding time and may be taken on a regular basis as a preventive measure to reduce the likelihood of coronary thrombosis or stroke. Side-effects include gastric irritation causing pain, nausea, vomiting, and bleeding. Aspirin tablets taken for the relief of toothache should not be placed on the mucosa adjacent to the offending tooth as ulceration will occur (**aspirin burn**). Aspirin has been implicated as a cause of *Reye's syndrome and should not therefore be prescribed to children under 12 years of age. 📷

assessor *n.* An independent person working within the National Vocational Qualification (NVQ) framework who ensures that a trainee dental nurse is competent in their area of work.

association *n.* **1.** A term used in statistics to describe two variables which have a known link or statistical dependence. A **positive association** exists when high values of one variable tend to be associated with high values of the other variable and vice versa e.g. smoking and lung cancer.

A **negative association** exists when high values of one variable tend to be associated with low values of the other variable and vice versa e.g. periodontal disease and frequency of toothbrushing. Association does not imply *causation. **2.** A recognized pattern of malformation not considered to be a *syndrome or an *anomalad.

asterion *n.* An anatomical landmark. It marks the junction of the *occipital, *parietal, and *temporal bones.

asthma *n.* A condition in which there is narrowing of the bronchial airways, which can change in severity over short periods of time. It is characterized by coughing, wheezing, and breathing difficulties. **Bronchial asthma** may be induced by a wide variety of causes including exposure to an *antigen, drugs (typically non-steroidal anti-inflammatory analgesics), air pollution, *anxiety, infection, and exercise. Signs and symptoms include breathlessness, *tachycardia, low respiratory flow rate, and *cyanosis of the lips and nail beds. If left untreated, the individual may develop **status asthmaticus** with possible respiratory arrest. Management is by the administration of oxygen and bronchodilators (e.g. salbutamol, ipatropium bromide via an aerosol or nebulizer). Avoidance of known allergens may help to reduce the frequency of occurrence.

astringent *n.* An agent that contracts or shrinks tissue by causing cells to precipitate protein from their surfaces. It is used to contract or harden tissue, reducing *bleeding or glandular secretion (e.g. from the *mucosa). Astringents such as aluminium chloride are often added to *gingival retraction cord to reduce gingival secretions.

ataxia *n.* An inability to coordinate muscle activity during voluntary movement.

atel- (atelo-) Prefix denoting imperfect or incomplete development. Examples: **atelocheilia** (of the lips); **ateloglossia** (of the tongue); **atelognathia** (of the jaw); **ateloprosopia** (of the face); **atelostomia** (of the mouth).

atheroma *n.* (*adj.* **atheromatous**) A thickening of the arterial wall due to the deposition of fat and fibrous tissue. It reduces blood circulation and can lead to *thrombosis or the formation of an aneurysm. It is associated with a high *cholesterol diet, refined sugar, obesity, smoking, and lack of exercise.

atherosclerosis *n.* A degenerative disease, principally of the aorta and its major branches, characterized by multiple *atheroma. It is one of the most frequent causes of death in the western world and is a common cause of *coronary thrombosis, strokes, and rupture of aneurysms.

atlas *n.* The first cervical vertebra (C1).

atomization device *n.* A piece of equipment used to convert a liquid into a spray, such as a nozzle attached to the end of a hypodermic syringe used for the delivery of intranasal *midazolam in the treatment of *status epilepticus.

atopy *n.* A hereditary or constitutional tendency to develop hypersensitivity reactions in response to low doses of *allergens, usually proteins, and as a consequence to develop typical symptoms such as allergic *asthma, hay fever, and atopic eczema.

atraumatic restorative treatment (ART) The process of removing *caries using hand instruments only and then restoring the tooth with an adhesive restoration. Restorative materials used are either glass ionomer *cement or *resin composite. It is particularly suitable for use in developing countries because of the need for minimum equipment and resources, allowing treatment to be delivered at low cost. ART may also be an effective method of treating root caries in elderly people, using chemically cured glass ionomer *cement. Hand instruments have been designed specifically for this method of restorative treatment.

 SEE WEB LINKS
- World Health Organization website providing practical information about undertaking ART.

atrioventricular node An area of specialized heart muscle located on the septal wall of the right *atrium close to the entrance to the right *ventricle. It receives electrical impulses from the *sinoatrial node and transmits them to the ventricles via the atrioventricular bundle. *See also* CARDIOVASCULAR SYSTEM.

atrium *n.* (*pl.* **atria**) The chambers of the heart which receive blood. The right atrium receives blood from the systemic circulation via the venae cavae: the left atrium receives blood from the lungs via the pulmonary veins.

atrophy *n.* A wasting or decrease in size of any organ, tissue, or cell of the body which is not sufficient to cause necrosis. It may occur in response to poor nutrition, lack of use (disuse or immobilization), reduction in blood supply, loss of nerve supply, chronic cell injury, or ageing.

atropine *n.* A drug that blocks the effect of the vagus nerve on the *sinoatrial and *atrioventricular nodes by antagonizing the neurotransmitter acetylcholine. It increases sinus node automaticity and aids atrioventricular conduction. It is used in cardiopulmonary resuscitation as a single bolus dose for patients in whom the heart no longer beats (asystole) or pulseless electrical activity (PEA) with a rate of <60 / min.

attachment *n.* 1. The means by which two objects are fastened together. 2. A mechanical device used to retain or stabilize a dental prosthesis. The **epithelial attachment** is the biological mechanism that joins the *junctional epithelium to the tooth. It is formed from the *reduced enamel epithelium. The junctional epithelium forms the *hemidesmosomal attachment of the gingival tissues to the teeth. The **attachment apparatus** includes the periodontal ligament, the cementum, and the alveolar bone. The **clinical attachment level** is the distance from the attachment of the periodontal tissues (junctional epithelium and gingival fibres) at the base of the *gingival crevice or sulcus (**attachment level**) to a fixed point on the tooth, usually the *cemento-enamel junction measured with a periodontal probe. With the development of chronic periodontitis, there is destruction of the crestal alveolar bone and apical migration of the crestal gingival fibres and junctional epithelium (**loss of attachment**). **New attachment** refers to connective tissue fibres attaching to previously diseased periodontal root surface; this is a desirable outcome following periodontal surgery. A *precision attachment is a prefabricated appliance used to retain a *bridge or partial denture (fixed or removable prosthesis).

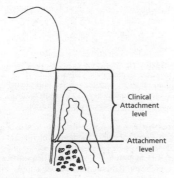

Clinical Attachment level

Attachment level

Attachment level

attention deficit hyperactivity disorder (ADHD) A childhood disorder characterized by inattentiveness, impulsiveness, and hyperactivity. It is three times more common in boys than girls. Treatment is usually with central nervous system stimulants and tricyclic antidepressants. Of dental significance is that there may be an interaction between the tricyclic antidepressants and *epinephrine used as a vasoconstrictor in a dental local *anaesthetic.

attrition *n.* The non-carious frictional tooth wear caused by tooth to tooth contact. Attrition, being a slowly progressive stimulus, results in the deposition of peritubular (intratubular) *dentine with sclerosis and obliteration of the tubular lumen. Tooth surfaces showing attrition often have a glassy appearance since, in comparison with intertubular dentine, peritubular dentine has smaller crystals and greater crystallinity and is thus considerably harder. Although it is considered a normal part of ageing, attrition may be exacerbated by *bruxism, loss of posterior tooth support, or developmental disturbances of tooth structure (e.g. amelogenesis imperfecta, dentinogenesis imperfecta). 📷

atypia *n.* (*adj.* **atypical**) Abnormality in the appearance of a cell. It may indicate the cell has an increased risk of becoming malignant. If atypical cells are seen in epithelial tissues the epithelium is described as **dysplastic** and this is graded into mild, moderate, and severe (atypical cells in the lower third, lower two thirds, or more than two thirds of the epithelium respectively). Epithelium that shows severe dysplasia has a high risk of turning malignant; that which shows mild dysplasia has a low risk.

atypical facial pain *See* FACIAL PAIN.

audit *n. See* CLINICAL AUDIT.

auricle *n.* 1. The externally visible cartilaginous part of the ear (pinna). 2. Part of each *atrium of the heart.

auscultation *n.* Listening for sounds within the body; it may be performed with the unaided ear or with a *stethoscope.

Austin retractor *n. See* RETRACTOR.

autoclave

n. A sealed pressurized vessel that uses the latent heat of steam to achieve effective *sterilization. All reusable invasive medical devices including dental instruments have to be cleaned, thermally disinfected, and sterilized prior to reuse. Autoclaves are often referred to as **steam sterilizers** in the healthcare setting. Steam sterilization is the preferred method for sterilizing reusable dental instruments. It is rapid and non-toxic, and can effectively destroy micro-organisms, including bacteria, fungi, and viruses, as well as bacterial and fungal spores, but will not necessarily destroy *prions. Sterilizers that have a pre-vacuum stage that actively removes air from the autoclave chamber are the most appropriate for sterilization for heat-tolerant dental instruments and other items, and should conform to current European Union Standards e.g. EN 285, EN 17665 EN 556 for large sterilizers and EN 13060 for bench top sterilizers. It is essential that trapped air is removed from the autoclave chamber as the air can prevent sterilizing conditions being achieved, hence the requirement for a pre-vacuum stage. **Class B** vacuum autoclaves (also known as porous load sterilizers) typically use a triple vacuum pulse at the start of the cycle and are appropriate for wrapped or porous loads. **Class S** vacuum autoclaves use a single vacuum pulse that removes enough air to permit sterilization of solid, hollow, and pouched instruments, but not porous or wrapped items. Porous load sterilizers provide an operating cycle which, as well as forced air removal, have a drying stage after the sterilization stage. When loading the sterilizer, instrument packs and other items to be sterilized should be arranged to facilitate free circulation of steam, and care should be taken not to over-fill the sterilizer chamber. Overloading the sterilizer chamber is a common cause of failure to achieve sterilization conditions. Sterilized packs should be allowed to dry inside the sterilizer before removing and handling. Many modern vacuum sterilizers have a post-sterilization drying cycle that facilitates the drying of packs. The operating cycle of a porous load sterilizer generally has five stages: air removal, steam admission, sterilization holding time, vacuum drying, and filtered air admission. Steam sterilization requires direct contact between saturated steam and all surfaces of the load at specific pressure, time, and temperature relationships. The highest

temperature compatible with the instruments/equipment to be sterilized should be used. The manufacturers' instructions for dental instruments purchased from the United States may specify steam sterilization cycles that are different from the standard cycle given in the table e.g. 132°C for ten minutes. In most cases these dental instruments can be processed through the standard cycle but confirmation should be obtained from the dental instrument manufacturer.

Many dental facilities use sterilizers without a pre-sterilization vacuum phase in which air is removed from the sterilizer chamber by steam displacement (i.e. downward displacement sterilizers). Downward displacement sterilizers are not appropriate for sterilizing wrapped loads of dental instruments and other items, or for items that contain a lumen e.g. dental handpieces, and should not be used for these purposes under any circumstances. Flash sterilizers rely on natural air displacement and should not be used for hollow devices or tubing, wrapped instruments, or other items. Boiling water sterilizers, hot-air ovens, ultra-violet light treatment, *hot salt sterilizers, *glass bead sterilizers, and *chemclaves are not appropriate for sterilizing dental instruments because their sterilization processes are difficult to validate. Best practice determines that all heat-tolerant reusable dental instruments, items, and equipment for use on patients should be packaged or wrapped prior to sterilization, and therefore the use of sterilizers without a pre-sterilization vacuum phase cannot guarantee proper sterilization. The manufacturers' instructions for correct use of sterilizers should always be followed and only trained competent personnel should use the equipment.

In order to ensure that a sterilizer is functioning properly and will consistently produce sterile loads, validation, maintenance, periodic testing, and record keeping are necessary. **Validation** is the documented procedure for obtaining,

Steam sterilization pressure, time, and temperature relationships

Minimum sterilization temperature	Steam pressure	Maximum permissible temperature	Minimum sterilization hold time	Dental instrument category
121°C	1.03 bar gauge	124°C	15 minutes	handpieces
134°C	2.30 bar gauge	137°C	3 minutes	dental instruments

recording, and interpreting the results needed to show that a process will consistently yield a product complying with predetermined specifications. It is comprised of commissioning (installation qualification and operational qualification), performance qualification, *autoclave periodic testing, and *autoclave revalidation. **Commissioning** is the process of obtaining and documenting evidence that the equipment has been supplied and installed in accordance with its specifications by the manufacturer, that it is safe to operate, and that it functions within predetermined limits when operated in accordance with the manufacturer's operating instructions. **Installation qualification** is the process of obtaining and documenting evidence that the equipment has been supplied and installed in accordance with its specifications by the supplier and that it is safe to operate. **Operational qualification** is the process of obtaining and documenting evidence that the equipment functions within predetermined limits when operated in accordance with the manufacturer's operating instructions. It consists of an air leakage test, a thermometric test, calibration, and a steam penetration test. Information from the installation and operational tests provide evidence that the sterilizer is functioning correctly. **Performance qualification** is required to show that sterilizing conditions are attained for typical loads and also test loads that are deemed by the user to be difficult to sterilize. Performance qualification is indicated for initial use of a new sterilizer or when the load profile changes (e.g. new instruments or equipment). It should be carried out by a suitably trained and qualified individual. These tests consist of air leakage tests (automatic), thermometric tests of all dental instruments to be processed, a steam penetration test (e.g. *Bowie and Dick), a load dryness test (only required for sterilizers with drying cycles), and microbiological tests (e.g. Spore tests). The performance qualification test protocol and data should be audited by the qualified person.

(⊕) SEE WEB LINKS

- Guidance on the operating of autoclaves from the University of Edinburgh.

autoclave periodic testing A programme of tests that are intended to show that the sterilizer's performance is continually satisfactory. The appropriate tests should be carried out at daily, weekly, and annual intervals.

A suitably trained person (usually the individual that operates the sterilizer on a daily basis) should draw up a schedule for periodic testing. After appropriate training the user should perform the daily tests. Many modern sterilizers have an integrated automated test facility that enables the sterilizer to perform some of the specialized weekly tests itself. The user can undertake these after appropriate training. Older sterilizers may require the services of a suitably qualified person to undertake weekly tests. A suitably qualified person should perform annual tests. Each cycle available to the user should be tested. If the sterilizer is not tested periodically it will not be possible to know if it is working correctly. Failure of a test implies that the sterilizer is not working to specification. The user should have a written procedure for handling test failures but, in all cases, the sterilizer must be withdrawn from service, the failure investigated, the cause rectified, and the sterilizer re-tested successfully before being used. The user has the ultimate responsibility for certifying that the sterilizer is fit for use. Sterilization cannot be confirmed by inspection and testing of the product.

autoclave revalidation One of the processes forming part of the validation procedure of a sterilizer (autoclave). Revalidation of each sterilizer should be undertaken quarterly to ensure the sterilizer is functioning correctly. A suitably qualified person should undertake this process and each sterilizer should be validated independently during annual tests. Revalidation should also be undertaken after sterilizer relocation, repair work, control function modifications, or when key component parts of the sterilizer are replaced or altered. On completion of each sterilization cycle parametric inspection must be undertaken to verify that the cycle has completed within defined, validated critical parameters e.g. 134°C to 137°C for 3 minutes. Most autoclaves can display or record key sterilization cycle parameters such as temperature, pressure, and time. Ideally, all sterilizers should be fitted with a recorder or a process evaluation system (EN 13060; EN 17665 [2006]; EN 285 [2006]). These systems provide a permanent record of daily tests and all production cycles, reduce time spent in performing daily tests, generate a unique cycle number that can be entered in the patients' notes to assist traceability, and eliminate the possibility of transcription errors. The recorder printout should be kept securely in the sterilizer logbook. Some types of cycle printouts (e.g. from thermal recorders) fade quickly and therefore special action may be required to preserve these records (e.g. photocopying). Many modern sterilizers can record cycle parameters in an electronic archive. A variety of other indicators can be used including chemical indicators and biological indicators. Chemical indicators should meet the requirements of appropriate standards (e.g. BS EN 867, ISO 11140) and should be used only for the process specified by the manufacturer. The manufacturer's instructions for use and storage should be followed. There are three main types, none of which prove that an autoclaved item is sterile. The first type (**process indicator**) is often printed on dental instrument sterilization pouches and bags and on autoclave tape. These sterilization indicator marks change colour (typically they darken in colour) when exposed to steam and serve only to distinguish processed items from unprocessed items. The second type of chemical indicator (**performance indicator**) are used as indicators for specific tests such as *Bowie and Dick steam penetration indicators used to monitor steam penetration into a test pack or a process challenge device. The third type of chemical indicator includes **integrating indicators** and **emulating indicators**. These indicators are intended to monitor the attainment of two or more critical variables in the sterilization process, either by a graduated response or a defined end point reaction.

Biological indicators are designed to show by the survival of a test micro-organism whether specified sterilization conditions have been attained. The most commonly used test micro-organisms are heat-resistant spores of the bacterium *Geobacillus stearothermophilius*. Biological indicators must meet the requirements of BS EN ISO 11138–1:2006. They are of limited value in routine sterilization process control because of the delay before the results are available and are restricted to a few special applications (e.g. in process validation) where they should always be regarded as additional to the measurement of temperature, pressure, and time.

(⊕) SEE WEB LINKS

• Provides information on decontamination in primary care dental practices.

autocrine *adj.* Describing the production by a cell of substances such as hormones which stimulate the cell itself.

autoimmunity *n.* A disorder in which the body fails to recognize some of its own components as 'self' and mounts an immune response against its own cells and tissues. It can result in diseases such as rheumatoid *arthritis, systemic *lupus erythematosus, *Sjögren's syndrome, and *pemphigus vulgaris.

automated external defibrillator A machine which analyses the underlying rhythm in a patient who has suffered a cardiac arrest. There are four possible rhythms: asystole, pulseless electrical activity, ventricular fibrillation, and pulseless ventricular tachycardia. If the rhythm can be treated with a direct current (DC) shock (ventricular *fibrillation or pulseless ventricular *tachycardia) the machine will generate the appropriate DC shock, which is delivered to the patient via special pads applied to the chest. There are two types of machine: **monophasic**, where the shock travels mono-directionally between the pads, and **biphasic** where the shock travels in both directions. 📷

autonomic nervous system That part of the nervous system that controls and regulates involuntary body functions (e.g. digestion, heart rate, and temperature regulation). It is divided up into the *sympathetic and *parasympathetic nervous systems.

autopolymerization *n.* The process whereby resin *monomers form large-chain molecules by chemical means without the need for light activation.

autosomal *adj.* Describing any chromosome that is not a sex chromosome and occurs in pairs in cells that have two sets of chromosomes (diploid cells).

autotrophic *adj.* Capable of growth without the need for an external food supply by synthesizing organic nutrients from inorganic substances such as carbon dioxide and nitrates.

auxiliary *n.* 1. A formally trained person who assists a professional undertaking professional services. Previously applied to members of the dental team other than the dentist but now replaced in the UK by the term *dental care professionals. 2. That part of an orthodontic appliance that enables forces to be applied to the teeth; it includes *ligatures, *elastics, *springs, and *separators.

avascular *adj.* Describing a lack of blood vessels (e.g. as in cartilage and enamel).

avulsion (evulsion) *n.* The detachment of a tooth from its socket due to trauma. It may be complete or partial. A completely avulsed tooth may be reimplanted. Prior to *reimplantation, the root surface should not be handled and the tooth should ideally be stored in a protective medium such as saliva or milk (dry storage rapidly damages periodontal cells).

axial *adj*. Relating to or parallel with the long axis of the tooth. The **axial wall** of a cavity lies nearest to the pulp parallel to the long axis of the tooth. *See also* TOOTH SURFACES.

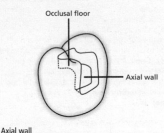

Occlusal floor

Axial wall

Axial wall

axis *n*. The second cervical vertebra (C2).

axon *n*. The fibre-like extension of a nerve cell (*neurone) that conducts electrical impulses away from the cell and onwards towards the next cell. Axons are typically 1μ in diameter but may extend to over a metre in length. In large nerves the axon has a myelin sheath interrupted by gaps called **nodes of Ranvier**.

azidothymidine (AZT) *n*. A retroviral drug used in the treatment of *HIV to delay the progression of the disease. Common side-effects include nausea, headache, and changes in body fat. Trade names: **Retrovir***, **Retrovis***.

azithromycin *n*. A macrolide antibiotic belonging to the azalide group. It may be prescribed as a *prophylactic antibiotic prior to invasive dental procedures in children who require antibiotic prophylaxis, as it is available in suspension form. It is taken orally; the most common side-effects are nausea, vomiting, and diarrhoea.

baby bottle caries *n. See* CARIES.

Bach flower remedies [E. Bach (1886–1936), English physician] A group of 38 flower remedies discovered by Dr Edward Bach in 1930. Rescue remedy, a combination of impatiens, cherry plum, clematis, rock rose, and star of Bethlehem, has been used orally by homeopathic dentists for the treatment of anxiety, shock, collapse, and stress. The evidence base for their effective use in the dental environment is currently lacking.

Bacillus *n.* A large genus of Gram-positive spore producing rod-like *bacteria e.g. *B. subtilis*, which produces the *antibiotic *bacitracin.

bacitracin *n.* A mixture of related cyclic *polypeptides produced by organisms of the licheniformis group of *B. subtilis*. Used systemically it is toxic, but used topically it is very effective in the management of skin, eye, or wound infections against Gram-positive cell walls. It is usually used in combination with polymyxin B or neomycin.

back-action clasp *n. See* CLASP.

bacteraemia *n.* The presence of bacteria in the blood, which is always abnormal as blood is usually a sterile environment. It can be a sign of infection but may also be transient following dental procedures such as *root planing or tooth extraction, or as a result of tooth brushing, flossing, or chewing. The condition is detected by blood culture in a microbiology laboratory and is treated with antibiotics. Antibiotic prophylaxis can be administered where contamination of the blood is anticipated.

bacteria *pl. n.* (*sing.* **bacterium**) Small micro-organisms lacking a distinct nuclear membrane (prokaryotes), most of which are unicellular. Most bacteria come in one of three basic shapes: spherical, rod-shaped, or spiral. Spherical bacteria (cocci) may exist in pairs (diplococci), clumps (staphylococci, e.g. *Staphylococcus aureus*) or chains (streptococci, e.g. *Streptococcus mutans*). Rod-shaped bacteria (bacilli, e.g. *Lactobacillus acidophilus*) can exist in chains (streptobacilli). Spiral bacteria may be curved or comma-shaped (vibrio), shaped as a thick rigid spiral (spirillum), or shaped in a thin flexible spiral (spirochete, e.g. *Treponema pallidum*).

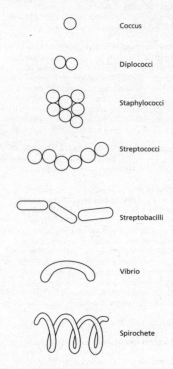

Coccus

Diplococci

Staphylococci

Streptococci

Streptobacilli

Vibrio

Spirochete

Bacteria: examples of bacterial shapes

Bacteria may be *aerobic or *anaerobic. They are ubiquitous in the environment and present in very large numbers on the skin, and in the digestive tract and oral cavity.

Further Reading: Roberts A. Bacteria in the mouth. *Dent Update* 2005;32:134–42.

bacterial endocarditis *See* ENDOCARDITIS.

bacterial toxin *See* TOXIN.

bactericide *n.* A substance that kills bacteria. Examples include disinfectants, antiseptics, and bactericidal antibiotics (e.g. quinolones and aminoglucosides).

bacteriology *n.* The branch of microbiology concerned with the study of bacteria. A person who specializes in the field of bacteriology is called a **bacteriologist**.

bacteriolysis *n.* The dissolution or disintegration of bacteria by a *bacteriophage, an enzyme, or other substance.

bacteriophage *n.* A virus (often referred to as a phage) that infects bacterial cells and either causes *lysis of the bacteria or forms a bacterial lysogen in which the virus genome inserts into the bacterial *deoxyribonucleic acid (DNA) and becomes dormant. Some bacteriophages carry genes for particular toxins that are produced by their bacterial hosts following lysogen formation (e.g. diphtheria toxin and scarlet fever toxin).

bacteriostasis *n.* (*adj.* bacteriostatic) Describing the process of retarding or inhibiting the growth of bacteria. *Compare* BACTERICIDE.

Bacteroides *n.* A genus of rod-shaped Gram-negative (*see* GRAM STAINING) anaerobic bacteria frequently associated with oral infections. They may be either motile or non-motile. *B. forsythus*, now classified in the *Tannerella* genus, is found in periodontal pockets in the presence of *periodontitis and has been implicated in disease progression. *B. gingivalis*, now classified in the *Porphyromonas genus, has been implicated in periodontal disease. *B. intermedius* has also been implicated in periodontal disease.

balanced diet *n. See* DIET.

balanced occlusion *n. See* OCCLUSION.

balancing *adj.* Describing equilibration or harmonization. **Balancing contacts** represent the contacts of the upper and lower teeth on the non-working side of a natural or artificial dentition. The **balancing side** is the side away from which the *mandible has moved during *mastication. A **balancing extraction** is the extraction of the same (or adjacent) tooth on the opposite side of the arch to preserve symmetry.

balsam *n.* An oily product obtained from the exudate of various trees and shrubs. It is a constituent of *Whitehead's varnish and some zinc oxide-eugenol cements. Because of its optical properties and purity, **Canada balsam** is used as a glue for conserving microscopic tissue samples.

BANA *n. See* BENZOYL-ARGININE NAPHTHYLAMIDE.

band *n.* 1. A **matrix band** is a thin metal or acetate strip used to form an artificial wall to a tooth during the placement of a restoration; it is often held in position by a *matrix band retainer. 2. An **orthodontic band** is a thin metal strip which encircles the tooth and is used to retain an orthodontic appliance; the band is closely contoured to the tooth using a **band adapter** or **band pusher** and cemented in position. The band is subsequently removed from the tooth on completion of treatment using **band remover** pliers; one beak rests on the occlusal or incisal surface while the other engages the border of the band.

bar *n.* 1. A piece of metal of greater length than width used as a connector in an orthodontic or prosthetic appliance. The bar may be situated lingually, labially, or palatally to join bilateral parts of a removable partial denture. 2. A shaped piece of metal used to stabilize mobile teeth.

barbiturate *n.* The earliest known of the sedative hypnotics which have now largely been superseded by benzodiazepines. They act on the *central nervous system by causing postsynaptic hyperpolarization. Their use ranges from sedation and hypnosis to anaesthesia and all have an anticonvulsant effect which can be used for the management of epilepsy. However, there is a significant problem with dependence and tolerance which severely restricts their usefulness. They readily cross the placenta and increase the risk of foetal abnormalities and are therefore contraindicated during pregnancy.

barodontalgia (aerodontalgia) *n.* Dental pain induced by a change in barometric pressure in an otherwise asymptomatic tooth. It may be experienced by pilots and mountain climbers during changes in barometric pressure. Possible causes of barodontalgia include caries, defective restorations, pulpitis, and pulp necrosis. Barodontalgia may also be due to referred pain from acute or chronic inflammation of one or more of the paranasal sinuses (**barosinusitis**) or acute or chronic traumatic inflammation in the middle ear space (**barotitis-media**). Fracture of restorations (**dental barotrauma**) has been reported to occur at high altitude, of which predisposing factors may include a leaking restoration or latent secondary caries underneath an existing restoration.

Further Reading: Zadik Y. Aviation dentistry: current concepts and practice. *Br Dent J* 2009;206:11-16.

Barrett's oesophagus [N. R. Barrett (1903-79), British surgeon] A condition in which there is a change in the oesophageal *epithelium from normal squamous to columnar due to damage caused by *gastro-oesophageal reflux. In severe cases, acid *erosion of enamel may be seen on the *palatal surfaces of the upper teeth and on the *occlusal and *buccal surfaces of the lower teeth. Patients have a greatly increased risk of developing adenocarcinoma.

barrier technique A protocol used in infection control to prevent microbiological cross-contamination between members of the dental team and the patient.

Bartholin's duct [C. Bartholin (1655-1738), Danish anatomist] A large duct that drains the anterior portion of the *sublingual salivary gland.

basal cell carcinoma (rodent ulcer) The commonest form of skin cancer; caused by sunlight. It occurs most commonly on the central part of the face and is characterized by a small slow-growing nodule which ulcerates and fails to heal. It can grow to a diameter of 1cm after about five years and is usually treated by surgical excision or cryotherapy.

basal lamina *n.* See EPITHELIAL ATTACHMENT.

basal layer *n.* A layer of cuboidal cells forming the innermost layer of the *epidermis or epithelium.

basal layer of Weil [L. A. Weil (1849-95), German dentist] A cell-free zone that develops below the odontoblast layer in the pulp at the time of tooth eruption.

basal metabolic rate (BMR) The amount of energy the body requires to keep functioning at rest to maintain vital functions such as circulation, respiration, digestion, and the maintenance of body temperature. The BMR is influenced by age, sex, and *thyroid activity and is generally higher in men than women.

base *n.* A compound that reacts with acid to form salt and water and releases hydroxyl ions in aqueous solution. The **cranial base** is that part of the facial skeleton which forms the floor of the cranial cavity. A **denture base** is the part of a full or partial denture that covers the soft tissues and is usually made of metal or resin or a combination of both. A **base lining** is a layer of material or cement used to insulate the *pulp in deep cavities or to eliminate undercuts. A **training base** is a temporary denture base usually made of resin used to allow a patient to be able to tolerate the bulk of a denture onto which additions can be made to allow progression to a denture once acceptance has been achieved.

baseplate *n.* A form representing the base of a denture which fits against the denture-bearing area of mucosa. It is used for making jaw *relation records by the addition of several layers of baseplate *wax to form an *occlusal rim. An **orthodontic baseplate** is usually made of resin, covers the soft tissues, and provides *anchorage for *springs, *clasps, and *archwires. A **stabilized baseplate** is a baseplate lined with a material to improve its fit and stability.

basic life support (BLS) The process of maintaining adequate ventilation and circulation as a holding operation until *advanced life support (ALS) is available. It involves assessing the patient to ensure there is no respiratory or cardiac activity and performing 30 chest compressions to 2 ventilations on the patient, to ensure that oxygen-rich blood circulates to the brain and myocardium until further treatment can be implemented to prevent irreversible brain damage. In dental practice, the term cardiopulmonary resuscitation (CPR) is more commonly used. The current guidance is available from the Resuscitation Council (UK).

Further Reading: Gill D. S., Gill S. K., Tredwin C. J., Naini F. B. Adult and paediatric basic life support: an update for the dental team. *Br Dent J* 2007;202:209-12.

SEE WEB LINKS
• The website of the Resuscitation Council which provides information on both basic and advanced life support.

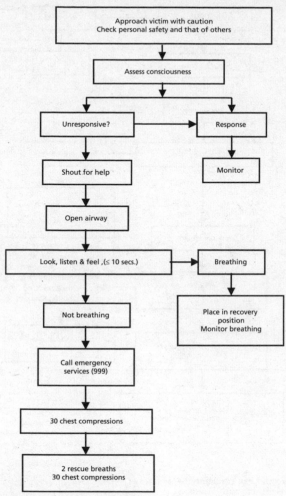

Adult basic life support

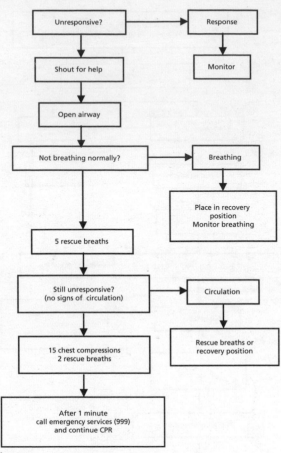

Paediatric basic life support

**basic periodontal examination (BPE)
(periodontal screening and recording
(PSR))** A periodontal *screening system which
identifies patients who require a more detailed
periodontal examination. It is carried out using
a *World Health Organization or *Community
Periodontal Index of Treatment Needs (CPITN)
probe using a probing force of 20–25gm. The
CPITN-E probe has one dark band 2mm in
width located 3.5–5.5mm from the probe tip;
the CPITN-C probe has an additional 3mm
dark band located 8.5–11.5mm from the
probe tip.

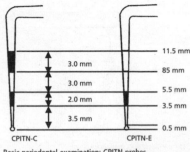

Basic periodontal examination: CPITN probes

BPE codes

Code	Signs	Management
Code 0	• probing depth 0–3mm • no bleeding on probing • no calculus or root roughness	oral hygiene reinforcement
Code 1	• probing depth 0–3mm • bleeding on probing • no calculus or root roughness	oral hygiene instruction; tooth debridement
Code 2	• probing depth 0–3mm • bleeding on probing • calculus or root roughness	oral hygiene instruction; tooth debridement
Code 3	• probing depth 3.5–55mm • bleeding on probing • calculus or root roughness	detailed periodontal examination required
Code 4	• probing depth >5.5mm • bleeding on probing • calculus or root roughness	detailed periodontal examination required
Code *	• loss of attachment (probing depth + recession ≥7mm) • furcation involvement	detailed periodontal examination required

The teeth in the mouth are divided into six mouth divisions or sextants (the third permanent molars are excluded). The probe is introduced into the *gingival crevice (sulcus) and walked around the buccal, labial, lingual, and palatal surfaces. Only the highest score for all the teeth in each sextant is recorded. The sextant score is recorded according to codes.

Sextants of the mouth using *FDI tooth notation

17–14	13–23	24–27
47–44	43–33	34–37

SEE WEB LINKS

• A policy statement on the recording of periodontal disease from the British Society of Periodontology.

basion *n.* The midline point on the occipital bone at the anterior border of the foramen magnum.

basophil *n.* A granular leukocyte with basic staining blue granules in the *cytoplasm. Its name is derived from its microscopic granular appearance when stained with basic blue dye.

Bass technique *n. See* TOOTHBRUSHING.

battered baby syndrome *See* CHILD ABUSE.

bayonet forceps *See* FORCEPS.

bed *n.* A surgically prepared recipient site for a *graft.

Bednar's aphthae [A. Bednar (1816–88), Austrian physician] Two patches or ulcers present either side of the midline on the surface of the hard palate in infants. They are caused by

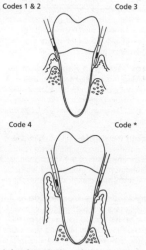

Codes 1 & 2   Code 3

Code 4   Code *

Basic periodontal examination codes

trauma, usually from sucking of the thumb and foreign objects, or pressure from the nipple.

beechwood creosote *n. See* CREOSOTE.

beeswax *n. See* WAX.

beetrode electrode An instrument used for measuring the *pH of dental plaque. The electrode tip has a diameter of 0.1mm which is small enough to measure interproximal sites.

Begg appliance [P. R. Begg (1898–1983), Australian orthodontist] A fixed *orthodontic appliance used to tip the crowns of teeth. It utilizes a round wire fitted fairly loosely into a channel at the top of the orthodontic bracket. It can produce both apical and rotational movement by using auxiliary springs or loops placed in the *archwire.

Begg bracket *See* BRACKET.

behavioural shaping (acclimatization) A procedure used to teach children to cope with dental treatment by a stage-by-stage exposure to dental procedures over several visits starting with the least traumatic.

Behçet's syndrome [H. Behçet (1889–1948), Turkish dermatologist] A condition of unknown aetiology characterized by *aphthous ulceration of the lips, tongue, buccal mucosa, and palate, together with ulceration of the iris and genital organs and/or skin. It is more common in men than women and there is a strong genetic link.

Bekhterev's reflex (nasal reflex) [V. M. Bekhterev (1857–1927), Russian neurologist] Stimulation of the mucosa of the nasal cavity, which produces contraction of the facial muscles on the same side of the face.

belladonna *n.* The alkaloid derived from deadly nightshade plant. This is a perennial herbaceous plant whose leaves, berries, and especially roots are highly toxic and hallucinogenic. It produces an atropine-like reaction by acting on the *parasympathetic nervous system and signs of poisoning include blurred vision, dilated pupils, loss of balance, confusion, and tachycardia. Its name is derived from the Italian, translating as 'beautiful lady' as historically it was used as eye drops to dilate the pupils and enhance beauty. The antidote is pilocarpine which is a sympathomimetic drug.

Bell's palsy [Sir C. Bell (1774–1842), Scottish physiologist] Paralysis of the facial nerve causing weakness of the facial muscles on one side of the face, an inability to close the eye, and possible loss of taste sensation or disturbed hearing. It is usually due to a viral infection and healing occurs without treatment. Rarely it may be due to a parotid neoplasm. *See also* RAMSAY HUNT SYNDROME.

bell stage *n.* The third stage of *tooth development. *See also* TOOTH GERM.

benign *adj.* 1. Describing a non-malignant neoplasm that does not spread to other parts of the body. 2. Any condition that does not produce harmful effects.

Bennett movement (shift) [N. G. Bennett (1870–1947), English dentist] The lateral movement of the *mandible produced when the mandibular condyles slide along the mandibular fossae during sideways jaw movement. The **Bennett angle** is the angle formed by the *sagittal plane and the path of the mandibular condyle during lateral movement when viewed in a horizontal plane.

benzocaine *n.* An ester local *analgesic derived from para-aminobenzoic acid. It is insoluble in water and therefore cannot be injected. It is used in dentistry as a *topical analgesic usually in gel or lozenge form to relieve painful symptoms caused by such conditions as *aphthous ulcers and *teething and as a means of obtaining surface analgesia prior to using a local analgesic needle.

benzodiazepine *n.* A group of compounds used to decrease emotional stress and *anxiety. One of these drugs (*midazolam) is routinely used for the management of dental anxiety and may also be administered buccally or intravenously for the emergency management of *epileptic seizures.

benzoyl-arginine naphthylamide (BANA) *n.* A bacterial enzyme used as a marker of bacterial growth in dental plaque and as a marker for the presence of *Porphyromonas gingivalis*, *Bacillus forsythus*, and *Treponema denticola*.

benzoyl peroxide *n.* 1. A chemical *photo-initiator incorporated into resin polymers to aid the initiation of polymerization. 2. An antibacterial preparation used in the treatment of acne and *fungal skin infections.

benzydamine hydrochloride *n.* A drug belonging to a group of medicines called *non-steroidal anti-inflammatory drugs (NSAIDs). It works by blocking the action of **cyclo-oxygenase**, thereby reducing inflammation and associated pain. It is used topically as a spray or mouthwash for inflammatory oral and throat conditions. Trade name: **Difflam**.

beta-blocker (beta-adrenergic blocker) *n.* An antihypertensive medication (e.g. atenolol, *propranolol), that prevents stimulation of the beta-adrenergic receptors at the nerve endings of the *sympathetic nervous system. It is used to treat high blood pressure and certain heart conditions by reducing the heart rate. Propranolol can cause dry mouth (*xerostomia), *lichenoid eruptions, and numbness of the perioral structures.

betamethazone *n.* A synthetic *corticosteroid which can be used systemically or topically. Because of its anti-inflammatory action it is used in the treatment of contact *dermatitis and oral *ulcerative lesions. A mouthwash can be made for topical use with betamethazone soluble tablets dissolved in water. Trade names: **Betnovate, Betnelan, Betnesol**.

betel quid *n.* A mixture of betel leaves (from the spice plant *Piper betle*), mineral lime (calcium oxide), and the areca nut chewed as a stimulant, *antiseptic, and mouth freshener. It may also be mixed with *tobacco. It is used extensively in south-east Asia and is associated with a substantial risk of submucous fibrosis and oral cancer.

bevel *n.* 1. An angle greater than 90° one surface makes when meeting another as a part of a cavity preparation. 2. A surface having a sloping or slanting edge. 3. *v.* To create a slanting edge or surface on a structure. An **external bevel** describes the blade placement angled towards the base of a periodontal pocket where the tip of the knife is apical to the neck of the blade when undertaking a *gingivectomy. An **internal bevel** incision is used in flap surgery and the tip of the scalpel is directed from the gingival margin towards the base of the periodontal pocket.

bias *n.* Any factor that distorts (or could distort) the true nature of an event, observation, or the results of a study. In a healthcare study, bias can occur due to systematic differences in the groups being compared (**selection bias**), in the care provided or exposure to factors other than the intervention of interest (**performance bias**), withdrawals or drop-outs of study participants (**attrition bias**), or how outcomes are assessed (**detection bias**). The **non-return bias (non-respondent bias)** can affect both a sample and a complete survey or questionnaire: the opinions or attitudes expressed by those who returned the survey may or may not represent the attitudes or opinions of those who did not return

the survey and it is impossible to determine which is true, since the non-respondents remain an unknown quantity.

In observational research, an **observer bias** is an example of a *confounding factor: observer bias can occur in that the observer, and thus their results, may be influenced by prior knowledge or experience of the situation, subjects, or participants under investigation. To protect against unintended differences in intervention and *control groups, those providing and receiving care can be *blinded so that they do not know the group to which the recipients of care have been allocated.

Design bias can be present in a *cohort study because of the way the subjects to be studied are selected and followed up, the way measures are taken, or the way data are analysed. It can occur in a questionnaire or survey because of the way the questions are phrased, selected, or asked.

Further Reading: Clarkson J., Harrison J. E., Ismail A. I., Needleman I., Worthington H. *Evidence based dentistry for effective practice.* Martin Dunitz, 2003.

bicuspid *n.* A *premolar tooth so named because it usually has two cusps. The adult dentition has eight bicuspids situated between the *canines and *molar teeth. They replace the primary first and second molars.

bifurcation *n.* The division into two parts such as the division of the roots of mandibular molar teeth.

bilateral *adj.* Occurring on or relating to two sides of the body, a tissue, or an organ.

bilophodont *adj.* Describing a tooth having two transverse ridges on its grinding surface as found in the tapir.

Bimler appliance (stimulator) [H. P. Bimler (1917–2003), German orthodontist] A removable *orthodontic appliance designed to induce tooth movement by the stimulation of reflex muscle activity. Also known as a **Bimler stimulator**.

bimodal *adj.* Referring to the description of a distribution of observations that has two *modes.

bimolar radiograph A variation of an oblique lateral radiograph which shows the teeth distal to the canines in both maxilla and mandible. It is commonly used diagnostically in children.

binangled *adj.* Describing an instrument, such as an enamel chisel, with two offsetting angles in its shank, thus providing access to a surface while maintaining an appropriate relationship to the handle.

Binder's syndrome A developmental condition, characterized by maxillo-nasal *dysplasia combined with other malformations including severe mid-facial retrusion, pseudo-mandibular or true mandibular prognathism, and hypoplastic frontal sinuses. Treatment depends on the severity of the malocclusion and may involve orthodontics or surgery. It was first defined by K. H. Binder in 1962 as a distinct clinical syndrome.

binomial *adj.* Consisting of or relating to two names or terms (e.g. $4x + 2y$).

bioburden *n.* The number of micro-organisms with which an object is contaminated. It is usually measured in colony forming units (CFU) per gram of product. **Bioburden testing** is performed to determine the number and nature of micro-organisms on a product prior to sterilization. *See also* PLAQUE.

biocompatibility *n.* (*adj.* **biocompatible**) The ability of a material, device, or appliance to be tolerated by living tissue. This is important for materials embedded in the tissues of the body such as dental *implants.

biofilm *n.* A complex aggregation of micro-organisms, especially bacteria, encased in a highly hydrated matrix of exopolysaccharide (EPS) excreted by the micro-organisms. Biofilms are usually found on solid surfaces exposed to an aqueous solution. Dental *plaque is an excellent example of a biofilm. Biofilms exhibit structural heterogeneity and are often permeated with pores or channels that facilitate the movement of water and nutrients. Formation of a biofilm starts with the attachment of free-floating micro-organisms (also known as planktonic micro-organisms) to a surface. This is followed by the attachment of other microbes and the production of EPS that holds the growing biofilm together. The biofilm grows through a combination of cell multiplication and recruitment of additional micro-organisms. Micro-organisms in a biofilm are protected by EPS from the actions of biocides and antibiotics and thus biofilms frequently exhibit increased resistance to these agents. Biofilms readily form on the surfaces of oral prostheses, such as dentures and orthodontic appliances.

biogenic *adj.* Produced by living organisms or biological processes.

biologic width A concept, first described by A. W. Gargulio in 1961, which established that the dimensional relationship between the crest of the alveolar bone, the length of the epithelial attachment, and the gingival sulcus depth is consistent. There is ongoing debate about the rational dimensions of the biologic width.

Further Reading: Gargulio A. W., Wentz F. M., Orban B. Dimensions and relations of the dentogingival junction in humans. *J Periodontol* 1961;32:361–7.

biomass *n.* The total quantity of living organisms at a given point in time, usually expressed in weight per unit area.

biomaterial *n.* A natural or synthetic material that is suitable for introduction into living tissue, especially as part of a medical device such as a dental *implant.

bionator *n.* A removable functional *orthodontic appliance designed to correct antero-posterior discrepancies between the *mandible and *maxilla. It was originally designed to modify tongue behaviour by means of a heavy wire loop on the palate. Some arch expansion is allowed by a buccal extension of the labial bow which holds the cheeks out of contact with the buccal segment teeth.

biopsy *n.* The removal of a specimen of tissue for microscopic analysis to aid the process of *diagnosis. Most biopsies of the oral cavity are either excisional or incisional. An **excisional biopsy** requires the removal of the entire lesion together with a margin of normal tissue. It is suitable for small benign lesions usually less than 1cm in diameter, such as papillomas, fibro-epithelial polyps, pyogenic granulomas, and hyperplastic tissue. Larger excisional biopsies are used to remove malignant neoplasms such as oral squamous cell carcinoma. An **incisional biopsy** removes only part of the lesion and involves an elliptical incision made to include normal as well as abnormal tissue to act as a reference. They should extend well into the underlying connective tissue; the length depends on the size of the lesion but as a general guide it is usually three times the width. Incisional biopsies are used to establish or confirm the diagnosis prior to definitive treatment and are appropriate for large or suspicious lesions such as chronic ulcers, lichen planus, squamous cell carcinoma, and bullous lesions. A **needle biopsy** involves aspiration of cells through a fine hollow needle. It is used for deep tissues such as lymph nodes, salivary glands, and soft tissue masses, or bony cysts that are not easily accessible. A **punch biopsy** is a type of incisional biopsy in which a small disc-shaped sample of tissue is removed using a sharp, hollow device.

Further Reading: Jephcott A. The surgical management of the oral soft tissues: 3. Biopsy. *Dent Update* 2007;34:654–7.

BIPP *See* BISMUTH IODOFORM PARAFFIN PASTE.

birth mark *See* NAEVUS.

biscuit *n.* Porcelain material after it has been initially baked and prior to glazing.

bisecting angle technique A method of taking a periapical *radiograph such that the x-ray tube is placed at 90° to a line bisecting the angle between the long axis of the tooth and the periapical film. The method is designed to reduce distortion of the radiographic image. Ideally it should only be used if the *paralleling technique is not possible.

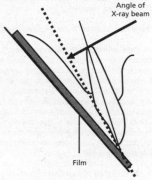

Bisecting angle technique

bisguanide antiseptic *n.* A group of broad-spectrum antimicrobial agents or biocides that are able to kill a wide range of micro-organisms by damaging their cell walls. The most common example with dental applications is *chlorhexidine gluconate. Chlorhexidine gluconate adsorbs onto oral surfaces and thus has a prolonged or residual effect (*substantivity).

bis in die Latin for twice a day. It is used in prescription writing and abbreviated to b.i.d. (bid) to describe the frequency at which a medicine should be taken.

bismuth iodoform paraffin paste (BIPP) An antiseptic material usually applied to ribbon gauze for packing into a cavity as a post-operative dressing. *See also* WHITEHEAD'S VARNISH.

bisphenol A-diglycidylether methacrylate (bis-GMA) *n.* A large

molecule methacrylate *monomer used in resin *composite material. It produces a viscous sticky resin which aids the flow of the material and reduces shrinkage. Contact dermatitis caused by residual bis-GMA monomer in resin composite restorations has been reported. *See also* TEGDMA (TRI-ETHYLENEGLYCOL DIMETHACRYLATE).

(bis-GMA) structure

bisphosphonates *n.* A class of drugs which inhibit the resorption of bone. They are most commonly used in the management and prevention of *osteoporosis in post-menopausal women, patients on long-term corticosteroids, and patients with malignant disease and an associated abnormally high concentration of calcium in the blood (**hypercalcaemia**). The drug is adsorbed onto the *hydroxyapatite crystals in bone and reduces the rate of bone turnover. They may be administered orally or by slow intravenous infusion. An important and increasingly reported side-effect of these drugs, whether taken orally or intravenously, is the risk of *osteonecrosis of the jaws. Frequently this follows extraction of teeth or trauma to the mucosa but has also been reported as a spontaneous finding. As yet there are no accepted guidelines as to whether patients taking these medications should be given prophylactic antibiotic cover prior to dental extractions. Should this become normal practice, the most likely antibiotic for prophylaxis is *clindamycin, owing to its spectrum of activity and excellent bone penetration.

Further Reading: McLeod N., Davies B., Brennan P. Bisphosphonate osteonecrosis of the jaws; an increasing problem for the dental practitioner. *Br Dent J* 2007;203(11): 641–4.
Malden N., Beltes C., Lopes V. Dental extractions and bisphosphonates: the assessment, consent and management, a proposed algorythm. *Br Dent J* 2009;206:93–8.

bite *v.* The action of bringing the mandibular and maxillary teeth into contact. A **close bite** describes a *malocclusion where there is an abnormally deep overlap of the incisors when the posterior teeth are in occlusion. An **open bite** is a form of malocclusion in which there is a failure of some teeth to meet in any mandibular position when the teeth of the jaws are brought into *occlusion. An open bite may be hereditary, due to external influences such as habits, or induced as part of orthodontic therapy. An **anterior open bite (AOB)** exists when there is no vertical overlap of the lower incisors by the upper incisors and when the anterior teeth fail to occlude in any position of the mandible. It may be in the midline, often produced by dummy sucking over a prolonged period of time, or to the side of the midline, typically seen due to prolonged digit sucking. An anterior open bite is often associated with a *tongue thrust. A **closed bite** is a decrease in the occlusal vertical dimension, usually resulting from excessive tooth wear or loss of posterior tooth support. An **edge-to-edge bite** exists where the mandibular and maxillary incisors occlude along their incisal edges and do not overlap. A **locked bite** occurs when lateral mandibular movements are restricted or prevented by the cuspal interference of the teeth. A **posterior open bite** exists when the posterior teeth on one side (unilateral) or both sides (bilateral) fail to come into vertical contact. It occurs more rarely than anterior open bite and the aetiology is less well understood. It can occur due to submergence of the primary molars or failure or arrest of eruption of the permanent buccal segment teeth; more rarely posterior open bite is seen in association with unilateral *condylar hyperplasia. A **scissors bite (crossbite, X-bite)** occurs if one or more teeth in the upper buccal segment is positioned so that its palatal cusp occludes buccal to the buccal cusp of a lower tooth: it can involve a single tooth or a complete quadrant, and can involve one side (unilateral) or both sides (bilateral) of the arch and be either anterior or posterior. 📷

bite block *n.* 1. A commercially available device usually made of rubber used to maintain the mouth open during prolonged treatment. *See also* MOUTH PROP. 2. An alternative name for an *occlusal rim.

bite fork *n.* A thin rigid U-shaped intra-oral extension of a *facebow to which an occlusal wax record is attached, to accurately locate the position of the maxillary teeth.

bite guard *n.* An acrylic resin appliance which covers the occluding surfaces of the teeth and provides a flat or modified platform allowing unobstructed movement of the mandible. A **reservoir bite guard** provides a slow release mechanism for artificial saliva in patients with *xerostomia.

bitemark *n.* The impression created by compression of soft tissue by the teeth. It is used as an important feature in *forensic dentistry analysis. Bitemarks typically present as semicircular injuries comprising two separate arcs, one for the upper teeth and one for the

lower. The severity of the injury is dependent on the force applied and the anatomical location.

Further Reading: Pretty I. A. Forensic dentistry: 2 Bitemarks and bite injuries. *Dent Update* 2008;35:48–61.

bite plate (plane) 1. A removable appliance that provides a flat biting surface covering the functional surfaces of the teeth to prevent their direct contact. 2. A temporary prosthetic appliance with a wax or resin occlusal rim used to record the vertical dimension and the intended position of artificial teeth on a partial or complete denture (registration plate).

bite raising appliance An appliance used to increase the vertical dimension between the mandible and the maxilla.

bite rim *See* OCCLUSAL RIM.

bitewing radiograph An intra-oral *radiographic film in which there is a central tab onto which the teeth can occlude in order to hold the film in position. The film is used to produce an image of the crowns of both mandibular and maxillary teeth for the primary purpose of diagnosing interproximal and secondary *caries beneath existing restorations. The film may be placed vertically (**vertical bitewing**) rather than horizontally to provide a more complete view of the root structure. 📷

Black G. V. (1836–1915) Greene Vardiman Black is considered to be one of the founders of modern dentistry. He began studying medicine at the age of 17 and in 1857 met Dr. J. C. Speer, who taught him the practice of dentistry. He researched many aspects of dentistry, including the composition of dental amalgam and the cause of dental fluorosis. He established the basic principles of tooth preparation including the idea of 'extension for prevention', which has only recently been superseded, largely due to the advent of adhesive restoratives. He devised a caries classification system which is still in use today (*see* BLACK'S CLASSIFICATION OF CAVITIES). He was appointed professor of pathology in the Chicago College of Dental Surgery. He was awarded a DDS by Missouri Dental School in 1877 and later an MD from Chicago Medical School. In 1897 he became the first dean of Northwestern University Dental School.

black hairy tongue *See* TONGUE, BLACK HAIRY.

Black's classification of cavities [G. V. *Black (1836–1915), American dentist] A classification based on the tooth type and the cavity location or tooth surfaces involved.

Black's classification of cavities

Class I	Cavities located in *pits or *fissures. These are located in the *occlusal surfaces of molars and premolars, the occlusal two-thirds of the *buccal surfaces of molars, the *lingual surfaces of upper incisors, and occasionally in the lingual surfaces of upper molars.
Class II	Cavities located in the proximal surfaces of molars and premolars.
Class III	Cavities in the proximal surfaces of canines, and incisors not involving the incisal angles.
Class IV	Cavities in the proximal surfaces of incisors or canines which also involve one or both of the incisal angles.
Class V	Cavities located in the gingival third of the *labial, buccal, lingual, or *palatal surfaces of any tooth.

Blake gingivectomy knife A surgical instrument used for the removal of gingival tissue. The handle is designed to hold a disposable scalpel blade of varying sizes and shapes which is secured in place by a screw tightened with the aid of an Allen key. *See also* PERIODONTAL INSTRUMENTS.

Blandin's gland [P. F. Blandin (1798–1849), French surgeon] A small anterior lingual gland situated at the base of the tongue on each side of the lingual fraenum (*US* frenum).

bleaching

n. The process of whitening teeth by the use of chemical oxidizing agents sometimes with the addition of light or heat. The active ingredient is usually *hydrogen peroxide, *carbamide peroxide, *sodium perborate, or chlorine dioxide. The procedure may be carried out on vital or non-vital teeth. The procedure of **vital bleaching** may be carried out in the home using soft plastic **bleaching trays**, which closely approximate to the teeth into which is placed a bleaching gel. It may also be undertaken by a dental professional in the surgery or clinic using a bleaching gel following the appropriate protection of the gingival tissues. All professionally applied whiteners that have the American Dental Association (ADA) seal contain 35% hydrogen peroxide. This latter method may be supplemented by light-activating units (**power-bleaching**) or *lasers. The side-effects can include post-operative tooth sensitivity or soft tissue irritation. Bleaching may exert a negative influence on restorations and restorative materials. The application of bleaching agents by those who are not dentists or *dental care professionals is subject to European and UK law. **Non-vital bleaching** can provide a conservative alternative to crowning or veneering a discoloured non-vital tooth which may or may not be root filled. Treatment involves the placement of a bleaching agent such as sodium perborate paste in the pulp chamber following the removal of any stained dentine, and sealing of the cavity for 1–2 weeks. The process may require repeating to achieve the desired shade change.

Further Reading: Pretty I. A., Ellwood R. P., Brunton P. A., Aminian A. Vital tooth bleaching in dental practice: 1. Professional bleaching. *Dent Update* 2006;33(5):288–90, 293–6, 299–300, 303–4.

bleb *n.* A blister or large vesicle.

bleeding *n. See* HAEMORRHAGE.

bleeding index *n. See* GINGIVAL BLEEDING INDEX; SULCUS BLEEDING INDEX.

blinding *n.* A method of removing conscious or unconscious *bias in clinical research. In a **single-blinding** experiment, the individual subjects do not know if they are in the control or experimental group. In a **double-blinding** experiment neither the individuals nor the researchers know who belong to the control or experimental groups. **Triple-blinding** occurs if the statistical analysis is also undertaken blind.

blister *n.* A swelling containing serum (watery fluid), blood, or pus formed within or just below the skin. Blisters usually occur in response to excessive friction, burns, or as a feature of certain diseases.

block analgesia *See* ANALGESIA.

block out The elimination of undesirable undercuts on a cast by the application of a temporary substance such as wax to the undercut areas, to leave only those undercuts essential to the planned prosthesis construction.

blood *n.* The fluid which circulates in the vessels of the circulatory system and provides transport for a large number of materials between the organs and tissues. It consists of blood cells suspended in a liquid medium, the *plasma. A **blood cell** is any of the cells present in the blood; they may be classified into three broad groups: red cells (*erythrocytes), white cells (*leucocytes), and *platelets (*thrombocytes).

A **blood clot** or thrombus is a solid coagulated mass formed inside or outside the circulatory system and consisting of the protein fibrin in which blood cells are trapped. **Blood coagulation (clotting)** is the conversion of liquid blood into a solid by means of the interaction of a number of factors, during which prothrombin is converted to thrombin. Thrombin acts as a catalyst for the conversion of fibrinogen to insoluble fibrin in which the blood cells are trapped. *See* COAGULATION. A **blood count** is a calculation of the number of blood cells per cubic millimetre. The **blood gas solubility coefficient** is a measure of the solubility of a gas, such as oxygen and carbon dioxide, in blood. Nitrous oxide has a low solubility in blood and is therefore excreted rapidly. **Blood groups** are the division of blood into types based on the compatibility of the red blood cells and plasma between different individuals. There are more than 30 blood group systems, of which two of the most important are the ABO system and the Rhesus system. The **ABO system** is based on the presence or absence of *antigens A and B: blood of groups A and B contains antigens A and B, respectively; group AB contains both antigens; and group O neither. Blood of group A contains antibodies to antigen B; group B contains anti-A antibodies; group AB has neither antibody; and group O has both. The blood group of a person determines whether they can be a donor or a recipient of transfused blood.

The ABO blood group system

Donor's blood group	Blood group of people from whom donor can receive blood	Blood group of people to whom donor can give blood
A	A, O	A, AB
B	B, O	B, AB
AB	A, B, AB, O	AB
O	O	A, B, AB, O

The presence of a group of antigens on the surface of red blood cells is the basis of the **rhesus blood group system**. Most people have the rhesus factor, i.e. they are **Rh-positive**; those people who lack the factor are termed **Rh-negative**. The lack of compatibility between the two groups is an important cause of blood transfusion reactions and blood disease of the new-born. **Blood plasma** is the fluid part of the blood in which the blood cells are suspended, consisting mostly of water and containing proteins, salts, hormones, waste products, nutrients, clotting agents, and antibodies. **Blood pressure** is the pressure of the

blood against the main arterial walls. The pressure is highest when the heart ventricles are contracting (*systole) and lowest when the ventricles are relaxing (*diastole). Pressure is measured by a *sphygmomanometer in millimetres of mercury. In a young adult at rest the average systolic blood pressure is 120mm and the diastolic blood pressure 80mg. The **blood sugar level** is the concentration of glucose in the blood. The blood sugar level is an important diagnostic investigation for diseases such as diabetes mellitus. *See also* HYPOGLYCAEMIA; HYPERGLYCAEMIA.

Bochdalek's ganglion [V. A. Bochdalek (1801–83), Czech anatomist] The ganglion formed by the junction of the middle and superior alveolar nerves situated in the maxilla above the root of the canine tooth.

Bodecker index [C. F. Bodecker (1880–1965), American oral histologist] The ratio of the tooth surfaces affected by caries and the total number of surfaces which could possibly be affected by caries. It is based on the assumption that each of the five surfaces of a tooth offers a risk of caries and that each surface is a unit. *See also* DMF INDEX.

bodies corporate A specific group of dental organizations which share the same type of legal entity. Prior to a 2005 amendment to the *Dentists Act 1984, which removed key restrictions, the number of bodies corporate was limited to 27. Any corporate body can carry out the business of dentistry provided that it can satisfy the conditions of board membership set out in the amended Dentists Act.

body mass index (BMI) The weight of a person (in kilograms) divided by the square of the height of that person (in metres). It is used as an indicator of whether or not a person is under- or overweight. In adults a BMI of less than 18.4 is considered underweight, 18.5–24.9 normal, 25–29.9 overweight, and greater than 29.9 indicates clinical obesity. The BMI may not be accurate for persons over the age of 60.

(((∰))) SEE WEB LINKS

• The NHS Direct web page that provides information on how to calculate BMI.

body temperature The temperature of the body, as measured by a thermometer. In normal individuals it is maintained at 37°C (98.4°F) by a small area in the base of the brain (hypothalamus). Body heat is generated by vital activities such as respiration, cardiac activity, circulation, and secretion and from the muscular activity of exercise and shivering. A rise in body temperature occurs in fever.

Bohn's nodules [H. Bohn (1832–88), German physician] Small, whitish or yellowish, asymptomatic *cysts filled with *keratin formed from remnants of odontogenic epithelium, which are particularly common in the new-born. They are located on the gingivae and normally disappear spontaneously during the first three months of life. Also known as Epstein's pearls.

Further Reading: Cambiaghi S., Gelmetti C. Bohn's nodules. *Int J Dermatol* 2005;44:753–4.

boil (furuncle) *n.* A localized swelling containing *pus and dead tissue usually at the site of a hair follicle. The most common causative organism is *Staphylococcus aureus.*

boiling-out The process of placing a *flask in boiling water in order to separate it into two halves so that the melted wax may be washed away leaving the denture teeth embedded in the investment plaster.

Bolam principle A test to determine the standard of care used by the legal profession to indicate that a practitioner has acted in accordance with a respectable body of medical opinion. It follows the judgement in a legal case of *Bolam* v *Friern Hospital Management Committee (HMC)* in 1957. The standard of treatment expected of a dentist is the standard of the ordinarily skilled and competent dentist in that particular dental specialty. At any one time there may be several responsible bodies of opinion in a particular field or area of expertise, and one should not be held to be negligent if one complies with any of these responsible bodies of opinion. *See also* BOLITHO.

Bolitho A legal judgement (*Bolitho* v. *City and Hackney Health Authority* 1997) that stated that a case cannot be defended on the basis of a current practice that is not reasonable or logical. *See also* BOLAM PRINCIPLE.

bolus *n.* A mass of food ready to be swallowed.

bonded amalgam *n. See* AMALGAM.

bonding *n.* The joining or attaching of two substances together by means of a chemical reaction or an adhesive, now extensively used in restorative dentistry. A **bonding agent** is a chemical agent used to provide a bond between two layers. **Bond strength** is measured in mega pascals (MPa) as the force necessary to break the adhesive bond per unit area. Bonding in restorative dentistry has evolved considerably during the latter part of the 20th century and is broadly divided into seven generations.

bonding to enamel is achieved by the removal of *hydroxyapatite and *enamel prisms using an acid, usually 37% *phosphoric acid, by the *acid-etch technique creating a micromechanical bond. Because dentine has a higher organic and water content than enamel, **dentine bonding** requires the use of a bifunctional monomer such as *HEMA (hydroxyethylmethacrylate). This has a hydrophilic terminal that can bond with the dentine surface and a hydrophobic terminal that can co-polymerize with the resin of the restorative material. Bonding systems are also used to stick orthodontic brackets onto the enamel surface. *See also* HYBRID LAYER; HYDROXYAPATITE.

Further Reading: Franklin P., Brunton P. Restorative materials. In *Clinical Textbook of Dental Hygiene and Therapy*, ed. R. S. Ireland. Blackwell Munksgaard, 2006.

The development of bonding systems

1st generation	Introduced in the 1960s to overcome polymerization shrinkage and excessive wear of restorative materials. Bond strength of about 1–3MPa.
2nd generation	Improved but still weak dentine adhesion by utilizing halophosphorous esters such as *Bis-GMA and *HEMA.
3rd generation	The introduction of acid etching of dentine to partially remove or modify the *smear layer. These systems usually used a hydrophilic dentine-resin primer.
4th generation	Involved the complete removal of the smear layer. Enamel and dentine were etched simultaneously.
5th generation	Simplified techniques introduced using a one bottle system incorporating both *primer and adhesive. The self-etching primer contained HEMA.
6th generation	An improved bond strength developed using a one-bottle etch and primer system.
7th generation	Further development of the 6th generation such that etching, priming, and adhesion are undertaken in one stage.

bone *n.* The hard mineralized connective tissue that forms the skeleton of the body. It has a matrix of calcium salts (mainly calcium carbonate and calcium phosphate), deposited around protein fibres. The matrix is deposited by the activity of *osteoblasts which become trapped in small hollows (**lacunae**) and cease laying down bone, becoming *osteocytes; these have a number of thin processes which extend from the lacunae through small channels within the bone matrix (**canaliculi**). The external layer of the bone (**compact, cortical,** or **lamellar bone**) consists of a hard mass of bony tissue arranged in numerous concentric circles with vascular channels (**Haversian canals**) running along the long axis of the bone.

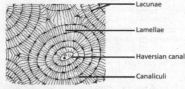

Lacunae
Lamellae
Haversian canal
Canaliculi

Compact bone tissue

Trabecular (**cancellous** or **spongy**) bone is found beneath the cortical bone and is made up of delicate bars and sheets of bone (**trabeculae**) which form a sponge-like network. Bone is subject to constant remodelling by *osteoblasts and *osteoclasts. **Alveolar bone** supports the teeth and is thin and compact immediately adjacent to the periodontal membrane whereas the bone between the tooth roots (interradicular) is less compact. The **crestal bone** is the most coronal part of the alveolar bone. When the teeth are lost, the alveolar bone undergoes *resorption. Bone can be classified according to its density, such as has been described by C. E. Misch in 1990.

Classification of bone density

Classification	Description
D1	Dense compact bone.
D2	Dense-to-porous compact bone with coarse trabecular core.
D3	Thin porous compact bone with fine trabecular core.
D4	Fine trabecular bone.
D5	Immature, non-mineralized bone.

bone defect A pattern of bone destruction which may be horizontal or vertical. It can involve 1, 2, or 3 walls.

bone file *See* FILE.

bone graft (augmentation) The use of bone or bone substitute material to replace diseased or missing bone. Bone graft materials include bone originating from within the body of the patient (autogenous bone), allografts, xenografts (*see* GRAFT), and inert foreign bodies used for transplantation into bone (**alloplasts**). Allografts do not contain live bone cells, unlike autogenous bone, but do contain proteins which encourage new bone formation. The donor sites for alveolar bone augmentation are the iliac crest of the hip (which affords large bone volumes), and the chin, mandibular ramus, and maxillary tuberosity, which afford more limited availability of volume but avoid external scarring.

bone morphogenic protein (BMP) A protein that induces the formation of bone and cartilage. It is composed of acidic polypeptides and is exposed in the cortical bone matrix when demineralized with hydrochloric acid.

bone sounding The process of probing anaesthetized tissue with a periodontal probe to establish the level of the underlying alveolar *bone.

Bonferroni correction [C. E. Bonferroni (1892–1960), Italian mathematician] A safeguard when using multiple tests of *statistical significance on the same *data thus controlling the overall *Type I error rate. Each test uses a criterion of significance (such as 0.05), which is divided by the number of tests conducted.

Bonwill triangle [W. G. A. Bonwill (1833–99), American dentist] A 4-inch equilateral triangle formed by lines joining the medial contact point of the mandibular central incisors and the centres of the mandibular condyles.

border moulding *See* MUSCLE TRIMMING.

border seal (facial seal) The seal produced by the contact of the lips and cheeks with the polished surface of a denture.

Botox *n. See* BOTULINUM TOXIN.

bottle brush A cylindrical brush usually used for cleaning bottles but adapted for use in dentistry for the removal of interproximal *plaque. The brushes are available in different sizes so as to provide an effective action in all interdental spaces.

botulinum toxin A potent neurotoxin protein produced by the bacterial species *Clostridium botulinum* and one of the most toxic proteins known. Although highly toxic, botulinum toxin is used in minute amounts to treat muscle spasms and as a cosmetic treatment for skin wrinkles. Dental applications include the treatment of masseteric hypertrophy, recurrent dislocation of the temperomandibular joint, chronic facial pain, and drooling. Trade names: **Botox, Dysport**.

Further Reading: Bhogal P. S., Hutton A., Monaghan A. A review of the current uses of Botox for dentally related procedures. *Dent Update* 2006;33(3):165–8.

bovine spongiform encephalopathy (BSE) A fatal, neurodegenerative disease in cattle commonly called 'mad cow' disease. It is caused by proteinaceous infectious particles or *prions that result in tissue degeneration in the brain and spinal chord. It is thought that the disease may be transmitted to humans by eating infected animals. In humans, BSE is known as new variant *Creutzfeldt-Jakob disease.

Bowie–Dick (Bowie and Dick) test An autoclave tape test for vacuum-assisted steam sterilizers devised by J. H. Bowie (1909–84) and J. Dick, and first described in 1963. It used a chemical indicator to detect the presence of air due to air leaks or inadequate air removal and steam penetration. The autoclave tape, through its steam sensitive indicator ink, changes colour at certain temperatures in the presence of moisture; a failure to change colour indicates the presence of air pockets and prevents the ink from undergoing a uniform colour change. The original test used 25–29 huckaback towels folded to give 8 thicknesses of cloth; strips of autoclave tape in the shape of a St Andrew's cross were then inserted at various intervals and the pack placed in a cardboard box or wrapped in fabric. Minimum safety factors for the Bowie–Dick test are defined within European Standards (ENs) and *International Standards Organization (ISO) standards.

Further Reading: Bowie J. H., Kelsey J. C., Thompson G. R. The Bowie and Dick autoclave tape test. *The Lancet* 16 March 1963:586–7.

box *n*. That part of a compound cavity preparation, excluding the occlusal portion, which has four cavity surfaces.

boxing *v*. The process of providing a provisional wall around the perimeter of an impression, usually of wax, to contain the material poured into the impression until it has set.

boxplot (box and whisker plot) *n*. A graphical representation of several characteristics from a set of observations. The *median is at the centre of the plot, which is surrounded by a box, the top and bottom of which represent the limits within which the middle 50% of observations fall (the *interquartile range). The whiskers are the two T-shaped lines which extend out of the top and bottom to represent the most and least extremes respectively.

B-point *See* CEPHALOMETRIC ANALYSIS.

brace *n*. A lay term used to describe any *orthodontic appliance, most commonly those with visible *wires, *bands, or *brackets.

brachy- A prefix denoting shortness. Examples: **brachycephallic** (short head), *brachydont, **brachyfacial** (short face), **brachyglossal** (short tongue), **brachygnathia** (short mandible), **brachyrhinia** (short nose).

brachycephalic *adj. See* CEPHALIC INDEX.

brachydont *adj*. Describing teeth that have short crowns relative to the total height of the teeth, such as the molar teeth of humans and anthropoid apes. *Compare* HYPSODONT.

brachystaphyline *adj. See* CHAMESTAPHYLINE.

bracing *n*. The process of providing rigid denture components (**bracing components**) to resist horizontal displacement forces generated during function by occlusal contact and the oral musculature surrounding the denture. The bracing components are placed against suitable vertical surfaces of the teeth and residual ridges. Bracing components on the teeth may be rigid parts of clasp arms or plates; bracing on the residual ridges and palate is achieved by major connectors and denture flanges. *See also* RECIPROCATION.

Further Reading: Davenport J. C., Basker R. M., Heath J. R., Ralph J. P., Glantz P. O., Hammond P. Bracing and reciprocation. *Br Dent J* 2001;190:10–14.

bracket *n*. An attachment on a fixed *orthodontic appliance. They are *bonded onto teeth with a *composite material. They consist of **tie wings** around which the *ligatures are tied, a **slot** into which the *archwire is placed, and a **base** that is curved to accurately fit the contour of the tooth.

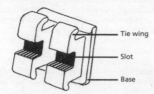

Orthodontic bracket

- Tie wing
- Slot
- Base

Most brackets have identification marks on their tie wings. They are usually made of stainless steel, plastic, or ceramic material. **Begg brackets** [P. R. Begg (1898–1983), Australian orthodontist] have a narrow vertical slot which corresponds to the archwire channel of the edgewise bracket; they only accept round wires and are retained with brass pins or *auxiliaries. **Ceramic brackets** are manufactured from monocrystalline or polycrystalline *alumina. They have good aesthetics and do not stain but have reduced fracture resistance and increased frictional resistance; the frictional resistance may be reduced by the use of metal reinforced or silica-lined archwire slots. Ceramic brackets are also extremely hard and may cause wear of opposing enamel surfaces and may increase the risk of enamel damage when *debonded due to the high bond strength. **Edgewise brackets** have a rectangular archwire channel with the largest dimension horizontally; they are used with rectangular or round wires. **Plastic brackets** are made of acrylic or polycarbonate; they have the disadvantages that they can stain and lack strength and rigidity during function. These disadvantages may be overcome by the use of reinforced composite material with a metal slot to increase rigidity. **Pre-adjusted brackets** have inbuilt tip, torque, and in/out adjustments, which reduces the need for complicated wire bending. **Self-ligating brackets** secure the archwire to the bracket by means of a sliding door (unlike edgewise brackets where the ligation of the archwire is via tie-wings) and may be active or passive; they have the advantages over conventional brackets of full archwire engagement, low friction between the bracket and the archwire, reduced time for archwire changes, and reduced chairside assistance. The **Damon system** is a passive self-ligation fixed appliance bracket system. **Stainless steel brackets** have none of the disadvantages of plastic and ceramic brackets but are less cosmetic. **Tip-edge brackets** incorporate a pre-adjusted system with a unique archwire slot; round archwires are used initially followed by rectangular archwires for later stages of treatment. 📷

Bradford Hill criteria [A. B. Hill (1897–1991), British medical statistician] A set of nine criteria used to determine the strength of an association between a disease and its supposed causative agent. They form the basis of modern medical and dental epidemiological research.

The nine Bradford Hill criteria	
Criterion	Explanation
Strength of association	The stronger the association, the more likely it is that the relation is causal.
Temporal relationship	Exposure always precedes the outcome.
Consistency	The association is consistent when results are replicated with different people under different circumstances and with different measurement instruments.
Theoretical plausibility	It is easier to accept an association as causal when there is a rational and theoretical basis for such a conclusion.
Coherence	The association should be compatible with existing theory, hypotheses, and knowledge.
Specificity	In the ideal situation, the effect has only one cause.
Dose response relationship	An increasing amount of exposure increases the risk.
Experimental evidence	Any related research that is based on experiments will make a causal inference more plausible.
Analogy	Sometimes a commonly accepted phenomenon in one area can be applied to another area.

brady- Prefix denoting slow. Examples: *bradycardia, **bradyglossia** (slowness of speech), **bradypnoea** (slow respiration).

bradycardia *n.* A slowing of the heart rate to below 50 beats per minute. **Sinus bradycardia** can occur in normal individuals such as athletes, young adults, or when a person is asleep, but it is also seen in patients with reduced thyroid activity, jaundice, hypothermia, or *vasovagal attacks.

bradykinesia *n.* Slowness of movement. It is a symptom of *Parkinson's disease.

bradykinin *n.* A plasma *polypeptide member of the kinin group of proteins which consists of nine *amino acids. It is a powerful *vasodilator and one of the mediators of an *anaphylactic reaction. It is thought to play an important role as a mediator of *inflammation.

branchial cyst *n. See* CYST.

Brännström's hydrodynamic theory A theory, first described by M. Brännström in 1966, which suggested that *dentine hypersensitivity is due to movement of fluid within the *dentinal tubules in response to mechanical, osmotic, and evaporative stimuli. Cold stimuli cause an outward flow of fluid and hot stimuli cause an inward flow.

Further Reading: Brännström M. A hydrodynamic mechanism in the transmission of pain producing stimuli through the dentine. In: *Sensory mechanisms in dentine*, ed. D. J. Anderson. Oxford: Pergamon Press, 1963; 73–9.

breathing, rescue An emergency procedure to ventilate the lungs of a person who has stopped breathing. The rescuer inflates the victim's lungs using an inflation device or by blowing expired air through the victim's mouth or nose. *See also* BASIC LIFE SUPPORT.

bregma *n.* An anatomical landmark where the sagittal suture and coronal suture meet.

Briault explorer See EXPLORER.

bridge *n.* An appliance attached to natural teeth or implants replacing missing, extracted, or unerupted teeth designed to restore function and usually aesthetics. A bridge may also be described as a fixed partial denture and, where it is retained by *precision attachments and is capable of being removed by the patient, a removable partial denture. A cantilever bridge is attached to an *abutment tooth at one end only. A bridge may be described as **fixed–fixed** where the *retainers at both ends of the bridge are cemented or *bonded to the abutment teeth, **fixed–movable** where only one end of the bridge is bonded to its abutment, or **removable** where the patient is capable of removing the entire bridge for cleaning or maintenance. The replacement tooth (*pontic) or teeth are attached to the abutment teeth by means of one or more *retainers. 📷

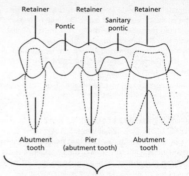

Five unit fixed bridge

Components of a bridge

Resin-bonded bridges, such as Maryland and Rochette bridges, require minimal tooth preparation. A **Maryland bridge** is retained by *acid-etch bonding of the abutment teeth; the retention is further improved by acid-etching of the metal surfaces in contact with the abutment teeth; the bridge may be cantilevered from the abutment tooth or be fixed at either side. A **Rochette bridge**, attributed to Alain L. Rochette, French physician and dentist, and originally used to splint periodontally involved teeth, is bonded to its abutment teeth using the acid-etch technique and the retaining metal surfaces are perforated to provide additional mechanical retention.

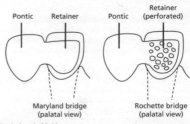

Resin-bonded bridges

Further Reading: St George G., Hemmings K., Patel K. Resin-retained bridges re-visited Part 2. Clinical considerations. *Primary Dental Care* 2002;9(4):139–44.

Barber M. W., Preston A. J. How successful are your resin-bonded bridges. *European Journal of Prosthodontics and Restorative Dentistry* 2008;16:2–9.

bridge remover device used for *debonding a temporary or permanently placed crown or bridge. A sliding hammer design utilizes a small hook which engages the restoration margin and then a weight is slid along the shaft in a series of short, quick taps to loosen the restoration. The forces must be directed along the path of removal to avoid damage to the underlying tooth. A wire may also be looped through the bridge *embrasure onto which a force can be applied. A number of potentially less damaging commercial products are available.

Further Reading: Addy L. D., Bartley A., Hayes S. J. Crown and bridge disassembly – when, why and how. *Dent Update* 2007;34:140–50.

Brinell hardness test [J. A. Brinell (1849–1925), Swedish engineer] A test used to measure the hardness of a metal using a tungsten carbide ball indenter. The **Brinell hardness number** is a numerical expression of the hardness of the material: the larger the indentation, the smaller the hardness number. *See also* KNOOP HARDNESS TEST; VICKERS HARDNESS TEST.

British Dental Association (BDA) The professional association and trade union for dentists in the UK, founded in 1880. It develops policies to represent dentists in the different spheres of clinical practice and teaching establishments.

British Dental Health Foundation (BDHF) A UK-based independent charity working to bring about improved standards of oral healthcare, both in the UK and around the world. It serves the public interest by improving awareness of, and access to, the means of maintaining better oral health, particularly among disadvantaged groups such as those on lower incomes, the disabled, the elderly, and ethnic minorities.

British Medical Association (BMA) A professional body and independent trade union for doctors dedicated to protecting individual members and the collective interests of doctors.

British National Formulary (BNF) A joint publication of the British Medical Association and the Royal Pharmaceutical Society of Great Britain. It is published under the authority of the Joint Formulary Committee. The Dental Formulary Subcommittee oversees the preparation of advice relating to drug management of dental and oral conditions and includes representatives of the British Dental Association. It includes information on the selection, prescribing, and administration of medicines and is updated every six months.

Further Reading: Wray D., Wagle S. M. S. A dentist's guide to using the BNF; Part 1 & Part 2 *Br Dent J* 2008;204:437–9, 487–91.

broach *n.* A fine tapered metal instrument used in *endodontic treatment. When smooth sided (**pathfinder broach**), it is used to locate the pulp canal and explore its structure. A broach with numerous barbs (**barbed broach**) is used to engage the pulp and facilitate its removal. The broach is usually introduced into the pulp canal using a hand-held **broach holder**.

bronchiole *n.* A subdivision of the bronchial tree that does not contain cartilage or mucous glands in its wall.

bronchus *n.* (*pl.* **bronchi**) One of the air passages that connect the *trachea to the *bronchioles and which contain cartilage and mucous glands. The trachea divides into two main branches, the left and right bronchi, which further subdivide to supply ten bronchopulmonary segments in each lung. Inhaled objects such as teeth or restorations are more likely to enter the right bronchus because of its more vertical location.

Browne's tube A small glass tube containing a red heat-sensitive dye used as a chemical indicator for sterilization. The dye changes colour to green after a defined period of time at a certain temperature but is not proof of sterilization. It was invented by Albert Browne Ltd in 1930.

brown tumour A lesion usually found within bone, which is characterized by accumulations of multinucleate giant cells in a vascular connective tissue. They are usually associated with primary *hyperparathyroidism and may be difficult to distinguish from other giant cell lesions of bone.

bruise (contusion) *n.* An escape of blood from ruptured blood vessels beneath the skin causing discoloration. It initially appears red, and then gradually changes to blue, then green, and finally yellow, as the haemoglobin is broken down as part of the healing process.

brushier (octocalcium phosphate) *n.* The mineralized element of *calculus during the first six months of its formation.

bruxism (occlusal neurosis) *n.* (*v.* to brux) An oral habit consisting of the non-functional involuntary rhythmic or spasmodic clenching or grinding of the teeth. It is usually an unconscious activity which may take place when the subject is asleep (**nocturnal bruxism**). It may be initiated by stress, fatigue, fear, or *occlusal irregularities. It has also been associated with neurological diseases, recreational drugs, and medication. Clinical features include extra-orally visible enlargement of the masseter muscles, linear *keratosis of the buccal mucosa corresponding to the occlusal plane of the posterior teeth, and scalloping of the lateral borders of the tongue. In severe cases (*brycomania), where grinding as well as clenching occurs, it may lead to abnormal wear patterns of the teeth, muscular problems, fractured cusps and restorations, periodontal destruction, and *temporomandibular joint dysfunction syndrome (TMD). Management of the condition includes the provision of a hard acrylic stabilization splint to protect the remaining tooth tissue. *See also* PARAFUNCTION.

brycomania (bruxomania) *n.* A severe form of *bruxism.

buccal *adj.* Relating to or adjacent to the cheek. The buccal surface of a tooth is the surface adjacent to the cheeks. *See also* TOOTH SURFACES.

buccal cavity *n.* 1. The cavity of the mouth which contains the tongue, teeth, and supporting structures and leads to the *pharynx. 2. A cavity located in the surface of a tooth related to the cheek.

buccal pad of fat A biconvex pad of fatty tissue situated between the masseter and the external surface of the buccinator muscles. It is more well developed in the new-born infant.

buccopharyngeal fascia The membrane that covers the muscular layer of the pharynx and is continued forward onto the buccinator muscle.

buck teeth A lay expression used to describe the prominent position of the upper anterior teeth in relation to the lower teeth (increased *overbite).

bud *n.* The first stage in *tooth development. *See also* TASTE BUDS.

buffer *n.* A liquid whose pH remains virtually unchanged by the addition of an acid or alkali. The saliva has a **buffering capacity** in reducing the demineralizing effect of acids on the teeth. Local *analgesic solutions usually contain **buffering agents** to stabilize the pH against body fluids.

bulimia nervosa *n.* An eating disorder in which large amounts of food are eaten followed by self-induced vomiting. It most commonly affects young girls but is increasingly seen in boys. The vomiting can lead to severe dental *erosion. Patients are often fanatical about oral hygiene, which can lead to toothbrush *abrasion and gingival recession. Disordered eating patterns may predispose to biochemical imbalances such as hypervitaminosis A, characterized by a yellow discoloration of the skin, and oral *mucosa. Treatment of bulimia is usually by psychotherapy, family therapy, and nutritional guidance. *See also* ANOREXIA NERVOSA.

Further Reading: Ashcroft A., Milosevic A. The eating disorders: 1 Current scientific understanding and dental implications. *Dent Update* 2007;34:544–54.

 SEE WEB LINKS
• The NHS Direct web page that provides information on bulimia nervosa.

bulla *n.* 1. A large vesicle (blister) containing fluid which is usually *serous exudate. 2. (in anatomy) A rounded bony prominence.

bunodont *adj.* Describing molar teeth with rounded or low conical cusps characteristic of omnivorous mammals. *Compare* LOPHODONT.

bunolophodont *adj.* Describing teeth in which the cusps are rounded and are linked by ridges (*lophs).

bunoselenodont *adj.* Describing molar teeth in which the inner cusps are in the form of blunt cones and the outer ones have longitudinal crescents.

Buonocore, Michael (1919–81) was born in Brooklyn and received bachelor's and master's degrees from St John's University. He then graduated from the Tufts Dental College. He served as a captain in the Army after the Second World War. In the 1960s his research into, and clinical evaluation of, plastic sealants led to a new development in adhesive dentistry. He is known for his innovative research on the preparation of the enamel surface with a weak acid to enhance adhesion of an organic plastic chemical sealant and the polymerization in situ of a sealant with ultraviolet light. He was chairman of the department of dental materials at the Eastman Dental Center, Rochester, USA.

bupivacaine *n.* A long-acting amino-amide local anaesthetic agent. Its clinical potency and its duration of action is approximately four times that of *lignocaine. It is commonly used as the anaesthetic agent in epidurals and spinal anaesthesia and after surgical procedures. It is available with or without adrenaline and is significantly more cardiotoxic than other local anaesthetics. Inadvertent intravenous injection can lead to *hypotension, *bradycardia, arrhythmias, and cardiac arrest. **Levobupivacaine** is the pure R-isomer of bupivacaine and is less cardiotoxic.

bur *n.* A rotary cutting instrument made of steel, tungsten carbide, or diamond grit used in a dental handpiece for cavity preparation and the trimming of restorations and other materials. They are described according to their size, shape, or function. An **end-cutting bur** only has cutting blades at the distal end of its head. **Finishing burs** have numerous fine cutting blades and can be barrel-, sphere-, or flame-shaped. A **fissure bur** has a cylindrical head with either parallel or tapering sides. A **goose (long) neck bur** has an elongated neck used to enlarge the coronal part of the root canal during endodontic therapy. An **inverted cone bur** has a truncated cone-shaped head with the largest diameter distal to the shank. A **round or rosehead bur** has a spherical head. A **trephine bur** has a hollow cylindrical or truncated cone-shaped head used primarily to remove a circular area of tissue.

Inverted cone tungsten carbide

Straight fissure tungsten carbide

Round/rosehead tungsten carbide

Wheel tungsten carbide

Tapering fissure tungsten carbide

Round-ended tapering fissure tungsten carbide

Cross-cut straight fissure tungsten carbide

Tapering diamond

Pear-shaped tungsten carbide

End-cutting

Flame-shaped finishing

Hollow trephine

Types of burs

Bur sizes and numbering system

Maximum diameter of bur head (in mm)	ISO code	UK sizes		
		Round	Flat fissure	Inverted cone
0.6	006	½		½
0.8	008	1	½	1
0.9	009		1	
1.0	010	2	2	2
1.2	012	3	3	3
1.4	014	4	4	4
1.6	016	5	5	5
1.8	018	6	6	6
2.1	021	7	7	7
2.3	023	8	8	8
2.5	025	9	9	9
2.7	027	10	10	10
2.9	029	11	11	
3.1	031	12	12	

burn *n.* Tissue damage to the skin or *mucosa caused by heat, sun-light, chemicals, electricity, friction, or nuclear radiation. A **first-degree burn** affects only the outer layer of skin (*epidermis) and is characterized by *erythema. A **second-degree burn** involves both the epidermis and the underlying tissues with the formation of *vesicles. A **third-degree burn** results in damage to the full skin thickness plus the underlying tissues, resulting in necrosis which may require skin grafting. The definition of a **fourth-degree burn** is controversial but it has been defined as occurring when charring of the submucous or *subcutaneous layers has taken place and the damage is irreparable.

burning mouth syndrome A condition characterized by a burning sensation (*dysaesthesia) which may affect the tongue (**glossodynia**), lips, or hard palate. The sensation may be present on waking and can get more severe during the day. The oral *mucosa appears normal and there are no precipitating factors. The aetiology is ill defined but *iron-deficiency anaemia, *vitamin B_{12} deficiency, *candidal infection, and *diabetes mellitus may be implicated.

burnish *v.* To smooth or polish a surface to obtain a high gloss finish or to improve the marginal adaptation of a material such as gold. It is achieved using a **burnisher** normally named according to its shape (such as ball, beaver-tail, fishtail, straight) or by the material on which it is used.

burn-out *n.* **1.** An area of excessive darkening (overexposure) on a dental *radiograph. **2.** The elimination by the use of heat of an investment *wax pattern prior to the investment mould receiving a casting metal.

Business Services Authority Formerly known as the Dental Practice Board. The authority is responsible for providing primary care trusts in England and local health boards in Wales with online payment systems that enable them to provide the data necessary to enable the division to make payments to General Dental Services (GDS) and Personal Dental Services (PDS), providers of National Health Service (NHS) dentistry. It was established in 2006 and is the main processing facility and centre of excellence for payment, reimbursement, remuneration, and reconciliation for NHS patients, employees, and other affiliated parties.

(⊕) SEE WEB LINKS

• The Business Services Authority website.

butt *v.* **1.** To bring any two flat-ended surfaces into contact so as to form a joint. **2.** To place directly against the tissues covering the alveolar ridge.

cacodontia *n.* The condition of having diseased or malformed teeth.

cacogeusia *n.* The sensation or illusion of an unpleasant taste, not related to the ingestion of specific substances and often caused by a neurological disorder e.g. epilepsy.

cacostomia *n.* A diseased or gangrenous condition of the mouth.

cadaver *n.* A dead body. A term usually used with reference to a body used for anatomical dissection.

CAD/CAM *See* COMPUTER-AIDED DESIGN/COMPUTER-AIDED MANUFACTURE.

café au lait spots Well defined pale brown or dark brown patches on the skin. They are present in up to 20% of the population.

Caffey's disease [J. Caffey (1895–1978), American paediatrician] A cortical bone overgrowth, particularly affecting the clavicles and mandible. It is self-limiting and usually appears before six months of age and disappears in childhood. It is characterized by fever and soft tissue swellings and is of unknown aetiology.

calcification *n.* The deposition of calcium salts in an organic matrix. It is part of the normal process of bone and tooth formation. **Ectopic oral calcification** occurs in the formation of *pulp stones and *salivary calculi. *See also* OSSIFICATION; MINERALIZATION.

calcific metamorphosis A reaction to tooth trauma resulting in partial or complete obliteration of the pulp chamber by secondary *dentine.

calcifying cystic odontogenic tumour (calcifying odontogenic cyst) A rare *benign cystic *neoplasm found in the mandible and maxilla of young adults.

calcination *n.* The process of heating a substance to remove water and create partial decomposition. It is part of the process in the manufacture of dental plaster and stone from gypsum.

calcitonin *n.* A *polypeptide hormone produced in the *thyroid gland which lowers the levels of *calcium and phosphate in the blood. It also inhibits bone resorption by reducing *osteoclastic activity.

calcium *n.* A metallic element essential for many metabolic processes and normal body development, particularly the *calcification of bones and teeth. The normal blood calcium level is 9–11.5mg/100ml and a deficiency can lead to *tetany. The normal dietary requirement is about 1gm per day, the principal sources being dairy products such as milk and cheese. Its uptake is aided by *vitamin D; where this vitamin is deficient the result can be *rickets or *osteoporosis. **Calcium carbonate** is an antacid used to neutralize gastric acidity. **Calcium fluoride** (CaF_2) occurs naturally as fluorspar which, when dissolved in water, releases fluoride ions. *See* FLUORIDATION. **Calcium hydroxide** is the active ingredient in a number of commercially produced cavity lining and pulp capping materials; it is used as a pulp capping material because of its antibacterial properties (it has a high alkalinity) and its ability to provide a favourable environment for the remineralization of the dentine. **Calcium salts** such as calcium carbonate and calcium phosphate are present in saliva and can precipitate in the form of salivary *calculi. **Calcium sulphate** and calcium phosphate are added to toothpastes as polishing abrasives.

calcium channel blockers Drugs that interfere with the movement of calcium ions across cell membranes. Calcium channel blockers block the influx of calcium ions through cardiac and vascular smooth muscle cell membranes. They affect myocardial cells, cells within the conducting system of the heart, and the cells of vascular smooth muscle. They reduce myocardial contractility and the propagation of electrical impulses within the heart which leads to vasodilation. Calcium channel blockers such as amlodipine and *nifedipine are used in the treatment of *hypertension, *angina, and arrhythmias; nifedipine can cause flushing, headaches, gingival *hypertrophy, and *hyperplasia similar to that produced by *phenytoin and *ciclosporin. Males are three times as likely as females to develop clinically significant overgrowth.

Further Reading: Gibson R. M., Meechan J. G. The effects of antihypertensive medication on dental treatment. *Dent Update* 2007;34:70–78.

calcium fluorapatite *n.* A mineral formed during the remineralization of *enamel when fluoride ions are present. The formation takes place according to the following equation:

$$Ca_{10}(PO_4)_6(OH)_2 + 2F^- = Ca_{10}(PO_4)_6(F)_2 + 2OH^-$$

calcium hydroxyapatite + fluoride ions = calcium fluorapatite + hydroxyl ions.

Calcium fluorapatite is more resistant to acid *caries attack than calcium hydroxyapatite. *See also* CARIES; FLUORIDE.

calcospherite *n.* A spherical zone of *hydroxyapatite formed during the mineralization phase of dentine formation (*dentinogenesis). Calcospherites eventually fuse together to form mineralized dentine.

calculogenesis *n.* The process during which calculi are formed.

calculus *n.* (*pl.* **calculi**) 1. A hard mass containing *calcium salts (calcium carbonate, calcium phosphate, magnesium phosphate) formed within the body and particularly found in the urinary tract, gall bladder, or salivary gland or duct (*salivary stone, sialolith). 2. A mineralized salivary deposit in an organic matrix found on the surfaces of teeth and dental prostheses. Calculus formation is always preceded by plaque deposition. It initially consists mainly of octocalcium phosphate (*brushier) but matures to hydroxyapatite after about 6 months. It forms most extensively on the teeth in relation to the ducts of the major salivary glands, namely buccal to the upper first and second molars opposite the *parotid duct, and lingual to the lower anterior teeth opposite to the *sublingual salivary ducts. Calculus tends to form most readily in alkaline saliva. **Supragingival calculus** forms at or above the gingival margin and is usually yellow in colour and clearly visible; the calcium salts are derived from saliva. **Subgingival calculus** forms below the gingival margin and is therefore less visible and best detected by probing. It is usually dark brown or green due to pigmentation by blood breakdown products; the calcium salts are derived from the gingival *crevicular fluid. Calculus is a local factor in contributing to periodontal disease because of its rough mechanically irritant surface and its ability to increase plaque retention. It provides a reservoir for many pathogenic micro-organisms. Calculus may be attached to the tooth in a number of ways: the *pellicle may act as an organic 'go-between' (most likely to occur on enamel), there may be direct attachment of the calculus organic matrix to the enamel, or there may be mechanical attachment, e.g. into surface defects in enamel, cementum, dentine, or restoration margins or surfaces. 📷

calculus surface index (CSI) A periodontal index used to measure the presence of calculus (supra- and subgingival) on the four mandibular incisors. The mesial, distal, labial, and lingual surfaces are examined and each tooth is assigned a number from 0 to 4 according to the number of surfaces on which calculus is recorded. The CSI is the total number of calculus-covered surfaces (maximum 16).

Caldicott report a review of patient-identifiable information chaired by **Dame Fiona Caldicott**, principal of Somerville College, Oxford, and commissioned by the Chief Medical Officer of England and Wales. The report, which was published in 1997, defined six key principles as to how confidential information should be managed within the National Health Service in the UK. These were: to justify the purpose for which patient-identifiable material is to be used; not to use patient identifiable information unless it is absolutely necessary; to use the minimum necessary patient-identifiable information; access to patient-identifiable information should be on a strict need-to-know basis; everyone with access to patient-identifiable information should be aware of their responsibilities; to understand and comply with the law.

(((⊕))) SEE WEB LINKS

• Report on the review of patient-identifiable information.

Caldwell–Luc operation [G. W. Caldwell (1834–1918), American surgeon; H. Luc (1855–1925), French laryngologist] A surgical procedure to create an auxiliary opening in the anterior wall of the maxillary sinus through the canine fossa, usually for improving drainage or for the purpose of removing pathological tissue from the maxillary *antrum such as thickened or infected antral lining or a *mucocoele.
A horizontal incision is made in the gingiva and a flap is reflected, which exposes the anteroinferior wall of the maxillary sinus. An opening through the bony wall is made into the sinus itself. It has been adapted for the removal of a tooth displaced into the maxillary sinus.

The bony defect created in the anterior sinus wall subsequently undergoes fibrous healing.

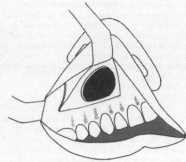

Caldwell–Luc operation

calibrated probe *n. See* PROBE.

calor *n.* Heat. One of the four signs of inflammation. *See also* DOLOR.

calorie *n.* The amount of heat required to raise one gram of water 1°C at 15°C. A kilogram calorie or large calorie (Kcal, Kg-cal, or Cal) is 1000 times greater than a calorie. The energy value of food is expressed in kilocalories.

calotte *n.* The *calvaria of the skull from which the base has been removed.

calvaria *n.* The *cranium without the facial bones attached.

Camper's line *n. See* ALA-TRAGAL LINE.

Camper's plane [P. Camper (1722–89), Dutch anatomist] *n.* A flat surface running from the tip of the anterior nasal spine (*acanthion) to the superior border of the tragus of the ears on the right and left sides.

camphorated parachlorophenol *n. See* PARACHLOROPHENOL.

camphorquinone *n.* A chemical added to resin composite to act as a polymerization initiator when activated by the presence of blue light (*photo-initiator).

Campylobacter *n.* A genus of Gram-negative, spiral, motile microaerophilic bacteria. They can have a curved, rod-like appearance. At least seven *Campylobacter* species have been identified from subgingival sites. *C. rectus* has been implicated as a periodontal *pathogen. *Campylobacter* is the commonest reported bacterial cause of infectious intestinal disease in England and Wales, of which *C. jejuni* and *C. coli* account for the majority of infections.

Further Reading: Macuch P. J., Tanner A. C. Campylobacter species in health, gingivitis, and periodontitis. *Journal of Dental Research* 2000;79:785–92.

campylognathia *n.* A curved deformity of the jaw. It is a rare congenital defect and may be associated with a cleft lip.

canal *n.* A tubular channel or passage. The **pulp canal** is that part of the root of a tooth which contains the pulp tissue; it is bounded by dentine. An **accessory root canal** is a lateral branch of the main root canal usually occurring in the apical third of the tooth root. The **mandibular (inferior dental) canal** extends from the mandibular foramen on the medial surface of the ramus of the mandible to the mental foramen and contains the mandibular artery and vein and the mandibular branch of the trigeminal nerve. **Nutrient canals** through which blood vessels pass are present in the alveolar bone of the mandible and maxilla.

canaliculus *n. (pl.* **canaliculi**) A microscopic canal linking the *lacunae of bone and cementum containing the filamentous processes of *osteocytes.

cancer *n.* A *malignant *neoplasm (including both *carcinoma and *sarcoma) which arises from the abnormal and uncontrolled division of cells and which invades and destroys the surrounding tissues. The primary neoplasm has a tendency to spread (*metastasize) to other parts of the body and establish secondary neoplasms. *See also* CARCINOMA; SARCOMA.

cancrum oris (noma) An opportunistic infection of the mouth occurring in children. It can spread from the *mucosa with initial gingival inflammation followed by rapid spread to extensive orofacial gangrene. The peak incidence is at 1–4 years of age and the infection is most common in sub-Saharan Africa. The condition is rare and is generally only found in cases of severe malnutrition. Cancrum oris may be preceded by diseases such as malaria, measles, severe diarrhoea, and necrotizing ulcerative *gingivitis. The acute stage responds readily to antibiotic therapy but the sequelae following healing can include functional and aesthetic impairment, which may require reconstructive surgery. 📷

Further Reading: Enwonwu C. O., Falkler W. A. Jr, Phillips R. S. Noma (cancrum oris) *Lancet* 2006;368:147–56.

Candida albicans A yeast (yeasts are classified as fungi) species frequently found as part of the commensal oral microbial flora and the female genital tract, having two distinct forms (dimorphic). The organism can exist as oval budding yeasts or as filamentous hyphae, of which the latter are frequently associated with tissue invasion. *C. albicans* is the most pathogenic species of the genus *Candida* and can cause infections when host immunity is impaired or when the normal microbial flora is disturbed, such as following broad-spectrum antibiotic therapy. *C. albicans* is an opportunistic pathogen and a frequent cause of infection of immunocompromised individuals, such as those infected with the human immunodeficiency virus (*HIV) or with acquired immunodeficiency syndrome (*AIDS).

candidiasis (candidosis) *n.* Commonly called thrush or yeast infection. A fungal infection caused by yeast species of the genus *Candida*, most commonly **C. albicans*. Candidiasis includes superficial infections, such as oral thrush, vaginitis, and nail infections, and potentially life-threatening systemic infections (also known as **candidemia**) of the blood, tissues, and organs. Over the last decade, several other *Candida* species have emerged as opportunistic pathogens, including *C. glabrata, C. tropicalis, C. krusei, C. parapsilosis,* and *C. dubliniensis.* **Oral candidiasis** may present in a variety of ways. Florid cases are characterized by white *hyperplastic patches on the oral mucosa, which can be wiped off, leaving a raw bleeding surface. This form is most common in the elderly and may be an indicator of underlying immune deficiency, such as *HIV infection or malignant disease. It sometimes presents as smooth red patches (**erythematous candidiasis**), particularly on the hard and soft palate and buccal mucosa, and this may be associated with long-term antibiotic therapy which disturbs the oral flora. It may also be seen on the palate under the fitting surface of a denture and at the angles of the mouth (*see* ANGULAR CHEILITIS). Candida may also grow in the surface of a fixed white patch (candidal *leukoplakia) and is associated with an increased risk of malignant change in such lesions. Systemic infections are most common in severely immunocompromised individuals, such as HIV-infected and AIDS patients, cancer patients, and transplant recipients. 📷

canine (cuspid or **eye tooth)** *n.* A single cusped tooth located between the *incisors and *premolars. There is one canine in the quadrant of each arch in both the *primary (deciduous) and *secondary (permanent) dentitions. The **canine fossa** is a depression on the mesial surface of the crown of the upper first premolar. There is a bony prominence over the root of the canine tooth on the labial surface (**canine eminence**).

The canines play a major role in the excursive movements of the mandible during masticatory function (**canine guidance**). The **canine relationship** is an important indicator when assessing a malocclusion. The relationship can be classified as **Class I**, where the tip of the upper canine occludes between the lower canine and first premolar; **Class II**, where the tip of the upper canine occludes between the lower lateral incisor and canine; and **Class III** if the tip of the upper canine occludes between the lower first and second premolars.

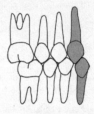

Class I

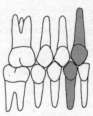

Class II

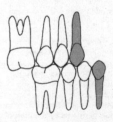

Class III

Canine relationship

canine, permanent mandibular *n.* The tooth located in the permanent *dentition of the *mandible between the lateral *incisor and

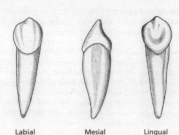
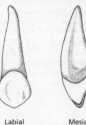
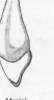
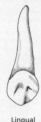

| Labial | Mesial | Lingual | | Labial | Mesial | Lingual |

Mandibular right canine   Maxillary right canine

Permanent canines

first *premolar. It has a crown that is narrower mesio-distally than the upper canine, and the incisal cusp is less pointed. The incisal edge is markedly rounded at the junction with the distal surface, and the labial surface is convex. The labial surface merges gradually with the distal surface, but the labial and lingual surfaces are inclined acutely to each other. There is no well-marked *cingulum on the lingual surface (unlike the upper canine); this is replaced by a ridge running from the incisal cusp tip to the cervical margin, bounded on either side by mesial and distal marginal ridges, thus creating two hollows. The mesial and distal surfaces are wedge-shaped and are longer than the upper canine. There is normally a single root, oval in cross-section and flattened on the mesial and distal surfaces with a groove in the long axis of the tooth on both surfaces. The *pulp chamber is narrower than in the upper canine but is of a similar morphological shape. There is normally only one root canal, although this is subject to considerable variation. *Calcification of the tooth begins at about 4–5 months after birth and the crown is normally complete by 6–7 years of age. The tooth erupts at about 9–10 years and the calcification of the root is complete at about 12–14 years.

canine, permanent maxillary *n.* The tooth located in the permanent *dentition of the *maxilla between the lateral *incisor and first *premolar. The crown has a pointed cusp and a convex labial surface which is ovoid in outline. The lingual surface has a bulky *cingulum and may be flat, convex, or slightly concave; a vertical ridge runs from the cingulum to the

apex of the incisal edge. The lingual surface is bounded by mesial and distal marginal ridges. The mesial slope of the incisal edge is shorter than the distal slope and the mesial surface of the crown is larger than the distal surface; both mesial and distal surfaces have a lingual inclination. There is a marked convexity at the junction of the incisal edge and the distal surface. The canine has a single root which is triangular in cross-section with rounded angles, creating labial, mesio-lingual, and disto-lingual surfaces, the latter two of which are frequently grooved along the long axis of the tooth. The *pulp chamber is oval in cross-section and is pointed towards the apex of the crown. There is normally only one root canal, although this is subject to considerable variation. *Calcification of the tooth begins at about 4–5 months after birth and the crown is normally complete by 6–7 years of age. The tooth erupts at about 11–12 years and the calcification of the root is complete at about 13–15 years.

canines, primary (deciduous) *n.* The teeth, two in each jaw, located between the lateral incisors and first primary molars. They have a similar morphological shape to the permanent canines but are smaller and much more bulbous. *Calcification of the primary canines begins at about 5 months of foetal life and the crowns are normally complete by 2 months after birth. The teeth erupt at about 16–18 months after birth, with the mandibular canines usually erupting first, and the calcification of the roots are complete at about 3 years of age.

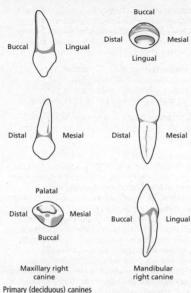

Maxillary right canine   Mandibular right canine

Primary (deciduous) canines

canker *n.* A colloquial name for *aphthous ulceration.

cannabis *n.* A plant genus which includes the species *Cannabis sativa* (hemp) whose dried leaves are known as **marijuana**. It is the most frequently used illicit drug in Australia. Cannabis abusers generally have poorer oral health than non-users, with an increased risk of dental caries and periodontal disease because of the associated *xerostomia. There can also be an increased stress response upon administration of local analgesic containing adrenaline.

Further Reading: Cho C. M., Hirsch R., Johnstone S. General and oral health implications of cannabis use. *Aust Dent J.* 2005;50(2):70–74.

Cannon's disease *See* NAEVUS.

cannulation *n.* The process of inserting a hollow tube (**cannula**) into a body cavity such as a vein.

cantilever bridge *See* BRIDGE.

cap *n.* 1. The name that describes a stage of *tooth development of the enamel organ (after the *bud stage and before the *bell stage). 2. An outmoded term for a baked porcelain crown. 3. A material applied directly or indirectly to the surface of the pulp (*pulp cap). 4. A lay term for any type of artificial *crown.

Capdepont syndrome [C. Capdepont (1867–1917), French dentist] An alternative name for dentinogenesis imperfecta.

capillary *n.* The smallest type of blood vessel in the body, with an approximate diameter of 5–20µm, which form networks in most tissues. They connect the arterial and venous side of the circulatory system, by means of arterioles which supply them with blood, and venules which drain them. The capillary wall is a single layer of epithelial cells which acts as a semi-permeable membrane, allowing the exchange of various substances including nutrients, metabolic waste products, and fluids and gases. Substances pass through the capillary wall by diffusion, filtration, and *osmosis.

capitation *n.* A system of financing in dentistry in which the dentist receives a fee per patient per defined period of time in exchange for the provision of specific dental services.

capitulum *n.* A small eminence on a bone by which it articulates with another bone, e.g. the capitulum of the humerus.

capnophilic *adj.* Describing the ability to survive in an atmosphere of carbon dioxide at a concentration exceeding that of air.

cap splint *n. See* SPLINT.

capsule *n.* 1. The cellular sheath or membrane surrounding an organ. A **joint capsule** is the tough fibrous sheath which surrounds a joint such as the *temporomandibular joint. 2. A slimy protective layer external to the cell wall of certain bacteria. 3. A soluble container used for the delivery of certain drugs or medicaments.

Carabelli's tubercle *See* TUBERCLE.

carat *n.* The degree of purity of *gold. Pure gold is 24 carat. 18 carat gold is 75% gold by volume mixed with other metals or alloys.

carbamazepine *n.* An anticonvulsant drug used in the treatment of *trigeminal neuralgia and *epilepsy and the management of chronic pain. It acts by reducing the influx of sodium ions during the transmission of a nerve impulse. Common side-effects include *nausea, dizziness, drowsiness, double vision, and muscular incoordination, and often these side-effects limit the therapeutic use of the drug. Rarely it can cause *leucopenia, thrombocytopenia, *agranulocytosis, and aplastic *anaemia. Other side-effects include cholestatic jaundice, *hepatitis, and acute renal failure. Haematological and biochemical monitoring of the blood is therefore important. Its use is contraindicated in patients with unpaced atrioventicular conduction abnormalities and those with a history of bone marrow depression. Trade names: **Tegretol, Epitol** (*US*).

carbamide peroxide An oxidizing agent consisting of *hydrogen peroxide compounded with urea which releases oxygen in contact with water. It has the chemical formula: $CH_6N_2O_3$. In dentistry it is used as a *bleaching agent. For home use it is usually in a 10–20% solution dispensed as a gel. Pure carbamide peroxide is soluble in water and contains approximately 35% hydrogen peroxide: it is a skin, eye, and respiratory irritant and can cause corrosive burns on contact with the gingivae or mucous membranes. *See also* BLEACHING.

carbohydrate *n.* Any one of a large group of organic compounds which contain carbon, hydrogen, and oxygen and provide a source of energy, such as sugars and starch. All carbohydrates are eventually broken down in the body to *glucose. With *fat and *protein they form one of the three main constituents of food. The storage form of carbohydrate when not completely broken down to glucose is *glycogen, which is stored in the liver and muscles. **Refined carbohydrates** refer to complex carbohydrates (starches) that have had the bran, hull, fibre and some nutrients removed from the grain during processing. They include such foods as white bread, white pasta, and some cereals. These foods are potentially *cariogenic and can produce a sudden and sharp increase in blood sugar (high *glycaemic index). *See also* DISACCHARIDE; MONOSACCHARIDE; POLYSACCHARIDE.

carbolized resin A sedative and antiseptic dressing containing resin, alcohol, and phenol. It has historically been used for the relief of pain on an exposed pulp.

carbon dioxide An odourless, colourless gas formed in the tissues as an end product of respiration and carried in the blood to the lungs where it is exhaled. An increase of carbon dioxide in the blood stimulates the nervous system to increase the respiratory rate, thus increasing the supply of oxygen and the elimination of carbon dioxide. Carbon dioxide *lasers are used for minor oral surgery and have been used experimentally for cutting tooth cavities.

carbonic acid *n.* A weak acid (H_2CO_3) formed when carbon dioxide dissolves in water. It is present in carbonated soft drinks and together with *citric and *phosphoric acid is responsible for their high acidity (approximately pH 2.8).

Carborundum stone *n. See* STONE.

carbuncle *n.* A collection of boils with multiple drainage channels draining pus onto the skin. It is usually caused by *Staphylococcus aureus*. Treatment is with antibiotics and sometimes also by surgery.

carcinogen *n.* A cancer-causing agent. Carcinogens include both ultra-violet and ionizing radiation, certain viruses, and chemicals such as tar in cigarette smoke.

carcinogenesis *n.* The process by which normal cells are transformed into malignant (cancer) cells.

carcinoma *n.* A *malignant *neoplasm (cancer) of epithelial tissue. Carcinomas histologically do not resemble the parent tissue to the same extent as *benign tumours. They frequently spread (metastasize) to other parts of the body, initially via the lymphatic system and latterly via the blood. They are generally classified according to their cell type, for example, carcinoma of glandular tissue (*adenocarcinoma) and squamous cells (**squamous cell carcinoma**). **Clear cell odontogenic carcinoma** is a rare malignant neoplasm of odontogenic epithelium, characterized by clear cells. Carcinoma of the *salivary glands is rare but **muco-epidermoid carcinoma** and *adenoid cystic carcinoma are the most common. **Nasopharyngeal carcinoma** is a rare malignant neoplasm arising from the mucosal epithelium of the *nasopharynx; it may be associated with the *Epstein–Barr virus, exposure to smoke, or chemical pollutants. A number of oral lesions, such as *leukoplakia and *erythroplakia, are considered to be possible precursors of oral carcinoma. The most common type of **oral carcinoma** is squamous cell carcinoma, arising in the squamous cells of the mucosal lining of the mouth and pharynx; risk factors associated with squamous cell carcinoma are all forms of *smoking, smokeless *tobacco, betal nut chewing, and alcohol use. The risk of oral carcinoma increases with age and is more common in men than women; the symptoms show wide variation and can include a painless swelling, a persistent ulcer, painless white or red patches, and difficulty in swallowing. Treatment is dependent on the nature and extent of the condition and may include surgery, radiotherapy, or chemotherapy. **Verrucous carcinoma** is a low grade variant of squamous cell carcinoma. It is characterized by raised warty white patches and rarely metastasizes. *See also* BASAL CELL CARCINOMA; LEUKAEMIA; MELANOMA; LYMPHOMA; ORAL CANCER.

cardiac arrest A complete cessation of heart function. It can result from a large number of causes including airway, breathing or circulatory problems, drugs, poisons, *myocardial infarction, circulatory collapse, *anaphylaxis, and *respiratory arrest. Ineffective pumping action of the heart can occur when the ventricles of the heart beat very rapidly (*fibrillation). Without prompt treatment, irreversible brain damage will occur. Management depends on the cause but initially is by commencing *basic life support.

cardiac muscle *n. See* MUSCLE.

cardiopulmonary arrest A failure of both the cardiac and respiratory systems.

cardiopulmonary resuscitation (CPR) *See* BASIC LIFE SUPPORT.

cardiovascular disease *n.* Any one of a number of pathological conditions that involve dysfunction of the heart and vascular system. These conditions include coronary heart disease, *atheroma, rheumatic heart disease, and systemic *hypertension. Studies have shown an association between *periodontal disease and an increased risk of *stroke and coronary heart disease, demonstrating the importance of minimized oral disease.

Further Reading: Ford P. J., Yamazaki K., Seymour G. J. Cardiovascular and oral disease interactions: what is the evidence? *Primary Dental Care* 2007;14:59–66.

cardiovascular system The heart together with the two networks of blood vessels, namely the systemic circulation and the pulmonary circulation. The vascular circulatory system between the right side of the heart, the lungs, and the left atrium is called the **pulmonary circulation**. The circuit of vessels between the left side of the heart, most of the body, and the right atrium is called the **systemic circulation**. It serves to provide the supply of nutrients and the removal of waste products from all parts of the body. Deoxygenated blood flows through the two largest veins (the superior and inferior venae cavae) into the right atrium; it then passes through the tricuspid valve into the right ventricle which then contracts forcing blood into the pulmonary arteries through the pulmonary valve to deliver it to the capillaries of the lungs. In the lungs the blood absorbs oxygen and gives up carbon dioxide via the capillaries surrounding the air sacs. Oxygen-rich blood from the lungs flows through the pulmonary veins into the left atrium of the heart; the blood then passes through the mitral valve into the left ventricle. On contraction of the left ventricle blood is forced through the aortic valve into the aorta and thence via the systemic arteries to all parts of the body except the lungs.

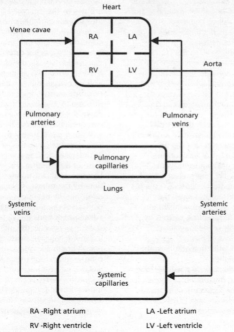

Heart

Venae cavae

RA | LA

Aorta

RV | LV

Pulmonary arteries

Pulmonary veins

Pulmonary capillaries

Lungs

Systemic veins

Systemic arteries

Systemic capillaries

RA -Right atrium   LA -Left atrium
RV -Right ventricle   LV -Left ventricle

Schematic representation of the cardiovascular system

Care Quality Commission Part of the UK parliament legislative programme included within the *Health and Social Care Act 2008. It is an integrated regulator for health and adult social care, bringing together existing health and social care regulators into one regulatory body, with tough new powers to ensure safe and high-quality services.

carer *n.* A person who provides support for another person in an unfunded or unpaid capacity. They are frequently responsible for oral hygiene practices of patients with physical or learning disabilities.

caries

n. (*adj.* **carious**) An infectious disease resulting in a progressive destruction of tooth tissue. It is the result of an interaction between bacteria from dental *plaque, *fermentable carbohydrates, and tooth tissue over a period of time and can only occur when all these factors are present. The rate of progression of caries is dependent upon the resistance of the tooth to carious attack which includes the chemical, structural, and morphological nature of the enamel surface and the cariogenicity of the environment of the tooth such as the diet, the nature of the plaque, and the consistency and constituents of the saliva. The exact process by which caries occurs is still the subject of much research. Potentially many micro-organisms may be involved in the caries process, although the most important are considered to be *Streptococcus mutans* and *Lactobacilli*. These organisms metabolize sugars found in the plaque or saliva and create local concentrations of acid in the inner layers of the plaque adhering to the tooth surface. This increases the *acidity (lowers the pH) on the tooth surface. When this reaches a critical level (pH 5.2–5.5 for enamel and pH 6.0–6.5 for dentine) sub-surface *demineralization starts to take place and *calcium and phosphates diffuse out of the enamel or dentine. If the pH rises again above this critical level, the process is reversed and *remineralization takes place. These fluctuations, caused by the metabolic activity of the associated biofilm, will cause loss or gain of minerals from the tooth, depending on the decrease or increase in pH respectively, cumulatively resulting in a net loss of minerals, dissolution of dental hard tissues, and the formation of a carious lesion (*see also* STEPHAN'S CURVE). This is represented by the equation:

$$[Ca_5(PO_4)OH \Leftrightarrow \Rightarrow 5Ca^{2+} + 3PO_4^{3+} + OH^-]$$

if the pH remains below the critical level for an extended period of time there is a marked loss of mineral below the tooth surface, resulting in the appearance of a *white spot lesion on the enamel. Microscopically, enamel caries starts as a wedge shape with the point towards the dentine and an intact outer layer of enamel about 20–50μm thick. The lesion is reversible at this stage. **Early childhood caries** describes caries in the teeth of infants or very young children; if severe it may be described as **severe early childhood caries** (S-ECC); alternative descriptions in common usage include baby bottle caries, bottle-mouth caries, and nursing bottle caries. **Enamel caries** tends to occur in areas of stagnation where the plaque is not readily removed, such as in tooth pits and fissures, interproximal areas, or around poorly contoured restorations. If the acidic condition persists, the lesion enlarges and as it progresses into dentine it spreads laterally along the amelo-dentinal junction to involve a large area of dentine. The dentine may respond at this stage by retracting the odontoblast processes down the dentinal tubules towards the pulp and occluding the tubules by the increased formation of intertubular dentine (so called **tubular** *sclerosis). This effectively blocks the odontoblasts and the pulp from the advancing caries. **Dead tracts** form when odontoblasts die and the tubules become filled with air and debris. As the lesion enlarges the enamel surface collapses, resulting in cavitation; the lesion is now infected by bacteria; these are able to migrate down the dead tracts and destroy the mineral component of dentine by acid production and the organic matrix by enzyme action. This destruction results in the formation of **liquefaction foci**, which coalesce to form a **zone of destruction**. The progress of the bacteria down the tubules may be halted for a time by the tubular sclerosis, and the odontoblasts may produce reactionary dentine at the pulpal surface, but in rapidly advancing lesions this defence reaction is quickly overcome; the pulp will then become inflamed. **Nursing caries (baby bottle caries)** is early tooth decay produced in a baby by the routine night-time use of a feeding bottle containing fruit juice or a sugared solution. **Radiation caries** is a type of tooth decay induced by a dry mouth (*xerostomia) due to a reduction in salivary flow, following salivary gland damage consequent upon radiation therapy in the treatment of malignant tumours. It frequently affects the cervical margins of the teeth, incisal edges, and cusp tips. **Rampant caries** describes a sudden rapid carious destruction of many teeth, often involving tooth surfaces that are normally relatively caries-free; it is most commonly seen in the primary teeth of infants using a sugar coated comforter or bottle containing sugar solution, and in the secondary dentition of teenagers who have a high cariogenic diet and poor oral hygiene. **Root caries (cervical caries)** begins at the gingival margins of teeth on any of the root surfaces. As it spreads it undermines the enamel margins, resulting in further tissue breakdown. Soft carious dentine has a high bacterial content and indicates an active lesion and should be removed, but lesions with a hard surface which are often dark brown (**arrested caries**) indicate evidence of remineralization and, while aesthetically displeasing, do not represent active lesions. **Smooth surface caries** is a lesion which forms on the surface of the tooth not involving pits or fissures; it usually occurs interproximally below a contact area or at the neck of a tooth. The interrelationship between the aetiological factors of caries make the epidemiology complicated but it is well established that in the UK caries levels are highest in the poorer socio-economic areas of society, who tend to consume a greater proportion of refined carbohydrate in the diet. However, this is the converse in developing countries because the ingestion of refined carbohydrates is much less, due to their higher cost and limited availability. There is ongoing research into the development of a *caries vaccine. 📷

caries diagnosis The process of establishing the presence of dental caries. Methods used include visual examination, radiography (especially bitewing *radiographs), *transillumination, and electronic devices which measure the electrical impedence of enamel (such as the **DIAGNOdent®**). 📷

Further Reading: Zandona A. F., Zero D. T. Diagnostic tools for early caries detection. *J Am Dent Assoc* 2006;137(12):1675–84.

caries prevention Activities and methods designed to stop the initiation of caries. Measures include reducing the amount and particularly the frequency of sugary intakes in the diet, modifying the saliva, mechanical removal of the *plaque, and modification of the tooth surface by the use of *fissure sealants or the application of *fluoride, either in the water supply or topically by the use of fluoride toothpastes, gels, and mouthwashes.

caries test A means of assessing the susceptibility of an individual to caries. The test is based on studies showing that groups of individuals with high *Lactobacillus counts often had, or developed, more caries than groups with low counts. *Lactobacillus* counts as a caries predictor have shown variable results in individual cases and therefore, as a single test to screen for caries risk, it is of limited value; however, the test has been used to identify at-risk groups. The test may be undertaken at the chairside or in the laboratory.

caries vaccine A protein antigen designed to immunize against the development of dental caries. The protein antigen is derived from *Streptococcus mutans* or *Streptococcus sobrinus* and is aimed specifically at *Streptococcus mutans* surface antigens with the aim of reducing the adhesion to tooth surfaces.

Further Reading: Russell M. W., Childers N. K., Michalek M. S., Smith D. J., Taubman M. A. A caries vaccine? *Caries Res* 2004;38:230–35.

cariogenic *adj.* Describing any substance that induces caries (tooth decay).

cariogenicity *n.* The ability of a substance to induce the formation of caries (tooth decay).

cariostatic *adj.* Describing any agent that inhibits caries (tooth decay).

carious *adj.* Pertaining to caries or tooth decay.

Carisolv® *n.* The trade name for a non-invasive *caries removal system. The active ingredient is *sodium hypochlorite which dissolves the *collagen in organic material through chlorination of *amino acids, and allows it to be

Initial area of cavitation

Occlusal   Smooth surface

Arrested caries

removed using primarily hand instruments. *See also* ATRAUMATIC RESTORATIVE TREATMENT (ART).

carnassial *adj.* A tooth that is designed to tear flesh or bone. The carnassial teeth of flesh-eating animals include the last premolar on either side of the upper jaw and the first molar on either side of the lower jaw; they are also known as **sectorial teeth**.

carotene *n.* One of the orange carotenoid plant pigments, the most important of which is ß-carotene, found in milk and some vegetables, which is converted in the body to vitamin A.

carotid triangle A space containing the bifurcation of the common carotid artery bounded anteriorly by the superior belly of the omohyoid muscle, posteriorly by the anterior border of the sternocleidomastoid muscle, and superiorly by the posterior belly of the digastric muscle.

carpal tunnel syndrome A condition characterized by *paraesthesia, numbness and pain in the hand usually related to the thumb, index, and middle fingers. Along with other work-related repetitive actions which give rise to physically debilitating ailments, it is also known as **repetitive strain injury** (RSI) or **cumulative trauma disorder**. Although the prevalence is low, there is evidence that dental professionals, particularly hygienists, are at risk.

carrier *n.* A person who harbours the micro-organisms causing a particular disease without suffering from any of the signs or symptoms of infection, and who can transmit the disease to others.

cartilage *n.* Tough, flexible connective tissue consisting mainly of chondroitin sulphate produced by cells called *chondroblasts. There are three types of cartilage: **hyaline cartilage** found in the larynx, trachea, nose, and covering joint surfaces; **elastic cartilage** in the external ear and epiglottis; and **fibrocartilage** in the intervertebral discs and tendons.

caruncle, mandibular *n.* The small fleshy swelling that forms the opening of the duct of the *sublingual salivary gland bilateral to the *lingual fraenum.

carver *n.* A hand instrument used to contour plastic materials. They are most commonly used to carve inlay *wax, or amalgam alloy restorations before the amalgam alloy has reached its final hardness, or for carving or shaping composite restorations prior to final polymerization. They are manufactured in a variety of shapes to suit their purpose. A **Frahm carver** is double-ended with diamond-shaped pointed tips; **Hollenback carvers** are double-ended with angled flat lanceolate pointed working ends and are manufactured in a variety of sizes; a **Le Cron carver** has a pointed blade at one end and a discoid shape at the opposite working end; a **Roach carver** is double-ended with a flat pointed lanceolate blade in the long axis of the instrument at one end and a cup-shaped working tip at the other; a **cleoid discoid carver** is double-ended with a pointed spade shape at one working end and a disc-shape at the other; **Ward's carvers** are double-ended and are manufactured in a variety of shapes and sizes with either an angled pointed lanceolate working end or an angled rounded flat blade.

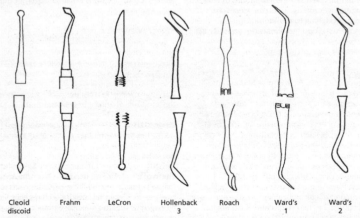

| Cleoid discoid | Frahm | LeCron | Hollenback 3 | Roach | Ward's 1 | Ward's 2 |

Types of carvers

case control study A research investigation which compares a group of people who have a disease with another group from the same population who are free from that disease. A case control study can identify risks and trends and suggest possible causes for disease. *See also* COHORT STUDY; CROSS-SECTIONAL STUDY.

casein phosphopeptide-amorphous calcium phosphate (CCP-ACP) A casein derived peptide, with added calcium and phosphate. It provides a phosphate and calcium reservoir when included within dental plaque and on the surface of the tooth. **Amorphous calcium phosphate (ACP)** is made by combining soluble salts of calcium and phosphorous. Calcium and phosphate ions are released when the *pH drops during an acid attack, to maintain *supersaturated surroundings with respect to *hydroxyapatite and as a result reducing *demineralization and increasing *remineralization. CCP-ACP has a buffering effect on the acids produced in dental *plaque and therefore has applications in the control of *caries, especially uncontrolled root caries. It can be delivered to the tooth surface in a variety of ways such as chewing gum, lozenges, topical crème, mouthrinses, toothpaste, and as an additive in glass ionomer cement restorative material. Trade names: **CPP-ACP™, Recaldent™, GC Tooth Mousse.**

cassette *n.* A container for holding an extra-oral x-ray film. It usually contains an intensifying *screen unless it is digital.

cast 1. *n.* An object formed by pouring liquid material into a rigid or flexible mould in which it subsequently hardens. 2. *v.* The process of throwing metal into a rigid mould such as in the production of a cast *gold inlay. An **altered cast** is a master cast that is produced from different impressions for different aspects of the cast. An example would be a master cast for a removable partial denture, where the record of anterior teeth was produced from one impression and the record of a posterior saddle area was produced from another impression, using a different impression technique. A **dental cast** is a positive reproduction of all or part of the mouth, usually in a hard material such as dental stone. A **diagnostic cast** is used for the purposes of diagnosis or treatment planning. A **duplicate cast** is an exact copy or replica of a cast. A **refractory cast** is made of material that will withstand the high temperatures of molten metal, such as in the construction of chrome cobalt *prostheses. A **split cast** is poured in two stages and is capable of subsequent separation by the use of a separating

medium such as petroleum jelly. A **working cast** is an accurate copy of a cast on which a casting such as an inlay can be modified without damage to the original master cast. A **cast core** is a metal casting, usually including a metal post extending into the root, which forms the structure on which an artificial crown is cemented. A **cast metal inlay** restores the shape and function of a tooth by replacing lost tooth tissue. *See also* INLAY.

casting 1. *n.* A metal object formed in a mould. 2. *adj.* The process by which a liquid metal is introduced into a mould. This can be achieved using a mechanical device such as an **air pressure casting machine** which forces the metal into the mould using compressed air, a **centrifugal casting machine** which utilizes centrifugal force to throw the metal into the mould, or a **vacuum casting machine** which removes all gases from the mould prior to casting. Potential problems with casting include dimensional inaccuracy, *porosity, contamination, rough surface, or incomplete casting. A **casting ring** is a metal tube in which a refractory mould is made to cast metal appliances or restorations.

catabolism *n.* The decomposition by the body of complex substances into ones of a simpler form with the release of energy. It is the opposite to *anabolism.

catalyst *n.* A substance that speeds up the rate of a chemical reaction but does not itself enter into the reaction and remains unchanged at the end of the reaction. *Enzymes are examples of biological catalysts.

cataphasia *n.* A speech disorder in which the same word or phrase is repeated several times in succession.

catecholamines *n.* A group of sympathomimetic compounds containing a benzene ring with adjacent hydroxyl groups (catechol) and an amine side chain. They include *adrenaline (epinephrine), *noradrenaline (norepinephrine), and dopamine, which are hormones released from the adrenal glands in response to stress.

categorical data Data that are classified into two or more discrete, non-overlapping categories e.g. age and gender.

catgut *n.* A natural material made from sheep's intestine and formerly used as a *suture material. Catgut is resorbable which avoids the need for its removal. Catgut has now been largely replaced by synthetic materials because of its tendency to cause tissue reaction.

catheter *n.* A hollow flexible tube that can be inserted into a cavity so that fluids may be removed or introduced.

cathode *n.* A negative electrode which in a dental x-ray tube usually consists of a helical tungsten filament with a molybdenum reflector to focus the electron beam on the anode.

catodont *n.* A person or animal possessing natural teeth in the lower jaw only.

CAT scan *See* COMPUTERIZED TOMOGRAPHY.

causal effect An association between two characteristics that can be demonstrated to be due to cause and effect: a change in one characteristic produces a change in the other.

causalgia *n.* An intense burning pain and marked sensitivity to touch in the distribution of an injured peripheral nerve. It is frequently at some distance from the site of injury.

causation *n.* A legal term used to define whether a medical or dental professional's actions or inaction created or contributed to a health problem. Not only must the claimant show that the defendant was in breach of his duty, but also that this breach led to the injury the claimant alleges. A causative link must be proved for the claimant to recover damages.

caustic *n.* Any substance that destroys, corrodes, or burns living tissue by chemical means.

cautery (thermocoagulation) *n.* (*v.* **cauterize**) The application of external heat to produce the searing or burning of living tissue. It is used to arrest *capillary bleeding or to remove small growths. It may be used to remove or recontour gingival tissue prior to taking an impression for a *crown or *bridge preparation. *See also* ELECTROCAUTERY; ELECTROSURGERY.

cavernous haemangioma *n. See* HAEMANGIOMA.

cavernous sinus *n. See* SINUS.

cavitation *n.* 1. The process by which *caries undermines the hard tissues of a tooth causing a cavity to form. 2. The result of passing ultrasonic waves through a solution creating the sequential formation and collapse of vapour bubbles (hydrodynamic turbulence). It can be used to remove contaminating material on the surface of instruments. Cavitation is also produced by the action of ultrasonic scalers when removing hard tooth deposits such as calculus. Cavitation has been used with an *irrigant to cleanse the root canal system when undertaking *endodontic therapy.

cavity *n.* 1. A hole in a tooth produced in response to *caries or non-biological tooth loss such as *abrasion or trauma. 2. A hole in a tooth prepared by mechanical instrumentation prior to the insertion of a restorative material. An **approximal cavity** is located on the *mesial or *distal surface of a tooth. A **compound** or **complex cavity** involves more than one tooth surface. The internal walls and margins of a cavity are defined according to their location. *See also* BLACK'S CLASSIFICATION OF CAVITIES.

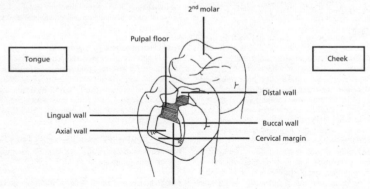

The walls of a mesio-occlusal cavity in a lower left first molar

cavity design The process of preparing a cavity for a restorative material. In a carious tooth it involves first gaining access to and removing the caries. The cavity design should be such as to protect the remaining tooth tissue and optimize the strength of the restoration. The shape and angulation of the surfaces of the cavity will be dictated by the choice of restorative material e.g. amalgam, resin composite, or gold.

cavity liner *n. See* LINING.

cavity, nasal *n. See* NASAL.

cavity, oral *n.* The region bounded anteriorly by the lips and posteriorly by the *soft palate. It contains all the oral structures including the teeth and supporting tissues and the tongue.

cavity varnish *n.* A solution of natural or synthetic resin (e.g. *copal resin) in an organic solvent of acetone, ether, or chloroform (that vaporizes after placement), which can act like a liner; it is used to seal the dentinal tubules and help prevent microleakage. It is placed in a cavity that is due to receive an amalgam restoration after any bases have been placed. Cavity varnish has now largely been replaced by dentine bonding resins as the liner of choice. Cavity varnish is not compatible with resin composite materials because it retards the setting reaction and has a detrimental effect on the bonding properties. Cavity varnish may also be used to protect the external surface of a newly placed *glass ionomer cement restoration from early moisture contamination.

cavosurface angle The angle related to a cavity preparation formed by the junction of the wall of the cavity with the surface of the tooth.

cebocephaly *n.* A rare craniofacial abnormality characterized by a small flattened nose with a single nostril situated below incomplete or underdeveloped closely set eyes.

cell *n.* The basic unit of any living organism that is able to grow and reproduce independently. Each cell consists of a lipid and protein **cell membrane**, which controls the passage of substances into and out of the cell, surrounding aqueous *cytoplasm which contains a nucleus, and various structures (**organelles**) specialized to carry out specific functions.

cell rests of Malassez [L. C. Malassez (1842–1909), French histologist] Epithelial cells in the periodontal ligament derived from *Hertwig's epithelial root sheath. They can proliferate in the presence of inflammation, possibly leading to *cyst formation.

cellulitis *n.* A diffuse, acute infection of the skin and subcutaneous tissues manifesting with pain, *erythema, and swelling of the tissue. There is usually an associated *trismus, inflammation of the cervical lymph nodes, and *pyrexia. Cellulitis usually develops quickly over the course of hours and is a response usually to streptococcal organisms. Cellulitis can spread to the tissue spaces on both sides of the floor of the mouth (*Ludwig's angina). Treatment involves removing the cause of the infection and providing drainage with additional use of *antibiotics, aimed at the causative organism, where appropriate.

The structures within a cell and their function

Structure	Function
Cytoplasm	It holds the structures of the cell in position.
Golgi apparatus	Stores, modifies, and transports proteins produced in the endoplasmic reticulum.
Lysosome	Enables the cell to utilize its nutrients by breaking down large molecules into smaller ones by using hydrolytic enzymes. It also breaks down the cell once it has died.
Mitochondria	Generate energy in the form of *adenosine triphosphate.
Nuclear membrane	Separates the nucleus and nucleolus from the rest of the cell contents.
Nucleolus	Responsible for the cell organelles e.g. ribosomes, lysosomes.
Nucleus	Carries genetic material in the form of chromosomes. It contains the nucleolus.
Ribosome	Interprets cellular information from the nucleus.
Endoplasmic reticulum	Concerned with the production and transport of proteins and lipids within and between cells. The smooth type lacks ribosomes.

cellulose acetate The acetate ester of cellulose used in the manufacture of matrix strips and temporary crown forms.

cellulose foam *n*. Oxidized regenerated absorbable cellulose sponge (which may also be in the form of a ribbon) applied to a wound or wound cavity to provide a matrix to aid *blood clotting (haemostasis). Trade name: **Surgicel**.

CE mark (officially **CE marking)** A visible declaration by the manufacturer (or their representative, importer, etc.) that the product which is marked complies with all the requirements of all the applicable **European Union** (EU) directives. The initials 'CE' do not stand for any specific words.

cement

n. A substance used in dentistry as a *luting material to secure a crown or inlay to a tooth or to act as a protective layer under a restoration. **Black copper cement**, which contains zinc phosphate and copper oxide, is used for restorations in the *primary dentition for its antibacterial effect on carious dentine. **Zinc polycarboxylate cement** is obtained by mixing carboxylic acid liquid with zinc oxide powder and is used as a restoration base for the cementation of cast restorations and orthodontic appliances. **Silicate cement** is a mixture of powdered acid-soluble glasses, made by the fusion of calcium, silicon, and aluminium oxides, added to *phosphoric acid. It has been used for the restoration of anterior teeth because of its aesthetic properties. **Zinc phosphate cement** is formed from an acid-base reaction made by mixing a powder consisting mainly of zinc and magnesium oxides with a liquid containing phosphoric acid, water, and buffering agents. The reaction creates heat (exothermic) and therefore mixing should be carried out on a cool glass slab to prevent a fast setting reaction; it is used for cementing cast restorations and as a base material under permanent restorations. **Zinc silico-phosphate cement** is a combination of silicate and zinc phosphate cement and is less translucent and less soluble than silicate cement but harder than zinc phosphate cement. **Zinc oxide-eugenol (ZOE) cement** consists of a powder containing zinc oxide, modified with rosin to reduce the brittleness, zinc stearate added as a plasticizer and zinc acetate to modify the setting reaction, and a liquid whose main constituent is eugenol, the purified derivative of *oil of cloves with olive oil added to improve plasticity. A small amount of water is essential for the setting reaction. ZOE cement is not as hard as zinc phosphate cement and is used as a sub-lining under permanent restorations or as a cavity temporary dressing material. To improve the strength and reduce the solubility of the cement, materials such as methyl methacrylate or alumina may be added (**reinforced zinc oxide-eugenol cement**); the liquid is a mixture of eugenol and ortho ethoxy benzoic acid (EBA). **Glass ionomer cements (GICs)** contain a polyalkenoic acid, most commonly polyacrylic, polyitaconic, or polymaleic acid, and an ion-leachable glass, usually calcium-alumino-silicate. The acid-base setting reaction takes place in three stages. During the *dissolution phase*, the polyalkenoic acid attacks the outer surface of the glass particles in the presence of moisture causing the release of fluoride, calcium, and aluminium ions. The *gelation reaction* occurs over several minutes, during which period the material becomes firm as the freed divalent calcium ions form ionic bonds with the negatively charged carboxyl ions on the poly-acid chains. The material is shaped and contoured during this stage. The final, *hardening phase* is completed over several days as the trivalent aluminium ions form more effective cross-links between adjacent chains. During the early part of this phase the material must be protected from contamination from oral fluids. The important advantages of glass ionomer cements are that they adhere to enamel, dentine, and base metals and they release *fluoride. Adhesion involves the penetration and embedding of poly-acid chains into the surface of the tooth *hydroxyapatite by displacing phosphate ions. They therefore have a variety of uses as a luting, lining, and a non-stress bearing restorative material in class III and class V *cavities in the *secondary dentition and as a posterior restorative material in the *primary dentition. The glass particle size tends to dictate the function of the material in that restorative glass ionomers contain larger particles than glass ionomers used as luting or lining materials. The adhesive and fluoride releasing properties make the cement useful for the *atraumatic restorative technique. The material is either hand mixed, where all the active ingredients are in a single powder which is mixed with water, or pre-capsulated. **Resin-modified glass ionomer cements (RMGICs, vitremers)** have been developed to overcome the disadvantages of moisture contamination problems, low flexural strength, and working time control problems found with glass ionomer cements. The acid-base setting reaction is similar to glass ionomer cements except that polymerizable groups and *HEMA monomers are additionally present on the poly-acid chains. The *polymerization process is largely an acid-base chemical reaction with initial photo-stabilization by means of an external light source. Resin-modified glass ionomer cements develop their strength more rapidly than GICs because of the resin component; however, this component provides no adhesion to dentine or enamel, and therefore *acid-etching is necessary to achieve bonding. More recently *cyanoacrylate esters have been used as an alternative to methacrylate because of their ability to adhere to both dentine and enamel. RMGICs are used as permanent restorative materials for situations where there is low occlusal stress, such as class III and class V cavities, and as lining materials under *amalgam and *resin composite restorations. Because of the tendency of HEMA to absorb water, RMGICs are unsuitable as luting cements for metal posts in root canals and all ceramic restorations, due to an expansion of about 4% creating excessive stress. *See also* CERMET; RESIN COMPOSITE; COMPOMER; GIOMER.

Further Reading: Cho S., Cheng A. C. A review of glass ionomer restorations in the primary dentition. *J Can Dent Assoc* 1999;65:491–5.

cementation *n.* The process of attaching a cast restoration or appliance to a tooth by the use of a luting agent or cement.

cementicle *n.* A calcified body lying in the periodontal membrane, either free or partially embedded in the *cementum and thought to be derived from degenerated *epithelial cells.

cement line The line of cement visible at the margin of a *crown or *inlay.

cementoblast *n.* A cell that takes part in the formation of *cementum. They are formed from the *dental follicle following the degeneration of *Hertwig's sheath. They form a single layer of cuboidal cells on the surface of the root *dentine.

cementoblastoma *n.* A rare *benign *neoplasm of *cementum. It usually affects patients under the age of 25 years. It is most often associated with the apices of

mandibular first molars and is not found in association with the anterior teeth. It presents radiographically as a well-defined, round radiopaque mass surrounded by a radiolucent rim, and is usually asymptomatic. The lesion obscures the lamina dura (*see* CEMENTOMA). Treatment is by surgical removal of the tooth and associated tumour.

cementoclasia *n.* The destruction of *cement by cementoclasts. It occurs normally as part of primary tooth exfoliation (shedding).

cementoclast *n.* A multinucleated giant cell similar to an osteoclast that destroys cementum.

cementocyte *n.* An inactivated *cementoblast which has become embedded within the *cementum matrix. It has protoplasmic processes which pass through the *canaliculi between the *lacunae.

cemento-enamel (amelo-cemental) junction (CEJ) *n.* The line at which the *enamel of the tooth *crown meets the cementum of the tooth *root. The area above this line constitutes the anatomical crown of the tooth. In about 60% of teeth the cementum overlaps the enamel, in about 30% of teeth the cementum and enamel meet exactly and in about 10% of teeth the cementum and enamel fail to meet, leaving an area of exposed dentine. In health, the *junctional epithelium is attached to the tooth surface in the region of the CEJ.

cementogenesis *n.* The process of cementum formation. *See also* CEMENTOBLAST; CEMENTUM.

cementoid *n.* A thin unmineralized layer present on the surface of developing cementum. Also known as **precementum** and uncalcified cementum.

cementoma *n.* This term is no longer used by the *World Health Organization (WHO) but it denotes an accumulation of cementum-like and bony material in the jaws associated with the *periodontal ligament. Such lesions were also known as cemento-osseous *dysplasias but are now classified as osseous dysplasias.

cementosis *n. See* HYPERCEMENTOSIS.

cementum *n.* A pale yellow calcified tissue providing a protective covering for the root surface to which the fibres of the periodontal membrane are secured. The embedded ends of the collagen periodontal fibres within the cementum form *Sharpey's fibres. Cementum is attached to the root dentine by a glue-like material, the hyaline layer. It is thicker towards the apical region of the root. It consists of approximately 65% inorganic hydroxyapatite, 23% organic collagen, and 12% water. It has no nerves and is insensitive to pain. When cementum first forms from the *dental follicle, it is acellular (**primary cementum**) and covers the root dentine. **Cellular cementum (secondary cementum)** has a structure similar to *bone with *cementocytes embedded in *lacunae which have cytoplasmic processes linking each other via *canaliculi. These processes are directed towards the *periodontal membrane from which they obtain nutrition. Cellular cementum is located mainly around the apical third of the root. Cementum formation (cementogenesis) continues throughout life and is dependent upon the functional needs of the tooth and any tooth movement which may occur, such as during *eruption or orthodontic tooth repositioning. Resorption of cementum can occur in response to excessive occlusal stress or orthodontic loading. Cementum usually slightly overlaps the enamel at the cemento-enamel junction but it can abut without overlap, or there may be a small gap between the two tissues; these variations can all occur on the same tooth. *See also* ANKYLOSIS; CONCRESCENCE; HYPERCEMENTOSIS.

central bearing device A device used to provide a central point of bearing or support between the arches of the maxilla and mandible. It is used to make intraoral or extraoral mandibular tracings. The point at which the stylus makes contact is the **central bearing point**.

central nervous system (CNS) The brain and the spinal cord. It is responsible for the integration of all nervous activities.

centre line relationship The association between the midline of the face and a vertical line drawn between the upper central incisors and the lower central incisors. A discrepancy between the upper and lower **dental centre lines** is measured in millimetres or as a proportion of the lower incisor width (e.g. ¼, ½, ¾, or full tooth). The relationship between the dental centre line and the midline of the face can be co-incident, where the two centre lines line up, or deviated, where there is a displacement either left or right.

centric occlusion *n. See* OCCLUSION.

centric relation The relationship of the mandible to the maxilla, independent of tooth contact, when the mandibular condyles are in their most superior and anterior position, resting on the posterior slopes of the articular eminences with the discs properly interposed. Centric relation can also be described as the position of the mandible relative to the maxilla, with the articular disc in place, when the muscles that support the mandible are in their most relaxed state. *See also* OCCLUSION.

Further Reading: Davies S., Gray R. M. J. Occlusion: what is occlusion? *Br Dent J* 2001;191:235–41.

centrifuge *n.* A device which makes use of the outward force exerted by a revolving body (**centrifugal force**). It is used in dentistry to force molten metal into a *casting.

cephalic index The ratio of the maximum width of the head to its maximum length measured in a horizontal plane multiplied by 100. It was devised by Anders Retzius (1796–1860) for use in anthropology. It is sometimes used for estimating the age of foetuses for legal or obstetric reasons. A cephalic index of 80 or more is called **brachycephalic** (broad skull); a measurement between 75 and 80 is **mesocephalic** (medium skull); below 75 is considered **dolicocephalic** (long skull).

cephalometer *n.* An instrument used for measuring the dimensions of the head.

cephalometric analysis The process of evaluating dental and skeletal relationships usually in lateral view by the use of measurements taken directly from the head or from *cephalometric radiographs and *tracings. Tracings can be made on which specific landmark lines and points are marked. The commonly used **cephalometric points and lines** include the Frankfort plane, maxillary plane, mandibular plane, and the upper, lower, and total *face height.

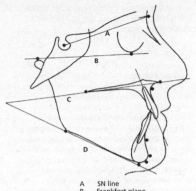

A   SN line
B   Frankfort plane
C   Maxillary plane
D   Mandibular plane

Cephalometric lines

A   Point A
ANS Anterior nasal spine
B   Point B
Gn   Gnathion
Go   Gonion
Me   Menton
Na   Nasion
Or   Orbitale
Pog Pogonion
Po   Porion
PNS Posterior nasal spine
S   Sella

Important cephalometric angles are the SNB, SNA, ANB, **upper incisor to mandibular plane (UiMx)**, **upper incisor to lower incisor (UiLi)**, and the **lower incisor to mandibular plane** (LiMd).

Cephalometric points

Commonly used cephalometric points and reference lines

Reference points and lines	Description
A point (A)	The point of deepest concavity on the anterior surface of the maxilla.
Anterior nasal spine (ANS)	The tip of the anterior process of the maxilla at the lower border of the nasal aperture.
B Point (B)	The point of deepest concavity of the anterior surface of the mandibular symphysis.
Gnathion (Gn)	The most anterior-inferior point on the chin.
Gonion (Go)	The most posterior inferior point on the angle of the mandible.
Menton (Me)	The lowest point on the mandibular symphysis.
Nasion (Na)	The point at which the frontal and nasal bones of the skull meet. It is a soft tissue landmark at the deepest point of the depression at the base of the nose in the midline and a hard tissue landmark at the most anterior point of the fronto-nasal suture.
Orbitale (Or)	The lowest anterior point on the lower margin of the orbit.
Pogonion (Pog)	The most anterior point on the mandibular symphysis (chin) in the midline.
Porion (Po)	The uppermost outermost point on the bony external auditory meatus.
Posterior nasal spine (PNS)	The tip of the projection from the posterior border of the horizontal plate of the palatine bones.
Sella (S)	The midpoint of the *sella turcica.
SN Line	A line connecting the midpoint of the sella turcica with the nasion. It represents the cranial base.
Frankfort plane	The line joining the porion and the orbitale.
Mandibular plane	The line joining the gonion and the menton.
Maxillary plane	The line joining the anterior nasal spine with the posterior nasal spine.
Functional occlusal plane	A line drawn between the cusp tips of the permanent molars and premolars (or primary molars in a mixed dentition).

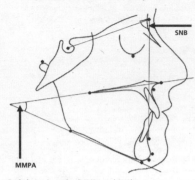

Cephalometric angles (MMPA and SNB)

Measurement	Average
Lower incisor to mandibular plane	93° ± 6° or 120° – MMPA
Inter-incisal angle	135° ± 10°
Lower incisor to APog line	+1 ± 2mm
Lower face height as % of total face height	55 ± 2%

The key features which can be identified are the relative size and position of the mandible and maxilla, and the steepness of the angle between the jaws and the angles of the upper and lower incisors to each other and to the skeletal base. Cephalometric radiographs can be taken at different stages of growth development and tracings of these superimposed on each other to show growth change. If no orthodontic treatment has been carried out then these changes will be due solely to growth.

cephalometric radiograph (lateral cephalogram) A diagnostic extra-oral radiograph characterized by a standardized relationship between x-ray source, subject, and *film position. The generally accepted distance between the centre of the subject and the x-ray source is 5 feet (152.4 cm). The distance between the subject and the film is usually 5 inches (12 cm); it is used to show jaw and cranial relationships.

cephalometry *n.* The study of the growth of the face, jaws, and skull by examination of standardized *radiographs.

cephalostat *n.* A specially adapted x-ray machine used for taking *cephalometric radiographs such that the subject's head and the film position can be accurately located in relationship to the x-ray machine. *See also* LATERAL CEPHALOGRAM.

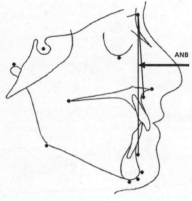

Cephalometric angle (ANB)

Cephalometric norms for Caucasians (Eastman Standard) have been defined.

Cephalometric norms for Caucasians (Eastman Standard)

Measurement	Average
SNA angle	81° ± 3°
SNB angle	78° ± 3°
ANB angle	3° ± 2°
Maxillary/mandibular planes angle (MMPA)	27° ± 4°
Upper incisor to maxillary plane	109° ± 6°

ceramics *n.* The process of shaping and firing inorganic non-metallic minerals at high temperatures. Dental *porcelains are an example of one group of these materials.

cerebellum *n.* The part of the metencephalon consisting of a vermis, flocculonodular lobe, and two hemispheres. It lies in the posterior cranial fossa. It is responsible for the coordination of movement and balance.

cerebral *adj.* Relating to that part of the brain known as the cerebrum. The **cerebral cortex** is the outer layer of the brain consisting of nerve cells and pathways responsible for cognitive function, including reasoning, mood, and perception of stimuli. **Cerebral hypoxia** occurs when there is a deficiency in supply of oxygen to the brain, even though there may be adequate blood flow. If mild it is characterized by symptoms of inattentiveness, poor judgement, and memory loss, but when severe it can lead to loss of consciousness and collapse. **Cerebral palsy** is a non-progressive neuromuscular disorder characterized by varying degrees of impairment. Sufferers have poor oro-motor control, and therefore high-volume chairside aspiration needs to be constant for dental procedures. Intravenous or oral sedation may be necessary because uncontrolled movements can jeopardize safe treatment.

cerebro-spinal fluid (CSF) A clear colourless fluid constantly being produced and resorbed which fills the ventricles of the brain and the central canal of the spinal cord. It has a protective and nutritional function for the central nervous system. An analysis of the contents can be diagnostic of certain pathological conditions.

cerebrovascular accident (CVA) A sudden and sometimes serious reduction in blood supply to the brain (ischaemia) which leads to a *stroke. There are two broad categories of CVA: **ischaemic CVA**, in which an area of brain tissue is completely deprived of blood supply due to a blood vessel blockage (this type is usually caused by a cerebral *thrombosis, *embolism or *atheroma in the arterial blood supply), and **haemorrhagic CVA**, where there is a bleed from a blood vessel supplying the brain (this type is usually caused by a ruptured aneurysm).

cerebrum (telencephalon) *n.* The largest and most developed part of the brain, divided into two hemispheres by the **longitudinal fissure**. Each hemisphere has an outer layer of grey matter (**cerebral cortex**) and an underlying outer white matter containing the **basal ganglia**. The cerebrum is responsible for the initiation and coordination of all voluntary activity and governs the functioning of the lower parts of the nervous system. It interprets sensory impulses such as sight, sound, touch, pressure, temperature, and smell.

Cerec® *n. See* COMPUTER-AIDED DESIGN/COMPUTER-AIDED MANUFACTURE.

cermet *n.* The name, derived from the contraction of the words ceramic and metal,

given to a group of glass ionomer cements to which metals such as silver and gold have been added. The metal particles are incorporated into the glass powder usually by using heat and pressure (sintering). Cermet is *radiopaque and has been advocated as a *core build-up material or as an alternative to *amalgam for *primary dentition restorations. These materials have been largely superseded by the resin modified glass ionomer cements. *See also* CEMENT.

cervical *adj.* Relating to the area at the neck of the tooth which forms the junction between the tooth root and the crown. *See also* TOOTH SURFACES. Cervical caries: *see* CARIES. The **cervical chain** represents a series of *lymph nodes arranged in three (superficial, deep, and posterior) serially linked chains which provide the lymphatic drainage of the face. A **cervical collar** is a leaded device used to protect the *thyroid gland from excessive radiation when taking dental *radiographs. A **cervical enamel projection** is an anatomical feature in which the cement enamel junction projects apically (the *periodontal attachment follows the projection). If the projection is in the area of a *furcation it increases the potential for rapid periodontal destruction in the susceptible individual.

cervical plaque index (CPI) An index to measure the accumulation of plaque at the cervical margins of tooth surfaces. The build-up of plaque is recorded at six cervical sites on each tooth i.e. mesio-buccal, buccal, disto-buccal, disto-lingual, distal, and mesio-lingual on a scale of 0 to 4 (0 = no plaque, 1 = up to 1mm thin plaque, 2 = more than 1mm thin plaque, 3 = up to 1mm thick plaque, 4 = more than 1mm thick plaque).

cetylpyridinium chloride A *quaternary ammonium compound included in some mouthwashes, toothpastes, lozenges, and throat sprays. It is an antiseptic that kills bacteria and other micro-organisms. It is effective in preventing dental plaque (*plaque control) and reducing gingivitis.

chalinoplasty *n.* An obsolete term used to describe the surgical correction of defects of the mouth and lips, especially of the angles of the mouth.

chamestaphyline *adj.* Describing an abnormally low and flattened palatal arch as defined by the palatal index. The palatal arch height may also be described as intermediate (**orthostaphyline**), or deep (**hypsistaphyline**). The palatal arch width can be of moderate width (**mesostaphyline**), having a *palatal index of 80 to 85. A narrow palate with a palatal index of up to 80 is described as **leptostaphyline** and a wide palate as **brachystaphyline** if over 85.

chamfer *n.* The marginal finish of a restoration which produces a bevel between the preparation wall and the cavosurface of the tooth.

chamomilla *n.* Homeopathic chamomile. A remedy which has been advocated for teething.

chart *n.* 1. A record of information relating to a patient's dental or medical history. 2. A diagrammatical representation of the surfaces of the teeth in both upper and lower jaws on which a patient's oral status and planned treatment can be recorded. A **bar chart** is a type of graphic display where *data are displayed in the form of bars that can be arranged vertically or horizontally. A **pie chart** is a circular graphic divided into sectors of a circle used to illustrate frequencies, percentages, or relative magnitudes.

Charters technique *n. See* TOOTHBRUSHING.

charting symbols *n.* Commonly accepted notations used on a clinical *chart or record to graphically represent the oral status and planned treatment of a patient.

Chayes attachment *n. See* PRECISION ATTACHMENT.

Cheatles forceps *n. See* FORCEPS.

check record An interocclusal record designed to allow the re-articulation of dentures (usually complete dentures) in order to facilitate occlusal and articulatory analysis and adjustment.

Chédiac–Higashi syndrome [Alexander Moisés Chédiac, Cuban physician (1903–), and Otokata Higashi, Japanese paediatrician] A rare childhood autosomal recessive immunodeficiency disorder. It is characterized by defective neutrophil function, abnormal skin pigmentation, and a susceptibility to infection which can lead to severe gingivitis, periodontitis, and aphthae. The disease is often fatal in childhood.

cheek *n.* The fleshy prominence either side of the face between the ear and mouth and below the eye. It is covered by skin externally and by

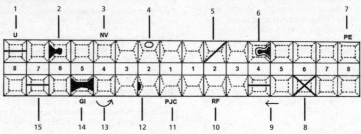

1. Tooth missing, unerupted
2. Disto-occlusal restoration
3. Non-vital tooth
4. Carious lesion
5. Tooth scheduled for extraction
6. Recurrent caries around restoration
7. Tooth partially erupted
8. Tooth recently extracted
9. Tooth drifted mesially
10. Root filling
11. Porcelain jacket crown
12. Restoration on distal surface
13. Tooth rotated
14. MOD gold inlay
15. Tooth missing

Common charting symbols

non-keratinized *mucosa internally except at the occlusal level, where there is a whitish horizontal line (linea alba). The cheek contains the duct of the *parotid gland (*Stensen's duct), exiting at the *parotid papilla and numerous minor salivary glands. Biting of the buccal mucosa (**cheek biting**) may occur as a result of a *malocclusion, alteration of the chewing cycle, or due to parafunction or a parafunctional habit.

cheilalgia *n.* Pain in the lip or lips.

cheilectropion *n.* Eversion of the lip or lips.

cheilion *n.* A *cephalometric point located at the angle (the corner or most lateral point) of the mouth.

cheilitis *n.* Inflammation of the lips which may present as acute, subacute, or chronic. **Atopic cheilitis** is a chronic condition characterized by dry eczametous lesions causing chronic *desquamation. Cheilitis may be caused by the action of excessive sunlight (**actinic cheilitis**). Cosmetic or chemical irritants can result in allergic contact cheilitis (**cheilitis venenata**). Inflammation of the submucosal glands of the lower lip (**cheilitis glandularis**) is characterized by progressive enlargement and eversion of the lower labial mucosa which, under environmental influences, can lead to erosion, ulceration, crusting, and sometimes infection; it can be a potential predisposing factor for actinic cheilitis and squamous cell *carcinoma. *See also* ANGULAR CHEILITIS.

cheilognathoschisis *n.* A developmental anomaly consisting of a *cleft lip and jaw.

cheilognathouranoschisis *n.* A developmental anomaly consisting of a *cleft of the lip, maxillary alveolar ridge, and palate.

cheilophagia *n.* Biting of the lips.

cheiloplasty (labioplasty) *n.* Surgical repair of injury or deformity of the lips (*cleft lip).

cheilorrhaphy *n.* The surgical repair of the lip most commonly for the repair of a developmental *cleft.

cheiloschisis *n. See* CLEFT.

cheilosis *n. See* ANGULAR CHEILITIS.

cheilotomy *n.* An incision in the lip.

chelating agent An organic chemical compound that forms complexes with metal ions. A chelating agent such as *ethylene diamine tetraacetic acid (EDTA) may be placed in a root canal to decalcify the walls and enable the root canal to be more easily enlarged.

cheloid *n. See* KELOID.

Chemclave *n.* The brand name for a chemical sterilizer which uses vaporized *alcohols, ketones, and *formaldehyde, and is steam heated to 127°C (261°F) under a minimum pressure of 20 pounds per square inch. This type of equipment is not appropriate for sterilizing reusable dental instruments as the process is difficult to validate. Reusable dental instruments should be sterilized in a vacuum steam sterilizer following appropriate cleaning and *decontamination. *See also* STERILIZER.

chemical cure *n.* The process of *polymerization of a *resin composite when all the ingredients are mixed. It is achieved without the use of an external light source.

chemoreceptor *n.* A cell or group of cells which respond to a chemical stimulus by initiating an impulse in a sensory *nerve.

chemotaxis *n.* The movement of a cell towards either a higher or lower concentration of a chemical substance.

chemotherapy *n.* The treatment or prevention of disease by the use of chemical substances. The term is generally restricted to the treatment of *malignancy using *cytotoxic drugs but could also be applied to the use of chemicals such as *chlorhexidine in the treatment of *gingivitis. **chemotherapeutic** *adj. See also* PLAQUE CONTROL.

cherubism *n.* An inherited condition, presenting in young children. It causes a bilateral swelling of the *mandible and maxilla, usually enhanced by upward-gazing eyes, *malocclusion, and abnormalities of the teeth. There is replacement of the bone with fibrous tissue containing multinucleate giant cells, resulting in multiple multilocular *radiolucencies.

chewing *n.* The movement of the mandible during *mastication. **Chewing tobacco** (smokeless tobacco) presents in shredded leaf form and is typically placed between the cheek and buccal mucous membrane. It allows nicotine to be absorbed through the mucosa which can lead to nicotine dependence. It is a known *carcinogen and can result in oral cancer, *leukoplakia, and *gingival recession.

chickenpox (varicella) *n.* A highly infectious contagious disease caused by the herpes virus (*varicella-zoster virus). It is characterized by fever followed by itchy vesicular lesions (which are easily broken), starting on the trunk and scalp and spreading to the face and limbs. Oral lesions may affect the oral mucosa, particularly the soft palate and fauces; the vesicles rupture early to produce small ulcers. The disease typically lasts 10 to 14 days but the virus may lie dormant in the sensory ganglia for years. It is reactivated spontaneously or by immuno-suppression and vesicles erupt on the skin following the branches of the sensory nerve affected. If the trigeminal nerve is affected, lesions may arise unilaterally on the skin of the face or affect the oral cavity. This is known as **shingles** (Herpes zoster) and typically lasts 10 to 14 days. Recovery may be complicated by post-herpetic neuralgia. *See* HERPES.

Chievitz's organ [J. H. Chievitz (1850–1901), Danish anatomist] A small structure located within the soft tissue overlying the angle of the mandible. It consists of multilobulated epithelium and has no direct connection with the parotid gland or the oral cavity. Although its function is uncertain, it may act as a mechanoreceptor and be involved in swallowing, mastication, and speech. Awareness of this structure is important to avoid unnecessary surgery. It is also known as the **juxta-oral organ**.

child abuse (battered baby syndrome) The description of a clinical condition in young children, usually under three years of age, who have received **non-accidental injury** or violence on one or more occasions by an adult in a position of trust. Bruising occurs in over 80% of cases, particularly to the head, face, or neck.

Further Reading: Harris J, Sidebotham P, Welbury R, Townsend R, Green M, Goodwin J, Franklin C. 'Child protection and the dental team: an introduction to safeguarding children in dental practice'. Committee of Postgraduate Dental Deans and Directors (COPDEND UK), Sheffield, 2006.

(⊕) SEE WEB LINKS
- The American Academy of Pediatric Dentistry guidelines on child abuse.
- British Society of Paediatric Dentistry advice for the dental professional.
- Child Protection and the Dental Team website.

children's dental health survey A review carried out every ten years since 1973 to provide information on the dental health of children in the United Kingdom and other EU countries. It measures changes in oral health since the last survey and provides information on children's experiences of dental care and treatment and their oral hygiene. *See also* ADULT DENTAL HEALTH SURVEY.

(⊕) SEE WEB LINKS
- The findings of the 2003 Children's Dental Health Survey.

chin *n.* The anterior portion of the mandible formed by the *mental protuberance.

chip syringe *n. See* SYRINGE.

chiropractic *n.* A specialty focusing on the non-surgical diagnosis, treatment, and management of neuromuscular skeletal conditions by means of manipulation of the spine and related structures.

(⊕) SEE WEB LINKS
- The website of the British Chiropractic Association.

chisel *n.* A hand instrument designed for cleaving bone or enamel. It is bevelled on one side only and the shank may be straight or angled. A **bone chisel** is a single-ended instrument with a long handle and a square end which can be struck by a mallet. A **Coupland's chisel**, often referred to as an elevator, has a sharp curved working tip, available in three sizes in line with the long axis of the instrument. It is used to elevate and separate a tooth from its periodontal membrane; it was designed by Douglas Coupland in the early 1930s, initially as a set of 8 or 12 chisels. A **Wedelstaedt chisel**, first described by E. K. Wedelstaedt in 1907, has a blade that is continuous with the shank, has no constricting neck, curves rather than angles into the shank, and is manufactured in varying widths with either a reverse or regular bevel.

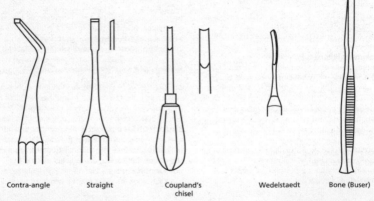

| Contra-angle | Straight | Coupland's chisel | Wedelstaedt | Bone (Buser) |

Types of chisels

chi-square test A statistical test used for estimating how closely an observed distribution matches an expected distribution or for estimating whether two random variables are independent (i.e. whether two categorical variables forming a *contingency table are associated).

chlophenamine (chlopheniramine) *n.* An *antihistamine which helps reverse *histamine-mediated *capillary dilatation. It is used orally, to treat allergies such as hay fever and rhinitis, and intravenously as a second-line treatment in *anaphylaxis. Trade name: **Piriton**.

chloral hydrate *n.* An oral sedative-hypnotic producing *central nervous system (CNS) depression and formerly used as a pre-operative sedative for dental treatment but now no longer recommended. Repeated doses increase the potential for excessive CNS depression. Trade names: **Aquachloral, Novo-chlorhydrate, Somnos**.

chlorhexidine gluconate *n.* A member of the *bisguanide group of antiseptics used as a mouthwash, gel, spray, varnish, or *irrigant. It is effective at inhibiting *plaque regrowth and the development of *gingivitis. It has a bitter taste and can deposit an extrinsic brown stain on the teeth. Trade names: **Corsodyl, Peridex, PerioGard**. It has been incorporated into a biodegradable hydrolysed gelatine chip (trade name: **Periochip**) which biodegrades when placed in a *gingival pocket, releasing the active ingredient over a period of about 10 days.

Further Reading: Kolahi J., Soolari A. Rinsing with chlorhexidine gluconate solution after brushing and flossing teeth: a systematic review of effectiveness. *Quintessence Int* 2006;37(8):605–12.
Cosyn J., Wyn I. A systematic review on the effects of the chlorhexidine chip when used as an adjunct to scaling and root planing in the treatment of chronic periodontitis. *J Periodontol* 2006;77(2):257–64.

chloroma (myeloblastoma) *n.* A solid collection of leukaemic cells occurring outside the bone marrow. It is composed of immature *malignant white blood cells and is a manifestation of acute myeloid *leukaemia. Although rare, chloromas may be seen in any tissue or organ including the skin and gingivae, where they may appear as asymptomatic raised nodules or plaques sometimes with a greenish tinge; they are observed more frequently in children and young adults.

chloropercha *n.* A mixture of chloroform and *gutta-percha. Used as a method of *root canal obturation in which gutta-percha points are partially dissolved in chloroform to form a plastic mass.

chlorpromazine *n.* A phenothiazine antipsychotic drug used in the treatment of severe *anxiety and *schizophrenia. A common side-effect is *xerostomia (dry mouth), which may result in an increased *caries incidence.

choanae *pl. n.* **(posterior nasal apertures)** The paired posterior opening of the nasal cavity into the nasopharynx.

choking *n.* Partial or complete obstruction of the *airway. It can occur in the dental chair due to fluid or a foreign body blocking the entrance to the *trachea. In the conscious patient, coughing normally clears the problem but this may require the aid of back blows, or chest or abdominal thrusts (*Heimlich manoeuvre). In the unconscious patient the airway is first re-established before commencing cardiopulmonary resuscitation (*see* BASIC LIFE SUPPORT).

(((•))) **SEE WEB LINKS**
• Further information on the management of choking from the Resuscitation Council (UK) website.

cholesterol *n.* A lipid-like material (sterol) which is an essential component of cell membranes but is also found in the blood in combination with a number of lipoproteins. It is made mainly in the liver and also consumed in food products. The normal level of cholesterol in the blood is 140–300 mg/100 ml (3.6–7.8 mmol/l). An elevated concentration in the blood (**hypercholesterolemia**), in association with high levels (over 4.4mmol/l) of low-density lipoproteins (LDL) and low levels of high-density lipoproteins (HDL), is associated with an increased risk of *atheroma, atherosclerosis, and cardiovascular disease. **Cholesterol clefts** (formed from the breakdown of cells) in association with foreign body giant cells may be found in chronic apical *granulomas, radicular *cysts, and inflamed dentigerous cysts.

choline salicylate *n.* A non-steroidal anti-inflammatory *analgesic. It inhibits prostaglandin synthesis. It is used in a gel form for topical application for the treatment of discomfort during *teething. Trade name: **Bonjela, Arthropan, Teegel**.

chondro- *n.* A prefix signifying *cartilage.

chondroblast *n.* A cell that originates from a mesenchymal stem cell and produces the matrix of *cartilage. Once the matrix is formed around the chondroblast, the cell is referred to as a **chondrocyte**.

chondroitin sulphate *n.* A mucopolysaccharide that forms an important constituent of *cartilage, *bone, skin, *teeth, and connective tissue.

chondrosarcoma *n.* A malignant *neoplasm of cartilage.

choristoma *n.* A mass of histologically normal tissue occurring in an abnormal location. Cartilaginous choristomas of the oral mucosa are rare, usually occurring on the tongue and less frequently on the soft palate and gingiva. They are normally covered by integral mucosa and can occur at any age.

Christensen's phenomenon
[C. Christensen, Danish dentist and educator] A gap occurring in the natural dentition or between the opposing posterior flat occlusal rims when the mandible is protruded (posterior open bite). It can lead to instability in full dentures unless compensating curves are incorporated into the dentures.

chromium–cobalt alloy *n.* See COBALT–CHROMIUM ALLOY.

chromosome *n.* One of the thread-like structures in the nucleus of a cell which contains genetic material (*see* DEOXYRIBONUCLEIC ACID) in the form of *genes. Chromosomes come in pairs, and a normal human cell contains 46 chromosomes— 22 pairs of autosomes and two sex chromosomes. 23 pairs are of maternal and 23 are of paternal origin.

chronic *adj.* (*n.* **chronicity**) 1. Describing a disease of long duration, usually of gradual onset, such as chronic gingivitis or chronic periodontitis. *Compare* ACUTE. 2. Describing a type of inflammation characterized by the presence of macrophages, lymphocytes, and plasma cells.

chronological hypoplasia *n.* See HYPOPLASIA.

chuck *n.* 1. Part of a turbine handpiece which retains a friction grip *bur. 2. An adjustable tool forming part of a lathe used to hold rotary instruments.

cicatrization *n.* The conversion of granulation tissue to scar tissue during the process of wound healing.

ciclosporin (cyclosporin, cyclosporine) *n.* An immunosuppressant drug used to treat, or prevent the rejection of, transplanted organs or tissue. As a side-effect it can cause gingival *hyperplasia similar in clinical appearance to that produced by *phenytoin-associated gingival

enlargement. It can be used as a mouthwash for the treatment of resistant oral ulceration. 📷

cigarette smoking *See* SMOKING.

ciliated *n.* Possessing hair-like processes, large numbers of which are found on columnar epithelial cells lining parts of the upper respiratory tract.

cingulum *n.* 1. A small protuberance in the cervical third of the lingual or palatal aspect of the crown of an incisor or canine tooth. A depression is usually created coronally to the cingulum, known as the **cingulum pit**. 2. A group of association fibres of white matter found in the cingulated gyrus of the cerebrum.

circle of Willis [T. Willis (1621–75), English anatomist] A circle of arteries linking the internal carotid arteries to the vertebrobasilar system lying around the sella turcica on the inferior surface of the brain.

circulatory system *See* CARDIOVASCULAR SYSTEM.

circumferential matrix band *See* MATRIX BAND.

circumferential probing *See* PROBING, CIRCUMFERENTIAL.

circumferential wiring A method of jaw fixation following fracture of the mandible. Stainless steel wire is passed around the lower border of the mandible from within the mouth, with the ends exiting into the oral cavity; the ends are then tied over a splint or existing denture.

circumvallate papilla (vallate) One of a variable number (usually 8–14) of mushroom-shaped projections on the dorsum of the *tongue, forming a row anterior to and parallel with the *sulcus terminalis. They are approximately 1–2mm in diameter and are surrounded by a trough containing *taste buds and serous glands (Von *Ebner's glands). They are innervated by the glossopharyngeal nerve.

cirrhosis *n.* A chronic degenerative disease of the liver in which the normal cells are replaced by scar tissue and fat, impairing its function. It can be caused by excessive alcohol (*alcoholism), viral infections such as *hepatitis, or an obstruction of bile flow.

citric acid A colourless crystalline organic acid found naturally in citrus fruits. It is also added to canned foods and some carbonated drinks to improve the flavour by increasing the acidity. This can result in erosion of the teeth if there is contact over a frequent or prolonged period of time. *See also* STEPHAN'S CURVE. Citric acid has also been used at the time of surgery to 'condition' periodontally involved root surfaces in order to expose connective tissue in the cementum and promote tissue healing and re-attachment.

Civatte body [A. Civatte (1877–1956), French dermatologist] *n.* A pink globular mass formed from degenerating epithelial cells, often found in *lichen planus and lichenoid reactions.

clamp *n.* 1. A surgical device used to achieve compression. 2. A device used to retain *dental (rubber) dam (**dental dam clamp**) around the neck of a tooth to obtain moisture isolation. Clamps are manufactured in a variety of shapes with jaws that correspond to the anatomical contour of the tooth. They may also be wingless or winged for location on the dental dam during placement.

| Butterfly | Wingless premolar | Winged premolar |

Dental dam clamps

Clapton's line [E. Clapton (1830–1909), English physician] A greenish discoloration of the marginal gingivae caused by chronic copper poisoning.

clasp *n.* Any hook or band used to attach a removable *prosthetic or *orthodontic appliance to a natural tooth. **Orthodontic clasps** are used to retain removable appliances. **Ball-ended clasps** engage the interproximal undercut but give minimal retention and may prise the teeth apart. A **Plint clasp** engages the undercut area under the tube assembly on a molar band.

A **Southend clasp** is usually made from 0.7mm stainless steel wire and utilizes the undercut beneath the contact area between two incisors. Clasps for prosthetic appliances are usually made of metal but can be made of a hard flexible resin. **Cast metal clasps** made of *cobalt–chromium alloy are stiff, easily distorted, and liable to fracture, but can be cast as an integral part of the denture framework. **Wrought-metal clasps** are usually made of *stainless steel but *gold clasps are more flexible, easy to adjust but prone to distortion. Clasps provide direct retention by engaging the undercut portion of a tooth. A **reciprocal clasp arm** is usually placed occlusal to the height of contour of the tooth so as to reciprocate any force produced by an opposing clasp arm on the same tooth. Clasps are broadly described by their shape or their position; they may approach the undercut area from an occlusal direction (**occlusally approaching**), such as the **G, E, back action and ring clasps**, or they may approach from the gingivae (**gingivally approaching**), such as the **T or L Roach clasps** [F. E. Roach (1868–1960), American dentist]. A **ring (circumferential) clasp** encircles the tooth by more than 180° and engages the undercut area on the crown of the tooth. *See also* CRIB.

| G-type | E-type | Ring-type |

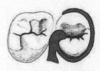

| Back action | L roach | T roach |

Types of clasp

Classification of conditions of the periodontium

Gingival disease		Periodontal disease
Dental plaque associated	Non-plaque induced	
Plaque-related only	Specific bacterial origin	Chronic periodontitis
Modified by systemic factors	Viral origin	Manifestation of systemic condition
Modified by medications	Fungal origin	Necrotizing periodontal disease
Modified by malnutrition	Genetic origin	Abscesses of the periodontium
	Manifestations of systemic conditions	Periodontal-endodontic lesions
	Traumatic lesions	Developmental or acquired conditions
	Foreign body reactions	
	Not otherwise specified	

Armitage G., Development of a classification system for periodontal diseases and conditions. International Workshop for a Classification of Periodontal Diseases and Conditions. *Annals of Periodontology* 1999; 4:1:1–6.

classification of conditions of the periodontium A means of categorizing the disease processes involving the periodontal tissues. Classification systems are used for most diseases and help clinicians to design appropriate therapeutic strategies based on evidence from appropriately conducted clinical trials. Classification provides the local and international healthcare community with a means of communication. A number of periodontal classification schemes have been proposed, modified, and updated as knowledge of the pathobiology of periodontal disease has improved; they may be grouped according to whether there is either periodontal or only gingival involvement.

classified worker A radiation worker who is likely to receive more than 6mSv of radiation per year while carrying out their work. It is highly unlikely that any dental related workers would be classified workers. Classified workers require compulsory personal monitoring and annual health checks.

claudication *n.* Cramp-like pains in the muscles. **Jaw claudication** is characterized by pain in the jaw or ear while chewing; it is caused by a deficiency in arterial blood supply, most commonly caused by temporal *arteritis.

cleft *n.* A longitudinal fissure. **Cleft lip (cheiloschisis, hare lip)** is a cleft deformity of the upper lip which may be unilateral or bilateral. Unilateral clefts occur most commonly on the left side. It results from the failure of fusion of the embryonic maxillary and medial nasal processes around the fifth to sixth week of intrauterine life. A **cleft palate** occurs where there is failure in the fusion of the *palatal shelves.

The cause of both conditions is multifactorial and can include environmental factors that affect the foetus, a genetic disposition, and drugs such as *vitamin A and *heroin (*cocaine). In some cases a cleft may occur as part of a syndrome, such as a small *mandible, and in others it may occur on its own. Cleft lip/palate is one of the most common *congenital abnormalities,

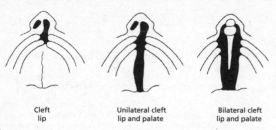

Cleft lip   Unilateral cleft lip and palate   Bilateral cleft lip and palate

Cleft lip and palate

occurring in about 1:700 live births in the UK. Early diagnosis can now more readily be achieved using ultrasonic scanning. Treatment is surgical and the use of intra-oral plates in babies to minimize the extent of surgical intervention is controversial. A **gingival cleft** is a vertical fissure in the gingiva. A **Stillman's cleft** [P. R. Stillman (1871–1945), American periodontologist] is a narrow slit-like or triangular-shaped fissure of the gingival tissue extending from the gingival margin. It may be associated with trauma but is not necessarily diagnostic of occlusal trauma; it can often progress to more extensive gingival recession: the cleft may be associated with a bony *dehiscence. A **transverse cleft** is an area of destruction caused by bacterial action in carious dentine which lies at right angles to the dentinal tubules.

cleft classification A number of classification systems have been defined. The **Kernahan 'striped Y' classification**, first described by D. A. Kernahan in 1971, uses the symbolic letter Y in which the upper arms of the Y represent the primary palate and the base represents the secondary palate, of which the most anterior segment represents the lip; the affected segments are darkened to give a visual representation of the type and extent of the cleft. The **Veau classification**, first described by V. Veau in 1931, classified clefts into four categories: Veau Class I is an isolated soft palate cleft, Class II is a hard/soft cleft palate, Class III is a unilateral cleft lip and palate, and Class IV is a bilateral cleft of the lip and palate.

cleidocranial dysplasia (cleidocranial dysostosis) *n.* A rare congenital disorder of bone characterized by abnormalities of the clavicles, skull, and dentition. Delayed eruption of the permanent dentition may also be a feature.

Further Reading: Nayar S., Bishop K. Cleidocranial dysplasia – a late diagnosis. *Dent Update* 2006;33(4):221–2, 225–6.

clenching *n.* The pressing and clamping of the jaws and teeth together. It may be frequently associated with acute nervous tension or physical effort.

cleoid *adj.* Shaped like a pointed spade or claw. *See also* CARVER.

climacteric *n.* The period of hormonal change that precedes the menopause, marked by a decreased production of oestrogen and progesterone, and declining sexual activity and fertility in men.

clindamycin *n.* A lincosamide antibiotic used to treat or prevent serious bacterial infections such as bacterial *endocarditis. It is effective against Gram-positive and Gram-negative

bacteria and has excellent bone penetration. Its use in treating dento-alveolar infections is increasing. Side-effects include nausea, vomiting, and diarrhoea. The risk of pseudomembranous colitis is no higher for clindamycin than amoxicillin but should be stopped if signs of pseudomembranous colitis develop. Trade names: **Dalacin, Cleocin C**.

clinical attachment level (CAL) The distance from the cemento-enamel junction to the junctional epithelium as measured with a periodontal probe. A fabricated *stent can also be used for sequential records of CAL, especially in research studies.

clinical audit The systematic analysis by any member of the dental team of an area of clinical dental healthcare to ensure that best practice is being carried out. It is usually described as a cyclic or spiral process in which an area for audit is identified, measured against a professionally recognized standard, and improvements introduced if the recognized standard is not being met; the audit topic is then measured again against the original standard, or a new standard if the original one is no longer considered acceptable.

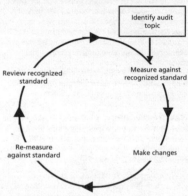

Clinical audit cycle

Further Reading: Miller A. G., Dowler F. Making the most of audit. *Dent Update* 2005;32:47–54.

clinical dental technician *See* DENTAL TECHNICIAN.

clinical effectiveness *See* EFFECTIVENESS.

clinical governance A framework through which organizations, such as the UK **National Health Service** (NHS), are accountable for continuously improving the quality of their services and safeguarding high standards by creating an environment in which excellence in clinical care will flourish.

Further Reading: Maidment Y. G. Clinical governance. What is it and how can it be delivered in dental practices? *Primary Dental Care* 2004;11(2):57–61.

clinical record A paper-based or electronic form that contains the medical or dental history of a patient including any radiographic or image data.

clinical root That part of the tooth attached by the *periodontal ligament to the alveolar bone and not exposed to the oral cavity.

clinical trial A research study designed to provide extensive data that will allow for statistically valid evaluation of treatment or interventions on a group of individuals. The study compares outcomes in the group of participants receiving the test material or treatment with a comparable group (control group) receiving either the standard treatment or a *placebo. *See also* BLINDING.

clinical waste Contaminated and non-contaminated refuse material produced during any clinical dental activity. Disposal of clinical waste is subject to strictly regulated procedures. **Special or hazardous waste** includes mercury, dental amalgam, cytotoxic or *cytostatic prescription medicines, x-ray developer, and fixer solutions and in the UK is controlled by the *Hazardous Waste Regulations (2005).

clonus *n.* A series of muscular contractions in response to a stretch stimulus.

closed bite *n. See* BITE.

closed reduction A process by which jaw bone fragments are manipulated into their normal position without surgically incising the mucosa or skin. The fractured bones are stabilized using rods and pins.

close support dentistry A teamwork approach to the process of undertaking clinical practice, using chairside assistance to improve efficiency and quality of care. Also known as **four-handed dentistry**. The operator and dental nurse are both seated with the patient in a supine position; the treatment area is designed so that all necessary instruments and materials are easily accessible to the seated team. The operator's seated position is such that the back is vertical, the top of the thighs slope at 15° to the floor, and the patient's mouth is at the operator's focal distance. The operator's location is usually between 10 and 11 o'clock relative to the patient's head; the dental nurse's position is at between 2 and 3 o'clock, within easy reach of all the required instruments

and equipment. A method of *instrument transfer between the operator and dental nurse is used to improve safety and efficiency. 📷

Clostridium *n.* A genus of Gram-positive, *obligate anaerobic, spore-forming, rod-shaped *bacteria that includes some important pathogens as well as common free-living species. Four species are responsible for disease in humans including *C. perfringes*, which causes gas gangrene; *C. botulinum*, which produces botulinum toxin, a powerful neurotoxin responsible for the symptoms of botulism. An extremely dilute form of botulinum toxin is used to treat facial muscle spasm; *C. tetani*, which produces tetanus toxin, a powerful neurotoxin responsible for the symptoms of tetanus or lockjaw; and *C. difficile*, the most significant cause of pseudomembranous colitis, a severe infection of the colon that can develop after the normal intestinal microbial flora is eradicated following antibiotic treatment. *C. difficile* pseudomembranous colitis frequently occurs in hospitalized patients and can be treated with metronidazole.

clot *n. See* COAGULATION.

clotting factors *See* COAGULATION.

clotting time *See* COAGULATION.

coagulation *n.* The process of converting a liquid into a jelly-like mass. *See also* BLOOD. **Coagulation factors** are a group of complex substances found in blood plasma which are capable of converting blood from a liquid to a solid state. They are normally ascribed roman numerals from I to XIII as well as names. The absence of one or more of these factors can result in a failure of blood coagulation. *See also* FACTOR VIII; FACTOR IX; FACTOR XI; FACTOR XII; HAEMOPHILIA. The **coagulation time (clotting time)** is the time required for blood to change from a liquid to a solid form, normally 2–8 minutes.

(⊕) SEE WEB LINKS

• The medical biochemistry page of Indiana University School of Medicine, which provides a detailed description of blood coagulation.

cobalt–chromium alloy A very hard corrosion-resistant metal alloy of approximately 70% cobalt and 30% chromium, used primarily in the construction of metal castings for removable *prostheses (*dentures). The fusion temperature is high (1400°–1500°C) and casting is generally done with a high-frequency induction furnace, using phosphate or silicate-bonded *investment material.

cocaine *n.* A crystalloid alkaloid derived from the leaves of the coca plant or prepared synthetically. Formerly used as a dental local *analgesic but because of its unpredictability and addictive properties it has been replaced by safer synthetic alternatives. It is still used topically as an anaesthetic in ear, nose, and throat surgery. It is both a central nervous system stimulant and an appetite suppressant. It leads to feelings of euphoria and increased energy levels. The vasoconstrictive activity of cocaine can have a potentially lethal effect when recently taken, prior to using epinephrine impregnated retraction cord or receiving a local analgesic containing *epinephrine due to the increased risk of *hypertension. The vasoconstrictive effect can result in local *ischaemia in chronic users, which in turn can lead to oronasal perforations (perforation of the nasal septum and hard palate) and severe alveolar bone loss. An additional side-effect of chronic use is *xerostomia, giving rise to an increased risk of *caries. Cocaine users may present with erosion of the buccal tooth surfaces, due to the abrasive effect of applying the drug using a digital rubbing action. Intravenous cocaine users have an increased likelihood of having *hepatitis or *HIV infection. *See also* DRUG.

Further Reading: Brand H. S., Gonggrijp S., Blanksma C. J. Cocaine and oral health. *Br Dent J* 2008;204:365–9.

((⊕)) SEE WEB LINKS
• Information on the health hazards of cocaine.

coccus *n.* (*pl.* **cocci**) Any bacterium which is spherical in shape. They may be arranged in pairs (*diplococci), chains (*streptococci), or clusters (*staphylococci).

Cochrane, Archibald Leman (Archie) (1908–1988) He was born in Galashiels, Scotland and obtained his medical degree in 1938. During World War II he worked as a medical officer and became a prisoner of war in 1941. In 1948 he joined the Medical Research Council's Pneumoconiosis Research Unit in South Wales and became Director in 1960. Here he undertook studies in dust exposure in the coal mines and the associated disability it caused. In 1960 he was appointed Professor of Tuberculosis and Diseases of the Chest at the Welsh National School of Medicine and in 1969 received a CBE for services to medicine. In 1972 he became the first president of the Faculty of Community Medicine (subsequently the Faculty of Public Health) and in 1973 received an honorary doctorate from the University of York. Archie Cochrane is best known for his enthusiastic advocacy of *randomized controlled trials and the importance of these in determining effective health care interventions. His ideas eventually led to the development of the **Cochrane Library database**

of systematic reviews, the establishment of the first UK **Cochrane Centre** in Oxford in 1992 and the founding of the international *Cochrane Collaboration in 1993.

Cochrane collaboration An international organization of researchers, practitioners, and consumers that aims to help people make well-informed decisions about healthcare issues by preparing, maintaining, and promoting the accessibility of systematic reviews of healthcare interventions. The reviews are published in the Cochrane database of systematic reviews, one of the components of the Cochrane Library.

((⊕)) SEE WEB LINKS
• The Cochrane Library database.

codeine *n.* A crystalline alkaloid derived from morphine and used as an *analgesic. It is one of the few opioids that is effective when taken by mouth and is useful in the management of mild to moderate pain. It acts centrally on the opioid receptors in the central nervous system and has approximately 8% of the potency of *morphine. It is often used in combined analgesics with *paracetamol or *aspirin. It is also effective at relieving coughing (antitussive) and is therefore found in many cough medicines. Side-effects include nausea, vomiting, constipation, dizziness, and drowsiness.

coeliac disease An inflammatory bowel disease associated with sensitivity to gluten found in wheat and other grains. Oral lesions include *aphthous ulceration.

coenzyme *n.* An organic non-protein substance that combines with an enzyme to promote the enzyme's activity. People with periodontal disease have been shown to have low levels of **coenzyme Q10** (CoQ10). However, the use of CoQ10 supplements to aid tissue repair requires further research.

Further Reading: Watts T. L. P. Coenzyme Q10 and periodontal treatment: is there any beneficial effect? *Br Dent J* 1995;178:209–13.

Coe-Pak® *n. See* DRESSING.

coffer dam *See* DENTAL DAM.

Coffin spring *See* SPRING.

cohere *v.* To stick together, unite, or form a solid mass. Pieces of *gold foil cohere when malleted together (*cold welding).

cohesion *n.* The intermolecular force by which the particles of a body are united throughout the mass, whether like or unlike.

cohesive gold foil *See* FOIL.

cohort study (longitudinal study) An observational study of a group of people either by studying existing data (**retrospective cohort**) or by examining data for a defined period of time or until a specific event occurs (**prospective cohort**).

col *n*. A valley-like depression which connects the *gingival papillae situated in the *interproximal space between two teeth. It lies below, and conforms to the shape of, the interproximal contact. It is covered by non-keratinized *epithelium. The col is considered an important site for the initiation of chronic periodontitis.

cold curing resin *n. See* RESIN.

cold sore *n. See* HERPES.

cold welding The property of welding two materials together under high pressure or vacuum without the addition of heat. It is exhibited when two pieces of uncontaminated *gold foil are malleted together at room temperature.

collagen *n.* (*adj.* **collagenous**) An insoluble protein that is the primary constituent of *connective tissue, cartilage, ligaments, skin, and *bone. **Collagen fibres** are relatively inelastic but have a high tensile strength.

collagenase *n*. An *enzyme that breaks down *collagen. When it occurs in the *dermis it results in ageing of the *skin. Collagenase is produced by bacteria associated with aggressive *periodontitis.

collet *n*. 1. A collar such as that part of a prosthesis which acts as a collar round the neck of a tooth. 2. A cone-shaped *chuck used for holding cylindrical items in a lathe.

collimation *n*. The elimination of divergent x-rays by using a metal tube, cone, or diaphragm (**collimator**) to produce a narrow beam directed specifically at the radiograph. Collimation gives the final shape and size of the x-ray beam. Legally in the UK the beam must be no more than 6cm in diameter.

colloid *n*. A suspension of very fine particles in a dispersion medium (e.g. *alginate hydrocolloid impression material).

collutorium (collutory) *n*. A mouthwash or gargle.

colophony (rosin) *n*. A substance distilled from gum rosin consisting mainly of abietic acid added to many dental materials such as periodontal dressings, impression materials,

cements, adhesives, and varnishes to improve the adhesive properties. It is a contact sensitizer which may initiate a contact dermatitis or stomatitis.

Further Reading: Sharma P. R. Allergic contact stomatitis from colophony. *Dent Update* 2006;33(7):440–42.

Colorado stain The name given to the white, yellow, and brown flecks of fluoride tooth mottling (*fluorosis) when first identified in residents of Colorado Springs, USA.

colour coding *See* FILE.

columella *n*. The central, lower portion of the nasal septum which divides the nostrils into right and left.

coma *n*. A state of profound unconsciousness in which an individual is incapable of sensing or responding to external stimuli and internal needs.

comforter *n*. A device used for an infant to suck or bite on as an artificial substitute for the mother's breast nipple. Dipping comforters in sugar significantly increases the risk of caries, especially at bedtime, because the secretion of salivary buffers decreases during sleep.

command cure (command set) A method of curing resin-based materials by means of a light source under the control of the operator.

commensal *n*. A micro-organism living on or in the body that is not pathogenic and may confer beneficial effects on the host. Commensal micro-organisms can cause infections in immunocompromised individuals.

Commission for Health Improvement (CHI) *See* HEALTHCARE COMMISSION.

Committee on Medical Aspects of Food and Nutrition Policy (COMA) A food standards advisory committee which was disbanded in March 2000 and replaced by the **Scientific Advisory Committee on Nutrition (SACN)** to advise the UK health departments and the Food Standards Agency on matters relating to food, diet, and health.

communicable disease Any disease that can be transferred from one individual to another by direct or indirect contact. Also known as **contagious disease**.

Community Dental Service (CDS) A salaried dental service funded within the UK *National Health Service which provides dental care for patients who have difficulty obtaining treatment in the *General Dental Service and who require treatment on referral which is not available in the General Dental Service.

Community Periodontal Index of Treatment Needs (CPITN) *n.* A screening method used to establish periodontal treatment priorities for children or adults in a group. *See also* BASIC PERIODONTAL EXAMINATION.

compactor *n.* 1. A condensing instrument used to aid the process of joining or packing a material e.g. gold *foil restorations. 2. A rotary instrument used to condense a *gutta-percha cone or introduce *calcium hydroxide into a root canal. The **McSpadden compactor®**, introduced by John McSpadden in 1978, has the design of an inverted Hedstrom *file, that is, with the blades turned towards the tip instead of towards the shaft; it softens the gutta-percha, forcing it ahead of and lateral to the compactor shaft.

comparative need *See* NEED.

compensating curve The curvature of the occlusal plane of dentures, created to permit balanced *occlusion, to compensate for the paths of the mandibular condyles as the mandible moves from centric to eccentric positions. *See also* CURVE OF SPEE.

compensating extraction *n.* The extraction of the same tooth on the same side in the opposing arch in order to prevent the development of a malocclusion.

competent lips *See* LIP.

complement *n.* A complex system of at least 20 serum *proteins, present in normal serum, which interact with one another to support the *antigen–antibody reaction by *lysis and *phagocytosis of invading organisms.

complementary medicine Various forms of medicine that are considered as complementary to conventional medicine. These include *acupuncture, *osteopathy, *homeopathy, *aromatherapy, and reflexology. Some of these forms of treatment are used in dentistry but there is limited provision for them within the confines of the National Health Service.

complete denture *See* DENTURE.

compliance *n.* The extent to which a patient follows the recommendations of a healthcare professional with respect to advice, medication, or other treatment.

compomer *n.* A poly-acid modified *resin composite which has an ion-leachable glass filler and *monomers which will polymerize to create a matrix onto which some acidic side chains are grafted. They may be used as an alternative to resin composites for the restoration of the *primary dentition since they have the advantage of *fluoride release. They require an *adhesive agent to create a retentive micromechanical bond to tooth structure.

composite *n. See* RESIN COMPOSITE.

compound *n. See* IMPRESSION COMPOUND.

computer-aided design/computer-aided manufacture (CAD/CAM) The process of creating product designs using computer software and using computers to program these designs into the equipment that will actually manufacture the products. CAD/CAM is used in dentistry to construct inlays, veneers, bridges, implants, and core structures or *copings from blocks of metal, ceramic, or resin-based material. It enables materials to be used, such as aluminium oxide and zirconium oxide, which would otherwise be impossible to manipulate using conventional techniques. The restorations are milled from an image of the prepared tooth or teeth gained from an optical or mechanical scanner which is then stored electronically. This technique frequently eliminates the need for taking preliminary impressions. The CAD/CAM milling device prepares the restoration by milling the block of material to fit the previously stored image of the preparation; the occlusal morphology may be ground out from a preselected pattern. Milling may be undertaken either as a wet or a dry process and using a device with 3, 4, or 5 axes of movement. The restorations can be cemented during the same visit in which they are prepared. Trade name: **Cerec®**. CAD/CAM also has applications in oral surgery with the construction of customized surgical templates that allow for precision implant placement, and the potential for less extensive surgery.

Further Reading: Lee M., Yau H. T. CAD/CAM use in the dental laboratory. *Dent Today* 2006;25(9):88, 90, 92–3.
Palin W., Burke F. J. Trends in indirect dentistry: 8. CAD/CAM technology. *Dent Update.* 2005;32(10):566–72.
Beuer F., Schweiger J., Edelhoff D. Digital dentistry: an overview of recent developments for CAD/CAM generated restorations. *Br Dent J* 2008;204:505–11.

computer-aided learning (CAL) Computerized programs used to develop interactive teaching, learning, and assessment in locations potentially distant from, and without direct contact with, the teacher.

Further Reading: Rosenberg H., Grad H. A., Matear D. W. The effectiveness of computer-aided, self-instructional programs in dental education: a systematic review of the literature. *J Dent Educ* 2003;67(5):524–32.

computerized tomography (CT) A diagnostic imaging procedure that uses a combination of *x-rays and computerized technology (formerly known as computed axial tomography or CAT scans). Horizontal and vertical images or slices are built up to create a three-dimensional image. A CT scan image can distinguish between different body tissues. CT delivers a high dose of *radiation to patients. A **cone-beam computerized tomography** (CBCT) scanner uses a cone-shaped x-ray beam rather than a conventional linear fan beam to provide images of the bony structures of the skull. CBCT provides an undistorted dimensional view of the jaws, and is faster (10–40 secs.) and provides stronger indication of bone quality than plain-film CT. CBCT also allows the creation in real time of images in the axial plane and two dimensional (2D) images in the coronal, sagittal, oblique, or curved image planes (multi-planar reformation). Dental indications for CBCT include the evaluation of the jaws prior to implant placement, the evaluation of bone pathology, the assessment of relevant structures prior to orthodontic treatment, and the fabrication of a 3D biomodel of the face and jaws.

Further Reading: Macleod I., Heath N. Cone-beam computed tomography (CBCT) in dental practice. *Dent Update* 2008;35:590–98.

concha (turbine bone) *n.* (*pl.* **conchae**) One of the bony structures within the nasal cavity. There are four named concha: the highest nasal concha, and the superior, middle, and inferior conchae.

concrescence *n.* The fusion of the roots of two teeth united by *cementum.

concretion *n.* A hard or solidified mass in or on tissues or organs, such as pulp stones, salivary calculi, and calculus.

concussion *n.* 1. A change in mental status caused by trauma. It is accompanied by confusion, loss of memory, and sometimes, loss of consciousness. 2. Injury to the supporting tissues of a tooth without displacement.

condensation *n.* 1. The act of compacting a restorative material such as *amalgam into a cavity. 2. The process by which water vapour changes to a liquid.

condensation curing *n. See* POLYMERIZATION.

condenser (plugger) *n.* A hand instrument with a flat serrated tip or face used for compressing *amalgam (amalgam condenser) or *gold foil into a tooth cavity. The shape of the face may vary according to the shape of the cavity and is usually round, oval, or rectangular (**box condenser/plugger**). A **mechanical condenser** (automatic mallet) provides a controlled blow produced by hand, dental engine, or compressed air. A **Hollenback condenser** [G. M. Hollenback (1886–1973), American dentist] is a pneumatic device which provides a controlled condensation pressure of variable intensity up to 300 strokes per minute.

condensing osteitis *n. See* OSTEITIS.

conditioner *n.* A substance added to *dentine to remove the *smear layer and debris from a prepared cavity creating an improved bonding surface. A commonly used dentine conditioner is 10% *polyacrylic acid.

condylar guidance 1. The functional movements of the mandible as determined by the morphology of the mandibular condyles; it depends on the steepness of the articular eminence. 2. The mechanical device on an articulator designed to produce guidance in articulator movement, simulating that produced by the paths of the condyles in the temporomandibular joints.

condylar hyperplasia A persistent or accelerated growth of the mandibular condyle after the period when growth should be slowing or have ceased. It is of unknown aetiology and is characterized by facial asymmetry and often by a crossbite malocclusion and posterior open *bite: there may also be a *prognathic facial appearance with a shift of the midpoint of the chin to the unaffected side. Treatment can include condylectomy, *condyloplasty, and orthodontic therapy.

condylar process *n. See* MANDIBLE.

condyle *n. See* MANDIBLE.

condylion *n.* The *craniometric point at the tip of the mandibular condyle.

condyloma acuminatum *n.* A venereal *wart which may occur in the oral cavity. They present as pink soft papillary lesions.

condyloplasty *n.* A surgical procedure to alter the shape of the mandibular condyle.

cone-beam computerized tomography A technique that enables three-dimensional reconstruction, but using a cone beam to decrease the dose to the patient when compared to conventional *computerized tomography.

confidence interval An estimated range of values with a predicted high probability of covering the true population value. The 95% (p-value = 0.05) and 99% (p-value = 0.01) confidence intervals are the most commonly used. These mean the interval which includes the true value in 95% and 99% of cases, respectively.

confidentiality *n.* The non-disclosure of information, particularly related to the patient, except to another authorized person. It is seen as the patient's right and is enshrined in Article 8 of the European Convention on Human Rights. Guidance for dental professionals is provided by the registration authorities.

confluent *adj.* (*n.* **confluence**) Describing a merging or meeting together.

confounding factor A factor or variable which is the common cause of two events that may falsely appear to be in a causal relationship. It is a variable that is not the one in which the researcher is interested, but which may affect the results of the trial. For example, if people in the experimental group of a controlled trial are older than those in the control group, it will be difficult to establish whether a higher risk of death in one group is due to the intervention or the difference in ages: age is then said to be a confounding factor or a confounding variable.

congenital *adj.* Describing a condition existing at or dating from birth; acquired during development in the uterus and not through heredity.

coning off (cone-cut) An error in taking a radiograph where the film is incorrectly aligned with the x-ray beam. It is characterized by a blank area with a curved margin on the processed film.

connation *n.* Two teeth united together. More commonly referred to as *gemination or *fusion. It is caused by a developmental anomaly of the dental lamina. It occurs more frequently in the primary dentition (around 0.4–0.9%) than the permanent dentition (around 0.2%).

connective tissue The supporting framework of tissue derived from the mesoderm and consisting of amorphous ground substance, collagen, elastic fibres, and other cells and structures, depending on the degree of specialization. *Vitamin C is essential in the maintenance of healthy connective tissue.

connector *n.* That part of a partial denture or *precision attachment that links two major components. It can also contribute to support and retention. Connectors for upper partial dentures include anterior, middle, or posterior palatal *bars, *plates, horseshoes, or rings. Connectors

for lower partial dentures include lingual or sublingual bars or lingual plates.

conscious sedation *n.* *See* SEDATION.

consent *n.* Agreement that may be expressed or implied either verbally or in writing. Acquiescence does not necessarily constitute consent. Consent cannot be considered to have been agreed to if it is given by a person who by reason of age, mental condition, intoxication, or drug use, is unable to make a reasonable judgement as to the nature or harmfulness of the action or treatment, or if consent is induced by force, duress, or deception. Competent adult patients have a fundamental right to give or to withhold consent to treatment. For consent to be valid, the patient must have enough information to make a decision (**informed consent**).

(⊕) SEE WEB LINKS

• The General Dental Council (UK) document that outlines the principles of patient consent.

consultant *n.* A fully trained specialist in a branch of medicine or dentistry.

consultation *n.* 1. A meeting between the patient, a dentist, and possibly other interested persons to discuss, following appropriate examination, the dental needs of the patient and the proposed treatment. 2. A joint discussion between two or more dentists or health professionals to determine the diagnosis and possible treatment options for a particular patient.

contact *n.* The act of touching or meeting. The **balancing contact** is the contact made by an upper and lower denture on the side opposite to the working side and which helps to maintain the stability of the dentures. The **contact area** is the area of contact of approximal surfaces of adjacent teeth. The **initial contact** is the first point of contact made between opposing teeth. A **premature contact** is a deflective contact that interferes with the normal movement of the mandible. A **working contact** is a tooth contact on the side of the arch to which the mandible has moved.

contagious disease *See* COMMUNICABLE DISEASE.

contamination *n.* (in statistics) The inadvertent application of the intervention being evaluated to people in the *control group in a controlled clinical trial.

contingency table A table showing the cross-classification of two or more categorical *variables. The results are arranged in a grid, and the number of observations in each category is recorded in the cells.

continuing professional development (CPD) Education that is ongoing throughout the working life of the *healthcare professional. It is a mandatory requirement for all healthcare professionals registered in the UK with the *General Dental Council (GDC). To remain on the *Dental Register, the GDC define minimum CPD requirements, including specified core subjects.

continuous variable *n. See* VARIABLE.

contour lines of Owen [Sir R. Owen (1804–92), English anatomist] Incremental lines produced in dentine owing to disruption of the rhythmical pattern of dentine formation (*dentinogenesis).

contra-angle *adj.* Describing a double angle in the shank of an instrument which brings its working tip into line with the long axis of the handle.

contract *n.* A verbal or written agreement between two or more legally competent parties. A written treatment plan and charge estimate signed by the patient forms the basis of a legal contract. Written legal contracts are normally drawn up by two or more dentists working in partnership. A dentist agreeing to treat patients within the National Health Service will enter into a legal contract with the primary care trust. Employees working with a dentist will have a contract of employment which will include a job description, salary, sickness arrangements, disciplinary rules, pension provision, and termination procedure.

contraction *n.* The shortening of a *muscle in response to *nerve stimulation.

contralateral *adj.* Relating to or affecting the opposite side of the body or reference point. *Compare* IPSILATERAL.

contrast medium (contrast agent) A radiopaque substance introduced into an air- or fluid-filled structure so that it can be more easily visualized. In radiography a positive contrast medium such as barium sulphate increases the density of a structure, whereas gas acts as a negative contrast medium.

control *n.* A standard against which other conditions can be compared in a scientific experiment. A **control group** is the group of individuals participating in a clinical research study which does not receive the experimental treatment or intervention, but receives either the

currently approved standard treatment for the disease or an inactive substance (*placebo).

controlled area An area surrounding the x-ray tube and the patient of 1.5 m and not in direct line of the primary x-ray beam defined during a radiation exposure. No one other than the patient should be within the controlled area during an exposure.

Control of Substances Hazardous to Health Regulations (CoSHH) 2002 A legal framework in the UK, first drawn up in 1988, for controlling the exposure of the public to hazardous substances, including microbiological hazards, arising from work activity.

contusion *n.* A bruising injury that does not break the skin.

convenience form *n. See* FORM.

copal resin (copal ether varnish) An organic resin made from the sap of the Bursera tree used as a dentine desensitizing *cavity varnish, prior to inserting an *amalgam restoration. Copal resin has now been largely replaced by dentine *adhesive systems or *luting cements.

coping (thimble) *n.* A thin metal, resin, or ceramic cap covering a prepared tooth. A cast metal parallel coping is placed over an *implant abutment to make it parallel to other prepared natural teeth or implant abutments. A **transfer coping** is a cap usually made of metal or resin used to accurately position a *die in an *impression.

copolymer *n.* A *polymer resulting from the *polymerization reaction of two or more chemically different *monomers. They are used to improve the flow of resins. *See also* RESIN COMPOSITE.

copper *n.* A ductile and malleable soft reddish-brown metallic element. Many modern *amalgams contain high amounts of copper (**copper enriched alloy**), usually about 10–15%, to reduce corrosion and creep and increase strength. The copper acts to convert the γ2 phase to γ1 with the formation of a silver–copper alloy. *See also* AMALGAM. A **copper ring** is a thin-walled copper tube used to contain impression material or to act as a *matrix band. Copper poisoning can result in a line of purple discoloration in the gingivae (*Corrigan's line).

copy denture *See* DENTURE.

core *n.* The central part. A heavily broken-down tooth can be built up in either *amalgam

(**amalgam core**) or composite (**resin composite core**) to replace missing tooth substance and form a rigid and retentive base for a *crown restoration. The core may be retained by mechanical undercuts, *pins, or *adhesive systems. The core may be made of cast metal (**cast core**) and extend into the root of an *endodontically treated tooth for retention and then cemented prior to the placement of a crown (**cast post and core**).

Further Reading: Bateman G., Tomson P. Trends in indirect dentistry: 2. Post and core restorations. *Dent Update* 2005;32 (4):190–92, 194–6, 198.
Wilson P. H., Fisher N. L., Bartlett D. W. Direct core materials. *Dent Update* 2003;30(7):362–8.

core-vent implant system *See* IMPLANT.

corlan® pellet *n.* (trade name) *See* HYDROCORTISONE.

cornu *n.* (*pl.* **cornua**) A horn-shaped structure such as a pulp horn or the horn-shaped process of the hyoid bone.

coronal *adj.* Pertaining to the *crown of a tooth. A **coronal seal** protects the root canal system against the ingress of fluids and micro-organisms from the oral cavity.

coronary artery disease (CAD) *Atherosclerosis of the coronary arteries which may lead to *angina pectoris or infarction of the heart muscle. Periodontal disease and CAD share common risk factors of age, smoking, socio-economic status, and glycaemic control, and there is some evidence to suggest a possible association between periodontal disease and CAD.

Further Reading: Bahekar A. A., Singh S., Saha S., Molnar J., Arora R. The prevalence and incidence of coronary heart disease is significantly increased in periodontitis: a meta-analysis. *Am Heart J* 2007;154:830–37.

coronary thrombosis (heart attack) The formation of a blood clot (*thrombus) in the coronary artery restricting the blood supply to the heart, usually due to *atheroma. It is characterized by sudden severe chest pain which may spread to the arms and throat.

coronion *n.* The *craniometric point at the tip of the coronoid process of the mandible.

coronoid process *n. See* MANDIBLE.

corporate body *See* BODIES CORPORATE.

Corporate Manslaughter and Corporate Homicide Act 2007 An act of the UK parliament which came into force in April 2008 that introduced a new offence, across the UK, for prosecuting companies and other organizations,

including National Health Service (NHS) trusts and dental partnerships where there have been fatal consequences to an employee, patient, or member of the public due to a gross failing, throughout the organization, in the management of health and safety or of a duty of care.

Further Reading: Wells C., Thomas D. Deaths in the dental surgery: individual and organizational criminal liability. *B Dent J* 2008;204:497–502.

correlation *n.* A statistical term used to describe the association between two *variables. A **partial correlation** is a correlation between two variables when the effects of one or more related variables are removed.

correlation coefficient (in statistics) A measure of the degree to which two variables are linearly related (number between −1 and 1). A perfect linear relationship with positive slope between two variables will produce a correlation coefficient of 1. A perfect linear relationship with negative slope between two variables will produce a correlation coefficient of −1. A correlation coefficient of 0 means there is no linear relationship between the variables. **Pearson's correlation coefficient**, also known as the **Pearson product-moment correlation coefficient** (typically denoted by r), is a measurement of the strength of relationship between two variables (e.g. X and Y). It takes the value somewhere between −1 and +1: despite its name [K. Pearson (1857–1936), British mathematician], it was first introduced by Sir Francis Galton (1822–1911). **Spearman's correlation coefficient** [C. S. Spearman (1863–1945), English psychologist] is the same as Pearson's correlation coefficient but uses data that have been converted into ranked scores.

Corrigan's line [D. J. Corrigan (1802–80), Irish physician] A purple line along the gingival margin caused by chronic copper poisoning.

corrosion *n.* The deterioration of a metal by chemical or electrochemical reaction with its environment. **Amalgam corrosion** can occur in the oral environment because of an interreaction between chloride ions present in the saliva and the amalgam alloy, resulting in both anodic and cathodic reactions. The extent of the corrosion may be influenced by such factors as the composition of the alloy, the particle size and form, the mercury content, the nature of the gamma-2 phase, and the degree of surface finishing. **Corrosion products** at the amalgam–tooth interface are considered to seal the gap between the restoration and the tooth and minimize microleakage.

corticosteroids *n.* A term used to encompass glucocorticoids, mineralocorticoids, and androgens. All are secreted from the adrenal cortex under the influence of the hypothalamic–pituitary–adrenal axis. They have effects on glucose, protein and fat metabolism, sodium retention and potassium loss, anti-inflammatory effects, and immunosuppressive effects.

corticotomy (cortical osteotomy) *n.* Sectioning through the bone cortex leaving the remaining bone, periosteum, and vascular tissues intact. It is a technique that can be used on alveolar bone to assist in the orthodontic treatment of palatally impacted teeth by weakening the resistance of the bone during the application of orthodontic forces. It is particularly important in distraction osteogenesis (*osteodistraction).

cortisol *n.* A corticosteroid produced by the adrenal cortex, often referred to as the 'stress' hormone as it is produced in response to stress. Serum levels of cortisol vary on a diurnal basis and are highest early in the morning.

corundum (emery) *n.* A form of aluminium oxide used as an abrasive.

coryza *n.* A catarrhal inflammation of the mucous membrane of the nose due to the common cold, narcotic withdrawal, or hay fever.

cost–benefit analysis *n.* A study of the relationship between the service or production costs and the health gain achieved for an individual or group.

cost-effectiveness *n.* The minimum expenditure in terms of finance, time, and professional services necessary to achieve the healthcare required or deemed appropriate.

Costen's syndrome [J. B. Costen (1895–1962), American otolaryngologist] Symptoms of muscular trismus and referred pain associated with the *temporomandibular joint thought to be caused by a *malocclusion resulting from a loss of vertical dimension and reduced posterior occlusal support.

cost–utility analysis *n.* A specific type of cost-effectiveness analysis using quality-adjusted life years as the measure of effectiveness.

cotton wool *n.* The refined, bleached, and absorbent fibres from the seed of the cotton plant (*Gossypium herbaceum*) used for moisture control. It is frequently used in a cylindrical form (**cotton wool roll**) or in a loose form of cotton fibres (**cotton batting**).

counterbalancing *n.* (in statistics) Systematic changing of the order in which the experimental conditions are given. For example, if there are two conditions (X and Y), by counterbalancing, half of the participants would receive condition X followed by Y and the remaining participants would receive condition Y followed by X. The purpose of counterbalancing is to remove the systematic *bias produced by practice.

Coupland's chisel *n. See* CHISEL.

coupling agent A chemical substance capable of reacting with both the reinforcement and the matrix of a *resin composite. It may also bond inorganic fillers or fibres to organic resins to form or promote a stronger bond at the interface. Compounds of silicon and hydrogen (**silane coupling agents**) play an important stabilizing role in dental resin composites.

covariance *n.* A measure of how much two *variables change together. A covariate is a variable that has a relationship, or could potentially relate to, the outcome variable being measured.

cover screw *n.* A thin metal covering firmly screwed into an *implant after placement. In the two-stage technique, the implant and cover screw are covered by oral mucosa to allow *osseointegration of the implant to take place. When this has occurred, the implant is exposed, the cover screw removed, and a suitable abutment selected: also known as a healing coping. 📷

Cowden's syndrome [named after a person affected by the condition] A rare inherited condition characterized by benign lesions of the skin and mucosa, including facial papules and warty papules on the upper surfaces of the hands and feet. The oral lesions present as numerous 1–3mm smooth whitish spots on the gingivae and palate that join together to create a cobblestone appearance (papillomatosis). Patients have an increased risk of developing malignant *neoplasms of several organs including the breast, uterus, and thyroid.

Coxsackie A virus *See* HERPANGINA.

cracked tooth syndrome A hairline fracture involving the *occlusal surface of the crown of a tooth often extending into the root. The crack may involve the pulp or be confined to enamel and dentine. It is most common in heavily restored teeth but may occur following biting on a foreign body such as lead shot or bone. The symptoms are often poorly localized, making diagnosis problematical. It is often characterized by severe pain on occlusal contact, due to the flexure of the tooth, which usually lasts for the duration of the contact only; there may also be pain in response to thermal stimuli.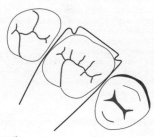

craniometry n. The technique of measuring the bones of the skull, which forms the basis of *cephalometric radiography. **craniometric** adj.

craniosynostosis n. The premature fusion of some of the cranial bones, usually before birth, preventing normal expansion of the skull. It results in abnormal facial and cranial development.

cranium n. That part of the *skull which houses and protects the brain. It consists of eight distinct bones united together. There are two paired bones, the parietal and temporal, and four single bones, namely the frontal, ethmoid, occipital, and sphenoid.

crazing n. A pattern of very fine cracks that may form on the surface of resin or porcelain.

creep n. The deformation of a material over a period of time. *Amalgam creep may result in cuspal fracture and is thought to be a cause of failure of *marginal ridges.

crenation n. 1. The scalloping of the margins of the tongue caused by the pressure against the lingual surfaces of the mandibular teeth. 2. The abnormal appearance of red blood cells in which the normally smooth margins appear wrinkled or irregular as a result of shrinkage in their volume.

creosote n. An oily liquid mixture of phenols obtained by the distillation of coal tar. **Beechwood creosote** is an antiseptic and mildly analgesic liquid and has been used for the disinfection of root canals during the non-vital pulpotomy of *primary teeth. It is placed on a pledget of cotton wool and sealed in the pulp cavity with zinc-oxide eugenol, usually for 1–2 weeks. This technique is no longer commonly used. *See also* FERRIC SULPHATE.

crepitus n. 1. A grating or crackling sound such as that produced by the worn articulatory surfaces of a joint or the rubbing of two fragments of a broken bone together. Crepitus is not uncommon in patients with *temporomandibular joint disorders. 2. A similar sound heard with a *stethoscope over an inflamed lung on inspiration.

crest n. An elongated ridge or linear projection usually applied to a bone e.g. the nasal crest of the maxilla, or to soft tissue e.g. *gingival crest.

cretinism n. A condition caused by a congenital lack of *thyroid hormone (hypothyroidism). Adults have symptoms of

lethargy, facial puffiness, and poor response to stress. Because treatment is with thyroid hormone, care should be taken when administering local anaesthetic containing *epinephrine.

Creutzfeldt–Jakob disease (CJD) A neurodegenerative disease resulting in a spongy degeneration of the brain and spinal cord. **Sporadic CJD** affects adults and produces initial symptoms of headache, tiredness, and weight loss. The disease can be spread by improperly sterilized instruments, grafts, and growth hormone products. **New variant CJD** has symptoms of involuntary movements progressing to dementia, and occurs in a younger age group. It has been linked to *bovine spongiform encephalopathy (BSE).

Further Reading: Scully C., Smith A. J., Bagg J. CJD: Update for dental staff. *Dent Update* 2006;33:454–60.

crevice n. A narrow opening or gap. The **gingival crevice** (gingival *sulcus) is a narrow gap between the free *gingiva and the *enamel of the tooth.

crevicular fluid (gingival crevicular fluid, sulcular fluid) A clear fluid containing antibodies, micro-organisms, plasma proteins, other therapeutic substances, and by-products of the inflammatory response that flows into the *gingival crevice (gingival sulcus). The flow increases and contains *cytokines when inflammation or disease is present.

crib n. A form of anchorage used in removable *orthodontic appliances. An **Adams crib** is a retention clasp, designed by C. Philip Adams, used to retain a removable appliance or prosthesis. It functions by engaging the mesial and distal undercuts on the buccal surface of a posterior tooth, usually the upper first molar.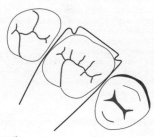

Adams crib

A **lingual crib** consists of an appliance with a wire framework placed lingually to the maxillary incisor teeth and designed to break habits such as thumb sucking.

cribriform *adj.* Perforated or sieve-like.

crisis *n. See* ADRENAL CRISIS.

cristobalite (crystobalite) *n.* A naturally occurring silicon dioxide used as a dental casting investment because of its capacity for thermal expansion and ability to withstand high temperatures. Cristobalite is formed from **tridymite** at 1471°C (2680°F) and melts at 1713°C (3115°F).

critical appraisal The process of assessing and interpreting evidence by systematically considering its validity, results, and relevance to clinical practice. The evidence may be derived from clinical observation, laboratory results, scientific literature, or other sources.

Crohn's disease [B. B. Crohn (1884–1983), US physician] A granulomatous disease that occurs in discrete areas in the small and large bowel, characterized by weight loss, diarrhoea, *anaemia, and intestinal pain. Oral symptoms include cobblestone appearance of the buccal *mucosa and *aphthous ulcers. In long-standing disease there may be *enamel hypoplasia.

Cronbach's alpha [L. J. Cronbach (1916–2001), American educational psychologist] (in statistics) A measure of the reliability of a scale or psychometric instrument.

crossbite (scissors bite, X-bite) *n. See* BITE.

cross-infection *n.* The transmission of a communicable disease, most commonly caused by an infectious micro-organism, either directly from one person to another by direct contact, or indirectly by contaminated instruments, equipment, surfaces, water, and air. A **cross-infection control policy** is a rational series of procedures designed to prevent work-related infections among dental healthcare personnel and support staff, and healthcare-associated infections among patients.

cross-infection control *n. See* INFECTION CONTROL.

cross-over trial A trial in which each of the groups in the study receive each of the treatments, but in a randomized order: each group will begin in one arm of the trial, but will, by design, cross over to the other arm or arms in turn.

cross-sectional study An observational research study in which data, such as disease data, are obtained at a single point in time from two or more samples. Also called a **prevalence study**. *See also* LONGITUDINAL STUDY.

cross-striations *n.* Incremental growth lines produced by daily deposits during enamel formation which are about 4μm thick.

Crouzon syndrome (craniofacial dysostosis) [O. Crouzon (1874–1938), French neurologist] A genetic disorder characterized by premature fusion of the skull sutures. It is similar to *Apert syndrome but without the deformation of the fingers and toes.

crowding *n.* An overlapping of the contact areas of the teeth. Potential causes include a tooth tissue discrepancy, such as disproportionally large teeth or a disproportionally small jaw, premature loss of the primary teeth that has allowed the adjacent primary teeth to drift into the space required for the permanent successors, and soft tissue pressures on the teeth leading to displacement. 📷

crown

n. **1.** That part of the tooth dentine which is covered by enamel (**anatomical crown**). **2.** That part of the crown that is clearly visible (**clinical crown**). **3.** An artificial covering cemented over a suitably prepared natural tooth. A **basket crown** is a form of three-quarter metal crown with a resin facing which was formerly used as a semi-permanent restoration for a fractured incisor. A **complete (full) crown** covers the entire anatomical surface of the clinical crown and may be of even thickness (**jacket crown**) or thin in cross-section with a tapered margin (**veneer crown, shell crown**). 📷

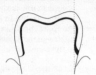

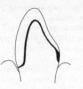

| All metal veneer posterior | Metal-ceramic posterior | Metal-ceramic anterior | Ceramic (jacket) anterior |

Types of crowns

A **dowel (post) crown** replaces the coronal portion of a tooth and is retained by means of a dowel or *post in the prepared *root canal of the tooth. A **partial veneer** or ¾ **crown** covers only part of the anatomical crown. A **veneered (bonded) metal crown** has one or more surfaces covered with a tooth-coloured material such as porcelain or resin; where porcelain is used it is fused to the metal (**metal–ceramic crown**). A **telescope crown** consists of a double metal crown in which two conical crowns are placed one over the other. **Temporary crowns** are usually made of resin or aluminium and are cemented with a soft cement, such as zinc oxide-eugenol, to facilitate easy removal. Heavily carious, damaged, or worn down primary posterior teeth may be restored either permanently or temporarily after appropriate preparation with **preformed metal crowns** usually made of stainless steel (*see also* HALL TECHNIQUE). Primary anterior teeth can be restored with **strip crowns** made from a preformed cellulose acetate crown former filled with resin or *resin composite. The incisal edge is reduced by 2 mm and then the proximal surfaces are reduced to produce a 15° taper with a shoulderless finish at the gingival margin; the labial and palatal surfaces are similarly reduced to remove any convexity. Where there is insufficient crown length for adequate retention, *crown lengthening may be indicated.

crown lengthening A clinical procedure undertaken by surgically removing or repositioning some of the marginal gingival tissue surrounding the crown of a tooth. It is indicated to improve aesthetics e.g. by correcting an uneven gingival contour or to facilitate restorative procedures such as increasing the crown height, accessing subgingival caries, or to relocate margins of restorations that are impinging on the *biological width. *See also* GINGIVECTOMY.

crown remover *See* BRIDGE REMOVER.

Crozat appliance [G. B. Crozat (1894–1966), American dentist] A removable orthodontic appliance, developed by Dr Crozat in the 1920s, to widen the dental arch without the extraction of teeth. It is made of precisely adapted wires soldered together.

crucible former *n.* The stand or base usually made of metal or resin onto which a sprued *wax pattern is placed. The shape of the base permits the smooth passage of molten metal during the casting procedure.

Cryer's elevator *See* ELEVATOR.

cryolite *n.* Sodium hexafluoroaluminate (Na_3AlF_6) often used as a *flux in the manufacture of silicate *cements.

cryosurgery *n.* The use of extreme cold in a specific location to remove diseased or unwanted tissue.

crypt *n.* The small cavity in the alveolar bone in which a tooth develops before eruption.

crystobalite *n. See* CRISTOBALITE.

culture 1. *n.* The growth of *micro-organisms, usually *bacteria, in a liquid or solid artificial medium (**culture medium**). 2. *v.* To grow micro-organisms in a culture medium.

curettage *n.* The removal of unwanted material from the walls of a hard surface. Removal of hard deposits on the root surface (**root curettage**) can lead to improved gingival health. **Periapical curettage** removes granulation tissue surrounding the root apex and any associated intra-bony *cyst lining. **Subgingival curettage** is the removal of inflamed tissue and the epithelial lining of a periodontal pocket. Curettage may be performed with hand instruments (*curettes) or ultrasonically.

curette (curet) *n.* A metal hand instrument with a sharp spoon-shaped blade used to undertake *debridement. The effectiveness of the working end of a curette is maintained by sharpening the blade face using a round stone or the side of the blade with a flat stone. A curette may also be defined by the area of use e.g. infrabony curette, subgingival curette. There are a number of different shapes of curette in common use in periodontal therapy. A **Barnhart curette** is a small bladed double-ended universal hand instrument with a rounded end used for removing subgingival calculus and plaque. The **Columbia universal curette** has a continuous blade with a cutting edge on both sides of the blade which curves around the toe and a flat face set at 90° to the lower shank; examples are the Barnhardt and Columbia. A **Gracey curette** (developed by Clayton H. Gracey in 1930) is curved in two planes to allow close adaptation to the root surface, with the blade sharpened on one side only and curved at an angle of 70° to the shank and with a rounded tip: the terminal shank is held against the surface of and parallel to the tooth and moved in a vertical direction; it is used for subgingival *curettage, particularly in deep narrow pockets. The **Gracey After Five** shank has a 3mm elongated terminal shank and the blade is 10% thinner than a standard Gracey blade. **Gracey mini five curettes** combine the longer terminal shank design with a 50% shorter blade. The **Langer curette** combines features from the Gracey and Columbia universal curettes.

curing *n. See* POLYMERIZATION.

curing light *n.* A hand-held unit that produces light in the visible spectrum within a specific waveband which initiates the *polymerization process by activating a *photo-initiator contained within *resin composite. The light waveband lies within the range of 400–500 nanometres (nm) at the blue end of the light spectrum. Ultra-violet light is no longer used because of safety issues. Lights with **light emitting diodes** (LEDs) that emit light at a waveband of 470nm may also be used. **Plasma arc curing lights** generate a high-voltage pulse and a reduced curing time, although this may be insufficient to cure all types of resin composite.

curve of Monson [G. S. Monson (1869–1933), American dentist] The curve of occlusion of natural teeth in which each cusp and incisal edge touches or conforms to a segment of the surface of a sphere 20.3cm (8in.) in diameter, with its centre in the region of the *glabella. *See also* COMPENSATING CURVE.

curve of Pleasure [M. A. Pleasure (1903–65), American dentist] A curve of occlusion which when viewed in the frontal plane conforms to a curve that is convex from the superior view, except for the last molars which reverse the pattern.

curve of Spee [F. von Spee (1855–1937), German embryologist] The anatomical curvature of the mandibular occlusal plane beginning at the tip of the lower *canine and following the buccal cusps of the posterior teeth, continuing to the terminal *molar.

Cushing's syndrome [H. W. Cushing (1869–1939), American neurosurgeon] A condition resulting from excess amounts of corticosteroid hormones. It is characterized by a rounded moon face, growth of body and facial hair, osteoporosis, an increase in body fat, and muscle wasting especially in the arms and legs. The syndrome may be due to overproduction of *adrenocorticotrophic hormone from a *pituitary or *adrenal tumour, or because of high-dose *steroids as used for *immunosuppression following transplantation. Patients undergoing dental surgery may be at risk of a steroid crisis.

cusp *n.* A pointed or rounded projection on the crown of a tooth. A cusp may be present additional to the normal crown morphology (**supplemental cusp**). The **cusp angle** is the angle made by the slope of the cusp and a vertical line bisecting the cusp, measured mesiodistally or buccolingually. A **stamp cusp** is a functional cusp that stamps into the *fossa of an opposing tooth. The stamp cusps of a lower premolar may have its tip in an *embrasure and have only the cusp shoulders in small fossae. *See also* TALON.

cuspal interference The undesirable contact of a cusp with an opposing tooth which may interfere with the normal *occlusion of the rest of the teeth.

cusp–fossa relationship *n.* The anatomical relationship between a stamp cusp and its *fossa.

cuspid *n.* An alternative name for a *canine tooth.

cuspidor *n.* A form of bowl or spittoon into which patients can expectorate.

cusp of Carabelli *See* TUBERCLE.

cutaneous *adj.* Relating to the skin.

cuticle *n.* 1. The epidermis of the skin. 2. A solid or semi-solid layer of material covering epithelium. 3. A layer of cells such as the outer layer of cells in a hair. The **primary cuticle** forms the remnants of the *enamel organ and oral *epithelium covering the enamel of a tooth following *eruption. The **secondary cuticle** is formed when the *ameloblasts are replaced by oral epithelium.

cyanoacrylate *n.* The generic name for a group of adhesive chemicals which rapidly polymerize in the presence of water. Cyanoacrylate is used as a soft *tissue adhesive and may also be blended with glass ionomer *cement to reduce the vulnerability of the glass ionomer to moisture and improve its adhesive properties.

cyanosis *n.* (*adj.* **cyanotic**) A blue discoloration of the skin or *mucosa, usually owing to deficient oxygenation of the *blood.

cyclamate *n.* An artificial sweetening agent about 30–50 times as sweet as *sucrose. It has been banned in the US and UK since 1969 because of its *carcinogenic potential.

cyclic neutropenia *n.* *See* NEUTROPENIA.

cyclosporin *n.* *See* CICLOSPORIN.

cylindroma *n.* An adenoid cystic *carcinoma that occurs within secretory glands, most commonly the major and minor salivary glands of the head and neck.

cynodontism *n.* Having teeth with small pulp chambers confined to the tooth crown as in mammals.

cyst

n. An abnormal cavity or sac usually lined with *epithelium and filled with gas, liquid, solid, or semi-solid material excluding pus. An **aneurysmal bone cyst** is a rare blood-filled cyst, more often found in the mandible than maxilla of young adults, which causes jaw expansion; it is treated by *curettage. A **dentigerous cyst** forms around the crown of an unerupted or *impacted tooth, usually mandibular third molars or maxillary canines. There is fluid accumulation between the crown of the tooth and the surrounding follicle and *reduced enamel epithelium which produces hydrostatic pressure causing *bone resorption. Cysts are often symptomless and discovered as an incidental radiolucency on a radiograph. A **dermoid cyst** (**dermoid**) is a developmental cyst lined by keratinized stratified squamous epithelium associated with skin appendages such as sebaceous glands and hair follicles. If no skin appendages are present it is called an **epidermoid cyst**; they are caused by inclusion of ectodermal tissue in the lines of fusion during the embryonic formation of the facial processes and may be found anywhere on the skin and occasionally in the oral cavity,

particularly below the tongue (sublingual dermoid cyst). An **eruption cyst** presents as a bluish swelling and forms over an erupting tooth, particularly in children. It usually disappears once eruption is complete although incision may be necessary. **Gingival cysts** are developmental in origin, arising either from basal cell extensions from overlying epithelium or from *odontogenic epithelial residues. They are particularly common in the new-born (*Bohn's nodules, *Epstein pearls) but relatively rare in adults. They invariably heal spontaneously in the new-born but may require excisional *biopsy in adults. An **incisive canal (naso-palatine duct) cyst** arises from epithelial remnants of the nasopalatine duct and lies in the incisive canal between the nasal cavity and the roof of the mouth. It is the most common maxillary development cyst and appears as a heart-shaped radiolucency in the midline between the central incisors. A **lympho-epithelial cyst** is a developmental cyst lined by epithelium with lymphoid tissue in the wall; also known as **branchial cysts** in the neck, they are found in the floor of the mouth as well. A **median cyst** is a rare cyst in the midline of the palate or mandible; most authorities agree that these are not distinct cysts but midline examples of other jaw cysts. A **mucous retention cyst** occurs when the duct of a gland, such as a salivary gland, becomes blocked, resulting in an accumulation of *saliva. It is relatively rare in comparison with a *mucous extravasation cyst, which is caused by rupture of a salivary gland duct due to trauma; saliva enters the tissues and becomes walled off by granulation tissue and infiltrated by macrophages and neutrophils. Both the mucous extravasation and retention cysts present as fluctuant blue swellings and the extravasation cyst is particularly common on the lower lip. Treatment is by surgical excision, including the associated minor salivary gland. A **nasolabial cyst** is a fluid-filled cavity lined with *epithelium, thought to originate from the embryonic *nasolacrimal duct; it is found near the base of the nostril, just above the *periosteum, or in the superior aspect of the upper lip. Treatment is by surgical excision. A **non-odontogenic cyst** is a cyst in which the epithelium is *not* derived from the tooth-forming tissues (e.g. nasopalatine duct cyst; nasolabial cyst). An **odontogenic cyst** is a cyst in which the epithelium *is* derived from the tooth-forming tissues. The residues include the *epithelial rest cells of Malassez, the *reduced enamel epithelium, or the *dental lamina (rests of Serres). Odontogenic cysts may be inflammatory in origin (e.g. radicular periapical cyst associated with a non-vital

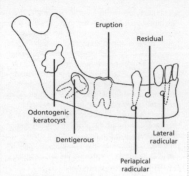

Cysts of the jaw

tooth) or developmental (e.g. lateral periodontal cyst, dentigerous cysts, odontogenic keratocyst) and are usually contained within bone. **Odontogenic keratocysts** differ from other odontogenic cysts in that they are lined by *keratinized epithelium. They increase in size because of epithelial proliferation rather than hydrostatic pressure, and tend to recur if not completely removed; they extend through the bone rather than causing expansion and are most common at the angle of the *mandible; they are not necessarily associated with a tooth, and tend to present radiographically as a multilocular radiolucency. A **paradental cyst** is an odontogenic cyst which occurs in association with the crown of a partially erupted tooth, most commonly the third molar. A **periapical (radicular) cyst** is associated with the apex of a tooth root with a non-vital pulp and is the result of spread of infection to the periapical tissues. The epithelial lining is derived from the remnants of cell rests of Malassez present in the periodontal ligament, and the wall is composed of chronically inflamed granulation and fibrous tissue. The cyst grows

owing to hydrostatic pressure of the cyst contents. The lesion appears as a unilocular radiolucency and usually disappears following root canal therapy but, if not, an *apicectomy may be required. A radicular cyst may remain after the tooth has been extracted (**residual cyst**). A **solitary bone cyst** can occur in the mandible of children and adolescents; it appears as a well-defined radiolucency and is lined by fibrous tissue with no epithelium; the cause is unknown.

cystic fibrosis An inherited disorder affecting the *exocrine glands, particularly the mucous secreting glands. Respiratory infection is a common complication and, in addition, oral signs can include tooth discoloration, enamel *hypoplasia, increased prevalence of *calculus, and *salivary gland enlargement.

cytokine *n.* A soluble protein or glycoprotein, released by cells, which modify the action of other cells. Cytokines are released by a wide variety of cell types and have a central role in the *immune system where they act as intercellular mediators in the generation of an immune response.

cytology *n.* The study of the structure and function of cells.

cytoplasm *n.* The jelly-like substance within the cell outside the nucleus.

cytostatic *adj.* Describing the inhibition or suppression of cellular growth and multiplication.

cytotoxic *adj.* Describing a substance that damages or kills cells. It is usually applied to drugs used in the treatment of *cancer.

Czermak's spaces [J. N. Czermak (1828–73), Austrian physiologist] Rows of irregular interglobular spaces following the outline of the dentine formed due to a developmental failure of *calcification.

D32/33 award The qualification that used to be required in order to become a fully trained **National Vocational Qualification** (NVQ) assessor for trainee dental nurses. The D32/D33 was replaced in 2003 with the A1 and A2 qualifications.

Dakin's solution [H. D. Dakin (1880–1952), American chemist] A dilute solution of *sodium hypochlorite and boric acid used as an *antiseptic.

Damon system *See* BRACKET.

dangerous drugs *See* MISUSE OF DRUGS ACT.

dappen dish (dappen glass) *n.* A small decagonal glass receptacle with a depression at both ends used to hold medicaments during operative procedures.

D'Arcet's metal [J. D'Arcet (1727–1801), French physician] An alloy of tin lead and bismuth which was historically used as a restorative material in its fused state. It was abandoned because of the high working temperature at which the metal fused (212°F; 100°C), which caused pain and pulpal damage and the shrinkage from the cavity walls on cooling. The metal has also been used in the past as a low-fusing die material.

Darier's disease [F.-J. Darier (1856–1938), French dermatologist] A rare genetic disorder of the skin characterized by a rash usually affecting the chest, neck, back, forehead, and groin. It may present with oral lesions consisting of coalescing white papules on the gingivae and palate.

dark zone An area of demineralized *enamel which is part of a carious lesion visible on ground sections of a tooth viewed under transmitted light. It lies between the outer intact layer and the deeper *translucent zone. Unlike the translucent zone, it represents an area of previous remineralization.

data *pl. n.* A collection of facts or organized information, usually the results of observation, experience, or experiment, or a set of premises from which conclusions may be drawn. Data may consist of numbers, words, or images.

Continuous data are observations made on a scale that has a natural zero and a well-defined unit of measurement, and can have an infinite number of values e.g. the weight of an individual. **Interval data** are measured on a scale of which the intervals are equal. **Nominal data** consist of observations classified into categories that are different in character and cannot be ordered e.g. blood types. **Ordinal data** consist of observations which have a common character and can be grouped into a limited number of categories that can be ordered in a series or rank e.g. a satisfaction survey. **Ratio data** are interval data that have an additional property in that the ratios are meaningful e.g. birth weight in kg. **Statistical data** are observations made on independent units or individuals.

Data Protection Act 1998 (in the UK) A British act of parliament that provides a legal basis for the privacy and protection of data of UK citizens and businesses. Users of data information are required to be registered. The act requires that personal data must be processed fairly and lawfully, for specific declared purposes, and in accordance with the rights of data subjects. It also states that data should not be transferred outside the European Economic Area without adequate protection. Patients who make a written application to see their medical or dental records must be provided with a copy within 40 days, together with an explanation of the content if they so wish and can demand to have inaccurate or misleading information amended. Disclosure of dental records to a third party can be resisted where there are grounds to believe that disclosure might be detrimental to the physical or mental health of the patient.

day-patient A person who is admitted to hospital for treatment, examination, or observation but who does not remain there overnight. *Compare* IN-PATIENT; OUT-PATIENT.

dead space volume 1. (anatomical) The amount of inspired air that occupies the airway passages and where no gaseous exchange takes place. 2. (physiological) The space relating to a reduction in the area for ventilation or perfusion.

dead tract *n*. An area of empty *dentinal tubules beneath a *carious lesion where the *odontoblasts have died and not laid down sclerotic dentine.

Dean, Trendley (1893–1962) An American dentist and epidemiologist who researched the effects of water fluoridation on tooth enamel. In 1931 he conducted a major research study for the National Institutes of Health (NIH) which demonstrated the link between a lower incidence of caries and water fluoridation. He created the Dean Index of *fluorosis classification.

debilitate *v*. To make feeble, to weaken.

debonding *n*. 1. The process by which orthodontic *brackets and associated *bonding resin are removed from the enamel surface of a tooth and the tooth is restored to its original condition. 2. The failure of the micromechanical bond between a resin restorative material and the enamel or dentine surface.

debridement *n*. (*v*. **debride**) 1. The removal of foreign or dead material from a wound to aid the healing process. 2. The removal of deposits on a tooth surface; root debridement (the removal of deposits on the root surface) should be contrasted with *root planing (the removal of deposits and the surface layer of cementum containing bacterial toxins).

decalcification *n*. The loss of *calcium or calcium salts from mineralized tissue such as enamel, dentine, or *bone.

decay *n*. See CARIES.

deciduous teeth The teeth constituting the first dentition. See PRIMARY DENTITION.

Declaration of Geneva The medical code of ethics first adopted in 1948 by the 2nd World Assembly of the World Medical Association in Geneva, Switzerland. It calls upon doctors and dentists not to allow considerations of age, disease, or disability, creed, ethnic origin, gender, nationality, political affiliation, race, sexual orientation, or social standing to influence their approach to patient care. It has replaced the Hippocratic oath.

decontamination *n*. A process or treatment that renders a medical device, instrument, or environmental surface safe to handle. It encompasses both cleaning and sterilization. The UK Department of Health document HTM 01-05 defines essential and best practice standards of care for instrument decontamination.

Further Reading: Decontamination Health Technical Memorandum 01-01 Department of Health 2008, available at http://www.dh.gov.uk/en/Publicationsandstatistics/Publications/PublicationsPolicyAndGuidance/DH_089245

decoronation *n*. The removal of the crown of a tooth.

decussation *n*. The crossing over of fibres from one side of the central nervous system to the other e.g. the decussation of the pyramids.

DEF (decayed, extracted, filled) index A dental *caries index applied to the primary dentition similar to the *DMF index used for the permanent dentition. See also DMF INDEX.

Defence Dental Service (in the UK) A tri-service organization which provides dental services to the Armed Forces through Royal Navy, Army, and Royal Air Force personnel and civilians to contribute to the operational effectiveness of the armed forces by achieving and maintaining, in the most cost-effective way, the dental fitness of its personnel stationed throughout the world. It also provides facilities for dental hygiene, therapy, and technology training.

((⊕)) SEE WEB LINKS

• The Defence Dental Services web site.

defibrillation *n*. The use of an electric shock to stop the rapid uncoordinated fibrillating movements of the heart and restore a normal rhythm. Defibrillation depolarizes most or all of the heart muscle simultaneously, allowing the natural pacemaking tissues to take over normal control of the heart. Defibrillation within 5 minutes of collapse gives the best possible outcome. The electrical impulse is provided by a **defibrillator**. Defibrillators have a power source which provides a direct current and a capacitor which is charged to a predetermined level and then discharged through two electrodes placed on the patient's chest. An **automated external defibrillator (AED)** is a type of defibrillator which detects the electrical activity in the heart and gives the rescuer automated instructions on what to do. The use of a defibrillator is part of *advanced life support.

degassing *n*. The process of removing unwanted gases trapped in a metal casting to improve the quality of the casting.

degloving *n*. The removal of an area of skin or mucous membrane to expose the underlying tissues. It may occur in response to trauma or by intentional surgery.

deglutition *n*. The process of swallowing by which food is transferred from the mouth to the *oesophagus. Food is forced backwards by voluntary movement of the *tongue followed by a reflex raising of the *soft palate to close the nasal passages and closure of the *larynx by the *epiglottis to prevent food entering the *trachea. Food enters the oesophagus and moves down towards the stomach by gravity and the muscular action of *peristalsis.

degrees of freedom A statistical term used to describe the number of values in the final calculation of a statistic that are free to vary. It is the number of categories or classes being tested minus 1.

dehiscence *n.* A defect shaped in the form of a fissure. It can occur as a cleft-like defect in the cortical bone of the jaw exposing the tooth root, particularly in the anterior region.

dehydration *n.* A loss or deficiency of water in the body or from tissues. **Gingival dehydration** can be the result of *mouth breathing and render the gingival tissues susceptible to *inflammation or infection.

dementia *n.* A *chronic or persistent disorder of behaviour due to organic brain disease. It is characterized by a decrease in intellectual function with changes in personality, mood, and behaviour. **Presenile dementia** occurs in young or middle-aged people. A common form of dementia is *Alzheimer's disease.

demi- Prefix denoting half.

demineralization *n.* A loss or removal of mineral salts from the tissues of the body. It occurs in *dentine and *enamel as part of the *carious process. Enamel starts to demineralize when the *plaque or saliva *pH drops below 5.5. *See also* STEPHAN'S CURVE.

demography *n.* The statistical study of human populations on a national, regional, or local basis, especially with reference to size and density, distribution, and vital statistics. It is used in dentistry to identify oral health needs and *risk factors for a given population.

demulcent *n.* A substance that protects the mucous membranes and relieves irritation. Demulcents form a protective film and are used in *mouthwashes to reduce irritation or inflammation in the mouth. *Gum tragacanth or milk can act as demulcents.

dendrite *n.* A branching process of a neuron that receives incoming messages from other nerve cells and transmits impulses to the body of the neuron.

dense bone island (idiopathic osteosclerosis) A localized area of *sclerotic bone occuring in the premolar or molar regions of the mandible. The cause is unknown.

dens evaginatus *n.* A developmental anomaly characterized by the occurrence of an extra cusp shaped as a tubercle projecting from the palatal or buccal surfaces (*talon cusp) of a tooth. In the anterior dentition, dens evaginatus is more commonly found on the palatal surface of the maxillary teeth. They are easily fractured exposing the pulp.

dens in dente (dens invaginatus) *n.* A developmental malformation of the teeth in which there is an invagination of the enamel giving the radiographic appearance of a 'tooth within a tooth'. It can be caused by the prolific growth of the *ameloblast and *odontoblast cell layers during tooth formation. It most commonly occurs on the palatal surface of permanent maxillary lateral incisors and presents as a blind channel opening on the *cingulum pit which is susceptible to caries. They may be described according to the extent of the invagination (Oehlers' classification, as described by F. A. Oehlers in 1957): **type 1** is an enamel-lined invagination occurring within the confines of the crown of the tooth, not extending beyond the *cemento-enamel junction; **type 2** is an enamel-lined blind sac which invades the root and which may or may not connect with the dental pulp; **type 3** is an invagination which penetrates through the root, perforating the apical area and forming a second foramen but with no immediate connection with the pulp. *See also* ODONTOMA.

Further Reading: Vaidyanathan M., Whatling R., Fearne J. M. An overview of the dens invaginatus with case examples. *Dent Update* 2008;35:655–63.

dent- (denti-, dento-) Prefix denoting the teeth e.g. **dentoalveolar** (relating to the teeth and supporting structures).

dental *adj.* Relating to the teeth.

Dental Access Centre A part of the UK primary dental care services within the *National Health Service which provide emergency care and occasional care to patients who are not registered with a dentist.

dental anxiety *n.* *See* ANXIETY.

dental anxiety scale A method of assessing the anxiety of an individual developed by Norman L. Corah, an American behavioural scientist, in 1969. The scale consists of four questions about different dental situations. Each question is scored from 1 (not anxious) to 5 (extremely anxious) so the range of possible scores is 4 to 20. Scores of 15 or more indicate profound anxiety. *See also* MODIFIED DENTAL ANXIETY SCALE.

Further Reading: Corah N. H. Development of a dental anxiety scale *J Dent Res* 1969;48:596.

Dental Auxiliaries Committee (in the UK) A committee of the *General Dental Council which deals with professional and disciplinary issues relating to *dental care professionals.

Dental Auxiliaries Regulations 1986 (in the UK) Regulations which provide for the enrolment and regulation of dental hygienists and dental therapists. These regulations were amended by statutory instrument in 2002. The amendments extend the work permitted to be carried out by dental hygienists to include removal of excess cement, taking impressions, administration of inferior dental nerve block anaesthesia, and replacing crowns which have been dislodged with a temporary cement. They are also permitted to carry out dental work on a patient under local or regional block anaesthesia administered by a registered dentist, or, provided there is a registered dentist in the room in which the dental work is carried out throughout the procedure, under conscious sedation.

dental care professional (DCP) A classification of healthcare professional in the UK, formerly known as professionals complementary to dentistry, which includes dental nurses, dental hygienists, dental therapists, dental technicians, clinical dental technicians, and orthodontic therapists.

dental chair unit (DCU) A complex medical device designed to provide the equipment and services necessary for the provision of a wide variety of dental procedures. It can include electric and air turbine handpieces, aspiration devices, and suction hoses. Because DCUs are used in the treatment of many patients during normal clinical activity, microbial contamination of specific component parts is an important potential source of *cross-infection and cross-contamination.

Dental Complaints Service (DCS) A mechanism run under the auspices of the *General Dental Council (GDC) in the UK to help dental patients resolve complaints about private dental care provided by a dentist or *dental care professional. It operates independently of, but is funded by, the GDC. If the staff of the DCS fail to achieve a satisfactory resolution, a local **dental complaints panel** may be set up which will make a recommendation. The panel consists of two lay members (chair and panellist) and a dental practitioner.

(⊕) **SEE WEB LINKS**
• The website of the Dental Complaints Service.

dental dam (rubber dam) A thin sheet of rubber which is pierced by a **dental dam punch** to allow the crowns of one or more teeth to protrude through and provide improved moisture control, operator visibility, airway protection, patient comfort, and infection control. It is manufactured in different thicknesses, colours, and sizes (usually 6-inch square), and may be made of latex or non-latex materials. It is normally supported by a **dental dam frame** and retained on the teeth by dental dam *clamps, floss, or rubber (latex or latex-free) strips. **Dental dam clamp forceps**, the tips of which engage in holes on the clamp, are used to place the clamp on the tooth and subsequently to remove it.

dental floss *n. See* FLOSS.

dental follicle *n.* A fibrous capsule which surrounds the *enamel organ during *tooth germ development. It eventually becomes the *periodontal ligament.

dental formula A method of describing the number and arrangement of teeth in man and animals using letters and figures. It is written as an expression of the number of each type of tooth in one side of the upper jaw over the number of teeth in one side of the lower jaw. The letters correspond to the type of teeth (I = Incisor, C = Canine, P = Premolar, M = Molar). Humans have two dental formulae, one for the primary dentition and one for the permanent dentition. The dental formulae for different animals varies according to diet and function.

Dental formulae of humans and some animals		
Species	Dental formula	Total number of teeth
Human (primary dentition)	I 2/2 C 1/1 M 2/2	20
Human (secondary dentition)	I 2/2 C 1/1 P 2/2 M 3/3	32
Dog	I 3/3 C 1/1 P 4/4 M 2/3	42
Horse	I 3/3 C 1/1 P 4/4 M 3/3	44
Sheep	I 0/3 C 0/1 P 3/3 M 3/3	32
Rat	I 1/1 C 0/0 P 0/0 M 3/3	16

dental health education *See* ORAL HEALTH EDUCATION.

dental health promotion *See* ORAL HEALTH PROMOTION.

dental hygienist A dental care professional statutorily registered in the UK with the *General Dental Council and working to the written prescription of a registered dentist. Their primary clinical remit is the prevention and treatment of *periodontal disease and dental caries by scaling and polishing teeth, applying prophylactic and antibacterial materials, *topical fluoride, and *fissure sealants, and delivering oral health advice. The clinical remit was extended in the UK following legislative changes in 2002, to include taking *impressions, administering inferior dental block *analgesia, temporarily cementing dislodged *crowns, and treating patients under *conscious sedation; these changes are subject to appropriate training. The clinical remit varies in different countries.

(((•))) SEE WEB LINKS
• The British Society of Dental Hygiene and Therapy website; it provides information on the current clinical remit of dental hygienists and therapists.

dental index *See* FLOWER'S DENTAL INDEX.

dental laboratory A location within or external to a dental practice or clinic where custom-made dental *appliances are fabricated which in the UK are manufactured to meet the requirements of the *Medical Devices Directive.

dental lamina *n.* A band of *epithelial tissue which connects the developing *tooth bud (*enamel organ) to the *oral epithelium. The dental lamina eventually disintegrates into small clusters of epithelium and is resorbed.

dental nurse A dental care professional who has received appropriate training to provide chairside assistance for the dentist which includes *aspiration, the preparation of materials, and the passing of instruments. As from July 2008, all dental nurses in the UK who have completed their professional training must be statutorily registered with the *General Dental Council. Dental nurses in the UK may undertake additional post-certification training in dental sedation, special care nursing, oral health, orthodontics, and radiology assessed by the *National Examining Board for Dental Nurses (NEBDN).

(((•))) SEE WEB LINKS
• The British Association of Dental Nurses website.

Dental Nurse Standards and Training Advisory Board (DNSTAB) A General Dental Council advisory body with representatives from dental nursing organizations such as the British Association of Dental Nurses and the National Examining Board for Dental Nurses. This body ceased to exist following the statutory registration of dental nurses in 2008.

dental panoramic tomogram (DPT) *n.* A tomogram or slice through the jaws which displays all the teeth and supporting structures on one film. Only structures within the focal trough will be visualized. The focal trough for a DPT is usually horseshoe-shaped. The image quality is always inferior to that of intra-oral films, and radiographic interpretation needs to take into account tomographic blur and ghost shadows produced by anatomical structures. Formerly known as an **orthopantomogram**.

dental papilla *See* PAPILLA.

Dental Practice Board *See* BUSINESS SERVICES AUTHORITY.

dental practice manager A person responsible for the administration of a clinic or practice. The **Dental Practice Managers Association (DPMA)** is an organization founded in the UK in 1993 to promote the training, career structure, and interests of those who are managing dental practices or clinics.

(((•))) SEE WEB LINKS
• The British Dental Practice Managers Association website.

dental public health The non-clinical specialty of preventing and controlling dental diseases and *oral health promotion, delivered to a target population or a community, on a regional or national basis rather than on an individual patient basis. It involves the *epidemiology of the causes and distribution of oral disease and the assessment of dental health needs and ensuring dental services meet those needs. It is also known as **public health dentistry**.

dental pulp *see* PULP.

dental record *See* CLINICAL RECORD.

Dental Reference Service (DRS) A part of the National Health Service which employs a team of experienced and calibrated dentists (**dental reference officers**) to monitor and advise on quality within the *General and *Personal Dental Services.

Dental Register A list of all dental professionals registered with the *General Dental

Council in the UK, who are thereby legally permitted to practise as a dentist, specialist, or a *dental care professional.

dental tape *See* TAPE, DENTAL.

dental technician A dental care professional who makes custom-made dental appliances including *dentures, *crowns, *bridges, *implants, and *orthodontic appliances. As from July 2008 all dental technicians in the UK must be registered with the *General Dental Council. **Clinical dental technicians** form a new class of dental care professional in the UK and are qualified dental technicians who have received additional training to develop their clinical skills; they are able to provide clinically a range of removeable complete and partial dentures without prior review by a dentist.

((⊕)) SEE WEB LINKS
- The British Dental Technicians Association website.
- The British Clinical Dental Technicians Association website.

dental therapist *See* THERAPIST, DENTAL.

dental unit water lines (DUWLs) Part of a *dental chair unit (DCU) used to provide water to cool and irrigate a variety of DCU-supplied instruments (i.e. turbine and conventional handpieces, ultrasonic scalers, and three-in-one air/water syringes), and tooth surfaces during dental procedures, as the heat generated during instrument operation can be harmful to teeth. DUWLs also supply water used by patients for oral rinsing during and following dental procedures and to rinse the DCU *cuspidor after oral rinsing. Water supplied by DUWLs is frequently contaminated with high densities of micro-organisms, especially bacterial species, due to the formation of *biofilm on the internal surfaces of the waterlines. The waterline network in a DCU consists of several meters of narrow-bore (i.e. a few mm) plastic tubing in which water stagnates when the DCU is not being used. Micro-organisms, in the DCU supply water, attach to the internal surfaces and form microcolonies that eventually give rise to multi-species biofilm. Water at the internal surface of DUWLs flows more slowly than water at the centre and thus there is little disturbance to any micro-organisms present. This allows the micro-organisms to multiply and disperse throughout the waterline network as planktonic forms. Micro-organisms from DUWLs

can be transferred directly into the mouths of patients during dental procedures and can be aerosolized during the operation of high-speed handpieces and ultrasonic scalers. The most common micro-organisms recovered from DUWL output water are aerobic heterotrophic Gram-negative environmental bacterial species, although pathogenic organisms such as *Pseudomonas aeruginosa, Legionella pneumophila*, and non-tuberculosis *Mycobacterium* species can also be present. The presence of high densities of micro-organisms in DUWL output water provides a potential risk of infection of dental patients and healthcare staff and is contrary to good *cross-infection control and prevention practices. Exposure to bacterial *endotoxin in DUWL output water poses additional potential adverse health effects. Biofilm in DUWLs can be effectively controlled by regular disinfection with disinfectants or biocides that effectively remove biofilm. A wide range of such agents are available commercially but only some have been shown to be effective in long-term studies.

Further Reading: Coleman D. C., O'Donnell M. J., Shore A. C., Swan J., Russell, R. J. The role of manufacturers in reducing biofilms in dental unit waterlines. *Journal of Dentistry* 2007;35:701–11.
Pankhurst C. L., Coulter W. A. Do contaminated dental unit waterlines pose a risk of infection? *Journal of Dentistry* 2007;35:712–20.
Walker J. T., Marsh P. D. Microbial biofilm formation in DUWS and their control using disinfectants. *Journal of Dentistry* 2007;35:721–30.

dentate *adj.* Describing the condition of having teeth. *Compare* EDENTULOUS.

dentia praecox Premature tooth eruption.

denticle *n.* 1. A small tooth or tooth-like projection. 2. A calcified mass found in the pulp chamber of a tooth also known as an **endolith** or pulp stone. It may be composed of irregular *dentine (**true denticle**) or an ectopic calcification of pulp tissue (**false denticle**).

denticulate *adj.* Finely toothed, serrated, or notched.

dentifrice *n.* A paste (*toothpaste), powder, or liquid used in conjunction with a *toothbrush to clean teeth and to act as a vehicle for bringing therapeutic agents into contact with the teeth. The constituents of a dentifrice relate to their function. *See also* FLUORIDE TOOTHPASTE, BLEACHING.

The main constituents of a dentifrice and their functions

Function	Example	Action
Abrasive	Sodium bicarbonate Calcium carbonate Sodium chloride Hydrated silica Diatomaceous earth Dicalcium phosphate	Removes plaque and extrinsic stain by abrasive or polishing effect.
Humectant (a substance that retains or attracts water)	Glycerine Sorbitol	Keeps toothpaste moist.
Binding agent	Carboxymethyl cellulose Hydroxyethyl cellulose Carrageenan (a polysaccharide from red seaweed) Cellulose gum	Improves the texture of toothpaste.
Detergent	Sodium lauryl sulphate (SLS) Sodium N-lauryl sarcosinate	Causes toothpaste to foam, assisting the removal of plaque and food debris.
Preservative	Formalin Alcohols Sodium benzoate	Improves the lifespan of the product.
Colouring and flavouring	Peppermint and spearmint Menthol Eucalyptus Aniseed Sodium saccharin Synthetic sugar-free fruit flavours	Improves acceptability of the product.
Water		Improves consistency.
Desensitizing agents	Strontium chloride Strontium acetate Potassium nitrate Potassium citrate	Reduces dentine sensitivity.
Anti-plaque agents	*Triclosan	Antibacterial and reduces plaque build-up.
Anti-calculus agents	Tetrasodium Pyrophosphate Ureate Zinc citrate	Reduces plaque mineralization.
Antacid	Bicarbonates	Raises the pH of plaque.
Fluoride	*Sodium monofluorophosphate *Sodium fluoride	Combines with calcium apatite to form caries resistant calcium fluorapatite.
Whitening agents	*Carbamide peroxide Sodium chlorite Sodium peroxodisulphate Sodium chlorate	Bleaches tooth enamel.

Further Reading: Netuveli G. S., Sheiham A. A systematic review of the effectiveness of anticalculus dentifrices. *Oral Health Prev Dent* 2004;2(1):49–58.

dentigerous *adj.* Containing or bearing teeth. Dentigerous cyst *see* CYST.

dentine (dentin)

n. The mineralized organic tissue that makes up the bulk of the tooth surrounding the *pulp, covered on the root surface by *cementum and on the crown surface by *enamel. It is pale yellow in colour and is harder than bone but not as hard as enamel or cementum. Dentine is 70% inorganic by weight consisting mainly of *calcium hydroxyapatite $[Ca_{10}(PO_4)_6(OH)_2]$ and 20% organic by weight consisting mainly of *collagen. The remaining 10% is water. Dentine is made up of many fine parallel *tubules (**dentinal tubules**) extending from the pulpal surface to the *amelodentinal junction. Each tubule contains an *odontoblast cell lying in a layer on the pulpal surface with the nucleus situated at the pulpal end of each cell. Each odontoblast cell has a process extending along the tubule and is surrounded by intercellular ground substance. Dentine may be divided into intertubular dentine and peritubular dentine. **Intertubular dentine** is the main product of the odontoblasts constituting the largest volume of the dentine; it consists of a fibrous network of collagen with deposited mineral crystals. The **peritubular** (**intratubular**) **dentine** forms a highly mineralized sheath about 0.5–1.0μ thick around the dentinal tubule consisting mainly of crystals of carbonated apatite together with a small amount of collagen. The peritubular dentine is sensitive to various external stimuli although sensitivity is not uniform in either teeth or individuals. *See* DENTINE HYPERSENSITIVITY. Dentine formation (*dentinogenesis) begins at about the 14th week of intrauterine life (late *bell stage) when the *inner enamel epithelium induces cells at the periphery of the *dental papilla to differentiate into dentine-forming columnar odontoblast cells. These cells secrete an unmineralized **dentine matrix** (**predentine**) as they retreat towards the pulp. When the predentine reaches a thickness of about 5μ *mineralization starts to occur with the formation of spherical areas of calcium hydroxyapatite (*calcospherites) which eventually fuse together to form the mineralized dentine layer (**primary dentine**), the outer layer being known as **mantle dentine** and the inner layer **circumpulpal** dentine. With age, more dentine continues to be laid down (**secondary dentine**) at the pulpal surface of the primary dentine, thus reducing the size of the pulp chamber. In response to caries, the odontoblasts lay down more dentine (**tertiary** or **irregular secondary dentine**) which contains fewer tubules and more mineral than primary dentine and appears transparent in ground section. It is therefore also known as **transparent** or **sclerotic dentine**. Tertiary dentine may be laid down by primary odontoblasts in response to a mild stimulus (**reactionary dentine**) or laid down by secondary odontoblasts derived from differentiated pulpal cells (**reparative dentine**). **Porotic dentine** in which the dentine becomes porous may occur in conjunction with *vitamin C deficiency. *See also* CARIES.

dentine adhesion The ability of a material to stick to dentine. Because traditional resin-based materials are *hydrophobic and dentine, which is 70% organic, is also primarily *hydrophilic, a bifunctional monomer such as *HEMA is used which has a hydrophilic terminal capable of intimately bonding with the dentine surface and a hydrophobic terminal which can co-polymerize with the resin component of the restorative material. The surface layer of the dentine is usually first *conditioned to remove the loose *smear layer and some of the mineral content, to expose the collagen fibres. The adhesive agent can then form a micro-mechanical bond around the exposed dentine surface (*hybrid layer).

Further Reading: Moszner N., Salz U., Zimmermann J. Chemical aspects of self-etching enamel-dentin adhesives: a systematic review. *Dent Mater* 2005;21(10):895–910.

dentine bonding *n. See* DENTINE ADHESION.

dentine bridge *n.* A thin layer of secondary dentine which forms over an exposed pulp or after a *pulpotomy creating a protective pulpal barrier. Formation is usually stimulated by the presence of *calcium hydroxide.

dentine dysplasia *n.* A defect in dentine development that is inherited as an autosomal dominant trait, affecting either the primary or the primary and permanent (secondary) dentitions. It is classified into two types. In type I the tooth crown has a normal appearance but there is no or rudimentary root development and incomplete or total obliteration of the pulp chamber; in type II the primary teeth have a brown or bluish discoloration with pulpal obliteration and the permanent teeth have normal sized roots with an enlarged, thistle-tube-shaped pulp chamber. Treatment involves the removal of pain, improvement of aesthetics, and protection of the posterior teeth from wear. *See also* DENTINOGENESIS IMPERFECTA.

dentine hypersensitivity

A condition often resulting in pain caused by exposure of dentine to external stimuli. Such stimuli may involve tissue loss and exposure of dentinal tubules (e.g. loss of enamel and cementum or gingival recession), opening up of dentinal tubules without tissue loss (e.g. by the removal of the smear layer during a restorative procedure, acid in dental plaque, diet, gastric reflux, agents in a dentifrice, or vital bleaching), by an inappropriate tooth brushing technique, or as a result of temperature change (e.g. cold drinks, ice cream, cold weather etc.). Dentine hypersensitivity is a common occurrence following root *debridement and *bleaching procedures. The mechanism transmitting the sensation through the dentine to the pulp is not thoroughly understood in spite of numerous research studies. Current theories include the belief that nerve fibres of the *pulp pass into the dentinal tubules (**innervation theory**), that *odontoblasts act as receptors, transmitting nerve impulses (**odontoblast receptor theory**), or that there is fluid movement within the dentinal tubules (**hydrodynamic theory**).

d

Treatment strategies for dentine hypersensitivity

Treatment strategies for dentine hypersensitivity

Level 1	Treatment applied at home by the patient: • oral hygiene instruction and dietary advice • home use of fluoride gels/mouth rinses • anti-hypersensitivity toothpastes
Level 2	In-office treatment to occlude the tubules: • gels, varnishes, *iontophoresis • primers containing hydroxyethyl methacrylate (*HEMA)
Level 3	In-office treatment to occlude and seal the tubules: • *glass ionomer and adhesive resin systems

In-office treatment

1A Varnishes and precipitants	Shellacs 5% sodium fluoride varnish 0.4% stannous fluoride, 0.14% hydrofluoric acid solutions 3% mono-potassium-monohydrogen oxalate 6% acid ferric oxalate calcium phosphate preparations calcium hydroxide
1B Primers containing hydroxyethyl methacrylate (HEMA)	5% gluteraldehyde 35% HEMA in water
2 Treatment agents that undergo setting or polymerization reactions	Conventional glass ionomer cements Resin-reinforced glass ionomers/compomers Adhesive resin primers Adhesive resin bonding systems

3 Use of mouth guards with various gels
4 Iontophoresis
5 *Lasers

Pashley D. H., Potential treatment modalities for dentine hypersensitivity: in-office products. In *Tooth wear and sensitivity: Clinical Advances in Restorative Dentistry*, ed. Addy, Embry, Edgar, Orchardson, 2000, London: Martin Dunnitz; 351–365.

Treatment strategies may be professionally undertaken or home-based by the application of desensitizing agents such as topical fluoride varnish, potassium chloride, strontium chloride, magnesium sulphate, calcium silicate, and strontium acetate.

Further Reading: Addy M. Dentine hypersensitivity: new perspectives on an old problem. *Int Dent J* 2002;5:367–75.

Canadian Advisory Board on Dentine Hypersensitivity. Consensus based recommendations for the diagnosis and management of dentine hypersensitivity. *J Can Dent Assoc* 2003;69(4):221–6.

dentine pin *n. See* PIN.

dentinogenesis *n.* The process of dentine formation. *See also* DENTINE.

dentinogenesis imperfecta A hereditary condition affecting the formation of *dentine. It can affect both primary and secondary (permanent) teeth. It is characterized by early calcification of the *pulp chamber and canals and dark opalescent yellow or grey discoloration of the teeth. Although the teeth are structurally normal on eruption, early loss of enamel leads to marked attrition. Three types are recognized: Type 1 is associated with weak and brittle bones (osteogenesis imperfecta); Type 2 dentinogenesis imperfecta only; and Type 3 a rare isolate found in North America. Treatment involves the restoration of function and aesthetics usually by means of *onlays or *crowns. *See also* AMELOGENESIS IMPERFECTA.

(((⊕))) **SEE WEB LINKS**

• Information on the genetic cause of dentinogenesis imperfecta from the US National Library of Medicine.

dentinogenic ghost cell tumour A rare malignant *neoplasm of *odontogenic epithelium and mesenchyme characterized by the formation of ghost cells and dentine-like material.

dentinoid *adj.* resembling dentine; calcified material that is associated with odontogenic epithelium. It may or may not contain tubules.

dentinoma *n.* Now not thought to exist. Most are considered to be *ameloblastic fibrodentinoma.

dentiparous *adj.* Tooth-bearing.

dentist *n.* A member of the dental profession who in the UK must be registered with the *General Dental Council.

dentistry *n.* The study, management, and treatment of conditions and diseases affecting the teeth, jaws, and oral structures. Sub-specialities are *dental public health, *endodontics, *implantology, *oral medicine, *oral surgery, *oral pathology, *orthodontics, *paediatric dentistry, *periodontology, *preventive dentistry, *primary dental care, *prosthodontics, and *restorative dentistry.

Dentists Act An act of parliament first introduced in 1878 to regulate the dental profession in the UK by introducing voluntary registration of dentists with the General Medical Council. A new act was passed in 1921 which made it mandatory for newly qualified dentists to register with the Dental Board of the UK. The Dentists Act 1956 established the *General Dental Council, which replaced the Dental Board. The Dentists Act 1984, together with the Dental Auxiliaries Regulations 1986, provided for the enrolment and regulation of dental therapists and dental hygienists. The Dentists Act 1984 (Amendment) Order 2005 introduced compulsory indemnity cover and allowed the General Dental Council to regulate the whole dental team, including dental nurses and dental technicians, and to take action in cases of poor professional performance.

(((⊕))) **SEE WEB LINKS**

• The Dentists Act 1984 (Amendment) Order 2005 Transitional Provisions Order of Council 2006.

Dentists Health Support Programme A confidential and independent UK organization (formerly known as 'The Sick Dentist Scheme'), formed to identify and support dentists who may be impaired by dependency or addiction to alcohol or other drugs through a system of investigation, verification, intervention, referral for treatment, post-treatment support, and monitoring.

(((⊕))) **SEE WEB LINKS**

• The National Clinical Assessment Service Resource Directory.

Dentists with Special Interests (DwSI) A category of dentists, defined by the Department of Health in the UK, working in the primary care setting who provide services which are in addition to their usual and important generalist role. The DwSI provides a service which is complementary to the secondary services but does not replace that provided by a dentist who has undergone the training required for entry to a specialist list. The DwSI is an independent practitioner who works within the limits of their competency in providing a special interest service, and who refers on where necessary. The DwSI may deliver a clinical service beyond that normally provided by a primary dental care practitioner or may deliver a particular type of treatment. Special interests may be demonstrated by dentists through completion of formal training programmes and/or experience-based evidence.

dentition

n. The arrangement of the teeth in the mouth. The **primary (deciduous) dentition** when complete consists of 20 teeth made up of two molars, one canine and two incisors in each quadrant. Eruption starts at about 6 months of age and is normally complete after 2–2½ years. Initial mineralization starts at about 4 months in utero with the maxillary incisors; the molars are the last of the primary teeth to complete root formation at about 3 years of age. The primary teeth are shed (exfoliated) from about 6–7 years, starting with the maxillary incisors, and total exfoliation is normally complete by about 13–14 years. During this period both primary and permanent teeth are present (**mixed dentition**). One or more permanent successors are sometimes absent leading to the primary teeth being retained into adult life. The **permanent dentition** consists of 32 teeth made up of three molars, two premolars, one canine, and two incisors in each quadrant. The first tooth to erupt is the first molar at about 6–7 years of age; it erupts behind the second primary molar. Eruption of the remaining teeth is normally completed by 14–15 years of age except for the third molars (wisdom teeth) which usually erupt between 18–25 years of age but can be considerably delayed. Eruption may be considerably delayed or prevented by

The development of the primary dentition

Arch	Tooth	Initial mineralization (months in utero)	Eruption date (in months)	Root completion date (in years)
	central incisor	4	7	1½
	lateral incisor	4½	8	2
	canine	5	18	3
Maxillary	first molar	5	14	2½
	second molar	6	24	3
	central incisor	4½	6	1½
	lateral incisor	4½	7	1¾
Mandibular	canine	5	16	3
	first molar	5	12	2½
	second molar	6	20	3

The development of the permanent dentition

Arch	Tooth	Initial mineralization	Eruption date (in years)	Root completion date (in years)
Maxillary	central incisor	3–4 months	7–8	10
	lateral incisor	10–12 months	8–9	11
	canine	4–5 months	11–12	13–15
	first premolar	1½–2 years	10–11	12–13
	second premolar	2 years	10–12	12–14
	first molar	birth	6–7	9–10
	second molar	2½–3 years	12–13	14–16
	third molar	7–9 years	17–21	18–25+
Mandibular	central incisor	3–4 months	6–7	9–10
	lateral incisor	3–4 months	7–8	10
	canine	4–5 months	9–10	12–14
	first premolar	1½–2 years	10–12	12–13
	second premolar	2 years	11–12	13–14
	first molar	birth	6–7	9–10
	second molar	2½–3 years	12–13	14–15
	third molar	8–10 years	17–21	18–25

impaction against an adjacent tooth, sometimes justifying *dentoalveolar surgery to remove the impacted tooth to prevent soft tissue infection, dental caries of the adjacent molar, or fracture of the jaw where facial trauma may be an occupational hazard e.g. contact sports, military personnel. *See also* PRIMARY DENTITION; PERMANENT DENTITION; SUPERNUMERARY TOOTH; SUPPLEMENTAL TOOTH.

dentoalveolar surgery Surgery involving the teeth and supporting structures including alveolar bone.

dentomycin *n. See* MINOCYCLINE.

dentulous *n.* Having natural teeth present in the mouth. *Compare* EDENTULOUS.

denture *n.* An artificial replacement (*prosthesis) for missing natural teeth and their supporting structures. A **complete denture** (full denture) replaces all the natural teeth and supporting structures in either the *mandible or *maxilla. It may be retained by a combination of muscular action and adhesion to the mucosal surface or by *endosteal or *sub-periosteal implants. A **copy denture** (**duplicate denture**) is a second denture intended to be a duplicate of the first denture, possibly including correction of discrepancies in the fitting surface, usually due to tissue change, or the occlusal surfaces, usually due to tooth wear (attrition). Copy dentures are particularly relevant for elderly patients who tolerate changes in the denture shape less readily. A **partial denture** replaces one or more but not all natural teeth and their supporting structures. It may be supported entirely on the soft tissues (**tissue-borne**) or entirely on the teeth (**tooth-borne**) or a combination of both. A denture may be made of resin only, usually *polymethylmethacrylate, or resin and metal where the metal is usually *cobalt–chromium alloy; the teeth are made of resin or *porcelain. A **skeleton denture** is mainly tooth-borne and has small size metal connectors leaving the mucous membrane and gingival margins largely exposed. An

immediate denture, which may be complete or partial, is constructed to replace teeth immediately after their extraction. Immediate dentures may be designed so that the replacement teeth are adapted to fit over the residual sockets on the alveolar ridge (open face) or with a buccal or labial extension of the acrylic resin base adjacent to the extracted teeth (flanged). A **spoon denture** is a form of upper partial denture supported entirely on the soft tissues (**tissue-borne**) such that the resin baseplate extends over the hard palate in the shape of a spoon and does not cover the gingival margins. A **swinglock denture** is a type of denture which has a labial retaining bar or flange which is hinged at one side of the mouth and locks at the other. The labial bar can be unlocked during insertion and locked after insertion. A denture worn for a limited period of time (**interim, provisional,** or **transitional denture**) is designed to restore aesthetics, function, or occlusal support, usually while tissue healing is taking place.

Further Reading: Lynch C. D., Allen P. F. The swing-lock denture: its use in conventional removable partial denture prosthodontics. *Dent Update* 2004;31(9):506–8.

(((⊕))) SEE WEB LINKS

• The Eastman Dental Institute self-assessment test on partial denture design.

denture-bearing area Those surfaces of the teeth and edentulous ridges covered by a denture.

denture cleanser A chemical powder, tablet, or liquid used to remove surface deposits and stains from removable dentures. Hard deposits may be removed by an effervescent action. Denture cleaning powders contain an abrasive which can result in excessive abrasion of the resin surfaces. Cleansing chemicals are usually *alkaline containing *sodium perborate, sodium bicarbonate, or sodium percarbonate. Solutions containing dilute phosphoric, hydrochloric, or acetic acid can damage the metal components of dentures. Household bleaching agents degrade the acrylic resin and can be detrimental to both denture fit and aesthetics. *Hypochlorite solutions are effective for acrylic dentures when immersed

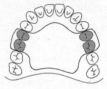

Tissue-borne

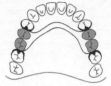

Tooth-borne skeleton

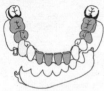

Swinglock

Types of removable denture

overnight, but if used with hot water are liable to cause bleaching. Some cleansers utilize the additional action of an *ultrasonic cleaning bath. Trade names: **Steradent**°, **Denclen**°.

denture construction The process of fabricating a denture which involves the dentist at the chairside and the dental technician in the laboratory. It is normally undertaken in a series of clinical stages which may include primary impressions for the purpose of constructing individually fabricated impression trays, secondary impressions taken in the individually fabricated trays, registration of the jaw relationship including the selection of the tooth shade and mould, trying in the denture with the teeth accurately located in a wax base, and finally fitting the finished appliance. Additional stages may be required for dentures which have a metal framework. Some stages may be omitted in the construction of immediate dentures. Between each clinical stage, the required denture construction is normally undertaken by a dental technician in the laboratory.

denture flask *n. See* FLASK.

denture granuloma *See* EPULIS.

denture repair The process of reuniting broken parts of a denture, usually by using a cold cure *polymethylmethacrylate denture base resin, commonly undertaken in a dental laboratory.

denture space That part of the oral cavity limited by the tongue, lips, and cheeks and the residual alveolar ridges, which the denture teeth and supporting structure should occupy.

denture stomatitis (denture sore mouth) An inflammatory condition of the *oral mucosa associated with the wearing of *dentures and the presence of *Candida* species. It is characterized by severe *erythema and *oedema of the denture-bearing area of the oral mucosa, occurring most frequently on the palate beneath a complete upper denture. Fungal infection may be evident in the form of asymptomatic white surface colonies. Risk factors associated with the condition are age-related chronic disease and drug therapy. Treatment is by improving denture hygiene, correcting any denture defects and the provision of antifungal therapy such as *nystatin.

denturist *n.* A dental technician specializing in making and fitting dentures as a direct service to the public rather than through a licensed or registered dentist. Denturists are not licensed to practise in some countries.

deoxyribonucleic acid (DNA) *n.* The genetic material for nearly all living organisms.

It is a large double-stranded helical molecule found within the nucleus of a cell. The **DNA probe test** is a method by which known periodontal *pathogens can be identified by comparing the DNA on the cell walls of bacteria in *plaque samples with reference DNA in the laboratory. It is designed to facilitate the choice of *antibiotic therapy.

Department of Health (DH) A government department responsible for healthcare policies and obligations which include the *National Health Service (NHS) and the promotion and protection of health for both individuals and the community.

dependence (drug dependence) *n.* The level of drug addiction or substance abuse at which severe physiological symptoms will occur if use of the drug is suddenly withdrawn. *See also* DRUG.

dependent variable *n. See* VARIABLE.

depolarization *n.* The rapid movement of charged particles across a semi-permeable membrane of a nerve or muscle cell to cancel out or reverse its testing potential and produce an *action potential. A nerve impulse is a process of rapid depolarization along the membrane of a nerve fibre.

depression *n.* 1. A mental state characterized by a pessimistic sense of inadequacy and a despondent lack of activity. 2. A pitted area on an anatomical structure such as a tooth. **Mandibular depression** is the lowering of the mandible caused by a rotational movement of the *temporomandibular joint.

dermatitis *n.* An inflammatory condition of the skin caused by outside agents. It most commonly affects the hands of dental personnel because of the use of gloves, soaps, and detergents (occupational dermatitis). *See also* LATEX ALLERGY. **Dermatitis artefacta (factitial dermatitis)** is a self-inflicted injury to the skin. It occurs more frequently in females than males with the majority of cases occurring in adolescence; it is usually associated with an underlying psychological problem. The lesions produced are commonly due to a sharp instrument, caustic chemicals, or burning. It can be associated with the oral tissues (**stomatitis artefacta**) or more specifically with the gingival tissues (*gingivitis artefacta). **Dermatitis herpetiformis** is an autoimmune blistering disorder affecting the skin and occasionally the oral mucosa. It is associated with gluten hypersensivity in the small bowel. *See also* COELIAC DISEASE. **Radiation dermatitis** is an inflammatory condition of the skin, usually seen as an undesirable side-effect of *radiation therapy for malignant tumours. It is initially characterized by a reddening of the skin, which may be followed by loss of hair, decreased sweating, swelling, ulceration, bleeding, and skin rashes.

dermatomyositis n. An uncommon autoimmune disorder characterized by skin rashes and muscular weakness. Oral manifestations may include localized areas of *desquamative gingivitis and lesions similar to *lichen planus.

dermatostomatitis n. See STEVENS-JOHNSON SYNDROME.

dermis n. A layer of dense connective tissue lying below the *epidermis. It contains nerve endings, blood vessels, and glandular tissue.

dermoid n. See CYST.

desensitization n. 1. A process by which the effects of a known *allergen are reduced by injecting gradually increasing amounts of the allergen over a period of time. 2. The reduction of *dentine hypersensitivity.

desensitizing agent A solution, gel, or varnish applied topically to a sensitive area of a tooth. See also DENTINE HYPERSENSITIVITY.

desiccate v. To dry by physical or chemical means. It can occur in *glass-ionomer restorations when isolated from contact with *saliva.

desmodontium n. See PERIODONTAL LIGAMENT.

desmosome n. Part of the protein cell structure specialized for cell-to-cell adhesion which resists shearing forces. They are found in simple and stratified squamous *epithelium such as the gingival epithelium. See also HEMIDESMOSOME.

desquamation n. The process in which the outer layer of *epidermal tissue or *mucosa is lost or removed by scaling. See also GINGIVITIS, DESQUAMATIVE.

detergent n. A synthetic water-soluble cleaning agent capable of reacting with and removing oil, grease, and suspended particles on a surface. Some detergents also contain an *antiseptic or *disinfectant.

determinants of health The factors which contribute to maintaining and improving health and wellbeing. These include individual lifestyle factors such as diet and smoking, social and community networks, and general socioeconomic, cultural, and environmental conditions.

detrition n. The wearing away by friction as in the *attrition of teeth.

developer n. An alkaline solution which converts sensitized silver halide crystals on a radiographic film to black metallic silver. It should be protected from daylight.

developmental tooth anomalies A variety of inherited or acquired disturbances of the teeth. Disturbances occurring early in tooth formation affect the shape, number, or size of tooth. See ANODONTIA; HYPODONTIA; SUPERNUMERARY TEETH. Those occurring later during hard tissue formation result in disturbances of tooth structure. See AMELOGENESIS IMPERFECTA; DENTINOGENESIS IMPERFECTA.

devitalization n. See PULP DEVITALIZATION.

dextran n. A soluble carbohydrate made up of branched chains of glucose units. It is a storage product of bacteria and yeasts. Dental *plaque is rich in dextrans. See also LEVAN.

dextrose n. A naturally occurring monosaccharide sugar similar to glucose found in honey and sweet fruits such as grapes.

diabetes n. (adj. n. **diabetic**) Any metabolic disorder characterized by excessive thirst and the production of large volumes of urine. **Diabetes insipidus** is a rare condition characterized by frequent and heavy urination, excessive thirst, and an overall feeling of weakness. It is caused by a deficiency of the *pituitary hormone *vasopressin (anti-diuretic hormone). Unlike diabetes mellitus, the blood sugar level is normal. **Diabetes mellitus** is a chronic metabolic disorder in which sugars are not metabolized to produce energy, due to a deficiency of the pancreatic hormone *insulin. The condition is characterized by thirst, loss of energy, excessive production of urine, and high blood sugar (*hyperglycaemia). Because of the breakdown of fats instead of sugars there is an excess of ketones in the bloodstream which can lead to **diabetic coma**. The features of oral significance are a decreased *salivary flow, leading to a susceptibility to *caries, tooth *erosion due to gastrointestinal disturbances, slow wound healing, and a potential for periodontal problems due to microvascular changes. Diabetes mellitus can significantly increase the loss of attachment of the periodontal tissues, which can begin as early as 6–11 years of age. Diabetes which occurs in childhood is known as **type 1** or **insulin-dependent diabetes mellitus** and is usually more severe than that beginning in later life; patients are dependent on insulin injections for survival. In **type 2** (**non-insulin dependent** or **maturity-onset**) diabetes mellitus, which usually occurs after the age of 40, the pancreas is capable of producing some insulin but it is insufficient to meet the body's requirements; alternatively, the body develops insulin resistance. Evidence suggests that *periodontitis is often more severe in patients with diabetes mellitus.

Further reading: Fiske J. Diabetes mellitus and oral care. *Dent Update* 2004;31:190–198.

diagnosis *n.* The process of arriving at the nature of a disease or condition from consideration of the patient's *signs and *symptoms and when appropriate, any additional diagnostic tests such as *radiographs, *biopsy, and blood or saliva analysis. The diagnosis of a condition or disease often involves comparison with other conditions which produce similar signs or symptoms (**differential diagnosis**).

diagnostic cast *n.* See CAST.

dialysis *n.* The process of separating out unwanted substances from a fluid using a semi-permeable membrane. This principle is the basis of filtering the *blood using an artificial kidney (**kidney dialysis**).

diamond *n.* A crystalline carbon substance used in particulate form as an abrasive material on rotary instruments for cutting or grinding, such as diamond-coated *burs and wheels.

diapedesis *n.* The migration of cells through the walls of blood capillaries. It is an important part of the inflammatory reaction of tissues to injury.

diaphragm *n.* 1. (in anatomy) A thin musculo-membranous layer or septum separating the abdominal and thoracic cavities. 2. (in dentistry) A thin metal covering over a tooth root usually forming part of an artificial crown. 3. (in radiography) A *collimation device, usually made of lead, with a small opening designed to restrict the size of the x-ray beam.

diarthrosis *n.* See JOINT.

diastema *n.* An unusually large space between two adjacent teeth. A **median diastema** is situated in the midline of the dental arch between the central incisors and is often *hereditary. A median diastema may be caused by small teeth in large jaws, missing teeth, a midline supernumerary tooth, proclination of the upper anterior teeth, or a prominent fraenum.

diastole *n.* (*adj.* **diastolic**) The period during the cardiac cycle when the heart muscle relaxes between two contractions and the chambers fill with blood. See also BLOOD.

diathermy *n.* See ELECTROSURGERY.

diatomaceous earth (kieselguhr) A naturally occurring sedimentary rock consisting mainly of silica, used as a filler and a polishing or abrasive agent.

diatoric *adj.* Describing an artificial porcelain tooth with holes at its base and extending into the body of the tooth through which the denture base material flows, serving as a mechanical means of attachment of the tooth to the denture base. Also called a **pinless tooth**.

diazepam *n.* A long-acting *benzodiazepine used to treat acute anxiety and as a *pre-medication. It can be given orally or by injection. It is metabolized by the liver and excreted by the kidneys. It has been used as an intravenous sedative and a hypnotic in dentistry since the 1960s but is now rarely used because of its very long *half-life.

dichotomous *adj.* Dividing into two distinct parts or classifications e.g. a dichotomous *variable.

die *n.* A positive reproduction of the form of a tooth or tooth preparation in a suitable hard substance on which inlays or crowns may be constructed. It is usually made out of metal or dental *stone. Dies are usually created in the dental laboratory by pouring the hard material into an impression; they are usually removable from within a *cast. **Die stone** is an alpha modified derivative of calcium sulphate hemihydrate formed by boiling gypsum in a 30% aqueous solution of calcium and magnesium chloride; this produces a hard material with compact particles capable of producing a high degree of accuracy during fabrication.

diet *n.* The nutritional intake of a person. A **balanced diet** contains the correct proportions of nutrients necessary to provide the essential requirements of the body. A balanced diet should include *proteins, *fats, *carbohydrates, *vitamins, *minerals, and water. When one or more essential nutrients are absent, or there is inadequate absorption from the gastrointestinal tract, *malnutrition can occur. Lysine (an essential amino acid) deficiency in the form of lysine decarboxylase activity has been implicated in mild gingivitis. A **cariogenic diet** is one high in refined carbohydrates or *non-milk extrinsic sugars (NMES). See also HIDDEN SUGAR. The diet may be monitored using a **diet diary**, a record of all food and drink consumed by an individual over a specified period of time. It is used as a basis for providing dietary advice, particularly where there is a high incidence of caries. The diary usually covers a three-day period, of which one day is a Saturday or Sunday. It provides a means of identifying the frequency, consistency, and quantity of caries-inducing foodstuffs and is most accurate when recorded contemporaneously.

dietary analysis The comparison of an individual's typical food intake against a defined set of dietary guidelines for the purpose of providing advice and guidance.

dietary reference values An estimate of the range of requirements of nutrients for a population or group. They are intended as guidance for the scientific basis of food counselling, meal provision, and food labelling.

dietician *n.* 1. A healthcare professional trained to provide advice and management on the nutritional intake of an individual or group. 2. (in America) An individual who meets the requirements of the **American Dietetic Association** (ADA).

Difflam *n. See* BENZYDAMINE HYDROCHLORIDE.

diffusion hypoxia *n. See* HYPOXIA.

digestion *n.* The process whereby food in the *gastrointestinal tract is converted into a form in which it can be absorbed by the body. It is both mechanical and chemical. The mechanical process starts in the mouth with *mastication involving the action of chewing, churning, and grinding ingested food. The chemical process starts in the mouth with salivary enzyme action but principally occurs in the stomach and small intestine.

digital imaging The process of producing an image in numerical form. Such images are used for the storage of clinical data such as radiographs (digital *radiography) and photographs. Digital images exist either as **vector graphics** (used mainly in professional graphics applications), storing information about the lines and colours of an image as a mathematical definition, or as **bitmap images** (used mainly on personal computers) composed of small rectangular blocks of colour (or greyscale) called **pixels**. Clinical digital images may be captured using a digital camera or video camera or may be digitized from a non-digital medium such as a referral letter using a device such as a scanner.

Further Reading: Turner J. Digital imaging: An update. *Dent Update* 2008;35:385–395.

digital radiography *See* RADIOGRAPHY.

digit sucking The habit of inserting a thumb or fingers into the mouth between the maxillary and mandibular teeth, most commonly practised

by babies and infants. It may result in a localized *malocclusion of either the primary or permanent dentition, usually resulting in an anterior *open bite, and in severe cases changes to the roof of the mouth. The malocclusion can also lead to a speech impediment. The habit is associated with comfort and relaxation and may be adopted to induce sleep. Digit sucking usually ceases naturally without external intervention prior to the eruption of the permanent dentition (between the ages of 2 and 4), but it can persist into adult life. 📷

Further Reading: Warren J. J., Slayton R. L., Bishara S. E., Levy S. M., Yonezu T., Kanellis M. J. Effects of non-nutritive sucking habits on occlusal characteristics in the mixed dentition. *Pediatr Dent* 2005;27(6):445–50.

diglossia *n.* A developmental condition in which the tongue is divided longitudinally for a certain distance, resulting in a bifid tongue.

digoxin *n.* A cardiac glycoside that increases heart muscle contraction and decreases the conductivity within the *atrioventricular node. It is used in the treatment of supraventricular tachycardias and especially for the management of atrial fibrillation.

dilaceration *n.* (*adj.* **dilacerate**) A distortion of the root of a tooth which has occurred during *tooth development. It occurs most commonly in the upper central *incisors as a result of trauma to the primary predecessors, causing them to be driven into the alveolus and striking against the underlying unerupted developing tooth.

dimensional change An alteration in the volumetric shape of a material, usually in response to a change in temperature or a chemical reaction e.g. the shrinkage of metal castings on cooling or the polymerization of resin.

diodontic implant *See* IMPLANT.

diphtheria *n.* An upper respiratory tract infection caused by strains of the facultatively anaerobic, Gram-positive bacterium *Corynebacterium diphtheriae* lysogenized with *bacteriophage encoding the diphtheria toxin gene. The disease is highly contagious and is characterized by sore throat, fever, and an adherent membrane on the tonsils, pharynx, or nose. A milder form of diphtheria is restricted to the skin. Diphtheria has been largely eradicated in developed countries through vaccination.

diphyodont *adj.* Describing the development of two successive *dentitions, one primary and another secondary (permanent), as found in most mammals including humans.

diplegia *n.* Paralysis affecting both sides of the body.

diplococcus *n.* Any of a group of non-motile spherical *bacteria that occur in pairs e.g. pneumococcus.

diplopia *n.* Double vision. It can be a complication following fracture of the *zygomatic bone and sometimes an unwanted side-effect of local anaesthesia in the upper arch.

diprotodont *adj.* Describing members of the marsupial order, which have two lower incisors.

direct inlay technique A method of constructing an inlay or casting by means of preparing a wax pattern taken directly into a tooth preparation in the mouth, as opposed to carving the wax pattern on a model made from a tooth impression.

disability *n.* The loss or restriction of functional ability or activity as a result of physical or mental impairment. The social model defines disability as the loss or limitation of opportunity to take part in the normal life of the community on an equal level with others owing to physical and social barriers. Under the *Disability Discrimination Act, a disabled person is described as 'a person who has or has had a physical or mental impairment which has a substantial and long-term adverse effect upon his or her ability to carry out normal day to day duties'. *See also* HANDICAP; IMPAIRMENT.

Disability Discrimination Act (DDA) 1995 A UK act of parliament which makes it unlawful to discriminate by actions or attitudes against people with disabilities in relation to employment, the provision of goods and services, education, and transport. Under the final part of the act, which came into effect in 2004, service providers such as dentists are required to assess obstacles and make reasonable adjustments to the physical features of their practices or clinics to overcome physical barriers such as the provision of ramps, lifts, and communication aids.

Further reading: Dougall A, Fiske J. Access to special care dentistry, part 1. Access. *Br Dent J* 2008;204:605–616.
Qureshi B, Scambler S. The Disability Discrimination Act and access; practical suggestions. *Dent Update* 2008; 35:627–635.

disaccharide *n.* A carbohydrate made up of two *monosaccharide units. The most common disaccharides are *lactose, *maltose, and *sucrose.

disc (disk) *n.* A thin flat circular object having abrasive particles on one or both surfaces used for smoothing or polishing. The abrasive particles are usually *carborundum, garnet, *diamond, or *silica.

disclosing agent A tablet or liquid which when applied to the tooth surface renders bacterial *plaque more visible. An erythrosine dye stains plaque red but two tone solutions stain older plaque blue and more recent plaque red. Aniline dye is thought by some authorities to be *carcinogenic and is not recommended, though the research data is inconclusive. Organic food colourants are also effective plaque disclosing agents. 📷

Further Reading: Kieser J. B., Wade A. B. Use of food colourants as plaque disclosing agents. *J Clin Periodontol* 1976;3(4):200–07.

disclosing wax *n. See* WAX.

disclusion *n.* The separation of the opposing *occlusal surfaces of the upper and lower teeth by movement of the *mandible.

discoid *adj.* Describing an object which is disc-like. Discoid hand *carvers with a disc-like blade are used for contouring *amalgam or removing *caries. *See also* EXCAVATOR.

discrete variable *n. See* VARIABLE.

disease *n.* Any illness or abnormal condition of the body with a specific cause (which may or may not be known), excluding physical trauma, that has recognizable *signs and *symptoms.

disease determinants The factors that influence a disease in an individual or population. They can be divided into social, environmental, and political (e.g. physical environment, social inequality, social support), behavioural and individual (e.g. *alcohol consumption, physical inactivity), clinical and physiological (e.g. high blood pressure, obesity), genetic (normal or abnormal genes), and health outcomes.

disinfectant *n.* An agent that destroys or removes *pathogenic organisms, not usually including bacterial spores, and is used in dentistry to clean surgical and other dental instruments and dental equipment such as chair, operating light, and work surfaces. Chemical disinfectants are used mainly to disinfect items of technical work such as dental impressions before sending them to the laboratory. Commonly used disinfectants can be broadly divided into alcohols such as ethyl and iso-propyl alcohol which require wet contact for at least 3 minutes, *quaternary ammonium compounds such as *cetylpyridinium chloride which are rapidly inactivated by organic material, and halogens, such as chlorine-containing agents, which are both bactericidal and virucidal but are corrosive to metals and inactivated by organic matter. Cetylpyridinium chloride is an active ingredient in some mouthwashes.

Further Reading: Bebermeyer R. D., Dickinson S. K., Thomas L. P. Chemical disinfectants in dental practice—a review. *Tex Dent J* 2005;122(10):1038–43.

disinfection *n*. The process of removing pathogenic organisms from instruments and equipment by the use of a *disinfectant. It may be achieved by using moist heat (washing and rinsing in water at 70°C–90°C (58°F–194°F) will kill most non-sporing micro-organisms), ultraviolet radiation, filtration, gases, and chemical disinfectants. Moist heat and chemical disinfectants are the most appropriate for clinical dental practice.

Further Reading: Bonsor S. J., Pearson G. J. Current clinical applications of photo-activated disinfection in restorative dentistry. *Dent Update* 2006;33(3):143–4, 147–50, 153.

disinfection, full mouth The process of removing all pathogenic bacteria from the mouth within a short space of time to reduce the risk of re-infection of treated periodontitis-affected sites. It involves complete root surface *debridement of all natural teeth present in the oral cavity, carried out within a 24-hour period, supplemented by *systemic antibiotic therapy. It is usually carried out over one or two clinical sessions and may be indicated for aggressive periodontitis and multiple periodontal abscesses. The evidence for the additional benefit of antiseptic use is currently inconclusive.

Further Reading: Eberhard J., Jepsen S., Jervøe-Storm P.-M., Needleman I., Worthington H. V. Full-mouth disinfection for the treatment of adult chronic periodontitis. *Cochrane Database of Systematic Reviews* 2008, Issue 1. Art. No.: CD004622. DOI: 10.1002/14651858.CD004622.pub2

Farman M., Joshi R. I. Full-mouth treatment versus quadrant root surface debridement in the treatment of chronic periodontitis: a systematic review. *Br Dent J* 2008;205:E18.

((⊕)) SEE WEB LINKS

• The NHS National Library for Health: a Cochrane systematic review of full mouth disinfection.

dislocation *n*. The displacement of one bone from its articulation with another bone. This is usually caused by trauma, but may occur spontaneously due to excess movement in a joint such as the *temporomandibular joint.

disocclude *v*. To grind the biting (occlusal) surface of a tooth or teeth so as to remove any contact with opposing teeth during mastication.

disposables *n*. Instruments, materials, or equipment designed to be used only once. They are widely used in dentistry to reduce cross-contamination.

distal *adj*. Furthest away from the midline of the dental *arch. *See also* TOOTH SURFACES.

disto- A prefix signifying *distal such as distobuccal, distoincisal, distolingual.

distocclusion *n*. A type of *malocclusion in which the mandibular teeth occlude *distal to their normal relationship with the maxillary teeth.

distomolar *n*. A *supernumerary tooth, usually rudimentary, located distal to a third molar tooth.

distraction osteogenesis A surgical technique which can be applied to facial and other bones to encourage new bone and soft tissue formation. An *osteotomy is carried out to produce a mobile or transport segment of bone and an appliance (distractor) is fitted which gradually applies traction to the transport segment over a period of several weeks encouraging new bone formation (*osteogenesis) in the gap created. The adjacent soft tissues are expanded simultaneously as the bone segment is transported. Distractor devices may be either intraosseous or extraosseous. The techniuqe can be used to generate more bone tissue and correct deficient alveolar ridges prior to the insertion of dental implants.

distribution *n*. (in statistics) An arrangement of values of a *variable showing their observed or theoretical frequency of occurrence. **Binomial distribution** is a calculation that measures the likelihood of an event taking place where the probability is measured between 0 (the event will certainly not occur) and 1 (the event is absolutely certain). A **frequency distribution** is a summary of the frequencies of the values or categories of a variable usually in the form of a table or graph. **Normal distribution** is a continuous, symmetrical, bell-shaped frequency distribution for variable data. **Poisson distribution** describes the number of events that occur in a certain time interval or spatial area. **Probability distribution** is represented by a frequency distribution curve of a particular variable from which it is possible to establish the probability with which particular values of that variable occur. **Uniform distribution** describes a distribution for which every value has the same relative frequency.

ditching *n*. A defect at the junction between a restoration and the tooth. It is often seen around the margins of longstanding *amalgam restorations due to material *corrosion. 📷

diuretic *n*. A drug that increases urine production by promoting the excretion of *mineral salts and water from the *kidneys.

diurnal *adj.* Active during daylight hours (daily). The opposite to **nocturnal**, meaning active during the night.

DMF index A means of classifying the disease state of the mouth by recording the number of teeth in the secondary (*permanent) dentition decayed (D), missing (M), or filled (F) and applying it to a sample population. So for example a DMF index of 4.6 in 16-year-olds will mean an average of 4.6 teeth are decayed, missing, or filled per child. It is a well-established index in dental epidemiology. This index may also be applied to the *primary (deciduous) dentition when the lower case letters are used, i.e. decayed (d), missing (m), or filled (f). The index may be modified to record the tooth surfaces as **DMFS** in the permanent dentition and **dmfs** in the primary dentition.

Dolder bar *n.* [E. J. Dolder, 20th-century Swiss dentist] A bar and sleeve attachment for providing additional retention of a removable partial denture (*prosthesis) or *overdenture. The sleeve may be ovoid, or pear-, or U-shaped, and is usually attached to the removable denture, the bar being attached to the cast *abutment restorations. The pear-shaped sleeve allows for both rotational and vertical movement. The U-shaped sleeve is entirely abutment-supported for maximum rigidity and strength.

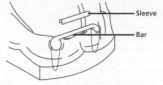

Dolder bar

dolich- (dolicho-) A prefix denoting long e.g. **dolichofacial** (long face), **dolichouranic** (long palate).

dolichocephalic *adj.* See CEPHALIC INDEX.

dolor *n.* Any kind of pain. One of the four signs of *inflammation, the others being *calor (heat), *rubor (redness), and *tumor (swelling).

domiciliary care Care provided by a dental professional for a patient in their home environment because of their inability to attend a clinic, dental practice, or mobile dental unit. For operative dentistry, specialized dental equipment, which includes a portable light, chair, aspirator, turbine, and handpiece motor, is usually required.

-dontic Suffix denoting of the teeth e.g. **endodontic** (relating to the tooth root).

dopamine *n.* A *catecholamine-derived *neurotransmitter that transmits messages from one *nerve cell to another in the nervous system. It is used in the treatment of shock, *hypotension, and low cardiac output. It also stimulates the release of *noradrenaline from nerve endings.

dorsal *adj.* Relating to the back of or posterior part of the body or an organ.

dorsum *n.* The upper or posterior surface of an organ or part of the body, e.g. the dorsum of the *tongue.

dose *n.* 1. A defined quantity of a *drug given to a patient. 2. (in radiography) The total *radiation delivered to a specific area of the body. **Radiation-absorbed dose** measured in *Grays refers to the amount of radiation absorbed by the part of the body exposed. **Equivalent dose** also takes into account the type of radiation used and is measured in *Sieverts. **Effective dose** takes into account the type of radiation and the part of the body irradiated; it is measured in Sieverts and allows dose comparisons between different procedures.

double blind trial A scientific study in which two or more groups of patients are subjected to different therapy regimes and neither the researcher (or observer) nor the patient are aware of which patients are in which group. *See also* BLINDING.

double teeth *n.* A developmental anomaly describing two teeth which appear to be joined together. *See also* FUSION; GEMINATION.

dovetail *n.* A cavity whose shape is flared, created to provide a retentive lock for a direct or indirect *restoration.

Down's syndrome (Down syndrome)
[J. L. H. Down (1828–96), British physician] A genetic abnormality in which an extra *chromosome 21 is present (**trisomy 21**). It is characterized by varying degrees of learning disability and multiple developmental defects. Patients have a characteristic flat face with slanting eyes. Of dental significance is a reduced *caries prevalence, possibly due to delayed tooth eruption, smaller or fewer teeth, or differences in *saliva composition. There is also an increased risk of *periodontal disease due to an altered immune response, reduced manual dexterity, and an open mouth posture resulting in a dry mouth (*xerostomia) and poor oral clearance of food.

doxycycline *n.* A *tetracycline antibiotic used in the treatment of periodontal disease because of its ability to inhibit the activity of *collagenase produced by bacteria. It may be prescribed in conjunction with subgingival scaling, root planning, or *debridement. It is contraindicated for patients sensitive to tetracyclines and children under the age of 8. The contents of the capsule can be diluted with water to form a mouthwash which is effective in the treatment of herpetiform ulceration. Trade name: **Periostat***.

drainage *n.* The emptying of fluid from a cavity or lesion by means of an external pathway. For example the drainage of *pus from a *periapical abscess through the *alveolar bone to the surface mucosa.

dressing *n.* 1. A protective covering for a wound to assist healing. 2. A temporary restorative material such as calcium hydroxide or zinc oxide *eugenol. A dressing may contain some form of medication; for example a zinc oxide eugenol dressing applied to the periodontal tissues following gingival surgery (periodontal *pack).

drifting *n.* The *migration of a tooth from its normal position in the dental arch. Drifting may be due to periodontal disease, loss of proximal support, loss of a functional opposing tooth, traumatic occlusal tooth relationships, or oral habits such as digit sucking. The extraction of a primary canine or molar may cause mesial drift of teeth distal to the space and distal drift of anterior teeth, with resultant displacement of permanent teeth and a movement of the centreline. *See also* SPACE MAINTAINER.

drill *n.* A rotary instrument used in a dental drive unit for cutting tooth or *bone. The cutting end may have a variety of shapes and is usually made of steel or tungsten carbide, or has a diamond grit coating. A **twist drill** has spiral grooves along its operating tip and is used prior to *pin placement. A **Gates–Glidden drill** is a type of endodontic *reamer with a long shaft and an elongated oval spiral cutting blade used to enlarge the coronal region of a root canal and improve access or for making a post hole. It has a blunt tip to prevent the lateral perforation of the root canal. It fits into a contra-angle *handpiece and is available in a variety of sizes and lengths.

(((●))) SEE WEB LINKS

• Provides information on the use of Gates–Glidden drills.

drug *n.* Any substance that affects the functioning of a living organism. The term medicine is sometimes preferred to provide a distinction between therapeutic drugs and narcotics or illegal substances. **Drug abuse** is the excessive or inappropriate use of drugs frequently taken for non-therapeutic reasons. Intravenous drug abusers have a likelihood of an increased incidence of *hepatitis B, C, and D, and possibly *HIV infection. Oral considerations for drug abusers are *bruxism, usually poor oral hygiene and therefore an increased risk of *caries and *periodontal disease, and an associated *xerostomia resulting in rampant caries. Patients taking *ecstasy may have tooth *erosion because of the dehydration which it produces encouraging them to have a high intake of carbonated drinks. Drugs placed in the buccal sulcus may have a direct erosive effect on the adjacent teeth and mucosa. **Drug dependence** *see* DEPENDENCE. **Drug interaction** is the different effect that one drug has when given at the same time as another. There may be an increased or decreased action of either or both drugs, or there may be an adverse reaction which is not normally associated with either drug when given on its own.

Drug Information Service An organization in the UK which provides information on drug therapy relating to dental treatment.

dry guard (dry aid) A disposable absorbent pad used to provide moisture control during intra-oral operative procedures. It is made from a variety of materials such as cardboard or an absorbent material enclosed in a permeable plastic cover. It is normally placed close to or over the opening of the parotid salivary duct.

dry mouth *n.* See XEROSTOMIA.

dry socket *n.* See ALVEOLITIS.

dual-cure composite See RESIN COMPOSITE.

dual impression technique See IMPRESSION.

duct *n.* A tubular canal which frequently carries glandular secretions.

duodenum *n.* The first part of the small intestine extending from the pylorus of the *stomach to the jejunum. It receives secretions from the liver via the gall bladder and the *pancreas.

duplicate cast *n.* See CAST.

duplicating material *n.* A material used in dental laboratories to produce a duplicate copy of a model or cast.

dye *n. See* DISCLOSING AGENT.

dys- A prefix denoting difficult, abnormal, or impaired e.g. **dyscephaly** (malformation of the facial bones).

dysaesthesia *n.* An abnormal or unpleasant sensation due to partial damage to sensory nerve fibres.

dysarthria *n.* A speech impediment induced by muscle spasticity, stroke, Parkinson's disease, or emotional distress. Speech is slurred but the language content and meaning are normal. There may also be difficulty chewing or swallowing.

dyscrasia *n.* An abnormal or physiologically unbalanced state of the body, particularly one due to abnormal metabolism or development.

dysgeusia *n.* The distortion or decrease of the sense of taste.

dysgnathia *n.* An oral abnormality which extends beyond the teeth to include either the maxilla or mandible or both. *Compare* EUGNATHIA.

dyskeratosis congenita *n.* An inherited condition which predominantly affects males. It is characterized by severe periodontal disease, white patches on the mucosa, and nail abnormalities.

dyskinesia *n.* Tremor or involuntary movement. It is a symptom of *Parkinson's disease.

dyslalia *n.* A speech disorder in which frequently children do not pronounce the sounds clearly or they replace one sound with another.

dyslogia (hypologia) *n.* Impaired ability to express ideas verbally resulting in disturbed or incoherent speech. Possible causes include *dementia and mental illness.

dysmasesis *n.* Difficulty in mastication.

dysostosis *n.* Defective bone formation. *Cartilage may be replaced by *bone in discrete sites. **Cleidocranial dysostosis** is characterized by defective formation or absence of the clavicles, defective formation of the *cranium, delayed tooth *eruption, the presence of *supernumerary teeth, or partial *anodontia. **Craniofacial dysostosis** has similar characteristics to cleidocranial dysostosis except that the clavicles are unaffected. **Mandibulofacial (faciomandibular) dysostosis** is a rare developmental malformation of the face and jaws in which the *mandibular body is underdeveloped and the teeth are consequently crowded and malpositioned. There is also *hypoplasia of the *facial bones.

dyspepsia *n.* A symptom of gastric discomfort after eating which may be accompanied by *nausea or vomiting.

dysphagia *n.* A condition in which *swallowing is either difficult or painful. It may be caused by diseases of the mouth, *pharynx, or *larynx, neuromuscular disturbances, or obstruction of the *oesophagus.

dysphemia *n.* A speech disorder characterized by stammering or stuttering. It is often of emotional or psychological origin.

dysplasia *n.* Abnormal development of tissues. It may imply potential malignancy in some tissues but not in others. **Anhidrotic ectodermal dysplasia (hypohidrotic ectodermal dysplasia)** is a group of inherited disorders involving all the structures which develop from *ectoderm. The most common forms are **anhidrotic X-linked**, affecting only males and **incontinentia pigmenti** affecting only females. The condition is characterized by frontal bossing (prominent forehead), dry skin (due to the absence of sweat glands), maxillary *hypoplasia, missing teeth, and teeth of abnormal shape, especially conical. Dental management is by orthodontics, restorative care, and careful attention to oral hygiene in order to retain the few teeth present. **Dentine dysplasia** *see* DENTINE DYSPLASIA. **Epithelial dysplasia** refers to abnormalities in the cells and differentiation of epithelium (*see also* ATYPIA). **Fibrous dysplasia** is a genetic, non-inherited disease in which a characteristic mutation leads to defects in osteoblast differentiation resulting in replacement of normal bone by cellular fibrous tissue in which immature woven bone is laid down. It characteristically occurs in young people and although it may affect any bone it particularly affects the maxilla in the head and neck region. **Monostotic fibrous dysplasia** affects one bone but **polyostotic fibrous dysplasia** affects multiple bones and may be associated with endocrine disturbances such as precocious puberty and skin pigmentation (**McCune–Albright syndrome**) [D. J. McCune (1902–76), US paediatrician; F. Allbright (1900–69), US physician]. Patients complain of increasing facial swelling and radiographically may show a radiolucency in the early stages which develops into an 'orange peel' radiopacity. Expansion usually ceases after cessation of growth and may be managed by surgical reduction. **Osseous dysplasia** describes a group of jaw lesions characterized by replacement of normal bone with fibrous tissue in which abnormal bone is laid down. **Periapical osseous**

dysplasia occurs beneath the lower anterior teeth and appears as a radiopaque area on a radiograph. **Florid osseous dysplasia** occurs in the posterior jaws in middle-aged women and may be bilateral.

dyspnoea *n.* Difficulty in breathing, affecting either or both inspiration or expiration.

dystrophy *n.* A disorder of an organ or tissue usually due to impaired nutrition of the affected part.

Eagle's syndrome A rare condition, first described by Watt Weems Eagle in 1937, in which there is an elongation of the *styloid process and calcification of the *stylohyoid ligament. It is characterized by *dysphagia, sore throat, and pain on chewing or turning the head. There may also be compression of the internal carotid artery.

earbow n. See FACEBOW.

early childhood caries See CARIES.

eating disorders n. pl. A group of dysfunctional nutritional disorders that includes *bulimia and *anorexia nervosa.

EBA cement See CEMENT.

Ebner's glands [V. von Ebner (1842–1925), Austrian histologist] A group of *serous glands found on the *dorsum of the *tongue anterior to the *sulcus terminalis at the base of the *circumvallate papillae.

Ebner's lines [V. von Ebner (1842–1925), Austrian histologist] Incremental growth lines, when viewed under a microscope produced in dentine during *dentinogenesis representing a daily growth pattern.

eburnation n. 1. An increase in bone density. 2. (in dentistry) The process whereby *dentine acquires a hard surface when *caries has been arrested.

eccentric adj. 1. Describing away from a central or reference position. 2. Describing a deviation from the normal or conventional.

ecchymosis n. A bruise caused by blood leaking from broken blood vessels into the tissues of the skin or mucous membranes. It appears as a bluish or red discoloration.

echinacea (purple coneflower) n. A nonspecific immunostimulant herbal extract which has been included in some *mouthwashes and *dentifrices for the treatment of *gingivitis. The research evidence to substantiate its effectiveness is currently limited. See also HERBALISM.

ecstasy (3,4-methylenedioxy-N-methamphetamine) n. A synthetic entactogen of the phenethylamine family whose primary effect is to stimulate the secretion of large amounts of serotonin as well as *dopamine and *noradrenaline in the brain, producing a sense of euphoria, decreased hostility, and an increase in energy. Of dental significance is the frequent presence of tooth *erosion because of the consumption of large quantities of carbonated drinks due to the extreme dehydration induced by the drug.

ectoderm n. The outermost of the three germ layers of the developing embryo, the other two being the *mesoderm and the *endoderm. It gives rise to the nervous system, sense organs, *epidermis, teeth, and *mucosa.

ectodermal dysplasia n. See DYSPLASIA.

ectopic adj. Occurring outside the normal anatomical location, e.g. an ectopic pregnancy is the development of an embryo outside the womb. The most commonly found ectopic teeth are mandibular first and third molars, canines, second premolars, and *supernumerary teeth.

ectostylid n. A small cusp or ridge of enamel present distal to the *protoconid on the disto-buccal aspect of the occlusal surface of a mandibular molar or premolar in certain mammalian or primate species.

eczema *n.* A common skin disorder characterized by itching, scaling, thickening of the skin, and *vesicle formation. It is usually located on the face, elbows, knees, and arms. Treatment is with topical or systemic *corticosteroids. **eczematous** *adj.*

edema *n. See* OEDEMA.

edentate *n.* Having no natural teeth.

edentulous *adj.* Describing having no teeth. *Compare* DENTULOUS.

edge strength *n.* Resistance of a material in an interface relationship to wear or fracture.

edge-to-edge bite *See* BITE.

edgewise appliance *n.* A fixed orthodontic appliance which uses a rectangular *labial archwire fixed to *brackets or *bands cemented onto individual teeth. The bracket is manufactured so that the rectangular archwire is inserted with its long cross-section horizontal instead of vertical.

Edlan–Mejchar Technique A mucogingival surgical technique to widen the band of attached *gingiva and deepen the vestibular *sulcus, described by A. Edlan and B. Mejchar in 1963.

EDTA *n. See* ETHYLENE DIAMINE TETRAACETIC ACID.

effectiveness *n.* The extent to which a specific intervention, when used under ordinary circumstances, does what it is intended to do. **Clinical effectiveness** is the extent to which an intervention does the patient more good than harm when assessed in a real-life situation rather than under ideal conditions.

effect size (in statistics) A standardized and objective measure of the magnitude of an observed effect. Measures frequently referred to include Pearson's correlations coefficient r, Cohen's d, and Glass's g.

efferent *adj.* 1. Referring to nerves that carry messages from the *central nervous system (brain and spinal cord) towards the muscles and glands in the body, i.e. *motor nerves. 2. Describing vessels or ducts that drain fluid from an organ. *Compare* AFFERENT.

efficacy *n.* The ability of a treatment or drug to produce the desired effect under ideal circumstances such as a clinical trial. *See also* EFFECTIVENESS.

Eikenella corrodens A Gram-negative, rod-shaped, non-motile, microaerophilic bacillus often found in the subgingival environment.

Ekstrand scoring system [K. R. Ekstrand, 20th-century Danish dentist] A method of using visual criteria to assess the depth and activity of occlusal caries.

Further Reading: Ekstrand K. R., Ricketts, D. N., Kidd E. A., Qvist V., Schou S. Detection, diagnosing, monitoring and logical treatment of occlusal caries in relation to lesion activity and severity: an in vivo examination with histological validation. *Caries Research* 1998;32:247–54.

elastics *n.* Small rubber bands used as auxiliaries to an *orthodontic appliance to provide a pulling force (traction). They may be used to provide traction within one arch (**intra-maxillary elastic**) or between the teeth of both jaws (**inter-maxillary elastic**). They are usually classified according to their size (⅛ inch to ¾ inch) and the force they are designed to deliver (2oz, 3.5oz, or 4.5oz). The positioning of the elastics determines the definitive tooth movements achieved. They require changing on a daily basis.

elastin *n.* A stretchable fibrous *protein that is the major constituent of the yellow elastic fibres of *connective tissue. It provides the elastic property of the skin.

elastomer *n.* A generic term which describes an elastic rubber-like polymer, capable of expanding and contracting and returning to original dimensions without fatigue, used for taking impressions. Elastomers include *silicone, *polysulphide, *polyether, and reversible and irreversible *hydrocolloids. **elastomeric** *adj.*

elastomeric module *n.* A small elastic band used to secure the *archwire into the archwire slot on a fixed orthodontic *appliance. They are quicker to place than wire ligatures but cannot be adjusted.

electro-acupuncture *n. See* ACUPUNCTURE.

electroanalgesia *n.* *Analgesia or *anaesthesia induced by an electric current. Pain is reduced by the electrical stimulation of a peripheral nerve. *See also* TRANSCUTANEOUS ELECTRICAL NERVE STIMULATION (TENS).

electrocardiogram (ECG) *n.* A paper recording of the electrical activity of the heart muscle used as an aid in the diagnosis of heart disease. The recording is made by an **electrocardiograph**.

electrocautery *n.* The application of a direct electric current to a wire loop or needle to heat it to red heat. It is used to cauterize tissue. Only the heated wire comes in contact with tissue, unlike in *electrosurgery where the patient is included in the circuit and the current enters the patient's body.

electrolyte *n.* A substance which, when in aqueous solution, produces ions and will conduct an electric current. Acids, bases, and salts are common electrolytes. In medical usage, electrolyte usually means the ion itself.

electroplating *n.* An electrolytic method of depositing metals such as silver and copper on the surface of a non-aqueous *elastomeric impression to produce an abrasion resistant working model or *die.

electrosurgery *n.* Surgery performed with instruments using high-frequency electrical currents in the radio transmission frequency band. Heat develops directly within the tissue cells over the entire surface of the electrode tip in contact with the tissues. Applications in dentistry include the removal of soft tissue lesions, the arrest of bleeding, and tissue cutting. It is not effective on hard tissues like enamel or bone. Electrosurgery may be either monopolar or bipolar. **Monopolar electrosurgery** has an active electrode tip, held in an insulated handpiece and designed for specific clinical indications such as incision, excision, *curettage, or coagulation, and a dispersive electrode in the form of a large flexible pad against which the patient lies. In **bipolar electrosurgery** both electrodes are mounted on a common handpiece and are of similar size. *See also* CAUTERY. 📷

elevator *n.* A bladed hand instrument used for engaging teeth or tooth roots in order to lever them from their alveolar sockets. There are many different designs of elevator developed to fit their function. An **apical elevator** has a small blade designed to remove a fractured or retained root from a socket; it is either straight or angled left or right. A **Cryer's elevator** [M. H. Cryer (1840–1921), American oral surgeon] is one of a pair of elevators with pointed tips used for elevating molar roots or removing interseptal alveolar bone. **Hospital pattern (Coleman) elevators** are available as left, right and straight versions all with broad serrated blades and heavy serrated hollow handles. A **Miller's elevator** has a narrow curved blade used to pass between the distal root of a lower second molar and the crown of an impacted third molar in order to assist in its extraction. A **periosteal elevator** has a handle and a thin slightly curved rounded blade and is used for

separating the *periosteum from the *bone when raising a mucoperiosteal flap: they are available in a variety of designs such as Howarth's, Syme's, Molt No. 9, and Hu-Friedy. A **Rowe's elevator** is used for elevating the zygomatic bone following traumatic displacement. **Warwick James elevators** [W. Warwick James (1874–1965), English oral surgeon] have small rounded working tips which may be in line with the shank (straight), or left and right used as a pair. **Winter's elevators** [G. B. Winter, contemporary American oral surgeon] are used for removing lower third molars and have a working tip similar to the Cryer's elevators but with a handle at right angles to the log axis of the instrument.

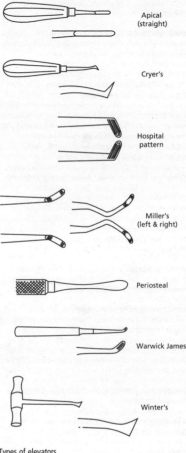

Apical (straight)

Cryer's

Hospital pattern

Miller's (left & right)

Periosteal

Warwick James

Winter's

Types of elevators

Elhers–Danlos syndrome [E. Elhers (1863–1937), Danish dermatologist; H.-A. Danlos (1844–1912), French dermatologist] A rare genetic syndrome caused by defects of collagen synthesis. Ten subtypes are described; aggressive periodontal destruction is associated with types IV, VIII, and IX. *See also* CLASSIFICATION OF CONDITIONS OF THE PERIODONTIUM.

Elyzol *n. See* METRONIDAZOLE.

embolus *n.* (*pl.* **emboli**) A detached intravascular solid, liquid, or gaseous mass such as a *blood clot, piece of tumour, fat, or air, that is carried by the bloodstream to a site distant from its point of origin, where it obstructs the flow of blood creating a blockage, the condition of **embolism**.

embouchure *n.* The use of the facial muscles and the shaping of the lips, tongue, and teeth to the mouthpiece of a wind instrument.

embrasure *n.* The space between two teeth created by the convexity of the surfaces. It may open onto the labial, lingual, buccal, palatal, or occlusal surfaces. An adequate **embrasure space** is an important consideration in the periodontal-restorative interface; it must be incorporated into fixed prostheses to facilitate oral hygiene procedures and maintain oral health. An **embrasure hook** provides stability for a *partial denture and is an extension into the embrasure above the *contact area. An **embrasure clasp** is part of a partial denture used where no *edentulous space exists, which, having passed through the embrasure, engages the undercut area of the tooth surface. An **occlusal embrasure** is the space between the curved proximal surfaces of the teeth which opens towards the occlusal surface.

embryology *n.* The study of the function, growth, and development of an organism from fertilization of the ovum to birth.

Emergency Dental Service (in the UK) Part of the National Health Service providing urgent dental advice and treatment outside normal surgery hours, to patients experiencing severe pain, bleeding, swelling, or trauma. It is funded as part of the Primary Care Trust (PCT) salaried services.

emergency drugs Medicines required in a dental surgery or clinic which conform to contemporary standards recommended by respected bodies for dealing with medical or dental emergencies.

emery *n. See* CORUNDUM.

eminectomy *n.* A surgical procedure to remove the articular eminence of the temporal bone. It is used most commonly to prevent recurrent dislocation of the temporomandibular joint.

EMLA cream A *eutectic mixture of 2.5% lidocaine and 2.5% prilocaine local anaesthetics (hence the name). It produces effective *analgesia of the skin and may be used prior to venous *cannulation and lumbar puncture. The presence of prilocaine can induce *methaemoglobinaemia. It is not recommended for oral use as the safe dosing amounts are unknown for mucosal application.

emollient *n.* A substance that soothes and softens the skin or *mucosa. It may be used as a base for more active drugs.

emphysema *n.* Air in the tissues. In **pulmonary emphysema** there is enlargement and damage to the air sacs (alveoli) of the lungs resulting in inefficient gaseous exchange. Emphysema is characterized by shortness of breath. **Surgical emphysema** can occur in the oral region when air is forced into a tissue space either by the injudicious use of the air syringe or by the water and air spray associated with a high-speed turbine; the presence of gas or air in the tissues gives a characteristic crackling feeling to the touch; the gas or air is easily absorbed once the leak or production has been arrested.

empirical *adj.* Describing experience based on observation rather than logic, reason, or proven scientific data.

enamel

n. The hard outer covering of the *crown of a tooth overlying the dentine. It is 96–97% inorganic, consisting of mainly *hydroxyapatite, 1% organic protein and 2–3% water (by weight). Enamel has a prismatic structure with millions of enamel prisms or **rods** which run from the surface of the dentine (*amelodentinal junction) to the external enamel surface. Each prism is made up of enamel crystallites which run parallel to the long axis of the prisms. Enamel is laid down by *ameloblasts in layers producing incremental growth lines with cross striations about 4μ thick marking daily growth patterns. **Enamel formation (amelogenesis)** begins immediately after the first layer of *dentine is formed when the *inner enamel epithelium differentiates into ameloblast cells. These columnar cells have their base attached to the *stratum intermedium and their opposite end has a pyramidal extension called the *Tomes process, through which the enamel matrix, consisting of calcium and phosphate ions, is secreted. Amelogenesis can be considered to be a two-stage process: the first stage is the **secretory stage** in which a pre-enamel protein-rich partially mineralized organic matrix is laid down; in the second phase, the **maturation stage**, the ameloblasts transport substances used in the formation of enamel. As maturation takes place, the organic component is reduced and the enamel crystallites increase in size. On completion of enamel formation the ameloblasts lose their Tomes processes and flatten off to form the *reduced enamel epithelium. This protects the tooth during *eruption and eventually becomes the *junctional epithelium. Incompletely calcified areas may appear microscopically as **enamel lamellae** extending as far as the amelodentinal junction. Enamel mineralization may stop or reduce during the period of birth and will often produce a distinct line of disruption (**neonatal line**) affecting only primary teeth and the first permanent molars; this can provide an important forensic landmark. Sometimes dentinal tubules can extend into the enamel (**enamel spindles**), most commonly beneath the cusps due to penetration by odontoblasts. Areas of incomplete enamel formation (**enamel tufts**) may occur extending from the amelodentinal junction and following the direction of the enamel prisms.

enamel bonding See BONDING.

enamel epithelium *n.* The cellular layer formed as part of the *enamel organ. The columnar cells of the **inner enamel epithelium** line the inner surface of the enamel organ and define the shape of the crown of the tooth. They eventually differentiate into enamel-forming cells (*ameloblasts). The **outer enamel epithelium** consists of a layer of cuboidal cells forming the external surface of the enamel organ. They maintain the shape of the enamel organ. The **reduced enamel epithelium** forms the remains of the ameloblast cell layer and protects the enamel during eruption. After eruption it becomes the *junctional epithelium.

enamel hypoplasia See HYPOPLASIA.

enamelin *n.* A protein secreted by *ameloblasts that forms an organic matrix. It plays a key role in the formation and growth of crystals in developing enamel. A defect in the gene which provides instructions for making enamelin, the

ENAM gene, can result in *amelogenesis imperfecta.

enamel infraction Microcracks in the thickness of the enamel often produced as a result of minor trauma.

enamel matrix derivative proteins (EMD) Proteinaceous materials associated with the development of acellular cementum, *periodontal ligament, and alveolar *bone.

enamel microabrasion (enamel abrasion) The process whereby compounds (usually a combination of acids and abrasives) are applied to the teeth in order to remove stain and discoloration in the superficial layers of the enamel. See also AIR ABRASION.

enameloma *n. See* ENAMEL PEARL.

enameloplasty *n. See* ODONTOPLASTY.

enamel organ *n.* Clumps of *mesenchymal cells formed from the *dental lamina at about 8 weeks of intrauterine life.

enamel pearl (enameloma) *n.* A developmental anomaly in which there is a small bead of enamel on the surface of a tooth root, usually in the bifurcation or trifurcation of the tooth on the *buccal surface. It occasionally is supported by dentine and very rarely contains pulp tissue. It can also be associated with a site of localized periodontal destruction. See also ODONTOMA.

enamel striae of Retzius [A. Retzius (1796–1860), Swedish anatomist] Incremental growth lines found in developing *enamel, which indicate weekly variation in *mineralization. They microscopically appear as a series of dark bands. Formed as a result of the constriction of the Tomes processes, they run obliquely from the *amelodentinal junction to the enamel surface, where they produce a series of grooves (*perikymata). The first 30–40 striae are obscured under the incisal edge. The average human incisor contains about 150 brown striae and the spacing between the striae represents about 7 days' growth; they have therefore been used for determining the age of death in contemporary humans and fossil hominids.

enamel stripping See REPROXIMATION.

endemic *adj.* Occurring frequently at a given location or in a defined population, applied generally to diseases.

endobasion *n.* A cephalometric point located in the midline of the most posterior point of the anterior border of the foramen magnum on the contour of the foramen. *See also* CEPHALOMETRIC ANALYSIS.

endocarditis *n.* Inflammation of the heart lining and valves. It is frequently caused by bacterial infection (**infective endocarditis, bacterial endocarditis**) or *rheumatic fever. It is characterized by fever, *embolism, and heart failure. **Subacute bacterial endocarditis (SBE)** occurs primarily after a *bacteraemia and can be a life-threatening complication in a patient with a history of rheumatic or congenital heart disease. It was previously thought that patients undergoing periodontal or surgically invasive dental treatment should receive antibiotic prophylaxis, but evidence based on systematic reviews suggests that this is unnecessary; there appears to be a greater risk from everyday procedures such as toothbrushing.

Further Reading: National Institute for Health and Clinical Excellence. Prophylaxis against infective endocarditis. Clinical guideline. 2008.

endocrine gland A ductless gland which manufactures *hormones and secretes them directly into the bloodstream (not through a duct). Examples include the *pituitary, *thyroid and *parathyroid, and *adrenal glands. *Compare* EXOCRINE GLAND.

endocytosis *n. See* EXOCYTOSIS.

endoderm *n.* (*adj.* **endodermal**) The innermost layer of the three germ layers of the early embryo (*see* MESODERM; ECTODERM). It develops into the gastrointestinal tract, lungs, and associated structures.

endodontic file *n. See* FILE.

endodontic implant *n. See* IMPLANT.

endodontic reamer *n. See* REAMER.

endodontics *n.* A specialty in dentistry that deals with the diagnosis, prevention, and treatment of diseases of the dental pulp and the tissues at the root apex. *See also* ROOT CANAL THERAPY.

endodontic stop *n.* A device attached to an endodontic instrument to control or indicate the depth to which it is inserted into a root canal.

endolith *n. See* DENTICLE.

endorphin *n.* One of a group of natural opioid biochemical compounds found in the brain derived from beta-lipotropin in the *pituitary gland. They have pain-relieving properties similar to morphine and are thought to be concerned with influencing the activity of the *endocrine glands.

endoscopy *n.* The procedure of viewing body organs or cavities using a flexible lighted tube (endoscope). **Periodontal endoscopy** involves the inspection of the subgingival tissues using a fibre optic endoscope attached to a specially designed dental instrument.

endosteal implant *See* IMPLANT.

endosteum *n.* A membrane consisting of a thin layer of connective tissue that lines the marrow cavity of *bone. It takes an active part in the repair of fractures.

endothermic *adj.* Describing a chemical reaction which results in the absorption of heat.

endotoxin *n.* A heat-stable lipopolysaccharide (LPS) component of the outer membrane of a wide variety of Gram-negative bacteria released when the organisms disintegrate or die. LPS consists of a polysaccharide chain and a lipid component, called lipid A. The polysaccharide chain is highly variable among different Gram-negative bacterial species and thus there are a wide variety of endotoxins. Endotoxins are highly toxic, capable of causing fever, malaise, respiratory distress, and even death. The lipid A component of endotoxins is responsible for the toxic effects.

enostosis *n.* A localized mass of proliferating *bone tissue within a bone. Radiographically it has a cotton wool appearance and can be distinguished from sclerosing *osteitis in that it is separated from the tooth by a few millimetres of normal bone. The lesions are usually multiple.

entoconid *n.* A cusp which develops lingual to the *hypoconid on a mandibular molar tooth.

entomion *n.* The craniometric point at the tip of the mastoid angle of the *parietal bone where it crosses the parietal notch of the *temporal bone.

Entonox® *n.* Trade name for a mixture of 50% nitrous oxide and 50% oxygen packaged and delivered from gas cylinders, used to produce analgesia without loss of consciousness.

enucleate *v.* Describing the process of completely removing an organ, tumour, or cystic lesion.

envelope of motion A three-dimensional range of mandibular movement which can take place during normal function. *See also* POSSELT'S ENVELOPE.

enzyme *n.* A protein that acts as a *catalyst, speeding up the rate at which a biological reaction takes place but without itself being changed or destroyed in the reaction.

eosin *n.* An acidic red dye used to stain biological material (e.g. cell cytoplasm) for examination under a microscope. It is commonly used with haematoxylin as part of an H&E stained section.

eosinophil *n.* A type of white blood cell with granular *cytoplasm (granulocyte) capable of ingesting foreign material. It is so called because of its characteristic brick-red stain with *eosin dye. Eosinophils play an important role in parasitic infections and allergic responses.

epactal *adj.* Supernumerary.

Epanutin *n. See* PHENYTOIN.

ependyma *n.* (*adj.* **ependymal**) The thin membrane that lines the ventricles of the brain and the choroid plexuses. It is responsible for helping to form cerebrospinal fluid.

ephelis *n.* (*pl.* **ephelides**) A flat red or light-brown spot on the skin or oral mucosa usually caused by an increase in pigmentation of the epithelium. It is of no pathological significance.

epi- Prefix denoting above or upon.

epidemic *n.* A sudden large outbreak of an infectious disease rapidly spreading among a population. The number of cases of the disease are clearly in excess of that which would normally be expected in a particular geographic area.

epidemiology *n.* A study of the occurrence, distribution, and control of disease in a population. It forms a basic part of dental public health.

epidermis *n.* The outer layer of the skin. The outermost layer of the epidermis is called the **stratum corneum (cornified layer)**, composed of flattened dead cells whose cytoplasm has been replaced by *keratin. Immediately below that is the area of living epidermal cells (*keratinocytes), which are continually replaced.

epidermolysis bullosa A group of genetically determined disorders affecting the skin and/or *mucosa, and characterized by blistering which heals slowly with scarring. A variety of forms exist which vary in severity; some are incompatible with life. Extensive scarring of the skin with deformities of the digits may occur and painful oral lesions may result in difficulty in swallowing. A rare autoimmune acquired form occurs in adult life. 📷

epiglottis *n.* A flap of elastic cartilage covered by *mucosa which protects the entrance to the *larynx during swallowing.

epilepsy *n.* (*adj.* **epileptic**) A disorder of brain function characterized by recurrent episodes of convulsive seizures. Most epilepsy is of unknown cause but there may be a genetic link or it may be associated with a number of acquired causes such as brain damage, stroke, brain tumours, or *cannabis use. Epilepsy may take the form of **tonic-clonic seizures** (formerly known as **grand mal**), where the patient senses an aura a few seconds before seizure, which is frequently with facial flushing, dilated pupils, rolling of the eyes, drooling the mouth, and raised blood pressure. In **partial epilepsy** the seizures take the form of **absences** (formerly called **petit mal**) and last a few seconds during which the patient appears vacant and staring. These may occur many times a day and are commonly seen in younger people. Some drugs used in the treatment of epilepsy, such as *phenytoin (now no longer the first choice of drug), can cause *gingival hyperplasia. Commonly used antiepileptic drugs are carbamazapine, lamotrigine, and sodium valproate. During a seizure in the dental surgery, the patient should be protected from potential damage from striking adjacent equipment resulting from the uncontrolled convulsive movements. *Status epilepticus is a potential medical emergency in the dental surgery.

epinephrine *n. See* ADRENALINE.

EpiPen (Trade name) *n.* A preassembled syringe containing 300 micrograms of adrenaline for intramuscular injection carried by patients at risk of *anaphylaxis for self or third-party injection.

epiphysis *n.* The end of a long bone which is initially separated from the **diaphysis** (the shaft) by *cartilage which disappears once bone formation is complete.

epistaxis *n.* Bleeding from the nose. The most common causes are trauma, high blood pressure, or infections such as the common cold. It may also be a symptom of an abnormality of the blood vessels or the blood clotting mechanism, or excess thinning of the blood following the use of *aspirin or other anticoagulant drugs.

epithelial attachment (junctional epithelium) A collar of non-keratinized epithelial cells forming the biological attachment to the tooth surface at the base of the *gingival crevice (sulcus) in the region of the cemento-enamel junction (CEJ). It is formed from the *reduced enamel epithelium. It contains very small rivet-like structures in the cell wall (**hemidesmosomes**) which link the **internal basement membrane** of the *junctional epithelium to the tooth surface. It consists of stratified squamous cells approximately 15–30 cells thick, coronally tapering to about 5 cells thickness apically. It plays an important role in periodontal health. The **external basal lamina** is a thin mat of extracellular matrix between the epithelial cells of the junctional epithelium and the gingival connective tissue. The **internal basal lamina** is a thin mat of extracellular matrix between the epithelial cells of the junctional epithelium and the tooth surface. The **long junctional epithelium** refers to the healing process in the dento-gingival junction following treatment of chronic periodontitis, especially root debridement. The junctional epithelium heals in the cleaned environment and forms a long band of epithelial cells attached to the tooth surface by a hemidesmosomal attachment.

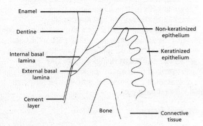

Epithelial attachment

epithelialization *n.* The process of growth of epithelium into an area that is normally covered by it as occurs during the normal healing process. This secondary intention healing occurs following external bevel *gingivectomy.

epithelial rest cells of Malassez [L. C. Malassez (1842–1909), French physiologist] The remains of the disintegrated *Hertwig's root sheath which persist into adult life and are situated between the collagen fibres of the *periodontal ligament.

epithelioid cell *n.* A modified *macrophage resembling an epithelial cell histologically and found in *granulomatous inflammation.

epithelium *n.* The tissue derived from embryonic *ectoderm and *endoderm which covers the external surface of the body and lines ducts and cavities (excluding the blood and lymphatic vessels). Epithelium is classified according to the number of cell layers and the shape of the cells. The cells rest on a **basement membrane** and may be in a single layer (**simple**), in several layers (**stratified**) or appear to be arranged in layers but actually share

a common basement membrane (**pseudo-stratified**). The cells of the epithelium may be **cuboidal**, **columnar**, or **squamous** (flat and scalelike) in shape. The oral *mucosa is covered by a layer of stratified squamous epithelium with varying degrees of *keratinization.

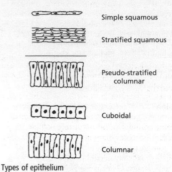

Types of epithelium

The columnar cell layer lining the inner surface of the *enamel organ (**inner enamel epithelium**) defines the shape of the crown of the tooth; eventually the cells differentiate into enamel-forming cells (*ameloblasts). **Junctional epithelium** *see* EPITHELIAL ATTACHMENT. The **outer enamel epithelium** forms the outer cuboidal epithelial cell layer of the *enamel organ which maintains its shape. The outer enamel epithelium meets the *inner enamel epithelium at the **cervical loop** forming *Hertwig's root sheath. The **reduced enamel epithelium** is the remains of the *ameloblast cell layer once enamel formation is complete; it protects the enamel during *eruption and eventually becomes the junctional epithelium.

eponym *n.* (*adj.* **eponymous**) A disease, structure, or species named after a particular person, usually the person who first described or discovered it, e.g. Bartholin's duct.

Epstein–Barr virus (EBV) [M. A. Epstein (1921–), English physician, and Y. M. Barr (1932–), contemporary English virologist] A *herpes family virus, also called human herpes virus 4 (HHV-4), associated with infectious mononucleosis (glandular fever) and Burkitt's lymphoma. It is also seen in the oral mucosa in hairy *leukoplakia. Most humans become infected with EBV, which is often asymptomatic.

Epstein pearls [A. Epstein (1849–1918), Bohemian paediatrician] These are synonymous with *Bohn's nodules.

epulis (*pl.* **epulides**) *n.* A non-specific name applied to tumour-like growths and swellings of the gingiva. They are usually but not always caused by trauma. A chronic mucosal hyperplasia (**epulis fissuratum**, denture granuloma, or denture-induced fibro-epithelial hyperplasia) can result from a low-grade irritation caused by the partial or full denture flange of an ill fitting denture; it is usually asymptomatic but there may be varying degrees of mucosal inflammation with some *erythema. The size of the lesion is variable but is characterized by folds of *hyperplastic connective tissue which may extend along the whole length of the flange area. Treatment is by surgical excision and correction or removal of the offending stimulus. A **fibrous epulis** is a localized overgrowth of fibrous connective tissue that may be caused by trauma from teeth, calculus, or an orthodontic appliance; it is typically slow-growing and mucosal coloured. A **pyogenic granuloma** (**vascular epulis**) is a red or purple soft swelling that is composed of granulation tissue; it bleeds easily and grows rapidly. It too is the result of trauma but typically occurs in pregnancy (**pregnancy epulis**) or during puberty as a result of hormonal changes. The pregnancy epulis usually occurs during the second or third trimester and is often associated with poor oral hygiene; it may be treated by oral hygiene instruction and surgical excision for cosmetic reasons or left until after childbirth when regression is frequently spontaneous; any causal irritation should be removed. A **giant cell epulis** (peripheral giant cell granuloma) presents as a dark red or purple swelling in the anterior part of the mouth. It is characterized by accumulations of multinucleated giant cells in a vascular connective tissue and may cause superficial resorption of bone; the cause is unknown but trauma may be a factor. A **congenital** (**granular cell**) **epulis** is a rare pedunculated swelling found only in the newborn and is of unknown aetiology; it usually occurs on the crest of the *alveolar ridge of the maxilla and can measure several centimetres in diameter. Histologically it consists of granular cells covered by flattened epithelium; treatment is by surgical excision. **Epulis granulomatosa** is a post-extraction sequel characterized by a tumour-like mass of inflamed granulation tissue associated with an extraction socket and sometimes a spicule of bone.

equilibration n. The restoration or maintenance of a state of equilibrium. **Occlusal equilibration** is achieved by selective grinding to modify the occlusal surfaces of the teeth and achieve occlusal harmony during normal masticatory function.

ergonomics n. The science of equipment design and location intended to maximize productivity by reducing operator fatigue and minimizing discomfort. An ergonomic environment is an important consideration in dental surgery or clinic design.

erosion

n. **1.** A superficial type of ulceration of the skin. **2.** The non-bacterial loss of tooth substance due to chemical agents. Acids are the most common cause, which may come into contact with the teeth from external (**extrinsic**) or internal (**intrinsic**) sources. Extrinsic sources include the diet.

Erosion: foodstuffs and their associated acids

Foodstuff	Associated acid
citrus fruits	citric
apples	malic
fruit drinks	citric, ascorbic, carbonic
acidic sports drinks	citric
wine	tartaric, malic
cider	malic
vinegar and pickled produce	acetic
sweets	citric, acetic
iron medicines	folic
acidic mouthwashes	malic
vitamin C	ascorbic

They also include occupational hazards e.g. from professional wine tasting and contact with factory acid fumes. Intrinsic acid sources include the gastric hydrochloric acid reflux associated with *bulimia and *anorexia or the gastric reflux from morning sickness occurring during pregnancy. Tooth loss is due to the binding or *chelation of the calcium in the teeth with the acid. While the pH of an acid source is an indicator of its erosive potential, a better guide is a measure known as the **total titratable activity**, which gives the capacity of a liquid to dissolve mineralized tissue. The clinical appearance can depend on the acid source and the mode of intake but generally extrinsic and intrinsic acids will erode the same tooth surfaces, mainly the palatal and occlusal surfaces. Excessive consumption of citrus foods, acidic sports drinks, wine, and beer can result in erosion of the labial surfaces of the upper anterior teeth and the occlusal surfaces of the upper and lower molars. Attempting to ameliorate such damage by drinking through a straw can result in enamel loss from the palatal surfaces of the upper teeth. Erosion in the permanent dentition appears as smooth, shiny, and rounded tooth surfaces with loss of developmental irregularities; incisal edges become thin and translucent giving a greyish appearance with a tendency to chip. The occlusal surfaces become concave and as dentine is lost a halo of enamel may remain as a rim around the eroded dentine. Erosion in primary teeth can be more rapid because of the decreased enamel thickness and is characterized by cup-shaped defects on the molars and a reduction in length of the incisors. Erosion may initially be asymptomatic but when more advanced can result in painful *dentine hypersensitivity to hot, cold, and sweet fluids. Erosion of enamel causes dissolution of the *hydroxyapatite fraction, creating a softened layer of up to 5μm in depth which is highly susceptible to *abrasion or *attrition; because of this, a delay of 30 minutes before toothbrushing after an acid attack is recommended. Treatment of erosion is by addressing the cause; the application of desensitizing solutions, pastes, or varnishes to minimize the symptoms e.g. *fluoride varnish, desensitizing *dentifrice; or by restorative measures to replace the enamel loss. 🔲

Further Reading: Bartlett D. W. Erosion and tooth surface loss. *Int J Prosthodont* 2005;18(4):300–01.

error bar (in statistics) A representation on a graph to show the error in a reported measurement. They often indicate one standard deviation of uncertainty, but they might also represent one standard error of the mean.

eructation *n.* Belching: the act of suddenly raising gas or air from the stomach.

eruption *n.* 1. A skin lesion in the form of a rash or blister. 2. The bodily movement of a tooth from its developmental position within the *alveolar process to its functional position in the oral cavity. Tooth eruption may be considered as passive or active. **Passive eruption** occurs where there is an apical migration of the *epithelial attachment resulting in an increased length of clinical crown often seen, without evidence of inflammation, in older people. **Active eruption** takes place when the tooth first enters the oral cavity and occurs as pre-functional and functional phases. During the **pre-functional phase** crown formation is completed and root formation begins. The overlying bone is resorbed by *osteoclastic activity and the *reduced enamel epithelium covering the enamel fuses with the *oral epithelium as the tooth emerges into the oral cavity to form the *epithelial attachment. The tooth continues to erupt in an axial direction

until it contacts (occludes with) the opposing tooth in the opposite jaw. The **functional eruptive phase** continues throughout life as the alveolar bone remodels in response to tooth movement and enamel wear. There is limited evidence to explain the mechanism creating the eruptive force but the following theories have been suggested: root growth generates a force beneath the tooth pushing it towards the oral cavity; bone resorption and deposition pushes the tooth out of the alveolar bone; traction of the periodontal fibres exerts a force on the tooth; cellular proliferation at the apical part of the pulp creates an eruptive pressure. The primary and permanent teeth erupt between approximately 6 months and 21 years.

Approximate eruption dates of primary teeth

Jaw	Tooth	Eruption date (in months)
maxillary	central incisor	7
	lateral incisor	8
	canine	18
	first molar	14
	second molar	24
mandibular	central incisor	6
	lateral incisor	7
	canine	16
	first molar	12
	second molar	20

Approximate eruption dates of permanent teeth

Jaw	Tooth	Eruption date (in years)
maxillary	central incisor	7–8
	lateral incisor	8–9
	canine	11–12
	first premolar	10–11
	second premolar	10–12
	first molar	6–7
	second molar	12–13
	third molar	17–21
mandibular	central incisor	6–7
	lateral incisor	7–8
	canine	9–10
	first premolar	10–12
	second premolar	11–12
	first molar	6–7
	second molar	12–13
	third molar	17–21

eruption cyst *n. See* CYST.

erysipelas *n.* An infection of the skin, especially the face, caused by B-haemolytic streptococci. It is characterized by redness and swelling usually with a sharply defined margin.

erythema *n.* (*adj.* **erythematous**) Diffuse or patchy redness of the skin or mucous membrane due to dilatation of the blood capillaries in the dermis. It may be physiological as in blushing, or due to inflammation or infection.

erythema infectiosum (slapped cheek disease, fifth disease) An infectious disease caused by the Parvovirus B19 virus infecting mainly children between the ages of 6 and 10. It is characterized by a bright red painless inflammation on one or both cheeks, sometimes spreading to a faint rash on the body, arms, and legs. It may be accompanied by influenza-like symptoms including a mild fever and aching joints. The infectious period is 4–20 days before the rash appears. Treatment is symptomatic and infection normally confers immunity.

erythema migrans *n. See* STOMATITIS.

erythema multiforme *n.*   An acute inflammatory self-limiting condition of the skin and/or *mucosa. It was first described by Ferdinand Ritter von Hebra, an Austrian dermatologist, in 1866. It is characterized by red macules (patches), papules (pimples), and sub-dermal vesicles (blisters) which develop into characteristic target lesions on the skin. Oral lesions are characterized by blood-filled blisters on the lips and intra-oral ulceration. The condition varies in severity from mild to severe (*Stevensen–Johnson syndrome) and may be recurrent; up to 70% of these are triggered by a preceding herpes viral infection. Other cases are associated with infections, collagen disease, drug sensitivities, *allergies, and pregnancy. 📷

erythematous candidosis *n. See* CANDIDIASIS.

erythrocine (erythrocin) *n.* A red dye used to disclose *plaque deposits on the tooth surfaces. It is used in both liquid and tablet form. *See also* DISCLOSING AGENT.

erythrocyte *n.* A red blood cell containing the oxygen-carrying pigment *haemoglobin. It is a biconcave disc about 7μm in diameter with no nucleus. There are normally about 5×10^{12} erythrocytes per litre of blood. Red cell production (**erythropoiesis**) usually takes place in

the bone marrow. The **erythrocyte sedimentation rate (ESR)** is an index of the degree of inflammation measured by the rate at which red blood cells settle in a test tube or pipette; generally the faster the blood cells settle the more severe the inflammation.

erythrodontia *n.* A reddish or reddish-brown discoloration of the teeth as may occur in **porphyria,** a rare metabolic disorder.

erythroleukoplakia *n. See* ERYTHROPLAKIA.

erythromycin *n.* An antibiotic derived from the bacterium *Streptomyces erythreus* which has an antimicrobial spectrum similar to *penicillin. It is poorly absorbed from and is irritant to the gastric mucosa. It is no longer recommended by the American Heart Association and the American Dental Association for the treatment of *bacterial endocarditis in patients allergic to penicillin. Trade names: **Erymax, Erythrocin.**

erythroplakia (erythroplasia) *n.* A condition defined by the *World Health Organization (WHO) as 'A fiery red patch that cannot be characterized clinically or pathologically as any other definable disease'. It has a high risk of malignant change and approximately 50% are carcinomatous at biopsy. It may be interspersed with white areas (**erythroleukoplakia**). *See also* LEUKOPLAKIA. 📷

Further Reading: Reichart P. A., Philipsen H. P. Oral erythroplakia—a review. *Oral Oncol* 2005;41:551–61.

erythroplasia *n. See* ERYTHROPLAKIA.

erythropoiesis *n.* The formation of red blood cells. This normally occurs in the blood-forming tissue of the bone marrow.

eschar *n.* (*adj.* **escharotic**) A thick scab or slough which forms as a result of damage to living tissue due to heat or a corrosive substance.

esophagus *n. See* OESOPHAGUS.

Essig splint A splint consisting of stainless steel wire, first described by Norman S. Essig, American prosthodontist, passed labially and lingually around a section of the dental arch and located in position by individual *ligature wires around the contact areas of the teeth. It is used to stabilize fractured or repositioned teeth and the associated alveolar bone.

Essix retainer A removable, vacuum-formed orthodontic appliance that fits over the entire arch of teeth and prevents the upper and lower teeth from making contact. It is used as part of orthodontic therapy primarily for retention, but may also be used for other functions such as to produce tooth movement, as a *bite plane, as a fluoride or bleaching tray, and in the treatment of *temporomandibular joint dysfunction syndrome.

ester local analgesic *n. See* ANALGESIC.

etching *n*. The process of removing some of the superficial *calcium in enamel or dentine to provide a micromechanical surface for the retention of *sealants or *bonding agents. The etching agent is usually *phosphoric acid gel. Plaque must be removed before etching as it is not penetrated effectively by the etching agent. Some bonding agents are self-etching and leave the *smear layer on the dentine; these usually produce less aggressive etching of enamel. *See also* ACID-ETCH TECHNIQUE.

Further Reading: Christensen G. J. Has the 'total-etch' concept disappeared? *J Am Dent Assoc* 2006;137:817–20.

ethics *n*. A code of professional standards that defines values and determines moral duties and obligations. An **ethics committee** is an independent group of medical, dental, and lay people who verify the integrity of a research study and ensure the safety, integrity, and human rights of the study participants. Research involving patients, staff, premises, or their records which is not considered part of normal clinical practice will normally require ethics committee approval.

Further Reading: Gelbier S., Wright D., Bishop M. Ethics and dentistry: 1. The meaning of ethics. *Dent Update* 2001;28:468–73.

ethmoid *n*. A bone of the neurocranium forming structures within the nasal cavity such as its roof, perpendicular plate, and the superior and middle *conchae. Air cells within the ethmoid bone form sinuses which drain into the nasal cavity.

ethyl chloride *n*. (C_2H_5Cl) A colourless liquid that boils at 12°C (54°F). When sprayed onto a mucosal surface it acts as a *topical analgesic of very short duration because of the superficial freezing produced by the rapid evaporation of the liquid: it may therefore be used to obtain analgesia when lancing an *abscess. Because of its cooling effect it may also be used when sprayed onto a pledget of *cotton wool to test for the *vitality of a pulp. Ethyl chloride is a potent inhalation anaesthetic.

ethylene diamine tetraacetic acid (EDTA) A *chelating agent used to aid root canal debridement. It functions by opening up the *dentinal tubules, softening the *dentine making it easier to remove, and lubricating the root canal.

etiology *n. See* AETIOLOGY.

eugenol *n*. ($C_{10}H_{12}O_2$) An allyl chain-substituted guaiacol which is a pale yellow oily liquid derivative of *oil of cloves. It is added to *zinc oxide in different specific ratios to form a paste for use as a temporary restorative material, as an *impression material, and formerly as a *base for a permanent restorative material.

eugnathia *n*. An abnormality of the oral cavity which is limited to the teeth and their immediate alveolar supports and does not include the jaws. *Compare* DYSGNATHIA.

eukaryotes *pl. n.* Organisms with complex cells, in which DNA is organized in tightly packed chromosomes within a membrane-bound nucleus. Eukaryote cells are generally much larger than *prokaryotic cells and have membrane-bound cell organelles. Eukaryotes include all animals, plants, and fungi, which are mainly multicellular and complex, and a variety of other groups of organisms called **protists** (e.g. protozoa), many of which are unicellular.

European Union Tissues and Cells Directive A directive of the European parliament and of the Council of the European Union which sets standards of quality and safety for the donation, procurement, testing, processing, preservation, storage, and distribution of human tissue and cells intended for human application. It was adopted by the European parliament on 7 April 2004. It requires everyone who procures, stores, or processes human tissue for human application to apply for a licence. *See also* HUMAN TISSUE ACT.

(⊕) SEE WEB LINKS

• General information and guidance on aspects relating to human tissues.

eutectic *adj*. Describing a mixture of two or more elements which has a lower melting point than any of its constituents, and which all crystallize simultaneously from the molten state.

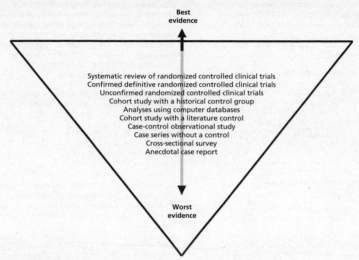

Best
evidence

Systematic review of randomized controlled clinical trials
Confirmed definitive randomized controlled clinical trials
Unconfirmed randomized controlled clinical trials
Cohort study with a historical control group
Analyses using computer databases
Cohort study with a literature control
Case-control observational study
Case series without a control
Cross-sectional survey
Anecdotal case report

Worst
evidence

Hierarchy of evidence

evaginated odontome *n.* *See* DENS
EVAGINATUS.

evidence-based dentistry A system of
practice that integrates clinically relevant
scientific evidence, clinical experience, and
the patient's treatment needs and preference,
taking into account the patient's oral and
medical condition and history. The strength of
the scientific evidence available can be ranked
in a hierarchical order and should be taken
into account when assessing its validity.

Further Reading: Richards D. Not all evidence is created
equal—so what is good evidence? *Evidence-Based Dentistry*
2003;4:17–18.
Evidence based dentistry for effective practice, ed. J. Clarkson et
al. Martin Dunitz, 2003.

(⊕) SEE WEB LINKS

• Levels of evidence defined by the Centre for
Evidence based Medicine.

evulsion *n.* *See* AVULSION.

examination *n.* Investigation of all or
part of the body for the purpose of
evaluating the state of health or disease.

In dentistry it can be both intra-oral and
extra-oral and may include visual inspection,
palpation, percussion, and measurement of
*mobility. Examination may also include
diagnostic *radiographs, laboratory tests, and
*biopsy.

excavator *n.* A hand instrument
primarily used for the removal of carious
dentine from a tooth cavity. The instrument
is usually double-ended and has a
sharp-edged spoon at each end which varies
in size and shape. It may also be used as a
*curette.

excipient *n.* A substance with no
pharmacological action that is combined with a
drug in order to render it suitable for
administration e.g. a drug taken in the form of
pills.

excision *n.* The act of cutting out or removing
an organ or tissue. **Radical excision** involves the
removal of not only the *lesion but also tissues
which may be remote from the site of the lesion.

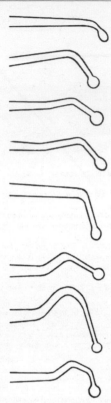

Types of excavators

excisional new attachment procedure (ENAP) A surgical procedure, first described by R. A. Yukna in 1976, in which the sulcular and junctional epithelium is resected. The aim of the procedure is to remove the diseased tissue and allow healing of the dentogingival and periodontal attachments.

excretion *n.* The natural removal of metabolic waste products, water, mineral salts, and carbon dioxide from the body. It occurs through the kidneys, lungs, and sweat glands.

exfoliation *n.* The natural physiological process of shedding the *primary (deciduous) teeth. The root of the primary tooth resorbs as the permanent tooth erupts from beneath it such that at the time of exfoliation only the crown of the primary tooth may be present. Premature

exfoliation may result in a loss of space for the permanent successor, resulting in a potential *malocclusion. Delayed exfoliation may be due to the absence of a permanent successor or to such conditions as *hypothyroidism, *hypopituitarism, ectodermal *dysplasia, or genetic disorders including osteogenesis imperfecta, *Down's syndrome, or *achondroplasia.

exocrine gland A gland which secretes via a duct onto the skin or *mucosa. *Compare* ENDOCRINE GLAND.

exocytosis *n.* A process by which secretory products, which are much too large to cross the *plasma membrane, are released from a cell via transport within *vesicles to the cell surface and subsequent fusion with the plasma membrane, resulting in the extrusion of the vesicle contents from the cell. The reverse of exocytosis is **endocytosis**, during which an invagination of the plasma membrane is pinched off to form a vesicle within the cell.

exodontia *n.* The practice of the planned removal of teeth from the oral cavity by a registered dental professional. *See also* TOOTH EXTRACTION.

exolever *n.* A modified *elevator for the extraction of tooth roots. It has a small rounded tip either in the long axis to the handle or angled left or right.

exophthalmos *n.* The protrusion of the eyeballs most commonly associated with overactivity of the thyroid gland.

exophytic *adj.* Describing a tendency to grow outward beyond the surface epithelium from which it originates.

exostosis *n.* A benign outgrowth of bony tissue on the surface of a bone or tooth root. *See also* OSTEOMA.

exothermic *adj.* Describing a chemical reaction that produces heat, such as the polymerization of resin and the hardening of zinc phosphate *cement. *Compare* ENDOTHERMIC.

exotoxin *n.* A soluble protein excreted by a micro-organism, most frequently by *bacteria. Exotoxins are usually (though not exclusively) heat labile, highly potent, and capable of causing major damage to the host by destroying cells or disrupting cellular metabolism. They can exert local and systemic effects. Exotoxins are produced by both Gram-positive and Gram-negative bacterial species. Some bacterial species can produce a wide range of different exotoxins (e.g. *Staphylococcus aureus*). Examples of diseases caused by bacterial exotoxins are *diphtheria (diphtheria toxin), botulism (*botulinum toxin), *tetanus (tetanus toxin), and cholera (cholera toxin).

expansion *n.* An increase in size, length, area, or volume. **Delayed expansion** occurs when *amalgam has been contaminated with water during *trituration or packing into a prepared cavity. An **expansion plate** is an orthodontic *appliance used to increase the width of the dental arch by buccal or labial movement of the teeth. **Thermal expansion** of an investment mould compensates for the thermal contraction of cast metal when it solidifies.

expectorant *n.* An agent that promotes the removal of mucous secretions and helps their expulsion through coughing, spitting, or sneezing.

experiment *n.* A scientific method of investigating research questions, solving problems, and evaluating theoretical assumptions. An experimental hypothesis predicts that experimental manipulations will have an effect or some identified *variables will relate to each other.

expert witness An individual who possesses specialized knowledge through skill, education, training, or experience beyond that of the ordinary person and can, during a legal case, provide the court with an assessment, opinion, or judgement within the area of his or her area of expertise. They are 'servants' of the court. An expert witness report addresses condition and prognosis, breach of duty, and causation.

expiratory reserve volume (ERV) The amount of air that can be forcibly exhaled after the end of normal exhalation.

explantation *n.* The removal of an *osseointegrated implant or *onplant such as an orthodontic implant placed to provide intra-oral *anchorage.

explorer *n.* Any dental instrument with a sharp point used to conduct a tactile examination of the tooth crown or root surfaces. It is used primarily to investigate carious lesions, hard surface deposits, and restoration margins. There are many different shapes, of which the most common are straight, half-moon, and Briault (double-ended with angled tips), designed to fulfil specific functions. *See also* PROBE.

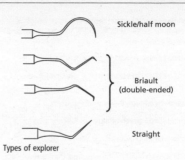

Sickle/half moon

Briault (double-ended)

Straight

Types of explorer

exposure *n. See* PULP EXPOSURE.

expressed need *n. See* NEED.

exsiccation *n.* Drying up, as may occur with a tissue deprived of an adequate water supply.

exsufflation *n.* The forced removal of secretions from the air passages by some form of manual or mechanical suction apparatus.

extension for prevention A restorative philosophy which advocated the extension of the margins of a cavity preparation into areas of the tooth considered unlikely to become carious because of their accessibility to cleaning. It was a concept proposed by G. V. *Black in 1891 and applied specifically to the materials available at the time. This philosophy has been heavily influenced by the advent of new restorative materials and techniques.

extent and severity index (ESI) A periodontal index used in *epidemiology to calculate and summarize the extent and the average severity of periodontal disease based on the degree of alveolar bone loss within the group being studied. It uses estimates of *periodontal attachment levels from probing measurements of 14 sites in one maxillary quadrant and 14 in the contralateral mandibular quadrant.

Further Reading: Carlos J. P., Wolfe M. D., Kingman A. The extent and severity index: a simple method for use in epidemiologic studies of periodontal disease. *J Clin Periodontol* 1986;13:500–05.

external bevel gingivectomy *See* GINGIVECTOMY.

external oblique ridge *n. See* MANDIBLE.

extirpation *n.* The complete removal or eradication of a tissue, organ, or growth. In endodontic therapy it is used to describe the complete removal of all vital pulp tissue.

extracoronal *adj.* Describing that which is outside or external to the body of a tooth such as an artificial *crown.

extraction *n.* See TOOTH EXTRACTION.

extraction instruments See ELEVATOR; FORCEPS.

extra-oral *adj.* Outside the mouth.

extra-oral anchorage *n.* See ANCHORAGE.

extra-oral traction *n.* See TRACTION.

extravasation *n.* The escape and spread of a body fluid, e.g. blood, from vessels into the surrounding tissues as a result of trauma, burns, inflammation, or allergy.

extrinsic tooth staining Discoloration originating from outside the tooth. Extrinsic stains include tobacco, red wine, tea, chlorhexidine mouthwash, and some metallic deposits encountered as occupational hazards. Extrinsic staining is usually successfully removed with mild abrasive toothpaste, or professionally, using an abrasive prophylactic paste. *Compare* INTRINSIC TOOTH STAINING.

Further Reading: Sulieman M. An overview of tooth discoloration: extrinsic, intrinsic and internalized stains. *Dent Update* 2005;32(8):463–4, 466–8, 471.

extrusion *n.* 1. Partial displacement of a tooth from its socket. If caused by external trauma, treatment involves repositioning the tooth in the socket under local anaesthesia using digital pressure followed by *splinting if there is alveolar bone fracture. Loss of *vitality is a common sequel. 2. The intentional pulling of a tooth into a more acceptable position, either in an occlusal or incisal direction. This may be carried out using *elastics linking a fixed or removable orthodontic *appliance to a hook cemented on to the crown of the tooth to be extruded.

exudation *n.* The slow outflow of a liquid (called the **exudate**) through the walls of intact blood vessels, usually as a result of inflammation such as a gingival *crevicular fluid exudate in chronic *gingivitis.

exuviation *n.* The shedding of an epidermal structure such as a primary tooth, the skin of a snake, or the shell of a crustacean.

facebow *n.* 1. A device used in dental prosthodontics to measure the positions of the *temporomandibular joints relative to the maxillary teeth so that such positions may be transferred to an *articulator. It essentially consists of two arms with calliper ends (condyle rods) that can be accurately adjusted to locate the axis of rotation of the mandible, together with a connecting structure which carries a *bite fork on which an impression of the occlusal surfaces of the maxillary teeth is located. The calliper arms make contact immediately anterior to the external auditory meatus, but may fit into it (**earbow**). The frame carrying the bite fork is capable of being adjusted relative to the two arms. 2. An orthodontic appliance used as extra-oral *anchorage for the posterior teeth during active orthodontic treatment. It is made of steel, is bow-shaped, and is inserted into tubes fixed on the molar teeth. The outer part of the bow protrudes from the mouth, presenting two hooked arms extending posteriorly over the cheeks which are attached to straps that pass around the neck or back of the head.

face height The vertical dimension of the face measured from the mid-point between the eyebrows and the base of the chin. It is divided into the **upper face height**, the vertical distance between the base of the nose and the mid-point between the eyebrows, and the lower face height, the vertical distance between the base of the nose and the base of the chin.

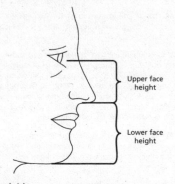

Upper face height

Lower face height

Face height

facemask *n.* A disposable barrier used to protect the oral and nasal mucous membranes of the wearer from inhaled spray, splashes, spatter, and aerosols. Face masks can also be effective against droplets being expelled into the environment by the wearer.

face shield *n.* A transparent barrier extending from the forehead to the chin protecting the face and eyes from aerosols, spatter, and debris generated particularly by *ultrasonic scalers and high-speed *turbines. 📷

facet *n.* A small flat surface on a bone or tooth. It usually indicates an area of tooth wear on a surface contacting another tooth or tooth restoration (*wear facet).

facial bone *n.* One of the 14 separate bones of the face that make up the jaws, cheeks, and nose. Six are paired, namely the maxilla, palatine, zygomatic, nasal, lacrimal, and inferior concha; the mandible and vomer are single unpaired bones.

facial index The relation of the length of the face to its width multiplied by 100. The length is measured from the nasion to the mental tubercle and the width is the maximum distance between the zygomatic prominences.

facial nerve paralysis (palsy) *See* BELL'S PALSY.

facial neuralgia *n. See* TRIGEMINAL NEURALGIA.

facial pain A generic description of pain of non-dental origin. It includes conditions such as trigeminal *neuralgia and post-herpetic neuralgia. **Atypical facial pain** (sometimes called **persistent idiopathic facial pain**) affects middle-aged women more than men and is characterized by continuous pain for months or even years. It is often described as gripping or vice-like. it affects the maxilla more than the mandible, and may cross the midline and other anatomical boundaries. There are no clear precipitating factors although patients are frequently depressed.

Further Reading: Woda A., Tubert-Jeannin S., Bouhassira D., Attal N., Fleiter B., Goulet J. P., Gremeau-Richard C., Navez M.L., Picard P., Pionchon P., Albuisson E. Towards a new taxonomy of idiopathic orofacial pain. *Pain* 2005;116 (3):396–406.

facial palsy See BELL'S PALSY.

facial seal See BORDER SEAL.

facies *n.* The appearance or facial expression of an individual. It is used to describe a facial expression suggestive, diagnostic, or indicative of a specific diagnosis or condition.

facing *n.* A tooth-coloured material, usually either porcelain or resin, used to provide a more aesthetic labial or buccal surface for a metal crown.

factitious *adj.* Artificially produced, either deliberately or by accident. Patients with factitious disorders produce or exaggerate the symptoms of a physical or mental illness. **Factitial gingival trauma** in children is often associated with finger or pencil sucking habits. **Factitious gingivitis** see GINGIVITIS ARTEFACTA.

factor analysis (in statistics) A *multivariate technique used to identify whether the *correlations between a series of *variables are due to their relationships with one or more latent variables in the *data.

Factor VIII (antihaemophilic factor) A blood-clotting factor normally present in the blood, a deficiency of which results in haemophilia A. It binds with *von Willebrand factor. See COAGULATION.

Factor IX (Christmas factor) A blood-clotting factor normally present in the blood, a deficiency of which results in haemophilia B (Christmas disease). See COAGULATION.

Factor XI A blood-clotting factor normally present in the blood, a deficiency of which can lead to excessive bleeding after surgery or trauma to the blood vessels. See COAGULATION.

Factor XII A blood-clotting factor normally present in the blood, a deficiency of which can lead to a prolonged clotting time. See COAGULATION.

facultative *adj.* Describing an organism that is capable of surviving under different or varying environmental conditions. See also ANAEROBE.

Faculty of General Dental Practice (UK) The Faculty of General Dental Practice (FGDP) is the academic home for general dental practitioners (GDPs) and dental care professionals (DCPs) in the UK. Part of the Royal College of Surgeons of England, it aims to promote excellence in the standards of patient care in general dental practice by encouraging involvement in postgraduate training and assessment, education, and research. The FGDP (UK) supports the career development of both GDPs and DCPs and recognizes the value of an integrated dental team in modern dentistry.

((((⊕)))) SEE WEB LINKS

• The Faculty of General Dental Practice (UK) website.

faint *n.* See SYNCOPE.

false negative A falsely drawn negative conclusion; in diagnostic tests it is a conclusion that a person does not have the disease or condition being tested, when they actually do. *Compare* FALSE POSITIVE.

false positive A falsely drawn positive conclusion; in diagnostic tests it is a result that indicates that a person has the disease or condition when in fact they do not. *Compare* FALSE NEGATIVE.

false (pseudo) pocket *n.* See POCKET.

familial *adj.* Describing a tendency to occur in more members of a family than would be expected by chance alone.

familial adenomatous polyposis (FAP) An inherited autosomal dominant disorder characterized by many thousands of glandular tissue *polyps throughout the colorectal part of the digestive tract. There is a very high risk of developing colorectal *carcinoma if patients are not treated with colectomy. Bone lesions of the mandible and maxilla and dental abnormalities such as impacted teeth other than third molars, *supernumerary teeth, congenitally missing teeth, and fused roots are present in more than 70% of individuals. It is also known as *Gardner's syndrome.

fascia *n.* (*pl.* **fasciae**) Layers of connective tissue of variable thickness. The **superficial fascia** is found immediately below the skin and **deep fascia** invests muscles, nerves, and other organs.

fasciculus (fascicule) *n.* A bundle of anatomical fibres such as muscle or nerve.

fasciitis *n.* Inflammation of the fascia due to bacterial infection or rheumatic disease. *See also* NECROTIZING FASCIITIS.

fat *n.* A substance that contains one or more *fatty acids and is the principal form of storing energy in the body. Fat serves as a cushion to protect organs, as a carrier of fat-soluble vitamins (*vitamins A, D, E, and K and carotene), and as an insulation layer under the skin. It is also involved in the maintenance of cell membranes.

fatty acids An organic acid that occurs naturally, either singly or combined, and consists of strongly linked carbon and hydrogen atoms in a chain-like structure. They are the constituents of many important *lipids such as triglycerides.

fauces *n.* The region between the oral cavity and the *pharynx. It is formed by the *tongue, *soft palate, and the **pillars of the fauces**. The two pillars are curved folds of tissue running from the palate to the base of the tongue. The anterior pillar is called the **palatoglossal arch** and the posterior pillar the **palatopharyngeal arch**. Between the two arches lie the palatine *tonsils.

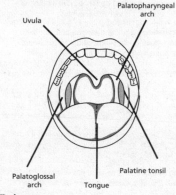

The fauces

Fauchard, Pierre (1678–1761) Fauchard was born in Brittany and trained as a surgeon in the French navy, which he left in 1700 to become a dentist in Angers, western France. In 1719 he established a practice in Paris and was the first person to use the title of surgeon–dentist (chirurgien–dentiste). He published the first dental textbook, 'Le Chirugien Dentiste ou Treatise des Dents' ('The Surgeon Dentist or Treatise on the Teeth') in 1728 (the first English translation was not published until 1946), in which he described 103 diseases of the teeth and oral cavity including pyorrhoea alveolaris. He introduced many new radical ideas, such as the treatment of patients in the chair (as opposed to the then conventional approach of lying them on the floor). He coined the term 'dental caries' and dismissed the idea of worms being the causative agent of dental decay. Because he appreciated the benefits of the judicious extraction of teeth to prevent malocclusion, he is regarded as one of the world's first orthodontic specialists. In his honour, in 1936 the Pierre Fauchard Academy was established. The academy maintains a 'Hall of Fame' that recognizes the achievements of over 7000 leading members of the dental profession.

Further Reading: Lynch C. D., O'Sullivan V. R., McGillycuddy C. T. Pierre Fauchard: the 'Father of Modern Dentistry'. *Br Dent J* 2006;201:779–81.

FDI *See* FEDERATION DENTAIRE INTERNATIONALE.

FDI tooth notation *See* TOOTH NOTATION.

febrile *adj.* Pertaining to a raised body temperature or fever.

Federation Dentaire Internationale (FDI) (World Dental Federation) A federation of National Dental Associations and, as such, its main roles are to bring together the world of dentistry, to represent the dental profession of the world, and to stimulate and facilitate the exchange of information across all borders with the aim of optimal oral health for all peoples.

fee *n.* Payment for professional services rendered. The **usual fee (customary, reasonable)** is the fee that an individual dentist most frequently charges for a specific dental service.

feldspar *n.* Any of a group of hard grey crystalline minerals that consist of aluminium silicates of potassium, sodium, calcium, or barium. A mixture of feldspar, quartz, and *kaolin is used in the manufacture of *porcelain denture teeth and in the construction of some porcelain crowns and inlays.

felt need *n. See* NEED.

felypressin *n.* A synthetic octapeptide which resembles the *pituitary hormone *vasopressin. It is a *vasoconstrictor which causes vascular smooth muscle to contract. It is included in dental *anaesthetic solutions in order to produce constriction of the venous vessels, thus reducing the rate at which the local anaesthetic is carried away by the bloodstream, and thereby extending the duration of the local anaesthetic to produce a deeper and more effective level of anaesthesia. Trade name: Octapressin*.

fenestration *n.* A procedure in which a hole is opened in the bone, e.g. alveolar fenestration in which access is gained to the apical root area through a window in the alveolar cortical plate. Fenestration can occur pathologically, producing a window-like defect in the cortical jaw bone to give an isolated area of exposed root surface. This lesion will be seen when the alveolar bone is exposed by flap surgery; it is associated with localized periodontal destruction.

fermentable carbohydrate *n.* An organic compound based on the general formula C_x $(H_2O)_y$, which is capable of being broken down by bacteria with the production of acid.

ferric oxide *n.* The impure form of naturally occurring iron oxide, used as a metal polishing agent and as a colouring agent in resins and ceramics. It is also known as jeweller's or red rouge.

ferric sulphate *n.* A chemical applied in aqueous solution to the pulpal surface of primary teeth to achieve *haemostasis in a *pulpotomy procedure. It is the active ingredient in some *gingival retraction cords.

Further Reading: Ibricevic H., Al-Jame Q. Ferric sulphate and formocresol in pulpotomy of primary molars: long term follow-up study. *Eur J Paediatr Dent* 2003 Mar;4(1):28–32.

ferrous sulphate *n.* An iron salt used in the treatment of iron deficiency anaemia. It may cause constipation or diarrhoea and will darken the colour of the stools. If in tablet form and dissolved sublingually it can result in mucosal ulceration.

Further Reading: Jones T. A., Parmer S. C. Oral mucosal ulceration due to ferrous sulphate tablets: report of a case. *Dent Update* 2006;33:632–3.

ferrule effect The protective effect achieved by the supra-marginal extension of the dentine coronal to the shoulder of a post and core crown preparation. This procedure creates a ferrule of dentine designed to reduce stress within a tooth.

Further Reading: Stankiewicz N., Wilson P. The ferrule effect. *Dent Update* 2008;35:222–8.

festoon 1. *v.* To shape and contour a denture base material to simulate the natural contour of the tissues including the gingival tissues replaced by the appliance. 2. *n.* The shape of a prosthesis which simulates that of natural tissues. 3. *n.* The vertical grooving of bone during osseous surgery. 4. *n.* Semi-lunar enlargements of the marginal gingivae (*see* MCCALL'S FESTOONS).

fetid *adj. See* FOETID.

fever *n. See* PYREXIA.

fiberotomy *n. See* PERICISION.

fibre *n.* 1. (in anatomy) A threadlike structure such as a muscle cell, a collagen fibre, or a nerve fibre. The free gingival and periodontal fibres of the *periodontal ligament (e.g. the apical, transseptal, and circumferential) are important in maintaining the integrity of the tooth interrelationship. 2. (in dietetics) Dietary fibre (roughage) is that part of food that cannot be digested and absorbed to produce energy; it is mainly found in vegetables, fruits, and cereals, and adds bulk to the diet.

fibre optic light A light source which uses flexible fibreglass to conduct light over long distances with little or no distortion. It may be used as an intra-oral light attached to a mouth mirror or handpiece.

fibre optic transillumination (FOTI) *See* TRANSILLUMINATION.

fibre reinforced resin composite *See* RESIN COMPOSITE, FIBRE REINFORCED.

fibrillation *n.* The disorganized random depolarization of muscle fibres of the heart producing a wriggling effect due to rapid, irregular, and unsynchronized activity. It prevents normal coordinated muscular contraction. **Atrial fibrillation** is a common condition found more frequently in elderly women and produces a fast irregular pulse rate. **Ventricular fibrillation** is a common cause of 'out of hospital' cardiac arrest.

fibrin *n.* An insoluble protein formed as the final product in *blood coagulation by the action of *thrombin on *fibrinogen.

fibrinogen *n.* A soluble protein found in blood *plasma that is acted upon by the *enzyme *thrombin to produce insoluble *fibrin as the final stage of *blood coagulation.

fibrinolysis *n.* (*adj.* **fibrinolytic**) The process of *fibrin breakdown by the enzyme **fibrinolysin** during the removal of small fibrin blood clots from the circulation.

fibroadenoma *n.* A benign tumour of epithelial origin containing recognizable fibrous tissue.

fibroblast *n.* A cell found in *connective tissue responsible for the production of *collagen fibres and *ground substance.

fibrocartilage *n.* A type of *cartilage in which there are dense bundles of fibres.

fibro-epithelial polyp *n. See* POLYP.

fibroma *n.* (*pl.* **fibromas** or **fibromata**) A non-malignant (benign) neoplasm of *connective tissue: they are rare in the oral cavity and most nodules of fibrous tissue are reactive *hyperplasia to trauma and not neoplasms. An **ameloblastic fibroma** is a circumscribed benign odontogenic neoplasm composed of cellular fibrous tissue resembling the dental papilla containing small islands of odontogenic epithelium. They are normally found in the mandible over unerupted molars of young patients and appear as a circumscribed *radiolucency; the soft tissue mass can cause expansion of the *bone cortex. Treatment is by conservative surgical excision. An **ossifying fibroma** (**cemento-ossifying fibroma**) is a well-demarcated lesion composed of cellular fibrous tissue in which calcification is laid down and which arises in the periodontal ligament of young individuals. They are most common in the posterior mandible and cause jaw expansion; radiographically they appear as a well-defined mixed radiolucency or radiopacity and are treated by surgical removal. An **odontogenic fibroma** is a benign odontogenic neoplasm of unknown aetiology derived from odontogenic connective tissue: it contains scattered islands of odontogenic epithelium and foci of calcification; treatment is by enucleation or curettage.

fibromatosis, oral (gingival) *n.* A rare benign overgrowth of fibrous tissue of hereditary or *idiopathic origin primarily affecting children and young adults. It is characterized by painless firm *hyperplastic tissue enlargement of the *gingivae which covers the teeth; there may also be associated gingival inflammation and bleeding where the oral hygiene is poor; one or more quadrants of the mouth may be affected. It is treated by wide excision (*gingivectomy), although it has a locally aggressive behaviour possibly leading to recurrence. The condition of fibrous gingival hyperplasia may also be drug-induced, e.g. by *phenytoin or *nifedipine, in which the hyperplasia occurs three or more years after the onset of drug use; treatment is by plaque control and may also include a change in drug therapy. **Symmetrical fibromatosis of the tuberosity** can occur in adults and is characterized by large, smooth, fleshy, hyperplasia of the tissues overlying the maxillary tuberosities; treatment is usually unnecessary unless there is interference with a denture fitting surface. 🖽

fibronectin *n.* A high molecular weight glycoprotein compound consisting of two disulfide-linked *polypeptides. It is found on cell surfaces, in connective tissues, in the blood, and in other body fluids. It may enhance the adherence of *fibroblasts to the tooth root surface.

fibrosarcoma *n.* A malignant tumour of *connective tissue of which the basic cell type is a *fibroblast. Although rare, they can occur in the oral region.

fibrosis *n.* (*adj.* **fibrotic**) A thickening and scarring of connective tissue due to excess collagen, usually as a result of chronic inflammation or injury. In oral submucous fibrosis, progressive fibrosis of the oral cavity leads to difficulty in opening (*trismus) and the lesion is regarded as *premalignant with an increased risk of oral cancer development. It is common in persons who chew paan or betel quid. **fibrotic** *adj.*

fibrous dysplasia *n. See* DYSPLASIA.

Fickling, Ben, CBE (1909–2007) A dental surgeon who played a pivotal role in the development of modern oral and maxillo-facial surgery. He designed several surgical instruments (*see* FORCEPS) and together with William Warwick James published 'Injuries of Jaws and Face' in 1940 and the translation of Le Fort's work into English. He was a founder member, and helped to write the constitution, of the British Association of Oral Surgeons and planned and inaugurated the Royal College of Surgeons' first higher examinations in general surgery. He was dean of the Faculty of Dental Surgery in the Royal College of Surgeons in England from 1968 to 1971 and was awarded the CBE in 1973.

fifth disease *n. See* ERYTHEMA INFECTIOSUM.

Filatov's spots [N. F. Filatov (1847–1902), Russian paediatrician] A synonym for Koplick's spots.

file *n.* A metal tool with a roughened surface or surfaces used for smoothing or shaping. A **bone file** is a hand instrument used to smooth a sharp or high bony surface during a surgical procedure. **Interproximal bone files** are double safe-sided instruments with either curved or straight tapering blades used for the reduction of interproximal bone during periodontal surgery. An **endodontic file** is a metal instrument used in endodontic procedures to *debride and shape the root canal system; they may be hand-held or mounted in a dental *handpiece. They are manufactured in different shapes and sizes to conform to the root canal structure. A **K-type-file** is made by twisting a square metal blank. A **Hedstrom file** is made by machining a continuous groove into a metal blank. A **K-flex file** is more flexible than a K-type-file and is made by twisting a rhomboid shape blank. A **flex-o-file** is more flexible than the K-type-file and is made from a triangular blank with a blunt tip. The *International Standards Organization (ISO) defines a **colour coding** related to the size of the file.

Endodontic file sizes		
Size	Tip diameter	International Standards Organization (ISO) colour
08	0.08	grey
10	0.10	purple
15	0.15	white
20	0.20	yellow
25	0.25	red
30	0.30	blue
35	0.35	green
40	0.40	black
45	0.45	white
50	0.50	yellow
55	0.55	red
60	0.60	blue
70	0.70	green
80	0.80	black
90	0.90	white
100	1.00	yellow
110	1.10	red
120	1.20	blue
130	1.30	green
140	1.40	black

Files have traditionally been made of steel but newer varieties are made of nickel titanium (NiTi) because of the metal's greater flexibility. **Finishing files** are used for preparing the apical third of a root canal and producing a variable taper.

filler *n.* An inert material added to *resin composite to increase strength and abrasion resistance. Filler particles are usually composed of quartz or glasses containing barium or strontium (added to give the resin radiopacity). Fillers provide a means of controlling various aesthetic features such as colour, translucency, and fluorescence. The filler particles may be large (**macrofilled**), small (**microfilled** or **nanofilled**), or a mixture of both (**hybrid**). *See also* RESIN COMPOSITE.

filler paste *n. See* PASTE.

filling *n. See* RESTORATION.

film *n.* A thin flexible piece of cellulose acetate coated with a light sensitive emulsion on each side.

film badge A device for monitoring and measuring the radiographic *dose retrospectively. Film badges are processed on a regular basis by the radiation safety office.

film holder *n.* A device for holding and stabilizing an intra-oral radiographic film.

film thickness 1. The depth of a layer of material such as luting cement, bonding liquid, or cavity liner applied to a surface. 2. The thickness of saliva between an appliance and the mucosal tissues.

fineness *n.* A method of describing the ratio of the primary metal in an alloy to any additives or impurities, expressed in parts per thousand of the pure metal. For example, a gold alloy containing 900 parts gold and 100 parts of impurities is 900 fine. *See also* CARAT.

finger rest Part of clinical dental operating technique in which the fingers of the non-working hand rest on the adjacent teeth or the fingers of the working hand to provide increased control or to provide a fulcrum for movement.

finger spreader A finely tapered, smooth-surfaced, flexible hand instrument used to laterally condense *gutta-percha points during *root canal therapy. The finger spreader is inserted between the canal wall and the gutta-percha point; after removal, a standardized accessory point coated with sealer is inserted into the residual space.

finger spring *n. See* SPRING.

finger sweep A method of removing a solid or semi-solid material from the mouth of an unconscious adult or older child.

finishing *n.* The process of removing excess material from a restoration or denture and creating a smooth surface contour. *See also* FILE; FINISHING.

finishing line A line marking the margin of a cavity or restoration where it meets the cavo-surface angle on the external surface of the tooth.

finishing strip *See* ABRASIVE.

first aid Emergency treatment given to an injured, wounded, or sick person before the services of a medical professional can be secured.

Fish, Sir Wilfred (1894–1974) Fish qualified in dentistry at the University of Manchester in 1914 and after the First World War joined the staff of the Royal Dental Hospital, London, where he was awarded a DSc for his research into the anatomical, physiological, and pathological factors that determine oral function and disorders. This led to the establishment of a periodontal clinic at the Royal Dental Hospital and the inauguration of the British Society of

Periodontology, of which Fish was the first president. He later became president of the Odontological Section of the Royal Society of Medicine and an honorary fellow of the society. He was dean of the Faculty of Dental Surgery of the Royal College of Surgeons of England from 1956 to 1959 and in 1964 he had conferred on him the first honorary fellowship of the Faculty of Dentistry of the Royal College of Surgeons in Ireland. He was elected to the Dental Board of the United Kingdom in 1939 and became its chairman in 1944. He was created CBE in 1947 and knighted in 1954. As the first president of the General Dental Council (GDC) in 1956, he oversaw the freeing of dentistry from medical administration. The Royal College of Surgeons of England has instituted a Wilfred Fish Research Fellowship and the GDC an annual eponymous lecture. He retired in 1961 but continued to contribute to discussions in dental journals until his death.

fissure *n.* 1. (in dentistry) A small groove found on the *enamel surface of a tooth. 2. (in anatomy) A groove or cleft e.g. the longitudinal cerebral fissure.

fissure bur *See* BUR.

fissured tongue *See* TONGUE, FISSURED.

fissure sealant *n.* A material bonded onto the enamel surface of teeth to prevent caries occurring in the pits or *fissures. It may be used on individuals who are assessed as being at high risk of dental caries. Materials used as fissure sealants are *resin composite or *glass ionomer. **Resin composite** is applied either as a thin unfilled resin or with a *filler added to increase the viscosity and wear resistance. Resin composite may be polymerized by either mixing a *catalyst and base together (**self- or chemical-cured**) or by using a light source to activate a *polymerization initiator such as *camphorquinone (**light-cured** or **command set**). The material is applied to the washed and dried tooth surface after the tooth has been first isolated and the enamel etched with *phosphoric acid to create a micromechanical bond. When the material has been fully polymerized, the occlusion is checked and any high spots removed. **Glass ionomer** has been used as an alternative to resin composite because it is less sensitive to the presence of moisture, bonds well to enamel, and releases *fluoride, providing a potentially *cariostatic effect; currently, however, more research is required to evaluate its long-term success in comparison to resin composite.

Further Reading: British Society of Paediatric Dentistry. Fissure sealants in paediatric dentistry: a policy document. *International Journal of Paediatric Dentistry* 2000;10:174–7.

fistula *n.* An abnormal tract or *sinus connecting two hollow organs or a hollow organ and the exterior. An **antral fistula** is a tract leading from a bone cavity e.g. a fistula between the maxillary antrum and the mouth (*oroantral fistula). An **alveolar fistula** connecting the alveolar bone to the mucosal surface is more commonly known as an alveolar sinus. A **blind (incomplete) fistula** has an opening at one end only. An **internal fistula** has no opening through the skin, unlike an **external fistula**, which does. A **salivary fistula** is an abnormal tract joining a salivary gland or duct either externally with the skin or internally with the mouth. *See also* SINUS TRACT.

fitness to practise A requirement by a regulatory body (the General Dental Council in the UK) for a registered dental professional to demonstrate a satisfactory standard of professional competence, conduct, and health. The Fitness to Practise Panel is independent of the General Dental Council (GDC) and consists of 76 members made up of dentists, lay members, and dental care professionals. The three GDC Practice Committees are the Professional Conduct Committee (PCC), the Health Committee (HC), and the Professional Performance Committee (PrPC).

Further Reading: Mathewson H., Rudkin D. The GDC-lifting the lid. Part 4: fitness to practice. *Br Dent J* 2008;205:95–9.

fixation *n.* 1. Immobilization of the parts of a fractured bone after trauma or a surgical procedure by means of wires, screws, plates, *elastics, or *splints until the healing process is complete. **Intermaxillary fixation** is a method of splinting a mobile mandible to the maxilla. 2. (in radiography) The removal of all the undeveloped salts of the film emulsion so that only the reduced silver remains to provide the permanent image.

fixative *n.* 1. Any substance used to glue or stabilize. **Denture fixative** is available in powder or paste form and reacts with saliva to develop adhesive properties, which aid the retention and stability of a denture. 2. A substance used to preserve histological tissue specimens for later examination e.g. *formalin.

fixed appliance *n. See* ORTHODONTIC APPLIANCE.

flange *n.* The *buccal, *labial, or *lingual part of a *denture base that extends from the necks of the teeth to the denture border.

flap *n.* A partially detached piece of tissue produced either as a result of trauma or surgically to repair a defect or to gain access to structures underneath e.g. a periodontal flap where surgical access may be required to treat a periodontally

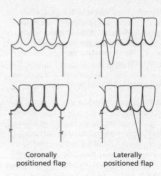

| Modified | Apically | Coronally | Laterally |
| Widman flap | positioned flap | positioned flap | positioned flap |

Flap design

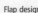

involved root surface, to remove a retained root, or to perform an *apicectomy. An **apically repositioned flap** is the repositioning of a periodontal tissue flap to reduce or eliminate gingival pocket depth or more commonly as a crown lengthening procedure to expose more tooth substance while maintaining the width of the attached *gingiva. Incisions are first made to outline the gingival tissue for its complete removal; a further incision is made distant from the area of recession preserving the papilla adjacent to the defect and a full thickness flap is positioned apically to expose the root surface and reduce pocket depth. For a **lateral sliding flap** the incised tissue is positioned laterally to cover the area of *gingival recession and sutured in position. A **coronally repositioned flap** is used mainly to cover exposed root surfaces during the treatment of *gingival recession. An **advanced flap** reaches its final destination without rotation or lateral movement. It is used mainly in periodontal reconstructive surgery. A periodontal flap may be modified with the removal of a superficial collar of the soft tissue wall of the pocket (**modified Widman flap**) by means of a scalloped inverse bevel incision made 1mm from the gingival margin with the knife blade aimed at the crest of the alveolar bone, followed by crevicular and horizontal incisions. It allows healthy connective tissue to contact the tooth surface in an attempt to improve post-surgical healing (this is a modification of the original Widman flap first described by Leonard Widman in 1918). The periodontal tissue should be plaque-free and not inflamed prior to flap surgery. (*See also* GINGIVECTOMY; GINGIVOPLASTY.)

A **pedicle flap** is a stem-shaped piece of tissue consisting of the full thickness of the skin epithelium and subcutaneous tissue attached by tissue from which it receives its blood supply. A **pericoronal flap** is a flap of gingival tissue partially covering an unerupted tooth, especially the lower third molar. *See also* GRAFT.

Further Reading: Saha S., Bateman G. J. Mucogingival grafting procedures—an update. *Dent Update* 2008;35:561–8.

flash *n.* An excess of acrylic resin squeezed out between the two halves of a denture *flask during processing. It can lead to an increase in vertical *dimension of the dentures if the two halves of the flask have not been completely closed.

flask *n.* A metal container in which either *plaster of Paris or artificial stone is placed for the purpose of compressing resin (**denture flask**) or *investment material for casting a metal restoration or appliance (**refractory flask**).

flasking *v.* The process of compressing resin into a *flask prior to curing (*polymerizing).

flexural strength The ability of a solid material to withstand bending before reaching the breaking point. It is usually measured in force per unit area.

flexure *n.* The quality or state of being elastically deformed or bent. It is an important property of many materials in dentistry such as restorative and appliance materials, retentive clasps, and endodontic instruments.

flora *n. See* ORAL FLORA.

Florida probe *n. See* PROBE.

floss *n.* Waxed or unwaxed thread or tape used to remove *plaque and food debris from the interproximal spaces between the teeth. The floss is placed in the gingival *crevice (sulcus) and, by pressure against the mesial or distal tooth surface, forms a C-shape. It is then withdrawn in a coronal direction. Floss is normally held between the fingers but there are a number of flossing aids to help the less dextrous or to gain access to less accessible areas. **Floss tape** is sometimes advocated for gaining access to tight interproximal spaces and may be made of *polytetrafluoroethylene (PTFE) to resist shredding and breaking. Floss is sometimes impregnated with *fluoride because of its *cariostatic properties, but its potential benefit requires further research. 📷

Further Reading: Hujoel P. P., Cunha-Cruz J., Banting D. W., Loesche W. J. Dental flossing and interproximal caries: a systematic review. *J Dent Res* 2006;85(4):298–305.

Flower's dental index [W. H. Flower (1831–99), English anatomist] A craniometric index indicating the comparative size of the teeth. It is the distance from the mesial surface of the first premolar to the distal surface of the third molar (dental length) multiplied by 100 and divided by the distance from the midline point on the anterior border of the *foramen magnum (basion) to the middle of the nasofrontal suture (nasion), the basinasal length.

fluconazole *n.* A triazole antifungal drug used in the treatment and prevention of *candidiasis and other superficial and systemic fungal infections. It is administered by mouth or intravenous infusion. Possible side-effects include nausea and vomiting. Trade name: **Diflucan**.

fluctuant *adj.* Describing the sensation of wave-like motion produced in a fluid-filled part of the body on applying light pressure with the fingers.

flumazenil *n.* A benzodiazepine antagonist used to reverse the effects of benzodiazepines. Trade names: **Anexate, Romazicon**.

fluorapatite *n.* A form of *hydroxyapatite in which *fluoride ions replace hydroxyl ions. It is slightly stronger and more resistant to acid than hydroxyapatite.

fluorhydroxyapatite *n.* The mineralized substance produced by the reaction between small amounts of *fluoride and *hydroxyapatite.

fluoridation

n. The process of adding *fluoride ions to the public water supply for the purpose of reducing the incidence of dental *caries. Fluoride may be present naturally in the water supply due to the presence of minerals such as fluorspar (calcium fluoride, $Ca F_2$); when dissolved in water, it releases fluoride ions according to the formula $CaF2=Ca^{++}+2F^-$. The concentration of free fluoride ions in water is measured by a **fluoride ion specific electrode**. Early

research carried out by Dr Trendley Dean (1893–1962), an American dentist in Grand Rapids, Michigan, USA, established that a fluoride concentration level of one part per million (1 ppm) was optimal in achieving a significant reduction in dental caries. Following this and further research studies, water fluoridation schemes have been introduced in the USA, the UK, and many other parts of the world. In the UK, the fluoride compound most commonly artificially added to the water supply is hexafluorosilicic acid (H_2SiF_6). This releases fluoride ions according to the formula: $H_2SiF_6 + 4H_2O \leftrightarrow 6F^- + Si(OH)_4 + 6H^+$. When the concentration of fluoride in the water supply exceeds 1 ppm, dental *fluorosis may occur. The only two compounds of fluoride permitted for artificial fluoridation in the UK are hexafluorosilicic acid and sodium hexafluorosilicate. In 1994 the *World Health Organization Expert Committee concluded that although water fluoridation was considered to be both safe and cost-effective as a public health measure, the technical operation of fluoridation systems should be monitored and recorded regularly and that there should be periodic surveys of dental caries and dental fluorosis. An expert systematic review of fluoride and health was carried out in 2000 by the National Health Service Centre for Reviews and Dissemination (NHS CRD) at the request of the chief medical officer of the Department of Health (**York review**). Its aim was to review the evidence on the positive and negative effects of population-wide drinking water strategies. From the evidence available, it concluded that fluoridation of drinking water supplies reduces caries prevalence; that a beneficial effect of water fluoridation was evident; that there was some evidence that water fluoridation reduces the inequalities in dental health across social classes in 5- and 12-year-olds, using the dmft/DMFT measure; that there was evidence of some dental fluorosis of aesthetic concern but that there was no evidence of an association between water fluoridation and bone fracture or cancer.

Further Reading: World Health Organization (1994) Fluorides and Oral Health. WHO Expert Committee on Oral Health Status and Fluoride use, WHO Technical Report Series, 846.WHO.

(●) SEE WEB LINKS

- The University of York Centre for Reviews and Dissemination: 'Fluoridation of drinking water'.
- The British Fluoridation Society website.

fluoride *n.* A salt of hydrofluoric acid, usually sodium, calcium, or stannous. Fluoride exists in inorganic and organic forms; the inorganic form yields fluoride ions. If ionic inorganic fluoride is present during tooth *mineralization or remineralization, it is incorporated into the tooth enamel to form calcium fluorapatite $(Ca_{10}(PO_4)_6(F)_2)$ according to the equation:

$$Ca_{10}(PO_4)_6(OH)_2 + 2F^- \rightarrow Ca_{10}(PO_4)_6(F)_2 + 2OH^-$$

Excessive ingestion of fluoride salts can result in **fluoride toxicity** in the form of *fluorosis, nausea, vomiting, calcification of ligaments, and cardiac or respiratory failure due to the rapid absorption by the body. The dose below which toxicity is unlikely is 1mg/kg body weight; to reach the 5mg/kg threshold (requiring hospitalization) a 5-year-old child weighing about 19kg would have to ingest 95 1mg fluoride tablets, or 95 ml of fluoride toothpaste, or 7.6 ml of 1.23% acidulated phosphate *fluoride (APF) gel. Fluoride has been added as a preventive measure to oral health aids such as dental *wood points or *floss. **Pre-natal fluoride** as a caries preventive measure is relatively ineffective as the placenta only allows a small amount of fluoride to cross into the foetus.

fluoride chewing gum A natural rosin or synthetic petroleum-based polymer containing a fluoride salt such as sodium fluoride. The fluoride is added for its *cariostatic effect. Additional ingredients include softeners such as glycerine and salivary stimulants. Non-cariogenic sweeteners such as xylitol and sorbitol may also be added.

fluoride drops A supplemental liquid form of *fluoride usually administered to children over the age of 6 months, at a dosage dependent on the age of the child and body weight. The success in reducing caries is largely dependent on patient compliance; this is generally poor in high-risk groups and therefore it is not considered to be an effective public health measure.

fluoride gel A topical gel form of *fluoride application. **Acidulated phosphate fluoride gel (APF)** is an aqueous solution derived from sodium fluoride acidulated with a mixture of sodium phosphate and phosphoric acid, which yields an effective fluoride ion concentration of 0.02%, and is used as a preventive measure to reduce caries. It is professionally administered by brushing on the teeth or placing in a tray which fits over the tooth arch. It is not normally given to children under the age of 6 years because of the risk of ingestion.

Further Reading: Richards D. Topical fluoride guidance. *Evid Based Dent* 2006;7(3):62–4.

fluoride milk A supplemental liquid form of *fluoride. It has been introduced in several countries and has the advantage that it can potentially reduce caries in areas of social deprivation.

Further Reading: Twetman S. Fluoridated milk may be beneficial to schoolchildren by helping prevent caries. *Evid Based Dent* 2005;6(4):88.

fluoride mouthrinse A topical form of *fluoride in an aqueous solution. The fluoride (usually sodium fluoride) concentration is in the approximate range of 200–900 ppm. There is a high risk of ingestion in young children.

Further Reading: Twetman S., Petersson L., Axelsson S., Dahlgren H., Holm A. K., Kallestal C., Lagerlof F., Lingstrom P., Mejare I., Nordenram G., Norlund A., Soder B. Caries-preventive effect of sodium fluoride mouthrinses: a systematic review of controlled clinical trials. *Acta Odontol Scand.* 2004;62(4):223–30.

fluoride salt A dietary form of *fluoride supplementation. It has been available in some countries, e.g. Switzerland, since 1955 and is considered cheap and effective for rural communities in developing countries. It is produced by mixing measured amounts of sodium fluoride and salt together; it can also be manufactured by spraying a solution of potassium fluoride onto the refined salt. It is less effective than some other methods as a preventive measure, since salt consumption is lowest in young children. It can result in a very variable intake and may be excessive in areas with *water fluoridation.

Further Reading: Marthaler T. M., Petersen P. E. Salt fluoridation – an alternative in automatic prevention of dental caries. *Int Dent J* 2005;55(6):351–8.

fluoride tablet A supplemental form of *fluoride. Tablets, usually containing sodium fluoride, must be chewable or bioadhesive in order to gain the topical caries reducing effect on tooth enamel. They are normally administered to children over the age of 6 months, at a dosage dependent on the age of the child and body weight.

Further Reading: Diarra M., Pourroy G., Boymond C., Muster D. Fluoride controlled release tablets for intrabuccal use. *Biomaterials* 2003;24(7):1293–300.

fluoride toothpaste A dentifrice to which a *fluoride salt has been added. The most common fluoride salts added are sodium fluoride and sodium monofluorophosphate. Fluoride is normally added within the range of 500–1500 parts per million with low fluoride toothpaste (<600 ppm) being recommended for low caries-risk children up to the age of 7 years. In Europe, the maximum concentration permissible in an over-the-counter toothpaste is 1500 ppm. Prescription-only toothpastes, containing 2800–5000 ppm fluoride, are available for the management of high caries-risk adolescents, adults, and the elderly. *See also* DENTIFRICE.

Further Reading: Davies R. M., Ellwood R. P, Davies G. M. The rational use of fluoride toothpaste. *Int J Dent Hyg* 2003;1 (1):3–8. Review.
Davies R. M., Davies G. M. High fluoride toothpastes: their potential role in a caries prevention programme. *Dent Update* 2008;35:320–23.

fluoride varnish A topical form of *fluoride (usually sodium fluoride) in a resin base. The concentration of fluoride may be as high as 22,600 ppm and there is therefore a potential risk of toxicity. It is professionally applied as a sticky yellowish or clear protective coating to the susceptible dried tooth surfaces in situations where the caries experience or risk is considered high. It hardens on contact with saliva. It is also used to reduce root *hypersensitivity. Contact with bleeding tissues may result in contact *allergy. Trade names: **Duraphat, Fluor Protector.**

Further Reading: Richards D. Fluoride varnish should be part of caries prevention programmes. *Evid Based Dent* 2006;7 (3):65–6.

fluoroaluminosilicate glass *n.* A family of glasses mixed with an ionic polymer (*polyalkenoic acid) which, when added to water, form *glass ionomer cement. They are formed by fusing together the oxides of silica, alumina, calcium, sodium, and others with fluoride salts such as cryolite and calcium fluoride. Strontium, barium, or lanthanum is added to make the glass *radiopaque.

fluorosis *n.* The effects of excessive fluoride intake characterized by mottled enamel. Fluorosis varies in severity from small white or opaque areas on the enamel surface to severe mottling causing aesthetic concern. *See* FLUOROSIS CLASSIFICATION. Fluorosis can occur when the level of fluoride in the water supply exceeds 2 ppm or from the use of fluoride supplements in areas where there is artificial water *fluoridation. Higher intakes can lead to systemic disease such as skeletal deformities. Most of the staining in mottled enamel is confined to the outer 50–100µm; therefore, if treatment is considered necessary, it is usually by means of aesthetic restorations, *veneers, or *crowns.

Further Reading: Khan A, Moola M. H, Cleaton-Jones P. Global trends in dental fluorosis from 1980 to 2000: a systematic review. *SADJ.* 2005 Nov;60(10):418–21.

fluorosis classification A system of defining the severity of chronic fluoride toxicity based on enamel defects. The most commonly used indices are the Dean Index [Dr Trendley *Dean (1893–1962), American dentist] and the Thylstrup–Fejerskov Index named after A. Thylstrup and O. Fejerskov. The Dean Index grades the enamel lesions according to the degree of severity described. The Thylstrup–Fejerskov Index uses a numerical classification.

The Dean fluorosis index

Criteria for Dean fluorosis index

Score	Criterion
Normal	The enamel represents the usual translucent type of structure. The surface is smooth, glossy, and usually of a pale creamy-white colour.
Questionable	The enamel discloses slight aberrations from the translucency of normal enamel, ranging from a few white flecks to occasional white spots. This classification is utilized in those instances where a definite diagnosis of the mildest form of fluorosis is not warranted and a classification of 'norma' is not justified.
Very mild	Small, opaque, paper-white areas scattered irregularly over the tooth but not involving as much as 25% of the tooth surface. Frequently included in this classification are teeth showing no more than about 1–2mm of white opacity at the tip of the summit of the cusps of the bicuspids (premolars) or second molars.
Mild	The white opaque areas in the enamel of the teeth are more extensive but do not involve as much as 50% of the tooth.
Moderate	All enamel surfaces of the teeth are affected, and the surfaces subject to attrition show wear. Brown stain is frequently a disfiguring feature.
Severe	Includes teeth formerly classified as 'moderately severe and severe'. All enamel surfaces are affected and hypoplasia is so marked that the general form of the tooth may be affected. The major diagnostic sign of this classification is discrete or confluent pitting. Brown stains are widespread and teeth often present a corroded-like appearance.

Source: Dean, 1942. As reproduced in 'Health Effects of Ingested Fluoride', National Academy of Sciences, 1993, p. 169.

The Thylstrup–Fejerskov index

Clinical criteria and scoring for the TF (Thylstrup–Fejerskov) index

Score	Criteria
0	Normal translucency of enamel remains after prolonged air-drying.
1	Narrow white lines corresponding to the *perikymata.
2	*Smooth surfaces*: More pronounced lines of opacity that follow the perikymata. Occasionally confluence of adjacent lines.
	Occlusal surfaces: Scattered areas of opacity <2mm in diameter and pronounced opacity of cuspal ridges.
3	*Smooth surfaces*: Merging and irregular cloudy areas of opacity. Accentuated drawing of perikymata often visible between opacities.
	Occlusal surfaces: Confluent areas of marked opacity. Worn areas appear almost normal but usually circumscribed by a rim of opaque enamel.
4	*Smooth surfaces*: The entire surface exhibits marked opacity or appears chalky white. Parts of the surface exposed to attrition appear less affected.
	Occlusal surfaces: Entire surface exhibits marked opacity. Attrition is often pronounced shortly after eruption.
5	*Smooth surfaces and occlusal surfaces*: Entire surface displays marked opacity with focal loss of outermost enamel (pits) <2mm in diameter.
6	*Smooth surfaces*: Pits are regularly arranged in horizontal bands <2mm in vertical extension.
	Occlusal surfaces: Confluent areas <3mm in diameter exhibit loss of enamel. Marked attrition.
7	*Smooth surfaces*: Loss of outermost enamel in irregular areas involving $\frac{1}{2}$ of entire surface.
	Occlusal surfaces: Changes in the morphology caused by merging pits and marked attrition.
8	*Smooth and occlusal surfaces*: Loss of outermost enamel involving $\frac{1}{2}$ of surface.

Source: Thylstrup and Fejerskov, 1978. As reproduced in 'Health Effects of Ingested Fluoride', National Academy of Sciences, 1993, p. 171.

(⊕) SEE WEB LINKS
- Information on dental fluorosis classification from the British Fluoridation Society.

Fluothane* *n. See* HALOTHANE.

flux *n.* Any substance that lowers the melting or softening temperature of the mix or compound in which it is present. In dentistry it is included in ceramic materials and used when soldering or casting metals to prevent oxidation and improve fluidity.

foaming agent *n.* A chemical substance added to toothpaste (*dentifrice) to lower the surface tension. It has the effect of loosening surface debris and thereby aiding removal by a *toothbrush. Examples of foaming agents are sodium lauryl sulphate (SLS) and sodium N-lauryl sarcosinate.

focal epithelial hyperplasia *n. See* HECK'S DISEASE.

focal infection The origin of an infection which may cause symptoms at a remote site.

focal palmoplantar and gingival hyperkeratosis *See* PAPILLON LEFÉVRE SYNDROME.

focus group A small group selected as a sample of a population to provide opinions and responses to a topic or issue presented in a group setting.

focus to skin distance (fsd) The distance between the focal spot of the x-ray tube (where x-rays are produced) marked with a red dot on the intra-oral x-ray head to the skin surface of the patient. For the long cone *paralleling technique the fsd must be at least 20cms.

foetid (fetid) *adj.* Having an unpleasant or foul smell.

foetus (fetus) *n.* (*adj.* **foetal, fetal**) The term used in human reproduction to describe an embryo after the eighth week of development until birth.

foil *n.* A very thin sheet of metal, usually gold, platinum, or tin. **Cohesive gold foil** is pure (24 *carat) gold which, when condensed at room temperature against another piece of foil, will cohere or weld to form one piece. It can be condensed in small pieces into a retentive cavity using a **gold foil mallet or condenser**. A **gold foil carrier** is a pointed instrument which can be used to pick up small pieces of gold foil and pass them through an annealing flame to remove any protective coating prior to placing them in a tooth cavity. **Platinum foil** is pure platinum in thin sheet form which, because of its high melting point, is used as a former during the fabrication of a porcelain *crown. **Tin foil** was used as an early 19th-century restorative material. *See also* GOLD.

Further Reading: Ferrier, W. I. *Gold foil operations*, University of Washington Press, 1959.

(((( ))) SEE WEB LINKS

• A historical paper describing the use of gold foil.

fold *n.* (in anatomy) The doubling back of two surfaces or membranes. The **mucolabial fold** extends from the alveolar mucosa of the *maxilla or *mandible to the *lip and in the midline forms the *fraenum. The **mucobuccal fold** extends from the alveolar mucosa of the mandible or maxilla to the *cheek. The **sublingual fold** is formed by the sublingual gland and is a crescent-shaped area in the floor of the mouth following the medial wall of the mandible.

folic acid (pteroylglutamic acid) A B vitamin that is important in red blood cell formation and is necessary to form essential body proteins and genetic materials. It functions as a coenzyme with vitamins B_6, B_{12}, and C. It is found in yeast, liver, and green vegetables. A deficiency can result in megaloblastic *anaemia and, if it occurs during the first three months of pregnancy, can result in congenital malformations due to neural tube defects leading to spina bifida or *anencephaly.

follicle (dental) *n.* 1. (in dental anatomy) A fibrous capsule which surrounds the *enamel organ of the developing *tooth germ. On eruption, it forms the *periodontal ligament. 2. (in anatomy) A small secretory sac or gland.

Fones' method (Fones' technique) *n. See* TOOTHBRUSHING.

Food Standards Agency (UK) An independent watchdog established to protect the public's health and consumer interests in relation to nutrition and food hygiene and safety.

food trapping The condition in which food particles are trapped or impacted between two teeth due to an *open contact, malocclusion, or a poorly contoured restoration.

foramen *n.* (*pl.* **foramina**) A natural opening or hole usually in bone. The **apical foramen** is the small opening at the apex of a tooth root through which nerves and blood vessels pass. The **foramen caecum** is a small depression on the dorsum of the *tongue situated at the apex of a V-shaped groove (*sulcus terminalis). The **foramen magnum** is a large aperture in the occipital bone in the base of the skull, through which passes the spinal cord. The **incisive (nasopalatine) foramen** is located in the midline, palatal to the maxillary incisors at the junction of the *premaxilla and *maxillae; it contains the nasopalatine blood vessels and nerve. The **mandibular foramen** is located on the medial aspect of the ramus of the *mandible and contains the inferior alveolar (dental) nerve and inferior alveolar blood vessels. The **mental foramen** is located on the lateral aspect of the body of the mandible, usually between the first and second premolar and inferior to their root apices. It is a circular opening through which pass the mental nerve and blood vessels. When teeth and associated alveolar bone are lost, the foramen may be located beneath the fitting surface of a denture base. See appendix B for full list of foramina of the skull.

forced expiratory volume (FEV) The volume of air that can be forcibly expelled in a defined period of time after full inspiration. It is a measurement of lung function.

forceps *n.* 1. A pincer-like instrument designed to grasp a tooth or tooth root so that it can be held firm and removed. 2. An instrument used for grasping and holding firm tissues or other objects. **Bayonet forceps** have elongated beaks with the hinge set at an angle to the handle designed for improving access for the extraction of maxillary third molars. **Cheatle's forceps** [Sir G. L. Cheatle (1865–1951), British surgeon] are long curved beaked stainless steel non-extraction forceps used frequently for handling instruments too hot to touch. **Dental extraction forceps** have many design variations related to the size, shape, and position of the tooth or tooth root to be extracted.

UPPER FORCEPS

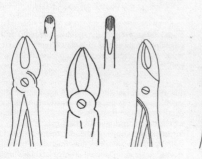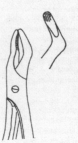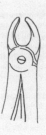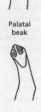

Palatal beak

Buccal beak

| Upper anterior | Upper premolar | Upper roots | Upper molar |

LOWER FORCEPS

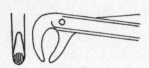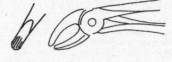

Lower anterior and lower premolar

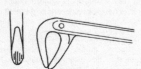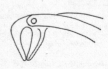

Lower anterior and lower roots

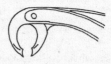

Lower molar

Types of forceps

Fickling's forceps [B. Fickling (1909–2007), English dentist] are used to grasp teeth and roots during minor oral surgical procedures; they are angled and have either toothed or non-toothed serrated jaws. **Haemostatic (mosquito) forceps** are used to grasp blood vessels in order to control

*haemorrhage. **Magill's forceps** [Sir I. V. Magill (1888–1975), British anaesthetist] are long angled and used for retrieving *foreign bodies causing airway obstruction in the mouth or throat in an unconscious patient. **Rongeur forceps** are short-bladed cutting forceps used for removing, trimming, or nibbling sharp edges of bone. **Dental dam clamp forceps** have small pointed beaks designed to engage in the holes of *dental dam clamps or retainers to facilitate their placement or removal. **Tissue forceps** are used to reposition skin and mucosa while suturing and may have toothed or non-toothed working tips.

Fordyce's spots [J. A. Fordyce (1858–1925), American dermatologist] Small creamy yellowish spots found on the mucosal surfaces of the *lips and *cheeks. They are produced by ectopic *sebaceous glands and are of no pathological significance.

foreign body n. Any abnormal object or substance found within the body.

forensic dentistry (forensic odontology) The appropriate handling, examination, and evaluation of dental evidence which will then be presented in the interest of justice. It includes the identification of human remains, particularly in mass fatalities, the assessment of *bitemark injuries, the assessment of cases of non-accidental abuse or injury, and age estimation.

Further Reading: Bushick R. D. Forensic dentistry: an overview for the general dentist. *Gen Dent* 2006;54(1):48–52.

(((●))) **SEE WEB LINKS**

• The British Association for Forensic Odontology website.
• The American Society of Forensic Odontology website.

form n. The shape or appearance of an object. The **convenience form** is the additional modification necessary to a cavity in order to gain access to it or to insert a *restoration. The **occlusal form** is the shape of the biting surface of a tooth. The **outline form** is the shape of a cavity defined by the cavosurface outline of the cavity. The **resistance form** is the shape given to a prepared cavity to enable the restoration to withstand displacement due to masticatory forces. The **retention form** is the shape of a prepared cavity designed to prevent displacement of a restoration in a direction opposed to masticatory forces.

formaldehyde n. A colourless flammable gas with a pungent smell. In aqueous solution it is used as a disinfectant and may also be applied to

the skin in the treatment of warts; its precursor is *paraformaldehyde.

formalin n. An aqueous solution containing 40% (by volume) formaldehyde and another agent, typically methanol. It is primarily used as a tissue fixative in pathology. It is a constituent in *formocresol.

formocresol n. A chemical compound containing 35% cresol and 19% *formalin in aqueous glycerine. It has been used to fix and disinfect pulp tissue during a *pulpotomy procedure for primary teeth; however, serious concerns have been raised over the potential toxicity and *cariogenicity of formalin and its possible blood-borne spread to distant sites. Its use in pulpotomies has now been largely replaced by alternative materials such as *ferric sulphate or *mineral trioxide aggregate (MTA).

formula n. See DENTAL FORMULA.

fossa n. 1. A hollow, pit, or depression e.g. on the enamel surface of a tooth. See also CANINE. 2. (in anatomy) A shallow cavity or depression in a surface. The **digastric fossa** is one of two depressions on the internal surface of the body of the mandible either side of the midline. The **mastoid fossa** is a depression on the lateral surface of the temporal bone. The **infratemporal fossa** is an irregularly shaped cavity situated below and medial to the zygomatic arch.

four-handed dentistry See CLOSE-SUPPORT DENTISTRY.

fovea n. (adj. **foveate**) A small pit or depression. The **palatine fovea** is one of two pits either side of the midline situated at the junction of the hard and soft palates made by minor palatine *salivary glands. The **pterygoid fovea** is a depression on the antero-medial side of the neck of the condylar process of the mandible and marks the site of attachment of the lateral pterygoid muscle. The **sublingual fovea (fossa)** is a shallow depression for the sublingual salivary gland on the inner surface of the mandible above the mylohyoid line either side of the mental spine. The **submandibular fovea (fossa)** is a shallow depression on the inner surface of the body of the mandible associated with the submandibular salivary gland.

fractionated radiation n. See RADIATION.

fracture n. Complete or partial breakage of a brittle material e.g. bone, tooth, resin, or metal. In a bone, there may be more than one fracture line (**comminuted fracture**) or the fractured surfaces may be exposed to the external environment (**compound fracture**). *See also* LE FORT CLASSIFICATION.

fraenectomy (frenectomy) *n.* The surgical removal of the fraenum including the underlying fibrous tissue. A **labial fraenectomy** is usually delayed until after the completion of orthodontic treatment, unless it prevents closure of a *diastema or shows evidence of trauma. A **lingual fraenectomy** may be undertaken if tongue movement is restricted in the older patient or to assist in speech development in young children. Failure to undertake a lingual fraenectomy may sometimes lead to periodontal problems in later life. 📷

fraenoplasty (frenoplasty) *n.* The surgical repositioning of an abnormally located *fraenum. It may be undertaken to include the removal of muscle attachments prior to the construction of a prosthetic appliance.

fraenotomy (ankylotomy, frenotomy) *n.* A surgical procedure involving cutting and releasing any fraenal attachment, especially that of the tongue. It is usually preferred to a fraenectomy in the treatment of tongue-tie in babies.

fraenum *n. See* FRENULUM.

fragaria vesca (wood strawberry) *n.* A homeopathic remedy which has a claimed ability to reduce calculus formation, although this is not currently substantiated by evidence-based research.

Fragile X syndrome A neuro-developmental disorder caused by a mutation on the X chromosome. It is second only to *Down's syndrome as a cause of learning disabilities. It only affects males and is characterized by high foreheads, unbalanced faces, and large jaws. Up to 80% of patients have heart valve involvement which may require antibiotic *prophylaxis for invasive dental procedures.

Frankel appliance [R. Frankel (1908–2001), German orthodontist] A removable functional orthodontic appliance which uses the oral and facial muscles to modify the growth of the jaws. It is made of a single block of *acrylic resin designed to posture the *mandible forwards and to open the bite. It is used to correct class II *malocclusions although may be modified to correct class III malocclusions.

Frankfort-mandibular plane angle (FMPA) The angle between the Frankfort plane and the mandibular plane.

Frankfort plane *See* CEPHALOMETRIC ANALYSIS.

Fraser competent *See* GILLICK COMPETENT.

F-ratio *n.* A test statistic used to determine whether the difference between two *variables is statistically significant or stable.

Freedom of Information Act 2000 An act of the UK parliament which gives individuals a general right of access to all types of recorded information held by public bodies, including dentists providing National Health Service treatment within the General Dental Services. It obliges dental practices routinely to make information available to the public and have a **freedom of information publication scheme**.

((⊕)) SEE WEB LINKS

• The website of the Information Commissioner's Office outlining details of the Act.

freeway space *n.* The distance between the *occlusal surfaces of the maxillary and mandibular teeth when the *mandible is in its physiological rest position.

fremitus *n.* 1. (in dentistry) The mobility seen or vibrations felt when the fingers are placed on the labial surfaces of the teeth and the patient gently occludes the teeth. 2. Vibrations perceived through the chest when a patient breathes.

frenectomy *n. See* FRAENECTOMY.

frenoplasty *n. See* FRAENOPLASTY.

frenotomy *n. See* FRAENOTOMY.

frenulum (frenum, fraenum) *n.* A fold of *mucosa which limits the movement of a tissue or organ. The **buccal frenulum** connects the tissues of the alveolar ridge with the cheek in the premolar region. The **labial frenulum** is situated in the midline and connects the mucous membrane of the lip with the alveolar ridge in the upper and lower jaws. The **lingual frenulum** is a thin vertical fold of tissue with attachments to the *tongue and the floor of the mouth; it may limit the movement of the tongue (tongue-tie or *ankyloglossia).

frequency (in statistics) *n.* The number of times an event occurs. A **frequency distribution** is a graph which plots the observed values on the horizontal axis and the frequency with which the value occurs on the data set on the vertical axis.

Frey syndrome [L. Frey (1889–1942), Polish neurologist] A rare neurological condition characterized by warmth, redness, and gustatory sweating (sweating in the anticipation of eating) of the area of the cheek adjacent to the ear. It follows trauma to the overlying skin or as a side-effect of parotid gland surgery. It is thought to be caused by post-traumatic crossover of sympathetic and parasympathetic innervation to the gland and skin, respectively.

frictional keratosis *n. See* KERATOSIS.

frit *n.* Wholly or partially fused *porcelain that has been plunged into water while hot which causes it to crack and fracture. This material (frit) is then ground to a powder and blended with opacifiers and pigments to make dental porcelain powders.

frontal bone *n.* The large cranial bone forming the front part of the cranium which includes the upper part of the orbits and extends to the junction with the parietal bones at the coronal suture.

frontal bossing *n.* An unusually large forehead, or a forehead with prominent bony *exostosis which is associated with many syndromes of the head and neck.

Further Reading: Gorlin R. J., Cohen M. M., Henneken R. C. M., *Syndromes of the head and neck.* Oxford Monographs on Medical Genetics, no. 42, fourth edition, 2001.

fronto-nasal process *n.* One of the five facial swellings formed from the *stomodeum at about four weeks of intrauterine life which eventually develops to form the forehead and nose.

fructose *n.* A simple (*monosaccharide) sugar occurring naturally in honey and some fruits, or by the metabolism of *sucrose during digestion. It is broken down in the body by *glycolysis to produce energy.

fulguration *n.* The destruction of unwanted tissue with a diathermy instrument. Also known as **electrofulguration**.

full mouth disinfection *See* DISINFECTION, FULL MOUTH.

full mouth rehabilitation Treatment intended to fully restore the function and aesthetics of the teeth in both dental arches by the use of individual restorations, implants, bridges, or prosthetic appliances.

fulminating (fuminant, fulgurant)
adj. Describing a condition or symptom that is of very sudden onset, severe, and of short duration. Fulminating conditions in the head and neck are usually caused by an *odontogenic or oropharyngeal infection; although rare, they are potentially fatal. They are characterized by extensive *necrosis e.g. *necrotizing fasciitis. Early diagnosis and aggressive treatment are critical for patient survival. The incidence of fulminating infection increases with age and most adult cases occur in patients with at least one underlying chronic illness e.g. *diabetes, *alcohol abuse, or poor nutrition.

functional appliance *n. See* ORTHODONTIC APPLIANCE.

functional impression *n. See* IMPRESSION.

functional occlusal plane *n. See* CEPHALOMETRIC ANALYSIS.

functional occlusion *n. See* OCCLUSION.

fungicide *n.* (*adj.* **fungicidal**) Any agent that destroys or inhibits the growth of a *fungus.

fungiform *adj.* Describing a shape like a mushroom.

fungistatic *n.* An agent that inhibits the growth of a *fungus. The commonly used azole group of antifungal drugs used to treat fungal infections in humans (e.g. fluconazole) are fungistatic.

fungus *n.* (*pl.* **fungi;** *adj.* **fungal**) Organisms with a distinct membrane-bound nucleus (eukaryotic) that belong to the kingdom Fungi. They are either **saprophytic** (living on dead or decaying tissue) or *parasitic on plants or animals. Several species of fungi are significant pathogens or opportunistic pathogens of humans such as *Candida albicans, aspergilli, and *Actinomyces

furcation *n.* The site of division of the roots in a multi-rooted tooth (bi- or trifurcation). The **furcation area** is the area of interradicular bone in the region of the tooth root furcation. A **furcation probe** is a double-ended hand instrument designed to help determine the extent of interradicular bone loss in the furcation area. Nabers furcation probe *see* PROBE. The presence of periodontal destruction in the furcation area reduces the long-term prognosis for tooth survival. Furcation involvement can be classified according to the extent of horizontal bone loss.

Classification of furcation involvement		
Degree	Involvement	Description
1	initial involvement	The furcation opening can be felt upon probing. The horizontal probing depth is less than one third of the bucco-lingual width of the tooth.
2	partial involvement	The horizontal loss of periodontal support exceeds one third of the width of the tooth, but does not extend to the other side of the furcation area.
3	through-and-through involvement	The probe passes through the entire dimension of the furcation.

furnace *n.* A type of oven for generating heat. An **inlay furnace** is used for heating up and eliminating the *wax from an inlay pattern which is surrounded by *investment material. A **porcelain furnace** is used for fusing ceramic material without being exposed directly to the heat source.

furuncle *n. See* BOIL.

fusiform *adj.* Cigar-shaped; larger in the middle and tapering at both ends.

fusion *n.* 1. (**synodontia**) The development of one large tooth from two *tooth germs which are in close proximity to each other. It involves the union between the dentine or enamel, or both, of the two developing teeth. Unlike *gemination, fused teeth have separate pulp canals. Fusion is often associated with a congenitally missing tooth. *See also* CONNATION. 2. A surgical procedure in which a joint is removed and the cut ends of the bones are held together with screws or clamps. 3. The uniting or joining together of two or more metals.

Fusobacterium *n.* A genus of filamentous, *anaerobic, Gram-negative non-spore-bearing *bacteria commonly found in the oral flora (e.g. *F. nucleatum*). Most species are *commensal but some are *pathogenic, such as *F. nucleatum* subspecies *fusiforme*, which is implicated in the aetiology of *necrotizing ulcerative gingivitis.

gag *n.* An instrument with jaws which are placed between a patient's teeth to prise and hold the mouth open, particularly during the extraction of teeth during a general anaesthetic; they are most commonly used when a mouth prop is being changed from one side of the mouth to the other. The **Ferguson gag** has jaws in line with the handles and a single-handed ratchet to allow the insertion of a *mouth prop.

gag reflex (pharyngeal reflex)
Normal reflex action caused by contraction of the pharyngeal muscles when the soft *palate or posterior region of the hard palate is touched or stimulated. It protects something from entering the oesophagus or trachea except as part of normal swallowing. It is used as a test for the integrity of the glossopharyngeal and vagus nerves. When excessive during dental procedures, it may need to be controlled by topical *analgesia, hypnosis, conscious *sedation, or acupuncture.

Further Reading: Packer M. E., Joarder C., Lall B. A. The use of relative analgesia in the prosthetic treatment of the 'gagging' patient. *Dent Update* 2005; 32(9):544–6, 548–50.

galactose *n.* A simple (*monosaccharide) sugar converted by *enzyme action to *glucose in the liver. It is a constituent of *lactose (milk sugar).

gallipot *n.* A small glazed receptacle used to contain ointments, solutions, or lotions.

galvanism [L. Galvani (1737–98), Italian physicist and physician] *n.* The production of an electric current when two dissimilar metals, such as *amalgam and *gold, are brought into contact with each other, usually with the *saliva acting as an *electrolyte; it can result in a sharp pain on initial contact.

Gamgee tissue [J. S. Gamgee (1828–86), English physician] *n.* A surgical dressing material consisting of a thick layer of absorbent cotton wool between two layers of absorbent gauze. It is also used as a throat pack.

ganglion *n.* (*pl.* **ganglia**) 1. (in anatomy) A knot or collection of nerve cells e.g. the trigeminal ganglion of the trigeminal nerve, the geniculate ganglion of the facial nerve, and the vestibular and cochlear ganglia of the vestibulocochlear nerve. There are four pairs of *parasympathetic ganglia in the head; these are the ciliary, pterygopalatine, submandibular, and otic ganglia. 2. An abnormal swelling on a tendon.

gangrene *n.* Death and decay of a tissue or part of the body due to deficiency or cessation of blood supply. The causes include disease, trauma, frostbite, severe burns, and blockage of major blood vessels. It may occur in the absence of infection (**dry gangrene**) or accompanied by putrefaction due to bacterial infection (**wet gangrene**), such as may occur in infected *pulp tissue.

Gardner's syndrome [E. J. Gardner (1909–89), US physician] An inherited condition characterized by multiple *osteomas, *cysts, and multiple *polyps in the colon. Multiple *supernumerary teeth are often associated with this condition.

gargle 1. *v.* To rinse the upper part of the throat (fauces) with a fluid through which expired air is forced to create a bubbling effect while the head is tilted backwards. 2. *n.* A medicated solution used for gargling.

gastric insufflation The blowing of air into the stomach which can result from over-enthusiastic inflation of the lungs during emergency pulmonary ventilation.

gastric juice The digestive secretions in the stomach consisting mainly of hydrochloric acid, pepsinogen (converted to pepsin by the acid), rennin, and mucin. Reflux of the gastric juices into the mouth can result in *erosion of tooth enamel because of the high concentration of *hydrochloric acid. *See* GASTRO-OESOPHAGEAL REFLUX DISEASE.

gastritis *n.* Inflammation of the mucosal lining of the stomach. **Acute gastritis** is characterized by gastric pain, anorexia, nausea, and vomiting. **Chronic gastritis** is frequently a symptom of underlying disease.

gastrointestinal tract The digestive tract which extends from the mouth to the anus and is approximately 8.3 metres long; it includes the mouth, pharynx, oesophagus, stomach, duodenum, jejunum, ileum, caecum, colon, and rectum.

gastro-oesophageal reflux disease (GORD) A condition in which the gastric contents are regurgitated back up into the *oesophagus and sometimes into the mouth. The chronic condition can result in oesophageal ulceration because of the low pH of the *hydrochloric acid. It may occur because of intra-abdominal pressure, such as obesity and late pregnancy, but can also be related to lifestyle factors such as *smoking and high alcohol intake. If dental *erosion occurs, it is usually evident on the palatal surfaces of the upper teeth and on the *occlusal and sometimes *buccal surfaces of the lower teeth.

gate control theory States that pain is a function of the balance between the information travelling to the spinal cord through large nerve fibres, which do not carry painful stimuli, and information travelling to the spinal cord through small nerve fibres, which do. It was first postulated by Ronald Melzack (1929–), Canadian psychologist, and Patrick Wall (1925–2001), English anatomist, in 1962. If the relative amount of activity is greater in large nerve fibres, there should be little or no pain. However, if there is more activity in small nerve fibres, then there will be pain.

Gates–Glidden drill *n. See* DRILL.

gauge *n.* An instrument used to determine measurements of an object, such as the bore of a needle. A **Willis bite gauge** is used to measure the *vertical dimension during the construction of a *complete denture; two measuring points are selected in the midline of the face, one related to the nose and one to the chin.

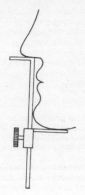

Willis bite gauge

An **undercut gauge** is a device attached to a dental cast *surveyor to measure the extent of the convexity of a tooth.

Further Reading: McCord J. F., Grant A. A. Registration: Stage II—intermaxillary relations. *Br Dent J* 2000;188;11:601–08.

gauze *n.* 1. Bleached cotton cloth of plain weave used for dressings, bandages, and intra-oral moisture control. 2. A thin silk, plastic, or metal woven mesh.

gel *n.* A colloidal jelly-like suspension. It is used as a vehicle for applying topical agents to the surfaces of the teeth, usually sodium or stannous fluoride in a glycerine base or chlorhexidine gel.

gelatin sponge *n.* An absorbable material inserted into a wound space to provide a structure to aid *blood clotting (haemostasis); it may be impregnated with an antiseptic or antibiotic. Trade name: **Gelfoam®**. *See also* CELLULOSE FOAM.

gemination (schizodontia) *n.* The partial development of two teeth from a single tooth bud following incomplete division; they appear clinically as double teeth. Unlike *fusion, the number of teeth in the arch is not reduced and there is a single root structure with an enlarged pulp canal. It most commonly affects the anterior teeth. *See also* CONNATION. ▣

gene *n.* The basic unit of genetic material located at a specific site on a *chromosome.

general anaesthesia *n. See* ANAESTHESIA.

General Dental Council (GDC) The statutory body that controls the practice of dentistry in the UK. Its aim is the protection of the public by the registration of dental professionals, overseeing mandatory recertification and defining and monitoring educational training standards. It consists of a chairman elected by council, 12 lay members appointed by the Appointments Commission on behalf of the Privy Council, and 12 registered members, made up of 8 dentists and 4 dental care professionals.

SEE WEB LINKS
• The General Dental Council website.

general dental practitioner (GDP) *n.* A person registered with a statutory authority (such as the *General Dental Council in the UK) to undertake the practice of *dentistry.

general dental services (GDS) A part of the National Health Service (NHS) dental service in the UK. The GDS was reformed in 2006 to become the nGDS in which all *general dental practitioners working within the NHS in England are required to enter into a service level agreement with a Primary Care Trust (Local Health Board in Wales and Scotland). Payment for the dental care provided is measured primarily in *units of dental activity (UDAs).

generalizability *n.* (in statistics) The application of general principles or conclusions to a specific instance. For example, if a statistical model generalizes it assumes that predictions from the model can be applied to a wider population from which the sample originally came.

General Medical Council (GMC) The statutory body that controls the practice of medicine in the UK.

SEE WEB LINKS
• The General Medical Council website.

general medical practitioner (GMP) A person registered with a statutory authority (the *General Medical Council in the UK) to undertake the practice of medicine.

genial tubercle (mental spine) *n. See* TUBERCLE, GENIAL.

genion *n.* The tip of the mental protuberance; a *craniometric point.

genioplasty *n.* A surgical procedure designed to reshape the contour of the *chin, usually by reduction or extension by augmentation with grafted *bone, *cartilage, or artificial material.

genome *n.* The total genetic information of a particular organism. The normal human genome consists of 3 billion base pairs of *deoxyribonucleic acid (DNA) in each set of 23 *chromosomes from one parent.

genomics *n.* The study of *genomes (including their molecular characterization) and the production of their gene products (proteins), their role in health and disease, and the effects of manipulation of these systems by agents such as pharmaceuticals and radiation.

gentamycin *n.* An aminoglycoside *antibiotic used to treat a wide range of bacterial conditions such as infective bacterial *endocarditis. It acts by inhibiting bacterial protein synthesis. Trade names: **Cidomycin, Genticin.**

gentian violet (methyl violet) *n.* A rosaniline dye used in an aqueous solution as an *antiseptic in the treatment of minor lesions of the oral mucosa. It is a *fungicide and is effective in the treatment of *Candida albicans infections (thrush). It is the active ingredient in *Gram's stain.

geographic tongue (benign migratory glossitis) *n. See* TONGUE, GEOGRAPHIC.

GERD *n. See* GASTRO-OESOPHAGEAL REFLUX DISEASE.

geriatric dentistry *See* GERODONTOLOGY.

German measles (rubella) A highly contagious viral disease. After an incubation period of 2–3 weeks, it is characterized by a widespread pink rash, *lymph node enlargement, sore throat, and a mild fever; there are flat red spots intra-orally. When rubella occurs in pregnant women it can result in severe malformations of the foetus.

germicide *n.* An agent capable of destroying micro-organisms, particularly those causing disease.

gerodontology (gerodontics) *n.* A specialized area of dentistry which deals with the *diagnosis, management, and treatment of dental conditions relating to the elderly. These include physiological and pathological age changes, disease and drug therapy, and the problems associated with the delivery of dental care. Dental conditions particularly relevant to the care of the elderly include root caries, tooth wear, and reduced adaptive capacity to the wearing of dentures. Oral health maintenance may be influenced by reduced manual dexterity and visual acuity. *See also* AGE CHANGE.

Further Reading: Milward M., Cooper P. Periodontal disease and the ageing patient. *Dent Update* 2005;32(10):598–600, 602–4.

ghost teeth *See* ODONTODYSPLASIA.

giant cell granuloma *See* GRANULOMA.

Gibson bandage [K. C. Gibson (1849–1925), US dentist] A bandage for stabilizing a fracture of the mandible.

Gillick competent A condition used in English law that defines a level of competence, demonstrated by a child under the age of 16 years, to *consent to treatment. Children under 16 can consent to treatment if they understand its nature, purpose, and hazards. That ability will vary with age, the child, and the nature of the treatment. To be able to consent, the child must understand the nature of the proposed treatment and fully understand and appreciate the consequences of the treatment, the alternatives, and the failure to treat. A dentist who judges the child to be 'Gillick competent' can disclose information to the parent only with the child's consent, regardless of parental responsibility. The name is derived from the name of the claimant in the case that established the principle (Gillick, 1985). The term **Fraser competent** is also used as an alternative term, after Lord Fraser who was the judge who ruled on the case.

Gillies' operation [Sir H. D. Gillies (1882–1960), New Zealand-born otolaryngologist] A technique for reducing fractures of the zygoma and the *zygomatic arch through an incision in the temporal region above the hairline. An elevator is passed blindly deep to the temporal fascia and the depressed bone.

Gillmore needle [Q. Gillmore (1825–1888), American engineer] A device which uses a penetration test to measure the difference between the initial and final setting time of dental cement. A ¼ pound needle is used for determining the initial set and a one pound needle is used for defining the final set.

Gilmer's splint [T. L. Gilmer (1849–1931), American oral surgeon] The immobilization of a fractured mandible using wire intermaxillary fixation involving the mandibular and maxillary teeth.

gingiva *n.* (*pl.* **gingivae**) Connective tissue and overlying keratinized *mucosa that immediately surrounds the teeth. The **attached gingiva** forms a strong protective cuff around the necks of the teeth and is tightly adherent to the underlying *connective tissue. At the apical aspect of the attached gingiva is the muco-gingival junction which separates the attached gingiva from the loose and more flexible *alveolar mucosa. Its external *keratinized layer of stratified squamous epithelium provides protection during masticatory function; it is characterized by a pale pink appearance with stippling, due to the fibrous attachment of the *epithelium to the *periosteum which prevents gingival movement. The **free gingiva** is the unattached coronal portion of the gingival margin which encircles the tooth to create a *gingival crevice (sulcus). The **marginal gingiva** is the most coronal part of the free gingiva.

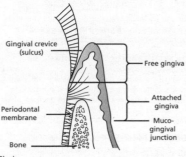

Gingiva

The gingiva between the teeth (**interproximal or interdental gingiva**) fills the space between two contacting teeth to form the *gingival papilla. The gingival blood supply is largely from the underlying periosteum and *anastomoses with the blood vessels of the *periodontal membrane. **gingival** *adj.* 📷

gingival abrasion *n. See* ABRASION.

gingival bleeding index A method of numerically recording the extent of gingival bleeding as a result of inflammation. Each tooth present is gently probed with a *periodontal probe at six sites (mesial, mid, and distal on both buccal and lingual surfaces): bleeding is scored as present or absent and the number of sites where bleeding is present is recorded. The number of sites where bleeding is recorded is divided by the total number of available sites in the mouth and multiplied by 100 to express the bleeding index as a percentage.

gingival cleft *n. See* CLEFT.

gingival crater *n.* A depression in the gingival papilla as a result of *necrosis of the tissue caused by necrotizing *gingivitis.

gingival crevice (sulcus) *n.* The space between the inner aspect of the free *gingiva and the tooth. It is normally 1–3mm in depth and deepest interproximally. The epithelium is non-keratinized. The gingiva is attached to the tooth at the base of the gingival crevice by the *junctional epithelium beneath which is a band of connective tissue/free gingival fibres. The gingival crevice produces a serum *exudate (gingival *crevicular fluid) which alters when disease is present.

gingival crevicular sulcus fluid *n. See* CREVICULAR FLUID.

gingival enlargement A swelling of the gingival tissues. There may be an increase in the size of the fibrous tissue cells (*hypertrophy) or an increase in their number (*hyperplasia). It can be drug induced e.g. by *phenytoin for the treatment of *epilepsy.

gingival fibres *See* PERIODONTAL FIBRES.

gingivalgia *n.* Pain in the gingival tissues.

gingival hyperplasia *See* HYPERPLASIA.

gingival index A method of recording the clinical severity of gingival inflammation. There are a large number of gingival indices used in current clinical practice: two commonly used gingival indices are modifications of the **Loe and Silness Gingival Index**, namely the **Mandel–Chilton Gingival Index** and the **Modified Gingival Index**. *See also* SULCUS BLEEDING INDEX.

Further Reading: Ciancio S. G. Current status of indices of gingivitis. *J Clin Periodontol* 1986;13:375–8.
Loe H., Silness J. Periodontal disease in pregnancy. I. Prevalence and severity. *Acta Odontologica Scand* 1963;21:533–51.
Loe H. The Gingival Index, the Plaque Index, and the Retention Index. *J Periodontol* 1967;38:610–16.
Marks R. G., Magnusson I., Taylor M., Clouser B., Maruniak J., Clark W. B. Evaluation of reliability and reproducibility of dental indices. *J Clin Periodontol* 1993;20:54–8.

gingival margin trimmer *See* MARGIN TRIMMER.

gingival overlay A removable resin overlay used to simulate lost gingival tissue and restore aesthetics, usually following gingival surgery on completion of healing.

gingival papilla A triangular extension of the free gingiva located interproximally between two contacting teeth. When viewed transversely, it resembles two peaks and a trough below the tooth contact area (interdental col). The structure of the gingival (interdental) papilla is dependent on the supporting alveolar bone and the integrity of the dental arch. Preservation of the papilla is important in aesthetic dentistry to avoid the appearance of a 'black triangle'. Inflammatory *necrotizing gingival conditions can result in the formation of an interproximal **gingival crater**.

gingival pigmentation A variation in gingival colour. It may be physiological and correlated to the complexion of the individual or *pathological e.g. the melanin pigmentation associated with *Addison's disease or the blue or black discoloration produced by *amalgam or depositions of heavy metals.

gingival recession The apical migration of the gingival tissues with exposure of the root surface. This is commonly age-related and occurs in response to periodontal attachment loss associated with *periodontitis. It may also be associated with thin gingivae, traumatic toothbrushing, or oral habits due to a disproportional size of the teeth in relation to the alveolar bone; it may sometimes occur as an unwanted side-effect following orthodontic treatment (*iatrogenic damage).

Further Reading: Baker P., Spedding C. The aetiology of gingival recession. *Dent Update* 2002;29:59–62.

gingival recession, classification A number of classification systems have been developed to more clearly describe the extent of gingival recession. The **index of recession (IR)** was introduced by R. G. Smith in 1997 and uses a two-digit code separated by a dash and preceded by the letter F for facial or L for lingual e.g. F3–4. The first digit represents the extent of horizontal recession and the second digit the extent of vertical recession. An asterisk present next to the second digit indicates involvement of the mucogingival junction.

g

Index of recession (IR)

The extent of horizontal recession

Score	Criteria
0	No clinical evidence of root exposure.
1	No clinical exposure of root exposure plus a subjective awareness of dentinal hypersensitivity in response to a one-second air blast is reported, and/or there is clinically detectable exposure of the cemento-enamel junction (CEJ) for up to 10% of the estimated mid-mesial to mid-distal distance.
2	Horizontal exposure of the CEJ more than 10% but not exceeding 25% of the estimated mid-mesial to mid-distal distance.
3	Exposure of the CEJ more than 25% of the mid-mesial to mid-distal distance but not exceeding 50%.
4	Exposure of the CEJ more than 50% of the mid-mesial to mid-distal distance but not exceeding 75%.
5	Exposure of the CEJ more than 75% of the mid-mesial to mid-distal distance up to 100%.

The extent of vertical recession

Score	Criteria
0	No clinical evidence of root exposure.
1	No clinical evidence of root exposure plus a subjective awareness of dentinal hypersensitivity is reported and/or there is clinically detectable exposure of the cemento-enamel junction (CEJ) not extending more than 1mm vertically to the gingival margin.
2–8	Root exposure 2 to 8mm extending vertically from the CEJ to the base of the soft-tissue defect.
9	Root exposure more than 8mm from the CEJ to the base of the soft-tissue defect.
*	An asterisk is present next to the second digit whenever the vertical component of the soft-tissue defect encroaches into the mucogingival junction or extends beyond it into alveolar mucosa; the absence of an asterisk implies either absence of mucogingival junction involvement at the indexed site or its non involvement in the soft-tissue defect.

Classification of papillary height

Classification of papillary height

Classification	Criteria
Normal	Interdental papilla fills embrasure space to the apical extent of the interdental contact point/area.
Class I	The tip of the interdental papilla lies between the interdental contact point and the most coronal extent of the interproximal cemento-enamel junction (CEJ) (space present but interproximal CEJ is not visible).
Class II	The tip of the interdental papilla lies at or apical to the interproximal CEJ but coronal to the apical extent of the facial CEJ (interproximal CEJ visible).
Class III	The tip of the interdental papilla lies level with or apical to the facial CEJ.

Miller's classification of marginal tissue recession

Classification of marginal tissue recession

Classification	Criteria
Class I	Marginal tissue recession that does not extend to the mucogingival junction.
Class II	Marginal tissue recession that extends to or beyond the mucogingival junction with no periodontal attachment loss (bone or soft tissue) in the interdental area.
Class III	Marginal tissue recession that extends to or beyond the mucogingival junction with periodontal attachment loss in the interdental area or malpositioning of teeth.
Class IV	Marginal tissue recession that extends to or beyond the mucogingival junction with severe bone or soft-tissue loss in the interdental area and/or severe malpositioning of teeth.

W. P. Nordland and D. P. Tarnow described a classification system for the loss of papillary height in 1998 which, together with the index of recession, is primarily used in epidemiological studies to describe the prevalence, severity, incidence, and aetiology of gingival recession.

A widely used clinical classification of gingival recession described by P. D. Miller in 1985 grades recession into four categories.

Further Reading: Smith R. G. Gingival recession: reappraisal of an enigmatic condition and a new index for monitoring. *J Clin Periodontol* 1997;24:201–5.

Nordland W. P., Tarnow D. P. A classification system for loss of papillary height. *J Periodontol* 1998;69:1124–6.

Miller P. D. Jr. A classification of marginal tissue recession. *Int J Periodontics Restorative Dent* 1985;5(2):9–13.

gingival retraction The laying back of the free gingivae to expose the gingival margin of a preparation using mechanical, chemical, or electrical methods. **Gingival retraction cord** is an absorbent string usually impregnated with a *haemostatic agent such as aluminium chloride, ferric chloride, or ferric sulphate, which is gently inserted into the gingival crevice (sulcus) to provide mechanical tissue displacement. Gingival retraction cord containing *epinephrine is contraindicated in patients with cardiac arrhythmias; viscous gels or pastes may be used as an alternative to cord. Electro-cautery and pulsed Nd:YAG *laser irradiation have been used to achieve gingival retraction.

Further Reading: Abdel Gabbar F., Aboulazm S. F. Comparative study on gingival retraction using mechano-chemical procedure and pulsed Nd = YAG laser irradiation. *Egypt Dent J* 1995;41(1):1001–6.

gingivectomy *n.* The surgical removal of excess gingival tissue. It can be an effective procedure in removing excess gingival tissue, such as that occurring with drug-induced overgrowth. An incision may be made with the tip of the blade of the knife directed at the base of the false *pocket and the neck of the blade apical to it, so as to make an external bevel incision (**external bevel gingivaectomy**); this procedure heals by secondary intention and does not provide access to the underlying bone. An external bevel gingivectomy is contraindicated where it would result in total excision of the attached gingiva or where infrabony pockets are present. An alternative technique, to preserve more of the gingival tissue, requires the tip of the knife to be at the base of the pocket apical to the neck of the knife (**internal bevel gingivectomy**); this procedure results in a flap which, when raised, gives access to the underlying bone. The healing is by primary intention when the flap margins are sutured. *See also* GINGIVOPLASTY; FLAP.

gingivitis

n. Reversible inflammation of the gingival tissue characterized by redness (erythema), swelling, false *pocket formation, and a glazed appearance with loss of stippling. Gingivitis may present with symptoms of bleeding and tenderness on brushing. Visual examination may show a red line at the gingival margin and initial swelling of the *interdental papillae and later the marginal gingiva. There is a tendency to bleed on gentle probing with a blunt *periodontal probe. The probing depth of the *gingival crevice does not exceed 3mm unless there is significant swelling of the gingival tissues to create a false pocket. The level of *gingival attachment remains unchanged with no loss of clinical attachment. Acute inflammation is seen in gingivitis of short duration; however, it may continue for months or years and result in a chronic condition. The most common cause of gingivitis is poor oral hygiene maintenance, resulting in accumulation of dental *plaque deposits. It may also be aggravated by local plaque retentive factors such as malpositioned or erupting teeth, or general factors including the hormonal changes occurring during pregnancy and *puberty (**hormonal gingivitis**). Improvement in dental plaque control results in resolution of the gingival inflammation. In early gingivitis there are an increased number of inflammatory cells in the gingival connective tissue and the *junctional epithelium becomes thicker. As the condition progresses there is a more dense infiltration of inflammatory cells with *plasma cells becoming more evident; *collagen loss increases due to the action of the enzyme *collagenase, and the lining of the *gingival crevice (sulcus) increases in thickness. 📷

gingivitis artefacta (factitious gingivitis) *n.* A self-inflicted lesion of the gingival tissues. It most commonly occurs on the gingival margin or papilla as an ulcer or localized stripping of the gingival margin from the tooth. It is usually due to irritation such as from a finger nail, pencil, or sharp object. *See also* DERMATITIS. 📷

gingivitis, desquamative *n.* A condition characterized by red, painful, glazed, and friable gingivae. It may be a manifestation of some muco-cutaneous conditions such as *lichen planus or a vesiculo-bullous disorder such as *pemphigoid. There is a loss of stippling and the gingiva may desquamate easily with minimal trauma (unlike plaque-induced gingivitis). It is more common in elderly females and affects mainly the buccal or labial gingiva. It does not respond well to traditional oral hygiene measures or conventional periodontal therapy alone.

Further Reading: Robinson N. A., Wray D. Desquamative gingivitis: a sign of mucocutaneous disorders—a review. *Aust Dent J* 2003;48:206–11.

gingivitis, necrotizing *n.* An ulcerative condition of the gingiva characterized by gingival bleeding, pain, and loss of the apices of the *interdental papillae, producing a punched out appearance. It is also known as **Vincent's gingivitis**, **Vincent's angina, Plaut–Vincent angina** [H. K. Plaut (1858–1928), German physician; J. H. Vincent (1862–1950), French physician], or **trench mouth**. In severe conditions the ulceration may spread to the throat and *tonsils with associated fever and malaise. A grey slough (**pseudomembrane**) is frequently seen on the gingival margins, together with tissue *necrosis causing a characteristically unpleasant *halitosis.

There is a cellular infiltrate of polymorphonuclear *leucocytes, *plasma cells, and lymphocytes. The aetiology is usually poor oral hygiene, often associated with stress or *smoking. Bacteria implicated in the condition are *Treponema vincentii, Fusobacterium nucleatum,* and *Prevotella intermedia.* Treatment is by correcting oral hygiene deficiencies, oxygenating *mouthwashes, and systemic *antibiotic therapy. If the treatment is inadequate, the acute condition may become chronic, developing into a chronic necrotizing *periodontitis. Necrotizing gingivitis is associated with *cancrum oris.

Further Reading: Minsk L. Diagnosis and treatment of acute periodontal conditions. *Compend Contin Educ Dent* 2006;27:8–11.
MacCarthy D., Claffey N. Acute necrotising ulcerative periodontitis is associated with attachment loss. *J Clin Period* 1991;18:776–9.

gingivitis, nephritic *n.* A form of gingivitis associated with kidney failure, characterized by white plaques on the gingivae (and other areas of the mouth), an ammoniacal odour, and increased salivation. *See also* STOMATITIS.

gingivoplasty *n.* The surgical reshaping and recontouring of the gingival tissues to improve the gingival form for cosmetic, physiological, or functional purposes. *See also* GINGIVECTOMY.

gingivostomatitis *n.* Inflammation of the gingival tissues and the oral mucous membranes. The condition can occur in response to viral infections, especially those that cause common childhood illnesses such as *herpes virus (**herpetic gingivostomatitis**) and Coxsackie viruses (*herpangina). It is characterized by yellowish or greyish ulcers on the gingivae, buccal mucosa, or the tongue. The condition is most common in children.

giomer *n.* A resin composite restorative material with active filler particles. It is a hybridization of glass ionomer and composite resin. Giomers contain pre-reacted surface or fully reacted glass-ionomer particles made of fluorosilicate glass that have been reacted with polyacrylic acid prior to being incorporated into the resin; these particles have been shown to be capable of sustained fluoride release. *See also* RESIN COMPOSITE.

glabella *n.* A smooth prominence on the midline of the *frontal bone between the eyebrows. It is an anatomical marker used in assessing the vertical proportions of the face.

gland *n.* An organ that produces secretions either for use in the body or for excretion. *Exocrine glands discharge their secretions by means of ducts e.g. *salivary and *sweat glands, and *endocrine glands secrete *hormones directly into the bloodstream e.g. the *pituitary and *thyroid glands.

glandular fever (infectious mononucleosis) An infectious disease most commonly of young adults caused by the *Epstein–Barr virus. Although it is a self-limiting disease, symptoms of swelling of the cervical lymph nodes, sore throat, fatigue, loss of appetite, and general malaise may persist for several weeks.

Glasgow coma scale (Glasgow coma score) A method of quantifying the level of consciousness in a victim following a traumatic injury. It rates three categories of patient response: the best eye opening, verbal, and motor response. The levels of response indicate the degree of impairment.

(((⊕))) SEE WEB LINKS
• The University of Leicester, Glasgow Coma scale explained.

glass bead sterilizer A method formerly used for sterilizing the working ends of *endodontic files and *reamers by placing them in a container containing glass beads heated to approximately 225°C (437°F) for a defined period of time. Glass bead sterilizers are ineffective against prions, and the effectiveness of the glass bead sterilizer for viral infection control has not been demonstrated unequivocally. The effectiveness of glass bead sterilizers is very difficult to validate. Current cross-infection control and prevention best practice requires that endodontic files are single-use items only and should not be processed for reuse under any circumstances. Many manufacturers of endodontic files specify that the items are for single use only.

glass ionomer cement n. See CEMENT.

glaze n. 1. A thin vitreous glossy layer of fused *porcelain which forms the final firing in the fabrication of a porcelain *crown. 2. A low-filled or unfilled resin applied to the surface of a restoration or temporary material to improve aesthetics and reduce the need to finish and polish; this material is also used to protect the surface of glass ionomer restorations after initial placement.

glenoid fossa n. A concavity in the *temporal bone at the root of the *zygomatic arch that receives the *mandibular condyle.

glial cell A cell which surrounds neurones in the central nervous system and provides supportive and nutritive functions. Glial cells are made up of oligodendrocytes, astrocytes, ependymal cells, and microglia. Glial cells make up approximately 40% of the total volume of the brain and spinal cord.

glossalgia n. A painful sensation in the *tongue. See also BURNING MOUTH SYNDROME.

glossectomy n. Total or partial removal of the *tongue.

glossitis n. Inflammation of the *tongue. It is characterized by swelling and a smooth appearance with possible tenderness and impaired speech, *swallowing, and *mastication. The whole surface of the tongue may appear smooth (**atrophic glossitis**) if all the filiform and sometimes the *fungiform papillae are lost. **Benign migratory glossitis** see TONGUE, GEOGRAPHIC. **Median rhomboid glossitis** is characterized by an asymptomatic smooth red nodular rhomboidal-shaped lesion located on the dorsum of the tongue in the midline, anterior to the circumvallate papillae; it is thought to be caused by a localized candidal infection. Glossitis can be due to a large number of causes including bacterial or viral infection, mechanical trauma (e.g. sharp teeth, restorations or appliances), burns, irritation from *alcohol or *tobacco, or *allergic reactions. The tongue appears pale if it is caused by pernicious *anaemia and fiery red if caused by *vitamin B deficiency. See also TONGUE, GEOGRAPHIC.

glossodynia n. See BURNING MOUTH SYNDROME.

glossoncus n. A swelling in one part or all over the tongue.

glossoplegia n. A unilateral or bilateral paralysis of the tongue.

glossoptosis n. A backward displacement of the tongue; a symptom of *Pierre Robin syndrome.

glossopyrosis n. A burning sensation of the tongue.

glossotrichia n. *Hairy tongue.

glottis n. The two vocal folds and the intervening space. The space between the vocal folds is known as the **rima glottidis**.

glove n. Protective hand covering used as a cross-infection barrier by healthcare professionals while performing dental procedures. Surgical gloves are single-use disposable, close-fitting, and thin to maximize operator digital sensitivity; the majority are ambidextrous and are made of *latex, vinyl, or *nitrile. The use of powdered gloves has been discontinued to reduce the risk of an allergic response. Reusable heavy-duty gloves are preferred for cleaning environmental surfaces or when scrubbing contaminated instruments, where operator digital sensitivity is less important.

glucagon *n.* A hormone produced by the *pancreas that increases the level of glucose (sugar) in the blood by acting on the liver to convert stored glycogen to glucose and release it into the circulation for immediate use. It has the opposite effect to *insulin.

glucose (dextrose) *n.* A simple sugar (*monosaccharide) which is an important source of energy for the body and the sole source of energy for the brain.

gluteraldehyde *n.* A germicidal *disinfectant used for the cold sterilization of instruments. Safer substitutes are now used in dentistry because of the risk of skin or respiratory system sensitization to both clinical personnel and patients, which can result in *dermatitis, *rhinitis, or *asthma. It was briefly used in the 1990s as a disinfectant in primary tooth *pulpotomy but its use was discontinued because of its toxicity. Heat-tolerant dental instruments should be sterilized by autoclaving in a vacuum steam sterilizer using a validated process, since cold sterilization is difficult to validate. Trade names: **Cidex, Totacide, Asep.**

glycaemic index (GI) *n.* A measure of the rate at which *glucose is absorbed through the intestine and its subsequent level in the *blood. *Carbohydrates are measured against pure glucose on a scale of 0 to 100, where pure glucose scores 100.

glyceryl trinitrate (GTN) *n.* A drug that acts as a *vasodilator; used to treat or prevent *angina. It is usually administered by mouth sublingually (where it is rapidly absorbed either as a spray or in tablet form), or used as a transdermal patch. Trade names: **Glytin spray, Nitrolingual Pumpspray.**

glycogen *n.* The principal form in which carbohydrate is stored in the body as branched chains of glucose units. It is stored mainly in the muscles and liver and is readily broken down into glucose. It is analogous to starch in plants.

glycolysis *n.* The oxidation of glucose. It may occur *anaerobically with the production of lactate (*lactic acid) or *aerobically with the formation of pyruvate. It occurs in the mouth when sugar and bacteria are present and therefore increases the risk of caries when occurring frequently. *See also* STEPHAN'S CURVE.

glycoprotein *n.* One of a group of compounds in which a *protein is combined with a *carbohydrate; examples are *mucin, certain enzymes, hormones, and antigens.

glycosialia (glycoptyalism) *n.* The presence of sugar in the saliva.

gnath- (gnatho-) A prefix denoting the jaw e.g. gnathoplasty (plastic surgery of the jaw).

gnathic index (alveolar index) A measurement of the relative protrusion of the jaw. It is expressed as a ratio of the distance from the *basion to the *nasion to the distance from the basion to the *prosthion multiplied by 100. A gnathic index of less than 98 is classed as *retrognathic (retruded jaw), 98–103 as *mesognathic (average or intermediate jaw), and greater than 103 as *prognathic (protruding jaw).

gnathion *n.* The lowest point on the midline of the mandible. It is a point used in certain cranio-facial measurements.

gnathodynamometer *n.* An instrument used for measuring and recording the muscular forces exerted when closing the jaws.

gnathology *n.* The study of the functional and occlusal relationships of the teeth and masticatory system as they relate to the temporomandibular joints.

gnathostat *n.* A jaw-positioning device used in a number of dental procedures such as radiology, facial photography, and *cephalometry. It is also used in orthodontics to accurately locate plaster casts.

gnathostatics *n.* A method of *prosthodontic and *orthodontic diagnosis based on defining the relationship between the teeth and certain cranial landmarks.

gnotobiotic *adj.* An environment which is micro-organism-free, such as the mouth of a baby at birth, or an environment associated with known or specified micro-organisms.

goitre *n.* An enlargement of the *thyroid gland creating a swelling in the neck. This may be due to lack of dietary iodine, a tumour, or over-activity of the thyroid gland (**exophthalmic goitre**).

gold *n.* A soft yellow, malleable and ductile, noble (chemically inactive) metal. It is used in dentistry either in its pure form (**gold foil**) or as an alloy usually with copper, platinum, palladium, or zinc to increase the hardness or, in the case of

Types of high-gold alloy

Type	Description	*Vickers hardness number	Use
I	Soft	40–70	Single-surface gold inlays
II	Medium	70–100	Most *inlays
III	Hard	90–130	Inlays, *onlays, full coverage crowns, short-span bridges
IV	Extra hard	130–160	Cast posts, long-span bridges, partial denture construction

gold solder, to lower the melting point. Three types of gold alloy are generally recognized: high-gold alloys (minimum 60% gold), medium-gold alloys (40–60% gold), and low-gold alloys (10–40% gold). Depending on the amount of silver, copper, platinum, and palladium added, high-gold alloys are classified into four types (*see* table). Gold alloys are classified by the **American Dental Association** (ADA) according to their *Brinell indentation hardness number: Type A alloy—soft (Brinell 40–75); Type B—medium (Brinell 70–100); Type C—hard (Brinell 90–140). Gold has also been added to glass ionomer cements (*cermets) to increase their strength. *See also* FOIL.

Goldenhar syndrome [M. Goldenhar (1924–2001), American physician] A congenital defect characterized by incomplete development of the ear (microtia), nose, soft palate, lip, and mandible. It is a variant of hemifacial *microstomia and additionally includes underdevelopment or lack of internal organs on one side of the body.

gold standard A method, procedure, or measurement that is widely accepted as being the best available, against which new developments should be compared.

gomphiasis *n.* Looseness of the teeth.

gomphosis *n.* A form of immovable joint in which a conical process, such as a tooth, fits into a socket allowing only limited movement.

gonion *n. See* CEPHALOMETRIC ANALYSIS.

GORD *n. See* GASTRO-OESOPHAGEAL REFLUX DISEASE.

Gore-Tex* *n.* The trade name for a thin porous fluoropolymer membrane used in *guided tissue regeneration.

Gorlin's syndrome (naevoid basal cell carcinoma syndrome) [R. J. Gorlin (1923–2006), US pathologist] A genetic condition characterized by disorders of the skin, bones, and nervous system, including developmental defects of the jaws such as the formation of *odontogenic keratocysts. There is a markedly increased risk of developing multiple *basal cell carcinomas.

gothic arch tracing A horizontal tracing resembling a gothic arch or arrowhead made by a tracing device, the apex of which represents the most retruded position of the mandible. *See also* CENTRAL BEARING DEVICE.

Gow-Gates block A technique to anaesthetize the inferior alveolar, lingual, and long buccal nerves by depositing local anaesthetic solution close to the head of the mandibular condyle under the insertion of the lateral pterygoid muscle. It was first described in 1973 by George Gow-Gates, an Australian dentist.

SEE WEB LINKS
• Contains a detailed description of the technique.

gown *n.* A protective garment worn by a medical or dental healthcare provider to prevent the spread of infection between the wearer and the patient. An additional impermeable protective covering is also recommended for invasive dentistry which might involve blood or saliva contamination.

Further Reading: Microbiology and cross-infection control. In *Clinical Textbook of Dental Hygiene and Therapy*, ed. R. S. Ireland. Blackwell Munksgaard, 2006.

Gracey curette *n. See* CURETTE.

graft *n.* An organ or piece of healthy skin, bone, natural or man-made biological tissue used to replace diseased or injured tissue or another organ. An **allograft (homograft)** describes an organ or graft tissue taken from another member of the same species. For alveolar bone augmentation, it may be harvested from cadavers in the form of demineralized freeze-dried bone; this acts as a scaffold into which new bone can grow, although it may not be free from the risk of infectivity. An **autogenous graft** is tissue derived from the body receiving the graft. The graft donor site is the site from which material is taken. Autogenous grafts may be derived intra- or extra-orally. A **free graft** is tissue completely detached from its donor site, unlike a **pedicle graft** where a portion of the graft remains attached to the donor site to maintain the blood supply, and the remainder is attached to the recipient site. A **full thickness graft** includes all the layers of the skin including blood vessels. A **split thickness graft** consists of sheets of superficial and some deep layers of skin. **Pinch grafts** are made up of several small pieces of donor skin placed on the recipient site, usually where there is poor blood supply. A **xenograft** is a living tissue graft that is made from an animal of one species to another of a different species and has been advocated for maxillary sinus grafting as in the *sinus lift procedure; the animal component is removed during processing to minimize the risk of infectivity. Soft and hard tissue grafts are commonly used in reconstructive management of periodontal destruction. Soft tissue free gingival, connective tissue, pedicle, and double papilla grafts are used to increase the zone of attached gingiva and to attempt coverage of the root surface in cases of gingival recession. Treatment of bony defects around periodontally involved teeth includes auto, allo, and xenografts. **Allogenic grafts** are pre-treated by freezing, radiation, or chemical agents. **Xenogenic grafts** include the use of bovine bone and *hydroxyapatite. *Alloplastic materials include hydroxyapatite, β tri-calcium phosphate, polymers, and bio-active glasses. A **graft versus host reaction** describes lesions which occur in patients who have had a bone marrow transplant and in which the transplanted white cells attack the host. In the oral cavity these resemble lichen planus. 📷

Gram staining (Gram's method) [H. C. J. Gram (1853–1938), Danish physician] A method of differentiating bacterial species into two groups (Gram-positive and Gram-negative) based on the properties of their cell walls. Gram staining has four sequential steps, the first of which involves applying a primary stain such as crystal violet to a heat-fixed smear of bacteria on a glass slide. The second step involves adding an iodine solution and the third step involves decolourization with alcohol or acetone. The final stage involves counterstaining with safranin or basic fuchsin. Gram-positive bacteria appear violet or blue and Gram-negative bacteria appear rose-pink.

granular layer of Tomes [J. Tomes (1815–95), English dentist] A narrow layer of granular or interglobular *dentine found in root dentine immediately adjacent to the *cementum.

granulation tissue A multicellular mass of tissue formed in response to injury. It contains many capillaries surrounded by fibrous *collagen and *fibroblasts and is an essential part of healing. It is most commonly seen in healing open wounds such as an extraction socket, where it may form an overgrowth beyond the confines of the socket.

granulocyte *n.* A white blood cell (*leucocyte) characterized by the presence of granules in the *cytoplasm. They are subclassified on the basis of the staining of the granules into *neutrophils, *eosinophils, and *basophils.

granulocytopenia *n.* Deficiency in the number of granulocytes in the circulating bloodstream. *See also* NEUTROPENIA.

granuloma *n.* (*pl.* **granulomata** or **granulomas**; *adj.* **granulomatous**) A specific type of chronic inflammatory response characterized by a localized accumulation of epithelioid *macrophages, multi nucleate giant cells, and *lymphocytes. These are formed in response to certain micro-organisms in specific infections (e.g. in tuberculosis, leprosy, syphilis), against foreign particles (e.g. retained sutures), or as part of the immune response (e.g. *Crohn's disease or sarcoid); this type of chronic inflammation is termed **granulomatous inflammation**. Granulomas associated with tuberculosis are characterized by central *necrosis (caseation). The term granuloma is also sometimes given to an accumulation of granulation tissue at particular sites and in these circumstances it should not be confused with granulomatous inflammation. For example, granulation tissue at the apex of a tooth (**periapical granuloma**) occurs in response to an infected or non-vital pulp and appears radiographically as a radiolucency with a well defined border. **Eosinophilic granuloma** is a localized form of *Langerhans cell histiocytosis typically occurring in bone. A **giant cell granuloma** is a lesion characterized by accumulations of multinucleate giant cells in a cellular haemorrhagic stroma which may arise on the gingivae (peripheral giant cell granuloma) (*see also* EPULIS) or within the jaws (central giant cell granuloma). In bone they appear as a multilocular radiolucency in young individuals and may cause pain and bone swelling. They are treated by curettage.

Histologically they cannot be distinguished from lesions caused by hyperparathyroidism (*see also* BROWN TUMOUR). A **pyogenic granuloma** has the same histology as a pregnancy granuloma (*epulis) but occurs in both males and females and in any location. It is characterized by a rapid growth of vascular *granulation tissue in response to plaque, calculus, or trauma such as the border of a denture (**denture granuloma**). Treatment is to remove the cause and excision if this fails to produce resolution. In pregnancy, excision may be delayed until after the baby is born. 📷

Graves' disease (thyrotoxicosis) [R. J. Graves (1797–1853), Irish physician] A condition produced by excessive amounts of *thyroid hormone in the bloodstream characterized by swelling in the neck (*goitre) and protrusion of the eyes (*exophthalmos).

Gray (Gy) [L. H. Gray (1905–65), English radiologist] *n.* The *International System of units (SI) measure of the amount of energy absorbed from the radiation beam per unit mass of tissue in joules/kg. One Gray is the dose of energy absorbed by a homogeneously distributed material with a mass of 1 kilogram when exposed to ionizing radiation bearing 1 joule of energy i.e. 1 Gy = 1 J/kg. One Gy is also equal to 100 *rads.

Greene–Vermillion index A simplified oral hygiene *index with a debris (*plaque) and *calculus component, first described by J. Greene and J. R. Vermillion in 1964. Six tooth surfaces are scored, four posterior and two anterior. Debris (plaque) is scored on a scale of 0 to 3.

The Greene–Vermillion index – debris component

Scores	Criteria
0	No debris or stain present.
1	Soft debris covering not more than one third of the tooth surface, or presence of extrinsic stains without other debris regardless of surface area covered.
2	Soft debris covering more than one third but not more than two thirds of the exposed tooth surface.
3	Soft debris covering more than two thirds of the exposed tooth surface.

Calculus deposits are scored for the same surfaces on a scale of 0 to 3.

The Greene–Vermillion index – calculus component

Scores	Criteria
0	No calculus present.
1	Supra-gingival calculus covering not more than one third of the exposed tooth surface.
2	Supra-gingival calculus covering more than one third but not more than two thirds of the exposed tooth surface, or the presence of individual flecks of sub-gingival calculus around the cervical portion of the tooth or both.
3	Supra-gingival calculus covering more than two thirds of the exposed tooth surface, or a continuous heavy band of sub-gingival calculus around the cervical portion of the tooth, or both.

The index values are calculated from the recordings of the calculus and debris scores. The debris scores are added together and divided by the number of surfaces scored for each person. For an individual score to be calculated at least two of the six possible surfaces must have been examined. A score for a group of individuals is obtained by calculating the average of the individual scores. The average group or individual score is defined as the **Simplified Debris Index (DI-S)**. The same process is used to obtain the calculus scores or the **Simplified Calculus Index (CI-S)**. To obtain the **Simplified Oral Hygiene Index**, the average group or individual calculus and debris scores are added together.

Further Reading: Greene, J. C., Vermillion, J. R. The simplified oral hygiene index. *Journal of American Dental Association* 1964;68:25–31.

(🌐) **SEE WEB LINKS**

• A description of a number of oral hygiene indices provided by the World Health Organization.

green rouge *n.* A fine polishing powder of chromium oxide used to polish chromium cobalt prostheses.

greenstick composition *n. See* IMPRESSION COMPOUND.

grey matter (grey substance) *n.* Darker coloured tissues of the spinal cord, cerebral cortex, and the outer layer of the cerebellum, composed mainly of the cell bodies of *neurones, branching *dendrites, and *glial cells.

grinding (selective) *n.* The process of correcting the occlusal surfaces of teeth, restorations, or prosthetic appliances by grinding at selected locations to improve the *occlusion and *masticatory function. It may be undertaken on an individual natural or artificial tooth or restoration to remove a premature contact (**spot grinding**); it is aided by the use of *articulating paper, wax, or marking materials. In an artificial dentition, occlusal correction may be achieved by placing abrasive material between the occluding tooth surfaces while the dentures make various excursions when mounted on an *articulator. **Tooth grinding** *see* BRUXISM; EQUILIBRATION.

grip *v.* To grasp tightly or to take a firm hold. The **palm grip** is a method of holding a hand instrument to give power to the working tip. The non-working end of the instrument is supported by the palm of the hand; the four fingers are bent around the instrument from one side, the thumb from the other side. When using the **pen grip**, the hand instrument is held between the tips of the thumb and forefinger and the lateral side of the last phalanx of the middle finger. This grip may be modified so that the instrument is gripped by positioning the tips of the first three fingers (forefinger, middle finger, and ring finger) and thumb against the instrument with the phalanxes bent (**modified pen grip**); the thumb and forefinger are positioned opposite each other.

ground substance *n.* The matrix of *connective tissue.

group function The simultaneous contact of a group of mandibular or maxillary teeth during progressive mandibular movements on the side to which the mandible is moving (the *working side), enabling the occlusal forces to be widely distributed.

guard bite *n. See* BITE GUARD.

guard mouth *n. See* MOUTH GUARD.

Guedel airway [A. E. Guedel (1883–1956), American anaesthesiologist] *n.* An oropharyngeal airway device used to maintain a patent airway by preventing the tongue from covering the *epiglottis. The airway is a rigid curved plastic tube with reinforcement and a flange at the oral end to withstand pressure from the teeth. It is manufactured in a variety of sizes from newborn to large adult and is usually indicated for unconscious patients because of the high probability of stimulating the gag reflex in the conscious patient. In adults, the airway is inserted into the mouth upside down and then rotated 180°, with the flared end resting securely against the oral opening. In infants the airway is inserted the right way up with the tongue held forward using a tongue depressor.

guide *n.* A device for directing the motion of an object. **Condylar guide** *see* CONDYLAR GUIDANCE. The **incisal guide** (**anterior guide**) is that part of an articulator on which the metal rod (**incisal guide pin**) attached to the upper member of the articulator rests to maintain the vertical dimension.

guided tissue regeneration (GTR) A method of reconstructive periodontal treatment aimed at providing conditions which aid the ingrowth of cells from the *periodontal ligament to form a new attachment, while excluding those from the oral *epithelium and the gingival connective tissue. An artificial membrane is

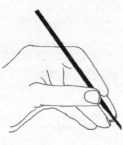
Pen grip

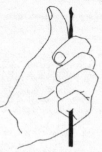
Palm grip

Hand instrument grip

placed between the cleaned root surface and the overlying soft tissue flap. Initially non-resorbable membranes made of cellulose acetate (trade name **Millepore***) or expanded *polytetrafluoroethylene (e-PTFE; trade name **Gore-Tex***) were used; these have been superseded by porcine collagen (trade name: **Bio-Gide***) and synthetic resorbable membranes such as polyglactin/polylactide (trade name: **Vicryl***), which have the advantages of reduced surgical time, less risk of damage to regenerated tissues, and better biocompatibility. **Guided bone regeneration** describes alveolar ridge augmentation or bone regeneration procedures.

Further Reading: Needleman I., Tucker R., Giedrys-Leeper E., Worthington H. Guided tissue regeneration for periodontal intrabony defects—a Cochrane Systematic Review. *Periodontol* 2005;37:106–23.

guideline *n.* A non-mandatory statement or set of statements of desired good, or best practice. **Clinical guidelines** are systematically developed statements designed to assist the clinician and patient in making decisions about appropriate healthcare for specific clinical situations; where possible they are based on scientific evidence but, where this is lacking, may be based on the opinion of respected bodies or individuals.

guide plane (guiding plane) *n.* 1. Part of an orthodontic appliance, having a predefined inclined plane that causes an alteration of the occlusal relation of the maxillary and mandibular teeth and permits their movement to a position not influenced by the cuspal surfaces of the teeth. 2. A plane developed on the occlusal surfaces of occlusion rims to position the mandible in *centric relation. 3. Two or more vertically parallel surfaces created on *abutment teeth to direct the path of insertion and removal of a removable partial denture.

gumboil *n. See* ABSCESS.

gumma *n.* A small granulomatous tumour characteristic of tertiary *syphilis. It may appear on the palate or tongue.

gum tragacanth *n.* A natural gum obtained from the dried sap of certain trees. It is viscous, odourless, tasteless, and water-soluble. When added to water it forms a gel and has therefore been used as an ingredient in denture fixatives and toothpastes.

Gunning splint [T. B. Gunning (1813–89), American dentist] *n.* A solid metal splint linking the *mandible and *maxilla together to provide fixation for a fractured mandible. A splint is provided for each jaw separately and wired into place. The two splints are then wired together producing a rigid fixation. In edentulous patients the individual dentures can be used as splints.

gustation *n.* (*adj.* **gustatory**) The sense of taste or the ability to taste.

gutta-percha (GP) *n.* A thermoplastic substance obtained from the dehydrated juice of certain sapotaceous trees. It is used as a temporary restorative material and to obturate root canals after *pulpectomy. **Gutta-percha points** are fine tapered cylinders of different sizes which are condensed into root canals following *pulp extirpation, either using heat or with the addition of a sealer. Because of their radiopacity they are also used for diagnostic purposes to measure *pocket depths or to locate a *sinus. Machines are commercially available which extrude thermoplasticized **injectable gutta-percha** into a root canal; although some contraction of the material may occur on cooling, the technique may be useful in the treatment of irregular root canal defects. Cores of metal or plastic may be coated with gutta-percha and used as carriers; they are pre-heated and pushed into the root canal to the correct length, and the core is then severed with a bur. A **gutta-percha baseplate** is a rolled sheet of gutta-percha combined with fillers and colouring agents used as a temporary base during denture construction.

gypsum *n.* A raw mineral consisting mainly of calcium sulphate dehydrate with carbonates. As a *cast (model) material it is dimensionally accurate and stable but has poor surface detail, low tensile strength, and poor abrasion resistance. *See also* PLASTER OF PARIS.

haemangioma *n.* A benign *hamartoma of blood vessels characterized by a purple or red slightly raised mark on the skin or mucous membrane. It is sometimes referred to as a birthmark or **port wine stain**. They may be composed of capillaries (**capillary haemangioma**) or large vessels (**cavernous haemangioma**). Excessive bleeding may occur following surgery. *See also* NAEVUS.

haematemesis *n.* The act of vomiting blood. It may occur as a result of swallowing blood or from bleeding in the oesophagus, duodenum, or stomach.

haematoma *n.* A localized accumulation of blood that forms in a tissue, organ, or body space as a result of a broken blood vessel, disease, or a *blood clotting disorder. It can occur as a result of puncturing a blood vessel when administering a nerve block injection to obtain local *analgesia.

haemoglobin *n.* The red pigment found in red blood cells (*erythrocytes). It is composed of a red iron-containing porphyrin (**haem**) linked to the protein **globin**. It is responsible for reversibly combining with oxygen in the bloodstream.

haemophilia *n.* (*n.* **haemophiliac**) A hereditary blood *clotting disorder caused by a deficiency of coagulation factors. **Haemophilia A** is due to a deficiency of *Factor VIII and **haemophilia B** is due to a deficiency of *Factor IX (Christmas factor). Haemophilia is characterized by excessive bleeding after trauma and sometimes spontaneously. Haemorrhage may appear to stop immediately after injury but intractable oozing with rapid blood loss soon follows. Bleeding into the tissues such as the brain, larynx, pharynx, joints, and muscles may occur. Prolonged bleeding after a dental extraction may be the initial presenting feature. The condition is an important risk factor for patients undergoing invasive dental procedures including the injection of local anaesthetic. Management is by Factors VIII and IX replacement therapy.

Haemophilus *n.* A genus of *Gram-negative, pleomorphic, coccobacilli bacterial species that are either *aerobic or facultatively *anaerobic.

The genus contains *commensal organisms and significant pathogens such as *H. influenzae*, which are found in the upper respiratory tract. They are also one of a number of pioneer organisms found in newly formed *plaque.

haemopoiesis (hemopoiesis, hematopoiesis) *n.* The process of formation, development, and differentiation of blood cells. All blood cells in adults are derived from bone marrow stem cells.

haemoptysis *n.* The coughing up of blood in the *sputum.

haemorrhage (bleeding) *n.* The internal or external escape of blood from a blood vessel. It follows immediately after surgery or tooth extraction (**primary haemorrhage**) and when excessive may be due to an excessively traumatic extraction, inflammation, or a blood dyscrasia such as *haemophilia. **Reactionary haemorrhage** occurs usually within 24 hours of a tooth extraction and is frequently due to disturbance of the blood clot. **Secondary haemorrhage** following tooth extraction is usually due to bacterial infection occurring 4–7 days after the extraction. Oral haemorrhage is treated by the application of a pressure pack for 20–30 minutes, which may be supplemented by *haemostatic drugs or *suturing of the tooth socket.

haemostasis *n.* The process of stopping the flow of blood or the arrest of haemorrhage.

haemostatic (styptic) *n.* An agent used to stop or prevent bleeding. Agents such as *fibrin sponge may be used to achieve *haemostasis following dental extraction. *Gingival retraction cord may be impregnated with a haemostatic agent such as aluminium or ferric chloride or ferric sulphate, to manage local bleeding around a subgingival preparation prior to taking an impression for a crown or bridge.

Hahnemann, Samuel (1755–1843) A German physician considered to be the first person to formulate the laws and philosophy of *homeopathy. He developed the philosophy of treating like with like (the law of similars), which is the foundation of modern homeopathy. He also postulated that by diluting remedies their medicinal properties were enhanced rather than diminished.

hairy leukoplakia See LEUKOPLAKIA.

hairy tongue See TONGUE, BLACK HAIRY.

half life The time required for something to fall to half its initial value. For example, the time it takes for one half of the original dose of a medication to leave the body or the time taken by certain materials to lose half their strength.

halitophobia *n*. An exaggerated fear of having bad breath. Also known as delusional *halitosis. It can have a significant impact on the personal or social life of the individual and in some cases may be symptomatic of mental illness.

halitosis (ozostomia) *n*. The condition of having bad breath. It can be caused by many conditions including recently eaten strongly flavoured foods, poor oral hygiene often with associated *periodontal disease, drug therapy such as paraldehyde, and diseases of the upper respiratory tract and stomach. The two practical methods for measuring halitosis are sensory (organoleptic) and instrumental, by measuring the volatile sulphur compound (VSC) levels.

Further Reading: Scully C., Rosenberg M. Halitosis. *Dent Update* 2003;30:205–10.

halitus *n*. Any exhalation such as of a breath or vapour.

Hall technique [N. Hall, Scottish dental practitioner] A method of restoring carious primary molars by the cementation of a preformed metal *crown without caries removal, tooth preparation, or the use of local anaesthesia. It has been shown to produce more favourable outcomes for pulpal health and restoration longevity than conventional restorations.

Further Reading: Innes N. P., Evans D. J., Stirrups D. R. The Hall technique is an effective treatment option for carious primary molar teeth. *Evidence-Based Dentistry* 2008;9:44–5.

halogen lamp *n*. A tungsten–halogen lamp containing halogen gases such as iodine or bromine used to polymerize restorative resin materials. It produces white light, which is filtered to produce blue light at a wavelength of 400–500nm and an energy level of approximately 400mW/cm^2. See also PLASMA LAMP.

halothane *n*. A potent liquid *anaesthetic agent administered by inhalation. It was first used in 1956 but has now been replaced by newer anaesthetic agents because of its potential to cause liver damage.

hamartoma *n*. A developmental abnormality in which all the tissue components are present but their organization or relative proportions, or both, are abnormal. **hamartomatous** *adj*. See also ODONTOMA.

hamulus *n*. A small hook-like projection. The **pterygoid hamulus** is a hook-like spine projecting from the posterior corner of the pterygoid bone, around which the tendon of the tensor veli palatini glides.

Hanau's quint [R. L. Hanau, contemporary American dentist] The five determinants or variables that affect occlusal contacts. They are the orientation of the *occlusal plane, the mandibular *condylar guidance, the *incisal guidance, the *cuspal angle, and the *compensating curve.

hand–arm vibration syndrome A condition characterized by finger numbness, and tingling or painful finger blanching triggered by cold. It is usually caused by hand-held vibration tools. It may be unilateral or bilateral and is initially episodic but may progress to become constant. It can be associated with *carpal tunnel syndrome. The prevalence is low but dental professionals such as *hygienists are considered to be at some risk. The treatment is symptomatic.

hand, foot, and mouth disease A highly infectious disease mainly affecting young children, characterized by a feeling of mild illness accompanied by usually painless mouth *ulcers (vesicular *stomatitis), particularly on the palate and lower lip, and blisters on the hands and feet. It is caused by the *Coxsackie virus A16.

hand hygiene The mechanical process of removing surface contaminants, including debris and micro-organisms, on the hands, as part of the prevention of cross-infection. A liquid soap preparation containing an antimicrobial agent (e. g. *chlorhexidine) is recommended for pre-operative surgical procedures. Hands should be thoroughly dried after washing to prevent the proliferation of bacteria and fungi. The use of alcohol-containing hand hygiene products have helped to improve overall hand hygiene because of their antimicrobial activity.

Further Reading: Boyce, J. M. Pittet, D.; Healthcare Infection Control Practices Advisory Committee. Society For Healthcare Epidemiology of America. Association For Professionals In Infection Control. Infectious Diseases Society of America. Hand Hygiene Task Force, 2002. Guideline for hand hygiene in health-care settings: recommendations of the Healthcare Infection Control Practices Advisory Committee and the HICPAC/SHEA/APIC/IDSA Hand Hygiene Task Force. *Infect Control and Hospital Epidemiology* 23, (12 Suppl), S3–40.

handicap *n.* A disadvantage, resulting from an impairment or a disability, that interferes with a person's efforts to fulfil a role that is normal for that person. Handicap is therefore a social concept, representing the social and environmental consequences of a person's impairments and disabilities (World Health Organization). *See also* DISABILITY; IMPAIRMENT.

(((🌐))) SEE WEB LINKS
- International classification of functioning, disability and health on the World Health Organization website.

handpiece *n.* An instrument used to hold rotary or reciprocating tools for cutting tissue, condensing materials, or removing surface deposits. It is connected by an arm, cable, belt, or tube to the power source. The handpiece head may be in line with the long axis of the shaft (**straight**) or be **right-angled** or **contra-angled**. Handpieces can be powered electrically using gears or by air or water turbine. The rotational cutting tool speed can also vary from approximately 100 rpm for electrically powered handpieces to 500,000 rpm for air turbines. Handpieces are not normally disposable and after use require to be detached, cleaned, decontaminated, and sterilized according to the manufacturer's instructions and local policy.

haplodont *n.* Having molar teeth with simple conical crowns and no tubercles, ridges, fissures, or cusps. They are found in some animals e.g. the northern fur seal.

Hapsburg lip (Hapsburg jaw) *n.* An over-developed lower lip often also associated with an over-developed lower jaw (*prognathism). It was a hereditary condition that affected members of the Hapsburg dynasty.

hapten *n.* A substance of low molecular weight capable of reacting with an antibody but which is too small itself to elicit an antibody response.

hard palate *n.* See PALATE.

hare lip *n.* See CLEFT.

Harvard citation system A referencing system which uses the author's name and date of publication in the body of the text; the bibliography is given alphabetically by author. There are many variations on the style. *See also* VANCOUVER CITATION SYSTEM.

Hashimoto's disease [H. Hashimoto (1881–1934), Japanese surgeon] *n.* Chronic inflammation of the *thyroid gland (**thyroiditis**) caused by viral infection or *autoimmune disease. It is characterized by firm swelling of the neck.

hatchet *n.* A hand instrument with a sharp straight cutting edge which may be beveled or bi-bevelled, similar to a *chisel. The broad side of the blade is parallel with the angle of the shank. It is used for removing or smoothing enamel edges during *cavity preparation.

Haversian canals [C. Havers (1650–1702), English anatomist] The longitudinally arranged canals in compact *bone that contain blood vessels and nerves.

Hawley retainer [C. A. Hawley, 20th-century American dentist] A removable orthodontic *appliance designed to passively stabilize the teeth after planned tooth movement is complete, to prevent relapse while the alveolar tissues complete their remodelling. It consists of a metal wire which surrounds the teeth, anchored to an acrylic resin plate which sits on the palate or floor of the mouth.

Hawthorne effect An observer effect in that the action of the observation of an action will in itself affect that action. For example, people in a clinical trial asked to brush their teeth in their normal way may do so more thoroughly because they know they are part of a clinical trial. The Hawthorne effect may be positive, similar to a *placebo, but usually has a negative effect, introducing *bias into an experiment. It may be an important factor affecting the application of clinical research to routine practice. The name comes from studies carried out at the Hawthorne Works in Chicago between 1924 and 1927.

Hazardous Waste Regulation Act (in England and Wales) A British act of parliament introduced in 2005, providing legislation on the appropriate disposal of hazardous or *special waste such as mercury, x-ray developer, and x-ray fixer solutions. All waste amalgam, whether collected by a separator or otherwise disposed of from the premises, is subject to the requirements of these regulations.

headcap *n.* A component part of orthodontic *headgear which uses the back of the head as a resistance force to produce distal and intrusive forces to the maxillary molars. It provides attachment for the intra-oral components of the *orthodontic appliance. It is often used for patients with an increased *vertical dimension. A **plaster headcap** is made of plaster of Paris and gauze and serves as a point of anchorage for *fixation and *traction appliances used for jaw and facial bone fractures.

headgear *n.* An extra-oral component of an *orthodontic appliance which encircles the head and provides *anchorage for an intra-oral appliance. It usually consists of a *facebow, *headcap, or *neckstrap, and some form of force mechanism such as a spring. It is normally worn at night and during part of the day. **Reverse headgear** consists of an external frame that rests on the forehead and chin which is attached, via elastics, to hooks on an upper fixed appliance; it is used to increase anterior anchorage or modify maxillary growth in an opposite way to conventional headgear.

healing *n. See* WOUND.

Health Act 1999 (in UK) A British act of parliament to amend the law about the *National Health Service, make provision in relation to arrangements and payments between health service bodies and local authorities with respect to health and health-related functions, and confer power to regulate any professions concerned (wholly or partly) with the physical or mental health of individuals. The act provides a mechanism to make certain changes to the statutory arrangements for professional regulation without the need to open the *Dentists Act to full parliamentary debate.

(⊕) SEE WEB LINKS
• The Health Act 1999 on the Office of Public Sector Information website.

Health and Safety at Work Act 1974 (in UK) A British act of parliament passed in 1974 defining legislation to protect all those at work, including all healthcare professionals, as well as members of the public who may be affected by the work activities of these people.

(⊕) SEE WEB LINKS
• The Health and Safety Executive website section on the Health and Safety at Work Act.

Health and Safety Executive (in UK) The enforcing authority, together with local government, for health and safety regulation. For example, certain accidents or adverse events occurring in the workplace must be reported to this body.

(⊕) SEE WEB LINKS
• The Health and Safety Executive website.

Health and Social Care Act 2008 A British act of parliament introduced to enhance the safety and quality of care and improve public health. Its policy areas include the *Care Quality Commission, professional regulation, public health protection measures, and health in pregnancy grant.

(⊕) SEE WEB LINKS
• The Department of Health web pages on the Health and Social Care Act.

health belief model States that behaviour change is not an instantaneous event but occurs as a series of clearly defined changes which are not final but part of an ongoing cycle of change. These behaviour changes are described as precontemplation, contemplation, ready to change, making a change, and maintaining a change. Maintenance may be impossible and the person may revert or relapse back to any of the previous stages. This model was first postulated by J. O. Prochaska and C. C. DiClemente in 1984.

Further Reading: Prochaska J. O., DiClemente C. C. Self change processes, self efficacy and decisional balance across five stages of smoking cessation. *Progress in Clinical and Biological Research* 1984;156:131–40.

healthcare *n. See* PRIMARY CARE; SECONDARY CARE; TERTIARY CARE.

Healthcare Commission (in UK) The independent regulator of *National Health Service (NHS) performance. The *Health and Social Care Act 2008 has replaced the Healthcare Commission with the *Care Quality Commission, which came into operation in April 2009. The Healthcare Commission checked that healthcare services were meeting standards in a range of areas, including safety, cleanliness, and waiting times; it had a statutory duty to assess the performance of healthcare organizations, award annual performance ratings for the NHS, and coordinate reviews of healthcare by others.

health centre (in Britain) A building usually owned or leased by a *Primary Care Trust or Health Authority that provides primary care services for ambulatory patients. These services may include dental as well as medical services.

Health Development Agency (in UK) A special health authority established in 2000 to develop the evidence base to improve health and reduce health inequalities. It worked in partnership with professionals and practitioners across a range of sectors to translate that evidence into practice. As a result of the Department of Health's 2004 review, the HDA was transferred to the *National Institute for Health and Clinical Excellence (NICE) on 1 April 2005.

(⊕) SEE WEB LINKS
• National Institute for Health and Clinical Excellence web page on the Health Development Agency.

health education The planned and managed process of giving an individual or population information to help achieve an improvement in health.

Health Education Authority (in UK) Established in 1987 as a special health authority to encourage *health education and *health promotion, and largely funded by the UK government's Department of Health. It was subsequently replaced by the *Health Development Agency, which became part of the *National Institute for Health and Clinical Excellence (NICE).

health needs assessment The process of establishing the health requirements of an individual or population. *See also* NEED.

health needs profiling A study of the positive and negative influences of health and lifestyle on a community so that the health or ill health of the community can be assessed.

health promotion The planned and organized process of encouraging and assisting in the improvement in health of a population. It includes raising knowledge about body function and disease prevention; raising competence in the use of the healthcare system, and raising awareness of the political and environmental factors influencing health.

Health Records Act *See* ACCESS TO HEALTH RECORDS ACT.

health risk assessment A method of identifying, comparing, and evaluating with the general population an individual's chance of getting a disease or dying of a specified condition. It is intended to draw a person's attention to the potential health consequences of a particular behaviour pattern or hazard.

Health Service Commissioner (Health Service Ombudsman) An official responsible to the UK parliament who provides a service to the public by undertaking independent investigations into complaints that government departments, a range of other public bodies in the UK, and the *National Health Service in England, have not acted properly or fairly, or have provided a poor service. The ombudsman can also investigate complaints about doctors, dentists, pharmacists, and opticians, including actions arising from their clinical judgement.

(⊕) SEE WEB LINKS

• The website of the Health Service Ombudsman.

health visitor A trained nurse with specialist qualifications in public health and *health promotion. Health visitors have an important liaison role with *oral health educators.

heart attack *See* CORONARY THROMBOSIS.

heartburn (pyrosis) *n.* Pain behind the breastbone usually caused by regurgitation of the acid stomach contents into the *oesophagus.

heart failure A condition caused by inadequate pumping action of the left ventricle of the heart. It results in increased blood pressure in the lungs and fluid accumulation in the tissues (*oedema). It is characterized by oedema of the legs and breathlessness even when not undertaking exercise.

heart rate The number of times the heart beats per minute. *See also* PULSE.

Heck's disease (focal epithelial hyperplasia) [J. W. Heck (1923–), American dentist] A rare type of oral mucosal wart characterized by flat-topped papules (pimples) without a stem (sessile) that are only slightly raised above the surface and are usually the colour of normal pink mucosa. They are caused by the human papillomavirus (HPV). Treatment is usually by removal using surgery, cryosurgery, or laser treatment, although they can regress spontaneously.

Heerfordt's syndrome *See* UVEOPAROTITIS.

Heimlich manoeuvre (abdominal thrust) [H. J. Heimlich (1920–), American surgeon] An emergency procedure to remove a blockage in the trachea to prevent asphyxiation, if treatment with up to five back slaps fails. The rescuer stands behind the casualty encircling him with their arms and grasping their hands together. The rescuer clasps one hand over the closed fist of the first hand and places them on the patient's abdomen, midway between the umbilicus and the xiphisternum. The rescuer then pulls upwards and inwards in a sudden sharp movement aiming to dislodge the obstruction. This action may be repeated up to five times.

Helsinki Declaration (accords) A proposal of ethical principles for the guidance of health professionals involved in medical or dental research involving human subjects. It was adopted by the World Medical Assembly in 1964. It formed the basis of the principles and practice of informed *consent, minimizing risk, safeguarding research subjects, and the adherence to an approved research protocol.

HEMA (hydroxyethylmethacrylate) *n.* A colourless liquid *monomer component of *resin composite restorative material. It can be harmful in contact with skin and can result in operator or patient *sensitivity; allergic reactions have been reported.

hematoma *n.* *See* HAEMATOMA.

hemi- Prefix denoting (in medicine) half or one side of a body or organ e.g. **hemilingual** (affecting one side of the tongue only).

hemidesmosome *n.* A button-like adhesion disc that connects the epithelial basal cells of the basal cell layer to the basal lamina. A *desmosome is a similar adhesion disc connecting two neighbouring epithelial cells.

hemifacial microsomia A congenital condition in which the structures of one half of the face are smaller and underdeveloped and are not the same as the other side. Treatment is by surgical correction to improve facial symmetry.

hemiplegia *n.* Paralysis of one side of the body. **Facial hemiplegia** affects one side of the face only.

hemopoiesis *n.* *See* HAEMOPOIESIS.

hemisectomy (radisectomy) *n.* The surgical division through the *furcation of a multi-rooted tooth so that a diseased or damaged root may be removed; it also involves the removal of the associated portion of the crown. *See also* APICECTOMY.

heparin *n.* An *anticoagulant that inhibits the action of *thrombin during blood coagulation. It is produced mainly in the liver and by some white blood cells.

hepatitis *n.* An *inflammation of the liver caused by viruses, toxic substances such as alcohol and *paracetamol, or immunological abnormalities. **Infectious hepatitis** is caused by viruses and is classified into five types known by the letters A to E. **Hepatitis A (endemic hepatitis)** occurs usually as a result of poor hygiene such as food and drink contamination; it is characterized by yellow discoloration of the skin (jaundice), fever, nausea, and vomiting after 15–40 days. Infection usually provides lifetime immunity; active immunization is preferable to temporary protection provided by immunoglobulin A. **Hepatitis B** (formerly known as **serum hepatitis**) is transmitted primarily by intimate contact with body fluids such as blood; it is characterized by fever, headache, general weakness, and jaundice after a 1–6 month incubation period; protection is by vaccination. **Hepatitis C** (formerly known as **non-A, non-B hepatitis**) transmission is similar to hepatitis B and the symptoms are as for hepatitis B, together with dryness of the eyes, fatigue, and sore bones. **Hepatitis D** is a defective virus and occurs only with or after hepatitis B; vaccination for hepatitis B also confers protection against hepatitis D. **Hepatitis E** is spread by poor hygiene

such as infected food or drink and can cause acute hepatitis. **Chronic hepatitis** can last for months or years, eventually leading to cirrhosis of the liver.

herbalism *n.* A form of traditional Chinese medicine that uses plants and plant extracts to treat a variety of conditions. It has been suggested that some herbs have an application in dentistry, such as *echinacea for the treatment of *periodontal disease. However, there is some concern over their safety because of the potential to interact with other drug therapies and the lack of evidence-based research to substantiate their beneficial claims.

Herbst appliance [E. Herbst (*fl.* 1930), German orthodontist] A fixed tooth-borne *functional orthodontic appliance used to treat Class II *malocclusions. Maxillary and mandibular fixed *splints are joined by a pin and tube apparatus to control the mandibular position.

Further Reading: Popowich K., Nebbe B., Major P. W. Effect of Herbst treatment on temporomandibular joint morphology: a systematic literature review. *Am J Orthod Dentofacial Orthop* 2003;123(4):388–94.

hereditary *adj.* Describing transmission from parents to their offspring.

hereditary gingival fibromatosis *n.* A rare autosomal dominant condition characterized by a diffuse generalized overgrowth of the gingivae, often resulting in delayed tooth eruption. In severe cases, the gingival enlargement may cover the crowns of teeth and cause functional and aesthetic concerns.

hereditary haemorrhagic telangiectasia *n.* *See* TELANGIECTASIA.

heroin *n.* A white crystalline powder which is a derivative of morphine. It is a powerful narcotic analgesic whose continued use can lead to dependence. Side-effects of dental significance are tooth grinding (*bruxism), reduced salivary flow (*xerostomia), and a craving for high-calorie foods and carbonated drinks. These, combined with a generally reduced level of oral hygiene, contribute to a high incidence of caries and periodontal disease.

herpangina *n.* An acute infectious viral disease in children caused by Coxsackie viruses. It is characterized by a sudden fever, acute ulceration, and vesicles of the soft palate and tonsillar area, about 1–2 mm in diameter and usually lasting 2–5 days; they break down to form greyish-yellow ulcers. Symptoms also include loss of appetite, difficulty in swallowing (*dysphagia), sore throat, and sometimes nausea and vomiting. Treatment is symptomatic.

herpes *n.* An acute inflammatory infection of the skin and *mucosa, resulting in collections of small blisters caused by **herpes viruses. Primary herpes (herpetic gingivostomatitis)** is caused by **herpes simplex virus type I** and is primarily transmitted by saliva; it affects mainly children and young adults. It is characterized by malaise, fever, enlarged lymph nodes, and blisters (vesicles) on the gingivae, palate, buccal mucosa, and tongue, which burst to form superficial ulcers with surrounding inflamed tissue. The disease is highly infectious and treatment is symptomatic since the disease usually resolves of its own accord after 10–14 days. Antiviral agents, such as *aciclovir, if prescribed in the early stages may limit the course of the disease. Primary herpes can occur as an asymptomatic sub-clinical disease. In about 30% of patients who have had primary herpes, the virus remains dormant in the ganglion of the trigeminal nerve. It can be reactivated by a number of agents such as sunlight, stress, and menstruation (**secondary herpes**) to cause vesicles on the lips (**cold sores, herpes labialis**). Antiviral agents prescribed in the stage immediately before vesicle formation, characterized by tingling of the lips (**pro-dromal phase**), may shorten the course of the disease, which otherwise lasts 10–14 days. **Herpes simplex virus type II** is mainly associated with **genital herpes** and is sexually transmitted. **Herpes zoster** is caused by the varicella zoster virus, resulting in **chickenpox** mainly in children. This condition is characterized by an itchy vesicular rash covering large areas of the skin, although only rarely do small mouth ulcers occur. The incubation period is about 21 days and the condition lasts 10–14 days. The virus may lie dormant and on reactivation can produce a characteristic rash (**shingles**) along the distribution of the nerve affected. It may occur on one side of the face or rarely in the mouth. 📷

herpetic whitlow *n. See* WHITLOW.

herpetiform *adj.* Describing a vesicular condition resembling herpes.

herring-bone pattern Distinctive markings produced on a radiographic film by the lead backing when the film has been exposed with the incorrect side facing the x-ray beam.

Hertwig's root sheath A layer of *epithelial cells formed from the downward growth of the *inner and outer enamel epithelium of the developing *tooth germ. Hertwig's sheath maps out the shape of the root. It atrophies once the

root is formed and any residual cells are known as the rest cells of *Malassez.

heterodont *adj.* Describing having teeth of different morphology, such as humans. The differently shaped teeth perform different functions. *Compare* HOMODONT.

heterogeneity *n.* The variability or differences in results between several studies of the same subject used in a systematic review.

heterograft *n. See* GRAFT.

heterotrophic *adj.* Describing organisms that require organic substrates for growth and development; being incapable of synthesizing their required organic compounds from inorganic sources.

hiatus *n.* An opening or aperture. A perforation through a bone or membranous structure e.g. the hiatus for the greater petrosal nerve and the hiatus for the lesser petrosal nerve.

hidden sugar *n.* Sugar present in food products which might not normally be expected to contain sugar, such as sauces and soups. These food products have a hidden *cariogenic potential.

hinge axis The axis of rotation of the mandibular condyles during the first few millimetres of mandibular opening. It is most commonly used for transfer to a semi-adjustable *articulator. The **terminal hinge axis** is the axis of rotation of the mandible when the mandibular condyles are in their most superior position in the *glenoid fossa.

Hippocratic oath [Hippocrates (460–377BC), Greek physician] A promise made by doctors and dentists in which certain ethical principles and guidelines are laid out. It was subject to a number of modifications until it was replaced in the UK by the *Declaration of Geneva.

Hirschfeld's canals (interdental canals) [I. Hirschfeld (1881–1965), American dentist] Channels in the alveolar process of the mandible and maxilla between the roots of the mandibular and maxillary incisors and the maxillary premolar (bicuspid) teeth, for the passage of blood vessels.

hirudiniasis *n.* A rare condition resulting from leeches attaching themselves to the skin or mucous membrane. It may occur in the mouth as a result of drinking infected water.

histamine *n.* A *biogenic amine involved in local immune responses and found in mast cells and basophils, and also in other tissues where it acts as a neurotransmitter. It causes dilation of blood vessels and contraction of smooth muscle and is involved in the modulation of sleep. It is released in large quantities after skin damage and in *anaphylactic and *allergic reactions.

histatin *n.* One of a group of histidine-rich *polypeptides with antibacterial and antifungal activity found in human parotid and submandibular gland secretions. They are capable of killing the common oral yeast *Candida albicans.*

histiocyte *n.* A large phagocytic cell that is enclosed within connective tissue. *See also* LANGERHANS CELL HISTIOCYTOSIS.

histogram *n.* A form of bar graph: a graphical representation of a frequency distribution showing the class intervals horizontally and the frequencies vertically.

histology *n.* (*adj.* **histological**) The study of the structure of normal tissues at a cellular level.

histopathology *n.* The study of the structure of diseased or abnormal tissues at a cellular level.

histoplasmosis *n.* A fungal infection caused by *Histoplasma capsulatum.* The *fungus may spread via the bloodstream and produce nodular, vegetative, or ulcerative lesions on the lips, tongue, palate, or oral mucosa.

HIV (human immunodeficiency virus) A retrovirus responsible for acquired immune deficiency syndrome (*AIDS). There are two types, HIV-1 and HIV-2. HIV-2 is related to HIV-1 but carries different antigenic components. Infection with HIV can cause marked *immunosuppression giving rise to specific oral conditions which include fungal infections, hairy *leukoplakia, *Kaposi's sarcoma, and severe *periodontal disease. **HIV gingivitis** is characterized by a fiery red band of gingival tissue that extends apically 2–3mm into the attached *gingivae. There may be spontaneous bleeding even in the presence of good plaque control. **HIV-periodontitis** is characterized by painful soft tissue ulceration and *necrosis of the periodontal tissues. It resembles acute necrotizing ulcerative *gingivitis except that the tissue damage extends further to involve the *crestal bone.

Further Reading: Frezzini C., Leao J. C., Cedro M., Porter S. Aspects of HIV disease relevant to dentistry in the 21st century. *Dent Update* 2006;33(5):276–8, 281–2, 285–6.

Hodgkin's disease [T. Hodgkin (1798–1866), British physician] A malignant disease of lymphatic tissue (*lymphoma). It is usually seen in young males and is characterized by enlarged *lymph nodes in the neck. Treatment is by

*chemotherapy and *radiotherapy. The side-effects of this treatment can result in *mucositis, discrete oral ulceration, and *xerostomia.

hoe *n.* A hand instrument with the cutting edge of the blade at right angles to the long axis of the handle. A **periodontal hoe** is used for removing *calculus and other deposits from the tooth surface; it has a straight cutting edge which does not conform to concave root surfaces. *See also* PERIODONTAL INSTRUMENTS.

holistic care *adj.* Describing an approach to patient care in which all the physical, mental, and social factors in the patient's condition are taken into account as an integrated system, rather than just the diagnosed disease or condition.

Hollenback carver *n. See* CARVER.

Hollenback condenser *n. See* CONDENSER.

homeopathy (homoeopathy) *n.* (*adj.* **homeopathic**; *n.* **homeopathist**) A system of alternative medicine which aims to treat like with like, developed by Dr Samuel *Hahnemann (1755–1843). It is based on the principle that diluting remedies enhances their therapeutic effects rather than diminishing them. Homeopathy is used as an adjunct to dental surgery to help alleviate pain, bleeding, anxiety, and inflammation, although its widespread use remains controversial because of the limited evidence-based research.

Further reading: Bhat S. S., Sargod S. S., George D. Dentistry and homeopathy: an overview. *Dent Update* 2005;32(8):486–8, 491.

homeostasis *n.* (*adj.* **homeostatic**) The ability of the body to maintain its physiological equilibrium (e.g. the circulatory system, body temperature, hormonal balance), despite variations in the external environment.

homodont *adj.* Describing having teeth all of the same shape such as an alligator (although they may differ from each other in size). *Compare* HETERODONT.

homogeneity *n.* (in statistics) The degree to which items are similar. This arises in describing the properties of a dataset: it measures the differences or similarities between the several studies.

homograft *n. See* GRAFT.

homozygous *adj.* Describing an individual or organism in which the members of a pair of genes that determine a particular characteristic are identical.

hook *n*. Part of an orthodontic appliance to which elastics are attached. A **crimpable hook** has an internal abrasive surface which, when crimped, increases the friction between the archwire and the hook.

Hopewood House The location of a *caries study undertaken on children in New South Wales, Australia, in 1953. The study involved 80 children brought up from birth to 12 years on a lacto-vegetarian diet virtually free of sugar and flour products. It concluded that children up to 12 years of age under close supervision were not protected from developing caries in subsequent years. This study, which was carried out before the Helsinki Declaration, would now be considered unethical dental research.

Further Reading: Lilienthal B., Goldsworthy N. E., Sullivan H. R., Cameron D. A. The biology of the children of Hopewood House, Bowral, New South Wales. I. Observations on dental caries extending over five years. *Med J Aust* 1953;20;40 (125);878–81.

hormone *n*. A chemical substance that is secreted by an *endocrine gland, such as the *adrenal, *thyroid, or *pituitary, into body fluids and transported to another organ or tissue, where it produces a specific effect on *metabolism.

Horner's syndrome [J. F. Horner (1831–86), Swiss ophthalmologist] A syndrome characterized by drooping of the upper eyelid (ptosis), constriction of the pupil (miosis), and the absence of sweating over the affected part of the face. It is usually unilateral and is caused by a disorder of the sympathetic nerves in the brainstem or neck region.

Horner's teeth [W. E. Horner (1793–1853), American dentist] *n*. Incisor teeth with horizontal grooves of *hypoplastic enamel.

hospice *n*. An institution that provides care, support, and treatment for the terminally ill.

hot salt sterilizer A small sterilizer containing salt heated to a temperature of 234°C (450°F), used for sterilizing endodontic burs and instruments immersed in the salt for 20–30 seconds. This type of equipment cannot be readily validated and is therefore no longer considered appropriate in clinical dental practice.

Howship's lacuna [J. Howship (1781–1841), English surgeon] *n*. small pit or groove in *bone that is being resorbed by *osteoclasts.

human immunodeficiency virus *n*. See HIV.

Human Tissue Act 2004 A UK act of parliament that covers the removal, storage, and use of relevant material from the deceased, and the storage and use of 'relevant material' (including teeth) from the living. It is supplemented by regulations operative from 2006. The act requires healthcare professionals to obtain patient consent if 'relevant material' is to be used for research, public display, transplantation, or obtaining scientific or medical information about a living person which may be relevant to any other person. Consent is specifically stated not to be required from living persons for 'relevant material' used for *clinical audit, education, performance assessment, public health monitoring, or quality assurance.

Further reading: Forsyth L., Woof M. The implications of the Human Tissue Act 2004 for dentistry. *Br Dent J* 2006;201:790–91.

SEE WEB LINKS
• The Human Tissue Act 2004 on the website of the Office of Public Sector Information.

Human Tissue Authority The competent authority that regulates the removal, storage, use, and disposal of human bodies, organs, and tissue from the living and deceased in the UK. It is the body responsible for licensing under both the *Human Tissue Act and the *EU Tissue and Cells Directive.

SEE WEB LINKS
• The Human Tissue Authority website.

humectant *n*. An agent that promotes the retention of moisture such as may be added to a *dentifrice to prevent it hardening on exposure to air.

Hunter–Schreger bands See SCHREGER'S LINES.

Huntington's disease (Huntington's chorea) [G. Huntington (1850–1916), US physician] A hereditary, progressive, degenerative disease of the central nervous system caused by a faulty gene that produces a protein called Huntingtin. It is characterized by an abnormal increase in motor function and activity, resulting in jerky involuntary movements (**hyperkinesia**) and an unsteady gait. Speech and swallowing can be impaired and *bruxism may be a feature. The hyperkinesia of the facial muscles can result in oral soft tissue trauma and fractured teeth, which are at risk of being inhaled. Drug therapy tends to produce a dry mouth (*xerostomia) leading to a high susceptibility to *caries and difficulty wearing dentures.

Hurler's syndrome (gargoylism) [G. Hurler (1889–1965), Austrian paediatrician] A hereditary disorder caused by a deficiency of an enzyme that breaks down

*mucopolysaccharides. It is characterized by learning disabilities, heart defects, dwarfism, and a gargoyle-like face with a depressed nasal bridge and bulging forehead. Treatment is by bone marrow transplant.

Hutchinson's incisors *n. See* INCISORS, HUTCHINSON'S.

hyalinization *n.* (in histology) A change in the tissues characterized by a homogenous, acellular, and avascular appearance. It may be seen in the *periodontal ligament due to prolonged occlusal trauma or excessive orthodontic forces.

hyaluronic acid *n.* A mucopolysaccharide found in large amounts in the *synovial fluid of joints. Topical application of hyaluronic acid gel to recurrent *aphthous ulcers may have an effect in providing a protective barrier and reducing the number of ulcers. Trade name: **Gengigel**.

Further Reading: Nolan A., Baillie C., Badminton J., Rudralingham M., Seymour R. A. The efficacy of topical hyaluronic acid in the management of recurrent aphthous ulceration. *J Oral Pathol Med* 2006;35:461–5.

hybrid layer (hybrid zone) *n.* The layer of dentine which has been *conditioned to remove the loosely adherent *smear layer and into which *adhesive resin has flowed to form a collagen/resin phase.

Further Reading: Nakabayashi N., Nakamura M., Yasunda N. Hybrid layer as a dentin-bonding mechanism. *Journal of Esthetic Dentistry* 1991;3:133–8.

hybrid resin composite *n. See* RESIN COMPOSITE.

hydrochloric acid *n.* A compound consisting of hydrogen and chlorine which is a natural secretion of the stomach. Refluxing of hydrochloric acid into the mouth in such conditions as *bulimia and *anorexia can result in extensive enamel *erosion. Enamel erosion due to hydrochloric acid fumes can be an occupational hazard. A mixture of hydrochloric acid and pumice can be used to remove *white spot lesions following orthodontic therapy.

hydrocolloid *n.* 1. An *agar-type gel used in the preparation of solid culture media for micro-organisms. 2. A type of impression material which changes from a liquid to a gel-like consistency; the change may be reversible or irreversible. A **reversible hydrocolloid** is a material composed principally of colloidal agar agar gel with water as the dispersing medium; it becomes fluid when heated to 40°C (which is compatible with the mouth) and reverts to a stiff gel-like consistency when cooled or chilled. As an impression material it has a high degree of

accuracy but requires specialized equipment; models need to be poured with minimum delay because of the long-term poor dimensional *stability. The physical state of an **irreversible hydrocolloid** is changed by a chemical reaction to an irreversible elastic state. *See also* ALGINATE.

hydrocortisone *n.* A corticosteroid similar to a natural hormone produced by the adrenal medulla. It may be used as a replacement when the body produces insufficient amounts. It has anti-inflammatory and immunosuppressive actions and may be used in the treatment of a number of conditions including arthritis, allergy, asthma, cranial arteritis, gastro-intestinal conditions, skin and blood disorders, and in the management of cancer. It has an application in dentistry since an *adrenal crisis can be induced by the stress of dental treatment. It can also be used in topical preparations for the skin or mucosa such as to reduce the painful symptoms of oral ulceration e.g. **Corlan*** (trade name) pellets.

hydrodynamic theory *See* BRÄNNSTRÖM'S HYDRODYNAMIC THEORY.

hydrofluoric acid *n.* A highly corrosive solution of hydrogen fluoride in water used for etching *porcelain and precious metals to create a retentive bonding surface.

hydrogen peroxide *n.* An unstable compound of hydrogen and oxygen. It is used in some mouthwashes because of its mechanical cleansing properties and its ability to produce oxygen and thus damage the environment of anaerobic infecting organisms such as those found in necrotizing *gingivitis. It may also be used as a tooth *bleaching agent.

hydrophilic *adj.* Describing having an affinity for water. Hydrophilic molecules in *adhesive restorative materials are capable of bonding to wet dentine. *Compare* HYDROPHOBIC.

hydrophobic *adj.* Describing having a lack of an affinity for water. *Compare* HYDROPHILIC.

hydroquinone *n.* 1. A reducing agent in x-ray film developing solutions. 2. An agent used in resin monomers to prevent *polymerization during storage. Its presence in acrylic dentures may give rise to a sensitivity reaction in denture wearers resulting in *stomatitis or allergic *cheilitis.

hydrostomia *n.* A condition characterized by excessive salivation and dribbling from the mouth.

hydroxyapatite *n.* A crystalline mineral compound which is a complex form of calcium

h

phosphate with the general formula $Ca_{10}(PO_4)_6(OH)_2$. It is the principal inorganic component of *bones and teeth. **Ceramic hydroxyapatite** is a synthetic form of natural hydroxyapatite used as a primary coating on dental *implants and some joint replacement prostheses to encourage bone growth onto the implant surface.

hydroxyethylmethacrylate *n.* See HEMA.

hygiene *n.* The science of health and methods of preserving it. **Oral hygiene** is the practice of maintaining cleanliness of the teeth, gingivae, and related oral structures. **Radiation hygiene** is the science of protecting individuals from injury by radiation.

hygienist *n.* See DENTAL HYGIENIST.

hygroscopic *adj.* Describing having the ability to absorb moisture. **Hygroscopic expansion** is exhibited by gypsum products after the initial set, when exposed to water; this has the effect of significantly increasing the setting expansion, which compensates for the contraction of the metal casting upon solidification.

hyoid bone *n.* A horseshoe-shaped bone found suspended in the *anterior triangle of the neck attached to muscles both superiorly and inferiorly, and to the *larynx and related structures.

hypalgesia *n.* An abnormally low sensitivity to pain.

hyper- Prefix denoting 1. Excessive, exaggerated, abnormally increased. 2. (in anatomy) Above.

hyperacusis *n.* Abnormally acute hearing or painful sensitivity to sounds.

hyperaemia *n.* An increased blood flow to an organ, tissue, or part of the body. It is a feature of the inflammatory response.

hyperalgesia *n.* An abnormal state of increased sensitivity to a painful stimulus, such as severe pain experienced in response to the insertion of a hypodermic needle. *Compare* ALLODYNIA.

hyperalveolism *n.* A condition in which the *alveolar process is normal in position in relation to the respective jaw base but is excessively high in a vertical dimension. *Compare* HYPOALVEOLISM.

hypercapnia *n.* The presence of an abnormally high concentration of carbon dioxide in the blood.

hypercementosis *n.* The excessive deposition of *cementum on the root of a tooth. It can be caused by increased or decreased forces on the root surface, *hyperpituitarism, *Paget's disease (when multiple teeth are often affected), or chronic infection in an adjacent area. Tooth extraction may be problematical because of the enlarged shape of the root in the apical area.

hyperdontia *n.* A condition in which either *supernumerary or *supplemental teeth are present.

hypergenia *n.* A condition in which the chin prominence is too high in a vertical dimension with respect to the rest of the facial skeleton but is normal in its height, projection, and width. *Compare* HYPOGENIA.

hypergeusia *n.* An abnormally acute sense of taste. It is also known as **gustatory hyperaesthesia**.

hyperglycaemia *n.* An excess of *glucose in the bloodstream such as occurs in *diabetes mellitus.

hyperkeratosis *n.* A thickening of the outer horny (keratinized) layer of the skin or mucous membranes. It commonly occurs in the oral mucosa due to trauma from teeth or dentures, but is also seen in *leukoplakia and other oral white patches such as *lichen planus.

hypermaxillism *n.* A condition in which the maxilla is too large in height due to an anomaly of the maxillary *alveolus. *Compare* HYPOMAXILLISM.

hyperostosis *n.* Excessive bone growth which may be associated with *exostosis and calcification of tendons or ligaments. The *mandible, clavicle, and ulnar are most frequently affected. *See also* VAN BUCHEM'S SYNDROME.

hyperparathyroidism *n.* Overactivity of the *parathyroid glands, usually as a result of a tumour. Large *cyst-like areas can be present on radiographs of the jaws due to bone *demineralization. Histologically they resemble central giant cell granulomas. *See also* BROWN TUMOUR.

hyperphagia *n.* An excessive ingestion of food beyond that which is necessary for basic energy requirements. It is a symptom of *Prader–Willi syndrome.

hyperpituitarism *n.* A condition caused by excessive production of hormones secreted by the *pituitary gland. Excessive production of growth hormone in adults results in *acromegaly. Changes of dental significance are precocious dental development, *osteoporosis, thickening of the facial and cranial base bony structures, and *hypercementosis.

hyperplasia *n.* An abnormal multiplication or increase in the number of normal cells in a tissue or organ. The affected tissue or organ increases in size but retains its normal shape. It usually occurs in response to an injurious agent or chronic irritation such as a fractured tooth crown. It may also be accompanied by cellular *hypertrophy. **Fibrous hyperplasia** is an overgrowth of fibrous connective tissue, usually in response to chronic trauma such as an ill-fitting denture (denture *granuloma). In the mouth it appears the same colour as the surrounding *mucosa. **Gingival hyperplasia** is an enlargement of the gingival tissues as a result of a cellular increase. Although it is often associated with inflammation, the tissues may appear a normal pink colour. Gingival hyperplasia is a possible side-effect of anticonvulsants e.g. *phenytoin, immunosuppressants e.g. *ciclosporin, and calcium channel blockers e.g. *nifedipine. **Papillary hyperplasia** describes multiple erythematous overgrowths on the palate caused by an ill-fitting denture. 📷

hypersensitivity *n.* 1. An adverse reaction to a substance which usually produces no adverse reaction in normal individuals. 2. An *allergic tendency. *See also* DENTINE HYPERSENSITIVITY.

hypertaurodont *n.* Describing a form of *taurodontism in which the pulp chamber extends partially or completely as far as the root apices.

hypertension *n.* An increase in arterial *blood pressure above the normal range. The cause may be known (**symptomatic hypertension**) or unknown (**essential hypertension**).

hyperthyroidism *n.* Overactivity of the *thyroid gland due to a tumour, glandular overgrowth, or *Graves' disease.

hypertonic *adj.* Describing a solution which has a higher osmotic pressure than another solution. Blood cells placed in hypertonic saline will shrivel as fluid passes from inside the cells through the cell membrane and into the saline solution. *Compare* HYPOTONIC; ISOTONIC.

hypertrophy *n.* An increase in the size of an organ or tissue due to an increase in the volume of the cells as opposed to an increase in their number. It is usually related to increased function e.g increase in the volume of a muscle following exercise. *Compare* HYPERPLASIA.

hyperventilation *n.* An abnormally prolonged and rapid breathing rate. It causes a fall in arterial carbon dioxide characterized by confusion, dizziness, numbness, and muscular cramp. It is usually caused by *stress, pain, or anxiety and may be associated with generalized anxiety disorders. *Compare* HYPOVENTILATION.

hypervitaminosis *n.* The condition resulting from the ingestion of excessive quantities of vitamins. An excess of the fat-soluble *vitamins A and D can be toxic and have a serious effect on calcium metabolism.

hyp- (hypo-) Prefix denoting 1. Deficiency, lack, or small size. 2. (in anatomy) Below, or beneath.

hypnosis *n.* An artificially induced sleep-like state in which the subject usually experiences a sense of deep relaxation with their attention narrowed down and focused on suggestions made by the therapist. Hypnosis is used in dentistry for pain management, stress-related disorders, obtaining *analgesia, salivation control, control of bleeding, treating dental *phobia, and to control the *gag reflex.

Further Reading: Roberts K. Hypnosis in dentistry. *Dent Update* 2006;33(5):312–14.

(((🌐))) **SEE WEB LINKS**
• The website of the British Society of Clinical and Academic Hypnosis, which incorporates the British Society of Medical and Dental Hypnosis.

hypo *n.* *See* SODIUM THIOSULPHATE.

hypoaesthesia *n.* A decreased sensitivity to painful stimuli.

hypoallergenic *adj.* Describing the characteristic of a substance or material possessing little or no allergy-producing symptoms, particularly in individuals with known sensitivities.

hypoalveolism *n.* A condition in which the *alveolar process is normal in position in relation to the respective jaw base but is excessively low in a vertical dimension. *Compare* HYPERALVEOLISM.

hypocalcaemia *n.* An abnormally low concentration of *calcium in the blood. It may be associated with *hypoparathyroidism.

hypocalcification *n.* An insufficient deposition of calcium salts in mineralized tissues (bones or teeth). When it occurs in enamel it is characterized by opaque white spots (*see also* FLUOROSIS). **Hypomineralized amelogenesis imperfecta** affects the primary and permanent dentitions and is characterized by soft chalky enamel which is rapidly lost, to expose the darker yellow coloured *dentine.

hypocementosis *n.* A reduction in the amount of *cementum. It may be seen in *cleidocranial dysplasia where there is failure of acellular cementum and *hypophosphatasia.

hypochlorous acid A weak but strongly oxidizing acid (HClO) produced by the reaction of chlorine and water and used as a bleaching agent, disinfectant, and chlorinating agent. It has been shown to be effective in controlling microbial contamination, reducing biofilm, and maintaining endotoxins at an accepted level in *dental unit waterlines. Trade name: **Sterilox.**

Further Reading: Bremer P. Disinfection of dental unit water lines. *NZ Dent J* 2006;102(1):18-19.

hypocone (tetartocone) *n.* The fourth, distopalatal cusp of a maxillary molar tooth.

hypoconid (tetartoconid) *n.* The distobuccal cusp of a mandibular molar tooth.

hypoconulid *n.* The distal cusp on the occlusal surface of a mandibular molar linked by enamel ridges to the *hypoconid and the *entoconid.

hypodermic *adj.* Below or under the skin e.g. hypodermic syringe.

hypodontia *n.* A decrease in the number of teeth compared to normal. It is sometimes called partial *anodontia. It is rare in the primary dentition but relatively common in the permanent dentition. The most frequent teeth to be missing are the mandibular second premolars, the maxillary lateral incisors, and the maxillary second premolars. It may be described as severe when six or more teeth are missing. Where the permanent tooth is missing, the primary tooth which it normally replaces is frequently retained into adult life but, having smaller roots, a retained primary tooth will usually be unable to survive many years of adult masticatory function. There may be a *hereditary trait but in most cases the occurrence is sporadic. Hypodontia is often seen in a number of members of a family and may be associated with other conditions such as ectodermal *dysplasia and orofaciodigital syndromes.

Further Reading: Gill D. S., Jones S., Hobkirk J., Bassi S., Hemmings K., Goodman J. Counselling patients with hypodontia. *Dent Update* 2008;35:344–52.

hypogenia *n.* A condition in which the chin prominence is too low in a vertical dimension with respect to the rest of the facial skeleton but is normal in its height, projection, and width. *Compare* HYPERGENIA.

hypogeusia *n.* A condition in which the sense of taste is abnormally diminished. It may be hereditary or acquired.

hypoglottis *n.* The under surface of the tongue.

hypoglycaemia *n.* A deficiency of *sugar in the bloodstream characterized by muscular weakness, confusion, dizziness, and sweating. It most commonly occurs in *diabetes mellitus and is usually due to *insulin overdosage or insufficient intake of carbohydrate.

hypognathous *adj.* Having a small or under-developed lower jaw.

hypohidrotic ectodermal dysplasia *n.* *See* ANHIDROTIC ECTODERMAL DYSPLASIA.

hypologia *n. See* DYSLOGIA.

hypomaxillism *n.* A condition in which the maxilla is too small in height due to an anomaly of the maxillary alveolus. *Compare* HYPERMAXILLISM.

hypomineralization *n.* A reduction in irregular deposits of calcium salts in either teeth or bone. Teeth with *fluorosis exhibit a subsurface hypomineralization of the enamel. **Molar incisor hypomineralization (MIH)** is the developmental hypomineralization of one or more permanent first molars associated with hypomineralization of the permanent incisors; the cause is unclear. The appearance can range from mild enamel opacities to enamel that is easily abraded on tooth eruption causing extensive hypersensitivity and often resulting in extensive carious lesions. Management is usually by sealants, restorative intervention, or extraction depending on the severity of the condition. *See also* HYPOPLASIA; AMELOGENESIS IMPERFECTA.

hypomyxia *n.* A condition in which the secretion of mucous is diminished.

hypoparathyroidism *n.* A decrease in *parathyroid gland function characterized by muscular spasm (*tetany), irritability, and muscle weakness.

hypopharynx *n. See* LARYNGOPHARYNX.

hypophosphataemia *n.* An inherited condition (also known as vitamin D-resistant rickets) in which there are abnormalities of dentine in addition to skeletal abnormalities. The pulp chambers are abnormally large and the pulp horns often extend to the *amelodentinal junction. Teeth are lost prematurely due to pulp *necrosis and periapical infection.

hypophosphatasia *n.* A rare inborn error of metabolism that results in reduced alkaline phosphatase in bone and serum. The condition is sometimes associated with premature and aggressive periodontal destruction as a result of the defective formation of bone and calcium. Teeth show cemental *hypoplasia or *aplasia and are often lost prematurely. Dentine formation may also be abnormal.

hypopituitarism *n.* Reduced activity of the pituitary gland causing dwarfism in children and fatigue and premature aging in adults.

hypoplasia *n.* (*adj.* **hypoplastic**) The defective or under-development of an organ or tissue such as the underdevelopment of parts of a tooth (**dental hypoplasia**). **Enamel hypoplasia** is a defect in either matrix formation or mineralization of enamel during *amelogenesis. It may be localized to one tooth or generalized to affect several or all teeth, the distribution being related to the extent of tooth formation at the time of the disturbance (**chronological hypoplasia**). Localized hypoplasia usually affects the upper central incisors as a result of infection or trauma to the primary predecessor. Hypoplastic enamel is characterized as yellow-brown, pitted, or irregular. It may also appear as isolated white opacities (*white spots), particularly on the upper central incisors. Chronological hypoplasia is largely as a result of systemic illnesses such as measles, mumps, and viral infections, resulting in a linear horizontal band of ridged or pitted enamel corresponding to the period of the infection. This mostly occurs during the first few months of life and is therefore most commonly seen affecting the permanent first molars, upper central incisors, lower lateral incisors, and canines. In the prenatal period, diseases affecting the mother can be significant. *See also* NEONATAL.

hypostomia *n.* A developmental anomaly characterized by an abnormal smallness of the mouth (*microstomia), in which the oral opening is a vertical instead of a horizontal slit.

hyposulphite *n. See* SODIUM THIOSULPHATE.

hypotension *n.* A condition in which the arterial blood pressure is abnormally low. It can be caused by excessive fluid loss, drugs, and conditions such as severe infections and allergic reactions. **Temporary hypotension** occurs during fainting (*syncope).

hypothesis *n.* A prediction made to explain certain observations or facts that require to be verified by further investigation.

hypothyroidism *n.* A decrease in *thyroid gland function characterized by *cretinism if present at birth and slow mental and physical activity, dry skin, and weight gain (*myxoedema) in adults; there may also be enlargement of the tongue. Patients with hypothyroidism respond poorly to stress such as dental surgery, and care should be exercised when administering local anaesthetic containing epinephrine.

hypotonic *adj.* Describing a solution on one side of a membrane where the *solute concentration is less than on the other side. *Compare* HYPERTONIC; ISOTONIC.

hypoventilation *n.* A condition in which breathing is abnormally shallow or slow, causing a high concentration of *carbon dioxide in the blood. It is characterized by *cyanosis. *Compare* HYPERVENTILATION.

hypoxia *n.* A deficiency of oxygen in the tissues. It can result in tissue death. It is a recognized side-effect of conscious *sedation using *benzodiazepines, which have the potential to cause respiratory depression. **Diffusion hypoxia** can occur at the end of conscious sedation using nitrous oxide/ oxygen. This is due to the low solubility of nitrous oxide in the blood and tissues resulting in a rapid outflow of nitrous oxide across the alveolar membrane when the incoming gas flow is stopped; this reduces the percentage of alveolar oxygen available for uptake. Diffusion hypoxia can be avoided by administering 100% oxygen for 2 minutes.

hypsistaphyline *adj. See* CHAMESTAPHYLINE.

hypsodont *adj.* Describing teeth with high crowns. It is a characteristic of the teeth of cows and deer which allows for wear and tear during function. *Compare* BRACHYDONT.

hysteresis *n.* The lagging behind of an effect when its cause varies in amount. It can be seen in reversible *hydrocolloids when the change from a liquid to a gel occurs at a different temperature from when it changes from a gel to a liquid. The degree of hysteresis in an *elastomer is the ability of the elastomer to return to its original shape after deformation.

-iasis Suffix denoting a diseased condition e.g. **elephantiasis** (a rare disorder of the lymphatic system caused by parasitic worms).

iatro- Prefix denoting medicine or doctors.

iatrogenic *adj.* Describing an unforeseen or unwanted side-effect of treatment provided by a health professional.

ibuprofen *n.* A proprionic acid derivative in the non-steroidal anti-inflammatory drug (NSAID) category. It binds extensively to plasma proteins and is rapidly absorbed following oral administration. It has *analgesic, anti-inflammatory, and *antipyretic properties and is used in the treatment of musculoskeletal, dental, and rheumatic pain. It is also a popular post-operative analgesic. Trade names: **Brufen, Fenbid, Junifen, Nurofen.**

ICON *See* INDEX OF COMPLEXITY OUTCOME AND NEED.

identification dot A small elevation or pimple on the corner of a radiographic film used to indicate the surface of the film facing the x-ray tube during exposure.

idiopathic *adj.* (*n.* **idiopathy**) Describing a disease or medical condition of unknown cause or which occurs spontaneously.

idiosyncrasy *n.* (*adj.* **idiosyncratic**) An unusual and unexpected sensitivity reaction by an individual to a particular food, drug, or cosmetic. Drug idiosyncrasy occurs when the standard dose causes an excessive response.

imbalance *n.* A disharmonious relationship between two or more functional systems, structures, or organs.

imbibition *n.* (*v.* **imbibe**) The absorption of liquid by a solid or a gel. For example, *glass ionomer cement undergoes imbibition of water during its early setting phase.

imbrication *n.* (in dentistry) Anterior teeth in the same arch which overlap each other. **Imbrication lines** are mesio-distal ridges on the cervical third of the labial surface of an anterior tooth associated with enamel incremental growth formation. *See also* STRIAE OF RETZIUS.

immediate denture *n. See* DENTURE.

immediate life support (ILS) *See* BASIC LIFE SUPPORT.

immobilization *n. See* FIXATION.

immune response (reaction) *n.* The bodily defence reaction of an organism that recognizes an invading substance (*antigen) such as a virus, fungus, bacteria, or transplanted organ, and produces an *antibody specific against that antigen. There are two types of immune response: B-lymphocytes (or B-cells) are responsible for **humoral immunity** producing free antibodies that circulate in the bloodstream; T-lymphocytes (or T-cells) are responsible for **cell-mediated immunity**.

immune system *n.* The organs and tissue responsible for *immunity. The **non-specific immune system** is made up of a primary barrier consisting of the skin and mucosa and a secondary barrier consisting of inflammatory cells and soluble factors. The third barrier is the **specific immune system** which includes the thymus, bone marrow, spleen, tonsils, and lymph nodes.

immunity *n.* The ability of the body to resist infection due to the presence of circulating *antibodies and white blood cells. **Natural (innate** or **non-specific) immunity** is a defence mechanism which includes natural, mechanical, chemical, and biological barriers to infection and which has no degree of memory or specificity; it is present at birth prior to exposure to infective agents. **Acquired immunity** is achieved in response to foreign *antigens in the body and involves the production of *antibodies which react specifically with the foreign antigen. **Active immunity** is achieved when the body's own cells produce and continue to produce appropriate antibodies in response to an infection or to artificial stimulation by the use of treated antigens to stimulate the body to produce its own antibodies (*immunization, *vaccination). **Passive immunity** is of short duration and occurs naturally at birth from maternal antibodies in the mother's milk (colostrum) and placental blood or by the injection of antibodies contained in antiserum taken from another immune person or animal.

immunization *n.* The production of *immunity by artificial means. It may be achieved actively or passively.

immunodeficiency *n.* A condition resulting from a reduced or deficient *immune response. This may be a **primary** condition due to a defect in the immune system or a **secondary** (or **acquired**) condition as a result of a disease process such as *AIDS.

immunoglobulins *n.* A group of structurally related serum proteins synthesized by *plasma cells which act as *antibodies.

immunosuppressant *n.* A drug or agent that reduces the *immune response. They are useful in maintaining the survival of transplanted organs or tissues which would otherwise be rejected and destroyed by the immune response, and for treating certain *autoimmune diseases such as rheumatoid *arthritis.

impaction *n.* The condition of being tightly wedged together. **Food impaction** can occur between the teeth due to an open contact, a poorly contoured restoration, or the plunger effect of opposing teeth. **Tooth impaction** occurs when a tooth is prevented from erupting into a fully functional position. The preventing agent can be another tooth, alveolar bone, or soft tissues. The most commonly impacted teeth are third molars, second premolars, and canines; the impacted tooth may lie in a variety of different positions. 📷

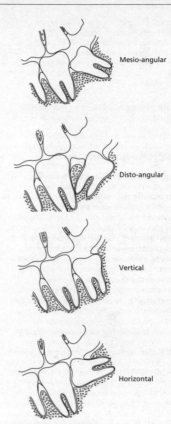

Mesio-angular

Disto-angular

Vertical

Horizontal

Types of impacted lower third molars

impairment *n.* Any loss or abnormality of psychological, physiological, or anatomical structure or function. It represents a deviation from a person's usual biomedical state. An impairment is thus any loss of function directly resulting from injury or disease. A social model defines impairment as the functional limitation within an individual caused by restricted physical, mental, or sensory activity. *Compare* DISABILITY; HANDICAP.

impetigo *n.* A superficial bacterial infection of the skin. It is characterized by small pus-filled blisters that form a yellow crust, usually around the nose and mouth. **Non-bullous impetigo** is caused by *Staphylococcus aureus* or *Streptococcus* species or both, is highly contagious, and occurs mainly in young children. **Bullous impetigo** is caused by *Staphylococcus aureus*, is less contagious, and can occur at any age. Treatment is usually by topical antibiotics.

impingement *n.* The unusually forceful application of food, teeth, foreign objects, etc. onto tissues, teeth, or prostheses.

implant

n. (in dentistry) A device specifically designed to be placed surgically within or on the mandibular or maxillary bone as a means of providing retention for a prosthetic replacement of one or more teeth. Implants may be broadly classified into three groups: **subperiosteal**, which rest on the surface of the bone beneath the *periosteum and mucosa; **transosteal**, which penetrate the inferior border of the mandible and project through the oral mucosa covering the edentulous ridge; and **endosteal (endosseous)**, which are embedded in the maxillary or mandibular bone and project through the oral mucosa covering the edentulous ridge. A subperiosteal implant used to be indicated when the bone had atrophied and the jaw structure was limited; however, it has now been superseded by the endosteal implant. A subperiosteal implant had a lightweight, individually designed, metal framework fitting over the remaining bone with metal posts that projected through the soft tissue into the oral cavity, providing the equivalent of multiple tooth roots; they were used in a limited area or, if all the teeth were missing, in the entire mouth to retain a complete denture. The potential contraindicating risk factors of this type of implant were bone resorption, injury to nerves causing *paraesthesia, fracture of the mandible, and soft tissue inflammation. An endosteal implant is placed directly into the jaw bone and the intraosseous part generally has a blade or root shape. Implant material is usually machined *titanium with a modified surface such as a titanium plasma spray (TPS) or *hydroxyapatite coating. Bioceramic materials are less commonly used. The **blade implant**, made of steel and used mostly for partially dentulous patients, was an endosteal implant developed in the late 1950s and was narrow bucco-lingually, with the blade following the arch of the jaw bone with openings or vents through which the bone could grow; it resulted in a connective tissue capsule around the implant rather than true *osseointegration with the surrounding bone. These implants have been superseded by titanium implants capable of true osseointegration following the work of Per-Ingvar Branemark, a Swedish orthopaedic surgeon, started in 1952. The **core-vent implant system** is an endosseous implant system in which the implant is made of titanium. The portion of the implant retained in the bone has a hollow vent and the part protruding above the soft tissues is machined to receive a prosthetic abutment. An **endodontic (diodontic) implant** is a metallic implant that extends through the root canal of a tooth into the periapical cortical bone to provide increased retention and decreased tooth mobility. It is used to stabilize and retain natural teeth and may be smooth, tapered, threaded, or have a porous surface. The intra-dental portion is cemented in position. The **IMZ (Intramobile Zylinder) implant** is an endosseous implant system introduced in 1987 and consisting of a cylindrical intra-bony element and a polyoxymethylene coated stress-breaking component, called an intra-mobile element, to allow implant connection to natural teeth. The **root-shaped endosteal implant** mimics the basic shape of the natural tooth root and is manufactured in a variety of shapes, sizes, and lengths. An endosteal implant requires at least 1mm of bone between it, the adjacent teeth, and the buccal and palatal alveolar plates.

A **self-tapping implant** is an endosteal implant which cuts its own path through bone tissue. The **staple implant** is an example of a transosteal implant which is retained by fixation screws tapped into the anterior region of the mandible from the lower surface to provide a number of pins penetrating the alveolar ridge and mucous membrane, to which a bar may be attached to retain a complete or partial denture. Implant placement may be undertaken either as a **one-stage technique** (early loading) in which the implant is placed into a new, healing, or healed extraction site and is visible above the oral mucosa immediately after placement (this avoids the necessity of a second surgical stage to expose the implant), or a **two-stage technique** in which the implant is placed into a new, healing, or healed extraction site and then covered by the oral mucosa so that it cannot be seen; at a second stage between one week and two months later (early loading) or after two months (conventional loading), allowing time for osseointegration to take place, the implant is uncovered and

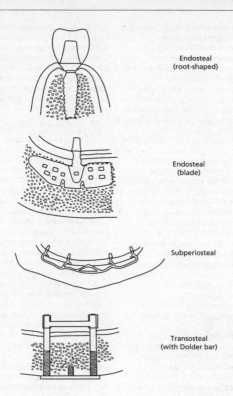

Endosteal
(root-shaped)

Endosteal
(blade)

Subperiosteal

Transosteal
(with Dolder bar)

Types of implants

intra-oral components added to allow the placement of one or more restorations. *See also* ABUTMENT. 📷

Further reading: Esposito M., Worthington H. V., Coulthard P., Thomsen P. Maintaining and re-establishing health around osseointegrated oral implants: a Cochrane systematic review comparing the efficacy of various treatments. *Periodontol* 2000 2003;33:204–12.

Bishop K, Addy L, Knox J. Modern restorative management of patients with congenitally missing teeth: the role of implants. *Dent Update* 2007;34:79–84.

implantology (oral) *n.* A specialist branch of dentistry concerned with the surgical insertion of materials or devices into the hard or soft tissues of the oral cavity for the purpose of providing support or retention for tooth restorations or a prosthetic appliance.

implant restoration A restoration placed on an implant designed to restore normal function, aesthetics, speech, and comfort. It may be

secured on the underlying implant by screw or cement retention, or a combination of the two. This allows the restoration to be removed for repair in the event of porcelain fracture, abutment fracture, or if the prosthesis needs to be modified such as when an implant has failed. The restorative prosthesis may consist of several units secured to a number of implants.

Impregum° *n.* The trade name for a *polyether impression material.

impression *n.* An imprinted mould of an object such as a tooth, arch of teeth, or edentulous ridge, obtained by pressing an *impression tray containing an *impression material over the target object, from which a positive reproduction of that object can be made. A **mucodisplacive (mucocompressive, functional) impression** utilizes a technique in which the denture-bearing area of the mucosa is loaded to produce a uniform reduction in volume which will be subsequently compressed during

denture wearing; the impression material used is of high viscosity such as *impression compound.
A **mucostatic impression** creates an impression of the denture-bearing tissues in their natural state and requires a low-viscosity impression material such as *plaster of Paris or *alginate. A **primary (preliminary) impression** is made for diagnostic purposes or for the construction of an impression in which a more accurate secondary impression can be taken; preliminary impressions may also be taken in order to construct a *model on which a custom-made impression tray can be fabricated for the purposes of taking a more accurate secondary impression. A **dual impression technique** is a method of taking an impression in layers using impression materials of different viscosities, chosen appropriate to the character and mobility of the soft tissues so as to provide differential compression. A **working (secondary** or **final) impression** is an accurate impression usually taken in a custom-made *impression tray used for making a master cast. A **sectional impression** is made in two or more parts. A **pick-up impression** is an accurate impression taken with an implant superstructure or one or more crown *copings in place so that they are included in the impression material; it provides an accurate impression of the oral mucosal tissue and the location of the metallic superstructure relative to the crown preparations or implants.

impression compound *n.* A material composed of fatty acids, shellac, glycerine, and filler used as a primary *impression material. When heated in a water bath at about 65°C (149°F) it becomes plastic and can be moulded in an impression tray and inserted in the mouth. The material becomes fairly rigid on cooling to mouth temperature and has low material flow at room temperature. It has a low thermal-expansion coefficient so that there is minimal dimensional change as the impression is cooled from mouth temperature and it does not adhere to moist oral tissue. It may be modified by the addition of an *alginate wash. Impression compound is usually used for taking primary impressions of the edentulous ridge prior to the construction of a custom-made *impression tray for complete *dentures. Impression compound is also available in sticks of various colours indicating different softening temperature ranges e.g. **greenstick compound (composition)**; these are used for impression correction and moulding the borders of custom impression trays, particularly around muscle attachments.

impression material *n.* Any substance used for making a negative mould of a structure. **Rigid impression materials** are inflexible and are usually used to take impressions of structures which have no undercut surfaces such that when removed the material is not required to be

deformed; such materials include *plaster of Paris, *impression compound, *zinc oxide, and *wax. **Elastic impression materials** are capable of deformation with minimal distortion; materials commonly used are reversible and irreversible *hydrocolloid, *silicone, *polyether, and mercaptan (*polysulphide). Syringable impression material may be used for obtaining an *occlusal record.

Further Reading: Stewardson D. A. Trends in indirect dentistry: 5. Impression materials and techniques. *Dent Update* 2005;32(7):374–6, 379–80, 382–4.

impression tray *n.* A rigid receptacle in which impression material is placed. Materials commonly used for impression trays are metal, *shellac, or resin. They are usually coated with tray adhesive immediately prior to use and may be perforated with 2–4mm diameter holes or made from metallic mesh to improve the adhesion of the impression material to the tray. **Stock trays** are rigid trays commercially manufactured in different sizes and shapes and usually made of resin or metal. **Edentulous stock trays** have a shape which conforms to the shape of the edentulous ridge of either the mandible or maxilla. **Dentate stock trays** have a box shape to accommodate the teeth in the arch. **Custom trays** are made from a primary cast and, because their shape conforms more closely to the shape of the teeth and tissues to give a more uniform thickness of impression material, it provides greater dimensional accuracy. Custom trays are usually made from shellac or resin. A **sectional tray** is used to take an impression of a specific area of the dental arch such as a quadrant or sextant.

IMZ implant system *n. See* IMPLANT.

incidence *n.* The number of occurrences of a disease, condition, or event within a defined time interval. The **incidence rate** is the number of cases of a specific disease, condition, or event diagnosed or reported during a defined period of time, divided by the number of people at risk for the disease.

incipient *adj.* In an initial stage; beginning to become apparent.

incisal *adj.* Relating to the cutting edge of an anterior tooth (incisor or canine). The **incisal edge** is the biting edge of an incisor or canine. The **incisal angle** is the angle between the incisal edge and the mesial or distal surface of an anterior tooth. The **incisal guide table** forms the base for the incisal guide *pin on an *articulator. **Incisal guidance** is the influence on mandibular movements caused by the contacting surfaces of the mandibular and maxillary anterior teeth during masticatory movements (eccentric excursions from centric *occlusion).

incision *n.* 1. The act of making a cut in body tissue. 2. The cutting action of incisor teeth.

incisor, permanent mandibular central *n.* One of two teeth which are the smallest in the permanent *dentition located between the mandibular lateral incisors either side of the midline. They replace the mandibular primary central incisor teeth. It has a convex labial surface with a flattened area in the incisal half. The lingual surface is concave, except above the cervical margin where it is convex. Unlike the upper central incisors, there is no well-defined *cingulum and no definite marginal ridges on the lingual surface. The mesial and distal surfaces of the crown are triangular in shape, to give a wedge-shaped appearance, and are almost at right angles to the incisal edge. On *eruption, the incisal edge has three small tubercles (*mamelons), which wear away to give a flat surface. It has a single root, oval in cross-section and flattened on the mesial and distal surfaces. The apical region may show some degree of bifurcation. The *pulp chamber has two mesial and distal pulp horns directed

towards the mesial and distal angles of the incisal edge. The root canal is subject to variation and may divide to give buccal and lingual canals. *Calcification of the tooth begins at about 3–4 months after birth and the crown is normally complete by 4–5 years of age. The tooth erupts at about 6–7 years and the calcification of the root is complete at about 9–10 years.

incisor, permanent mandibular lateral *n.* One of two teeth located between the mandibular central incisors and the canines in the permanent dentition. They replace the mandibular primary lateral incisor teeth. It is similar to the lower central incisor but is wider mesio-distally and therefore more fan-shaped. The lingual surface usually shows more definite mesial and distal marginal ridges. On *eruption, the incisal edge has three small tubercles (*mamelons), which wear away to give a flat surface. *Calcification of the tooth begins at about 3–4 months after birth and the crown is normally complete by 4–5 years of age. The tooth erupts at about 7–8 years and the calcification of the root is complete at about 10 years.

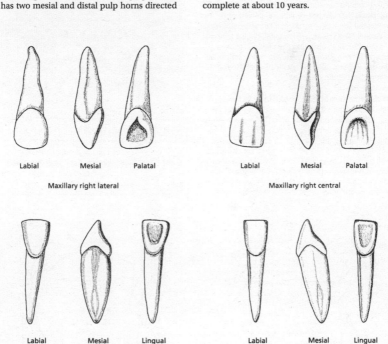

Labial   Mesial   Palatal

Maxillary right lateral

Labial   Mesial   Palatal

Maxillary right central

Labial   Mesial   Lingual

Mandibular right lateral

Labial   Mesial   Lingual

Mandibular right central

Permanent incisors

incisor, permanent maxillary central *n.*
One of two teeth located between the maxillary lateral incisors either side of the midline in the permanent *dentition. They replace the maxillary primary central incisor teeth. The crown has a convex labial surface slightly flattened incisally, usually with two slight vertical grooves close to the incisal edge. The labial surface merges more gradually with the distal than the mesial surface. The lingual surface is concave except for a pronounced convexity (*cingulum) towards the cervical margin. The lingual surface is triangular, bounded by mesial and distal marginal ridges extending from the incisal edge to the cingulum. Between the marginal ridges and the cingulum lies a lingual pit which may be partly divided by a central ridge. The mesial and distal surfaces are triangular in shape and are both inclined lingually. The angle formed by the incisal edge and the distal surface is much more rounded than the angle formed by the incisal edge and the mesial surface. The tooth has a single root, triangular in cross-section, tapering gradually towards the apex. The pulp chamber is triangular in cross-section with two pulp horns directed towards the mesial and distal incisal corners. There is usually only one root canal but it may be subject to considerable variation. *Calcification of the tooth begins at about 3–4 months after birth and the crown is normally complete by 4–5 years of age. The tooth erupts at about 7–8 years and the calcification of the root is complete at about 10 years.

incisor, permanent maxillary lateral *n.*
One of two teeth located between the maxillary central incisors and the canines in the permanent *dentition. The crown has a very similar morphology to the upper central incisor but is significantly smaller with a narrower mesio-distal width. The disto-incisal angle is more rounded than the upper central incisor, and below the *cingulum there is a well-defined fossa or pit. The root is a similar shape to that of the upper central

incisor and of almost equal length. The pulp chamber is triangular in cross-section, with two *pulp horns directed towards the mesial and distal incisal corners. There is usually only one root canal but it may be subject to considerable variation. The upper lateral incisor is the most common incisor tooth to be congenitally absent or show some degree of deformity, usually being conical or peg-shaped. *Calcification of the tooth begins at about 10–12 months after birth and the crown is normally complete by 4–5 years of age. The tooth erupts at about 8–9 years and the calcification of the root is complete at about 11 years.

incisor relationship The relation of the upper and lower incisors when in tooth contact (centric *occlusion). The British Standards Institute classify the incisor relationship as Class I, Class II division I or division II, and Class III.

Incisor relationship	
Class	Definition
Class I	The lower incisal edges occlude with or lie immediately below the cingulum of the upper incisors.
Class II division I	The lower incisal edge occludes behind the cingulum of the upper central incisors and the upper incisors are proclined.
Class II division II	The lower incisal edge occludes behind the cingulum of the upper central incisors, and the upper incisors are retroclined (the lateral incisors may be proclined).
Class III	The lower incisal edge occludes in front of the cingulum of the upper incisors.

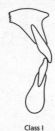 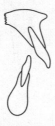 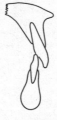 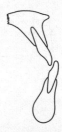

Class I   Class II div. I   Class II div. II   Class III

Incisor relationship

incisors, Hutchinson's [J. Hutchinson (1828–1913), English physician] *n.* Permanent incisors of abnormal shape in which the incisal edges are notched and narrower than the cervical region. The upper central incisors of the permanent dentition are most commonly affected. It is a symptom of congenital syphilis.

incisors, primary (deciduous) *n.* The first four teeth to erupt in the primary dentition located between the maxillary and mandibular canines. They are morphologically similar to their permanent successors; however, although smaller, their mesio-distal width is relatively larger when compared to the vertical height (axial length) of the crown to give them a more bulbous appearance. Unlike the permanent incisors, they do not have any tubercles (*mamelons) on the incisal edge on eruption. Relative to the size of the tooth, the pulp chamber is larger than in the permanent incisors and therefore the surrounding dentine is proportionally thinner. Calcification of the primary incisors commences at 4–5 months in foetal life and the crowns are normally complete by 2 months after birth. They erupt at about 6–8 months after birth and the roots are complete at 1–2 years. *See also* DENTITION.

inclination *n.* The angle of slope from a point of reference such as the eruption path of a tooth, the path of removal of a prosthesis, and the draw of a cavity preparation.

inclusion cyst *See* CYST.

incompetent lips *See* LIP.

incontinentia pigmenti (Bloch–Sulzberger syndrome) *n.* A rare genetic disorder characterized by pigmented skin, lesions of the eyes, skeletal abnormalities, *hypodontia, and enamel *hypoplasia.

incremental lines The growth pattern produced by the laying down of enamel during *amelogenesis. *See also* ENAMEL.

incubation period (latent period) 1. The interval between the exposure to an infection and the appearance of any symptoms. 2. (in bacteriology) The period of development of a bacterial culture.

incubator *n.* A piece of laboratory equipment consisting of a closed chamber used for the cultivation of bacteria or fungi on solid or liquid growth media. The temperature of the internal

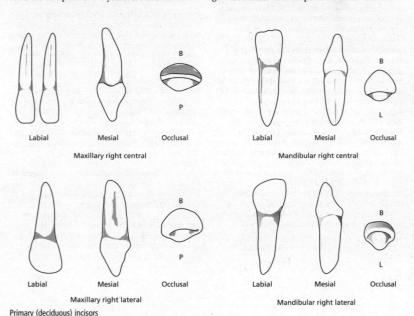

Labial	Mesial	Occlusal
		B / P

Maxillary right central

Labial	Mesial	Occlusal
		B / L

Mandibular right central

Labial	Mesial	Occlusal
		B / P

Maxillary right lateral

Labial	Mesial	Occlusal
		B / L

Mandibular right lateral

Primary (deciduous) incisors

environment can be regulated to optimize growth conditions for particular micro-organisms. Some incubators contain shaking platforms to increase the aeration of micro-organisms being grown in a liquid culture medium.

independent t-test (in statistics) A test that uses the t-statistic to establish if two *means obtained from independent samples differ significantly.

((((⊕)))) SEE WEB LINKS

• University of the West of England web page, giving an overview with an example.

independent variable *See* VARIABLE.

index *n.* 1. A mould or impression used to record the relationship of a tooth or teeth to one another or to a cast. 2. The formula expressing the ratio of one measurable value to another. An index may be defined as a numerical value describing the relative status of a population on a graduated scale with definite upper and lower limits designed to permit and facilitate comparison with other populations classified by the same criteria. Indices are used in health service research, epidemiological surveys, clinical trials, and also to diagnose disease and monitor the progress of treatment in individual patients. An index may be classified as reversible or irreversible, based on the direction in which its scores can fluctuate. It may be full mouth or partial mouth, depending on the area of the mouth examined. An index may assess only the presence or absence of the variable or it may assess the severity of the variable; it may relate the clinical finding to treatment need. A number of indices have been developed for use in epidemiology and clinical dental practice which include the *calculus surface index, *Community Periodontal Index of Treatment Needs, *DEF index, *DMF and dmf indices, *extent and severity index, functioning teeth index, *gingival bleeding index, *gingival index, *Greene–Vermillion oral hygiene and deposit index, *index of complexity outcome and need (ICON), *index of orthodontic treatment need (IOTN), *papillary marginal attached (PMA) index, peer assessment rating (*PAR) index, *periodontal disease index, *plaque index, and *tissue health index.

Further Reading: Young W. O., Striffler D. F. *The dentist, his practice and his community.* Philadelphia, Saunders, 2nd edition, 1989.

index of complexity outcome and need (ICON) An index developed to assess orthodontic treatment complexity. It provides a summary score based on the severity of the malocclusion and the difficulty of the proposed treatment from an examination of the pre-treatment study models. It incorporates features of the *Index of Orthodontic Treatment Need (IOTN) and the *Peer Assessment Rating index (PAR). Occlusal traits are scored and multiplied by their respective weightings.

ICON index variables	
Occlusal trait	ICON index weighting
IOTN aesthetic component	7
Upper arch crowding/ spacing	5
Crossbite	5
Overbite/open bite	4
Buccal segment relationship	3

A score of more than 43 is taken to indicate a demonstrable need for treatment. The index can be applied to the post-treatment models to assess treatment outcome; if the summary score is less than 31 the outcome may be considered to be acceptable.

index of orthodontic treatment need (IOTN) An index used to assess a patient's need and priority for orthodontic care, used in the UK as a basis for determining whether a patient should be accepted for treatment within the National Health Service (NHS) healthcare system. The index is based on an assessment of *malocclusion and has aesthetic and dental health components. The **aesthetic component** is based on a comparison of the malocclusion with ten centric view photographs graded from 1 to 10 to indicate a scale of increasing need for treatment based on psycho-social impairment. The **dental health component** defines the malocclusion into five grades determined by the potential harm that a particular malocclusion can have on the longevity of the dentition.

IOTN dental health component

Category		Description	Treatment need
Grade 1		Extremely minor *malocclusions including displacements less than 1mm	None
Grade 2	a	Increased *overjet 3.6–6mm with competent lips	Little
	b	Reverse overjet 0.1–1mm	
	c	Anterior or posterior *crossbite with up to1mm discrepancy between retruded contact position and intercuspal position	
	d	Displacement of teeth 1.1–2mm	
	e	Anterior or posterior open bite 1.1–2mm	
	f	Increased overbite 3.5mm or more without gingival contact	
	g	Prenormal or postnormal occlusions with no other anomalies includes up to half a unit discrepancy	
Grade 3	a	Increased overjet 3.6–6mm with incompetent lips	Moderate
	b	Reverse overjet 1.1–3.5mm	
	c	Anterior or posterior crossbites with 1.1–2mm discrepancy between the retruded contact position and the intercuspal position	
	d	Displacement of teeth 2.1–4mm	
	e	Lateral or anterior open bite 2.1–4mm	
	f	Increased and incomplete overbite without gingival or palatal trauma	
Grade 4	a	Increased overjet 6.1–9mm	Great
	b	Reverse overjet greater than 3.5mm with no masticatory or speech difficulties	
	c	Anterior or posterior crossbites with greater than 2mm discrepancy between the retruded contact position and intercuspal position	
	d	Severe displacements of teeth greater than 4mm	
	e	Extreme lateral or anterior open bites greater than 4mm	
	f	Increased and complete overbite with gingival or palatal trauma	
	h	Less extensive hypodontia requiring pre-restorative orthodontics or orthodontic space closure to avoid the need for a prosthetic appliance	
	l	Posterior lingual crossbite with no functional occlusal contact in one or more buccal segments	
	m	Reverse overjet 1.1–3.5mm with no recorded masticatory and speech difficulties	
	t	Partially erupted teeth, tipped and impacted against adjacent teeth	
	x	Existing supernumerary or supplemental teeth	
Grade 5	a	Increased overjet greater than 9mm	Very great
	h	Extensive hypodontia with restorative implications (more than one tooth missing in any quadrant) requiring pre-restorative orthodontics	
	i	Impeded eruption of teeth (apart from third molars) due to crowding, displacement, the presence of supernumerary teeth, retained deciduous teeth, and any pathological cause	
	m	Reverse overjet greater than 3.5mm with reported masticatory and speech difficulties	
	p	Defects of cleft lip and palate	
	s	Submerged deciduous teeth	

Further Reading: Ferguson J. W. IOTN (DHC): is it supported by evidence? *Dent Update* 2006;33(8):478–80, 483–4, 486.

induration *n.* The pathological hardening of a normally soft tissue or organ, especially the skin and mucous membranes.

industrial dentistry Dental care provided for employees within a specific company or industry. It may be specifically related to emergency care or to the effects of the working environment on dental health.

infant oral mutilation (IOM) The cultural practice involving the removal of an infant's healthy primary (deciduous) teeth, normally by traditional healers operating in rural communities. It is prevalent in many parts of Africa. It often leads to malformation of the underlying permanent dentition and can result in life-threatening infections.

 SEE WEB LINKS

• Dentaid web pages on IOM in Africa.

infarction *n.* The death of part or the whole of an organ or tissue caused by a reduction in blood supply due to the blockage of the arterial blood vessels by an *embolus or *thrombus. A small localized area of dead tissue produced by either an inadequate blood supply or obstructed venous outflow is known as an **infarct**.

infection *n.* The growth and multiplication of a parasitic organism (most commonly caused by micro-organisms including bacteria, fungi, and viruses) within the tissues of the body. The growth of normal *commensal flora (e.g. in the oral cavity or the intestinal tract) is not usually considered an infection. A **nosocomial infection** is acquired in a hospital or healthcare service facility, but secondary to the patient's original condition; it may be acquired in hospital but only appear after discharge. Examples of common nosocomial infections include pneumonia, urinary tract infections, and infections caused by meticillin-resistant *Staphylococcus aureus* (MRSA) or enterococci.

infection control The discipline concerned with preventing the spread of infections within the healthcare environment and with investigating and managing proven or suspected cases of *cross-infection within particular healthcare facilities. It is aimed at the prevention and the spread of pathogens between patients, from healthcare personnel to patients, and from patients to healthcare personnel in the clinical healthcare environment. Infection control and prevention form a vital component of healthcare in all healthcare facilities. Effective cleaning,

*decontamination, and sterilization of reusable invasive medical devices (i.e. most dental instruments used in the oral cavity) is an integral part of infection control and prevention in modern dental practice. *See also* STERILIZATION.

infectious mononucleosis *See* GLANDULAR FEVER.

infective endocarditis *See* ENDOCARDITIS.

inferior *adj.* (in anatomy) Describing something situated lower in the body in relationship to another structure.

inferior alveolar (dental) nerve block *n.* *See* ANALGESIA.

infiltration *n.* The abnormal entry of a substance (infiltrate) into a cell, tissue, or organ. The infiltrate may be an excessive amount of a substance normally present or a foreign substance.

infiltration analgesia *See* ANALGESIA.

inflammation *n.* The body's response to an area affected by trauma, infection, or invasion by a foreign substance; it may be either acute or chronic. **Acute inflammation** is the immediate defensive reaction to injury and is characterized by pain, heat, redness, swelling, and loss of function of the affected tissue or organ. The blood flow to the inflamed site is increased due to the dilatation of the local blood vessels. White blood cells enter the tissues and engulf the bacteria or other foreign substances. The accumulation of dead cells can result in the formation of *pus. Where healing does not occur following acute inflammation, **chronic inflammation** may ensue. This is characterized by infiltration of the tissues with *macrophages and *fibroblast cells. **Granulomatous inflammation** is a type of chronic inflammation characterized by the development of accumulations of epithelioid macrophages, lymphocytes, and multinucleate giant cells (*granulomas); this form of chronic inflammation can be seen as a reaction to tissue damage caused by foreign substances such as silica particles and suture materials, or in certain diseases such as tuberculosis and Crohn's disease. *See also* GRANULOMA. 📷

informed consent *See* CONSENT.

infrabony defect A periodontal pocket with its base apical to the crest of the *alveolar bone. Infrabony defects may have one, two, or three bone walls.

infrabulge *n*. The area of the crown of a tooth *cervical to an eminence determined by the path of insertion of a removable appliance.

infradentale *n*. The apex of the *septum between the mandibular central incisors. Because it is the most anterior point of the alveolar process of the mandible and is easily identified, it is a point used in *craniometry.

infraocclusion (infraclusion, infraversion) *n*. The process where a tooth fails to achieve or maintain its normal occlusal relationship with adjacent or opposing teeth. The tooth may also be referred to as **submerged**.

infraorbital *adj*. Describes the area immediately below or beneath the orbit of the eye.

infratemporal fossa An irregular space bounded laterally by the zygomatic arch and the ramus of the mandible, medially by the lateral pterygoid plate, anteriorly by the zygomatic process, posteriorly by the articular tubercle and the posterior border of the lateral pterygoid plate, inferiorly by the alveolar border of the maxilla, and superiorly by the squama of the temporal bone and the infratemporal crest on the greater wing of the sphenoid bone. It contains the *pterygoid venous plexus.

inhalation *n*. The breathing in of any airborne substance that may be in the form of gas, fumes, mists, vapours, dust, foreign bodies, or aerosols. Inhalation of foreign bodies such as teeth, crowns, inlays, and fragments of restorative materials are a potential hazard of dental treatment if the airway is unprotected.

Further Reading: Al-Wahadni A., Al Hamad K. Q., Al-Tarawneh A. Foreign body ingestion and aspiration in dentistry: a review of the literature and reports of three cases. *Dent Update* 2006;33(9):561-2, 564-6, 569-70.

inhalation anaesthesia *See* ANAESTHESIA.

inhalation sedation *See* SEDATION.

inion *n*. The most prominent projection in the midline on the posterior occipital protuberance; it is a *craniometric point which can be felt at the base of the skull.

initiator *n*. A chemical agent, such as dibenzoyl peroxide, added to a resin to initiate *polymerization.

injection *n*. The introduction into the body of a liquid by means of a needle and a syringe. Common routes for injection are into the skin (**intracutaneous, intradermal**), immediately below the skin (**subcutaneous**), into a muscle

(**intramuscular**), and into a vein (**intravenous**). An **intra-arterial injection** is where the injected fluid is placed within an artery and is a potential hazard, particularly with dental block analgesia. *See also* ANALGESIA.

Injex *n*. The trade name for a system of achieving local *analgesia without the use of a needle by means of a jet spray of local anaesthetic solution applied to the mucosa under pressure.

inlay *n*. A rigid restoration made to conform to the shape of the tapered prepared cavity, which is then retained in place with a *cement luting material. Inlays are normally made from cast *gold, *porcelain, or *composite resin. Inlays may be prepared by the **direct method** in which the pattern is carved or shaped within the mouth or by the **indirect method** in which an impression is taken of the tooth preparation and a model constructed on which an inlay pattern is then prepared. *See also* CAD/CAM. 📷

inlay furnace *n*. *See* FURNACE.

Inman aligner A removable orthodontic appliance developed by the Inman Orthodontic Laboratory, designed to align maxillary or mandibular incisors and canines. It uses piston-like components driven by nickel titanium coil springs.

Further Reading: Quereshi A. The Inman aligner for anterior tooth alignment. *Dent Update* 2008;35:377-84: 569-76.

inner enamel epithelium *See* ENAMEL EPITHELIUM.

innervation *n*. The nerve supply to a tissue or organ of the body.

inoculation *n*. The introduction of a small quantity of a disease-causing material such as a *vaccine for the purpose of inducing *immunity; it is a more general term for *vaccination.

inorganic *adj*. Being or composed of matter other than hydrocarbons and their derivatives, or matter that is not of plant or animal origin.

inostosis *n*. The in-growth of bony tissue replacing tissue that has been destroyed e.g. alveolar bone growing into cementum.

in-patient *n*. An individual who is admitted to hospital for medical treatment, examination, or observation and who has to stay for one or more nights. *Compare* DAY-PATIENT; OUT-PATIENT.

insalivation *n*. The mixing of saliva and other secretions with food in the mouth during eating.

insertion *n*. 1. The placing of a restoration in a tooth, a bridge on abutment teeth, or a prosthesis in the mouth; these normally have a defined *path of insertion. 2. The point of attachment of a muscle that is relatively moveable when the muscle contracts. *Compare* ORIGIN. 3. The act of introducing a needle into tissue.

inspissation *n.* The process of thickening a liquid (secretions etc.) by evaporation or dehydration.

instrument *n.* A tool, device, or implement. The parts of a **hand instrument** may be described as the handle or shaft, which is grasped by the operator's hand; the working end designed for a specific function, such as the reflective surface of a mouth mirror, the point of an explorer, or the cutting surface of a chisel; and the shank, which joins the working end to the shaft. A **plastic instrument** is used to manipulate any plastic restorative material.

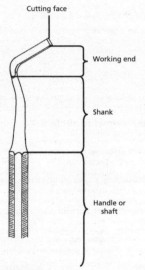

Parts of an instrument

instrument formula A method of defining dental hand instruments devised by G. V. *Black (1836–1915). It consists of three figures (sometimes four). The first figure denotes the width of the blade in tenths of millimetres; the second denotes the length of the blade in millimetres; and the third describes the angle of the blade in relation to the shaft and is measured in hundredths of a circle (centigrades). A fourth number is added if it is necessary to additionally

describe the angle of the cutting edge to the instrument shaft, such as for margin trimmers; the fourth number is entered in brackets as the second number of the formula.

instrument transfer The process of passing an instrument between operator and assistant. During **parallel instrument transfer**, the instrument being received by the assistant is hooked around the little finger and the instrument to be delivered is held between the thumb and first two fingers such that, at the point of exchange, both instruments are parallel to each other. Instruments are transferred with their working ends pointing in the direction of use and, for safety reasons, in the area around the sides and to the front of and below the patient's mouth (transfer zone).

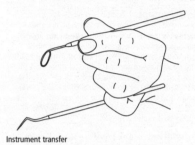

Instrument transfer

insufflation *n.* The act of blowing air, a gas, or powder into a body cavity such as the lungs. Examples are inhalation nitrous oxide *anaesthesia and mouth-to-mouth insufflation as part of *basic life support. It is a potential hazard when using air turbines for oral surgery.

insulin *n.* A hormone produced by the beta cells of the *islets of Langerhans in the *pancreas. It is involved with the regulation of glucose metabolism and acts by facilitating the entry of the glucose present in the bloodstream into the cells. This glucose is then converted into glycogen for storage. A deficiency gives rise to *diabetes mellitus which may be treated by insulin injections.

intensifying screen *See* SCREEN, INTENSIFYING.

intention *n. See* WOUND.

intercellular *adj.* Situated or occurring between cells.

intercondylar distance The distance between the vertical axes of two condyles.

intercuspal position (ICP) *n.* The complete *intercuspation of the teeth of the opposing jaws to give maximum *occlusion. *See also* CENTRIC RELATION.

intercuspation *n.* The cusp-to-fossa relationship of the mandibular and maxillary posterior teeth.

interdental brush *See* TOOTHBRUSH.

interdental canals *See* HIRSCHFELD'S CANALS.

interdental col *See* COL.

interdental papilla *See* PAPILLA.

inter-diffusion zone The retentive interface created within dentine by the penetration of an adhesive restorative resin. It lies between the applied *resin composite material and the deeper resin-free dentine.

interferon *n.* A substance produced and released by cells infected by a *virus, which inhibit viral multiplication and modify the body's *immune response.

interim denture *n. See* DENTURE.

interleukin *n.* A *cytokine produced by cells of the *immune system that function in the regulation of the immune response.

intermaxillary *adj.* Situated or occurring between the *maxillae. **Intermaxillary fixation** is the fixation of fractures of the maxilla by wiring or linking the two maxillae together. If the mandible is fractured the mandibular and maxillary arches may also be wired together to provide rigidity and stability.

intermaxillary traction *See* TRACTION.

internal bevel gingivectomy *See* GINGIVECTOMY.

internal derangement A condition of the temporomandibular joint defined in 1992 by the Consensus Conference for Temporomandibular Surgery as 'a localized mechanical fault in the joint which interferes with its smooth action'.

internal root resorption *See* OSTEOCLASTOMA.

international normalized ratio (INR) A measure of the efficacy of anticoagulant treatment. It compares the time taken for blood to clot between an anticoagulated patient and a normal control. Routine dental treatment including extractions can be undertaken on a patient whose INR is below 4. The dental practice procedures which require measurement of the INR for patients taking oral anticoagulants are endodontics, local anaesthesia, minor oral surgery, extractions, periodontal surgery, biopsies, and subgingival scaling. Additional local measures to ensure haemostasis, such as the application of haemostatic gauze and sutures, are recommended following extraction.

Further Reading: Perry D. J., Noakes T. J., Helliwell P. S. Guidelines for the management of patients on oral anticoagulants requiring dental surgery. *Br Dent J.* 2007;203:389–93.

(((🌐))) SEE WEB LINKS

• British Committee for Standards in Haematology provides guidelines for the management of patients on oral anticoagulants requiring dental surgery.

international qualifying examination (IQE) A test of the clinical skills and knowledge of overseas dentists (from outside the European Economic Area) who wish to apply for full registration with the *General Dental Council (GDC) of the UK. It is divided into three parts. Part A consists of a written paper and two oral examinations; part B is a series of practical exercises forming a simulated clinical assessment; and part C consists of two written papers and a clinical patient examination followed by an oral examination. This examination was replaced in 2007 by a new statutory examination, the **Overseas Registration Examination (ORE)**, which is in two parts; part one is a knowledge test consisting of two, three-hour written papers undertaken on a computer, and part two is made up of four elements: an objective structured clinical examination (OSCE), practical exercises undertaken on dental manikins, a diagnosis and treatment planning exercise, and an examination in medical emergencies. The GDC expects candidates to have spent an appropriate number of hours treating patients in the dental chair before applying to sit the examination.

International Standards Organization (ISO) A non-governmental organization, of which the **American National Standards Institute (ANSI)** is the US member, established to promote the development of standards to facilitate the international exchange of goods and services, and to develop mutual cooperation in areas of intellectual, scientific, technological, and economic activity. It has defined standards for dental equipment, instruments, and materials.

International System of Units [abbreviated SI from the French Système International d'Unités] SI is the modern form of the metric system and is generally a system devised around the convenience of the number 10. It was initiated in France in 1791 and was originally called the centimetre-gram-second (CGS) system and then the metre-kilogram-second (MKS) system. Since 1960 it has been called the SI system. It is the world's most widely used system of units.

interocclusal *adj.* Situated or occurring between the biting or occlusal surfaces of the opposing teeth.

interproximal *adj.* Describing the area situated or occurring between the *proximal surfaces of adjoining teeth. **Interproximal attrition** can occur due to the wearing away of the proximal surfaces of adjacent teeth associated with age or an abrasive diet. The space between adjacent teeth (the **interproximal space**) is divided into the region above the contact area (the *embrasure) and the septal space below the contact area.

interquartile range (in statistics) The limits within which the middle 50% of an ordered set of observations occur.

interradicular *adj.* Describing the area situated or occurring between the roots of a multi-rooted tooth. The **interradicular septum** is a thin area of bone within the tooth socket that is situated between the roots of a multi-rooted tooth occupying the **interradicular space**.

interstitial *adj.* (*n.* **interstice**) Relating to or situated in the small, narrow spaces between tissues or parts of an organ.

intervention study A study in which subjects are selected from one population and divided into two or more groups and subjected to different regimes (interventions) such as treatment or preventive measures. One group receives no intervention (**control group**) and is compared with the group or groups which receive the intervention (**study group** or groups) at the end of the study period.

intestine *n.* (*adj.* **intestinal**) The part of the *alimentary tract extending from the stomach to the anus. The first part is the **small intestine** divided up into the duodenum, jejunum, and ileum. The surface area of the small intestine is increased by the presence of many finger-like projections called **villi**. The second part is the **large intestine**, divided up into the caecum, vermiform appendix, colon, and rectum; the large intestine is mainly concerned with the absorption of water from the contents of the intestine.

intra-arterial injection *See* INJECTION.

intracellular *adj.* Situated or occurring within the cell.

intracoronal *adj.* Situated or occurring within the crown of a tooth. Intracoronal restorations do not extend beyond the normal tooth crown contour. An **intracoronal retainer** is one that relies on its retentive capacity being obtained from within the crown of the tooth.

intra-examiner variability *n.* The variation in recordings of the same situation, such as a clinical condition, made by the same examiner on two or more occasions.

intra-ligamentary analgesia *See* ANALGESIA.

intramuscular *adj.* Within the muscle. An intramuscular injection is made into a muscle.

intranasal sedation *See* SEDATION.

intra-oral *adj.* Situated or occurring within the mouth.

intra-oral camera A photographic device that utilizes a small hand-held wand to take digital video or still images inside the mouth. It provides many benefits, including the visualization of areas which would otherwise have poor visual access, the simulation of possible treatment options, the opportunity for personalized patient education, and the ability to transfer images to a computer for either real-time viewing or for storage as part of the clinical record.

intraosseous *adj.* Situated or occurring within the bone.

intraosseous analgesia *See* ANALGESIA.

intravascular *adj.* Situated or occurring within a vessel.

intravenous *adj.* Situated or occurring within a vein. **Intravenous cannulation** is the process of inserting a removable tube into a vein which acts as a passageway for the purpose of removing blood or administering drugs or fluids. **Intravenous sedation** *see* SEDATION.

intrinsic tooth staining Staining within the tooth as opposed to being on the surface (extrinsic). The common causes of intrinsic staining in vital (live) teeth are *tetracycline staining, *fluoride mottling, and inherited or acquired disorders such as *amelogenesis imperfecta. In non-vital (dead) teeth, intrinsic staining is usually the result of pulpal haemorrhage following trauma, a dead pulp (pulpal necrosis), or contamination of the dentine with blood breakdown products following *root canal therapy. Treatment is usually by *bleaching, *microabrasion to remove the discoloured tissue, or by covering the visible tooth surface with a *veneer or *crown. *Compare* EXTRINSIC TOOTH STAINING. 📷

Further Reading: Sulieman M. An overview of tooth discoloration: extrinsic, intrinsic and internalized stains. *Dent Update* 2005;32(8):463–4, 466–8, 471.

intrusion *n.* The axial displacement of a tooth. A tooth may be intruded into its tooth *socket due to a failure of the tooth to fully erupt, a pathological condition, trauma, or intentionally as part of orthodontic treatment. Intruded teeth with immature roots (open apices) are likely to erupt without treatment; intruded teeth with closed apices are likely to require orthodontic treatment or surgical repositioning and splinting in severe cases. Intrusion due to trauma may require surgical repositioning followed by flexible splinting for 1–2 weeks. *See also* LUXATION.

intubation *n.* The insertion of a tube into an orifice of the body. **Tracheal intubation** refers to insertion of a flexible plastic tube (endotracheal tube) through the larynx and into the trachea via the nose or mouth to protect the airway from the inhalation of foreign bodies and to provide mechanical ventilation by allowing air, gas, or vapour to pass into the lungs.

invaginate *adj.* Describing the folding back of one tissue into another tissue or part of the same tissue. It can occur during tooth development (*dens in dente).

invasive *adj.* Having a tendency to spread to neighbouring tissues. It is one of the cardinal features of *malignancy.

inverse square law The principle in radiology that states that the intensity of radiation from a point source will decrease with the inverse square of the distance from the point source, provided there is no absorption or scattering by the x-ray equipment.

invest *v.* To surround, embed, or envelop in an *investment material e.g. a wax pattern invested in a gypsum product.

investment *n.* The material used to surround the wax pattern of a restoration or prosthetic appliance prior to casting. Investment used for high-fusing alloys is bonded by a phosphate and a metallic oxide. *Gypsum-bonded investment is used for gold alloy casting and some low-fusing *cobalt-chromium alloys; this type of investment material is not generally used above 750°C (1382°F) as it breaks down.

Invisalign *n.* The trade name for an orthodontic technique using a succession of clear plastic arch aligners, similar to bleaching trays, which fit over all the surfaces of the teeth and which are designed to move the teeth in a controlled and predetermined direction. Each aligner is constructed to move the teeth 0.25–0.3mm and is changed on a two-weekly basis. The technique has the advantages of ideal aesthetics, improved oral hygiene, and good ease of use and comfort for the patient; the disadvantages include poor control over tooth movements, a lack of operator control, and an unsuitability for use in anterior–posterior discrepancies greater than 2mm.

in vitro *adj./adv.* Referring to a process or reaction occurring in an artificial environment, i.e. outside the body of a living organism, such as a laboratory. *Compare* IN VIVO.

in vivo *adj./adv.* Referring to a process or reaction occurring within the body of a living organism. *Compare* IN VITRO.

involucrum *n.* A sheath or layer of new bone growth outside existing bone seen in chronic *osteomyelitis. It is produced in response to infection and can contain a *sequestrum of *necrotic bone.

iodine *n.* An element required in small amounts for healthy growth and development. Because of its radiopacity it is used as a contrast agent for intravenous injection. In a 10% alcoholic solution it is used as a topically applied skin *antiseptic. Povidone-iodine is used as a *mouthwash.

ion exchange A theory of bonding to tooth substance in which the carboxyl groups of a glass ionomer bioreact with apatite in the tooth structure. The carboxyl groups bond with the charged surface of the enamel or dentine following dissociation of the calcium and phosphate ions.

Ionising Radiation (Medical Exposure) Regulations (IR(ME)R) 2000 Legislation that is concerned with patient protection. They replace POPUMET (Protection Of Patients Undergoing Medical Examination and Treatment) 1988. They provide new definitions of positions of responsibility for the employer, the IR(ME)R employer referrer, practitioner, and operator. The **IR(ME)R employer (legal person)** is responsible for radiation safety of the dental practice and for ensuring that staff conform to procedures and regulations relating to radiation safety. They are responsible for ensuring that staff receive appropriate training and updating. The **IR (ME)R referrer** is a registered doctor or dentist entitled to refer a patient for a medical exposure to a practitioner; the referer is responsible for ensuring sufficient clinical information is given regarding the need for a radiographic exposure to allow the practitioner to justify such an exposure. The **IR(ME)R practitioner** is a registered doctor or dentist who is entitled to justify the medical exposure. They should be adequately trained to allow them to take decisions and responsibility for the justification of every medical exposure. The **IR (ME)R operator** is a suitably trained individual who conducts any practical aspect of the medical exposure; this includes the positioning of the x-ray tube, the choice of exposure factors, and the developing of the image receptor.

Ionising Radiations Regulations 1999

Statutory legislation introduced by the UK parliament to cover the use of x-ray equipment in dental clinics or practices. When x-ray equipment is installed, it requires that the Health and Safety Executive are informed, a risk assessment is undertaken, a *radiation protection supervisor and *radiation protection adviser are appointed, operating staff are fully trained, and that local rules are written and visibly displayed.

ionizing radiation Energy in the form of waves or particles produced either by unstable atoms or from an x-ray generating device. Unstable atoms have an excess of energy or mass or both; in order to reach stability, these atoms emit the excess energy or mass in the form of radiation; gamma radiation and x-rays are examples of electromagnetic radiation.

ion-leachable glass See FLUOROALUMINOSILICATE GLASS.

iontophoresis n. A procedure that uses a low-voltage electric current to enhance the diffusion of ions into the tissues. Dental iontophoresis is used most often in conjunction with fluoride pastes and solutions in the treatment of *dentine hypersensitivity. Fluorides such as sodium and stannous fluoride are thought to decrease the permeability of dentine, possibly by the precipitation of insoluble calcium fluoride in the dentinal tubules.

IOTN n. See INDEX OF ORTHODONTIC TREATMENT NEED.

ipsilateral adj. On or affecting the same side of the body. Compare CONTRALATERAL; BILATERAL.

iron n. An element essential to life and to the transfer of oxygen in the body. Most of the iron in the body is stored in the *haemoglobin in the red blood cells. A good dietary source of iron is liver. A deficiency of iron may lead to *anaemia.

irradiation n. Exposure of a substance or the tissues of the body to ionizing radiation such as diagnostic dental x-rays or the gamma radiation of materials to render them sterile.

irreversible adj. Incapable of being reversed or returned to an original state such as an irreversible hydrocolloid *impression material.

irrigant n. A liquid used to wash away debris. It may have antibacterial properties such as *sodium hypochlorite and *chlorhexidine used as endodontic irrigants. In endodontics, an irrigant can have the added function of a lubricant to aid instrumentation.

irrigation n. The process of using a solution (*irrigant) to wash out debris from a wound, cavity, or root canal. **Subgingival irrigation** is used to deliver liquid, usually containing an antimicrobial agent, into the subgingival area to flush out any unwanted material or to inhibit the growth of micro-organisms.

ischaemia (US ischemia) n. (adj. **ischaemic**) Describing a deficiency of blood supply to a part of the body. **ischaemic** adj.

islets of Langerhans [P. Langerhans (1847–88), German physician and anatomist] Small groups of hormone-producing cells, distributed evenly throughout the *pancreas, which secrete directly into the bloodstream (endocrine glands). There are three main types of cells: alpha (α) cells, which secrete glucagon; beta (β) cells, which produce insulin; and D cells, which release somatostatin. The beta cells are destroyed in type 1 *diabetes.

iso- A prefix denoting equality, uniformity, or similarity.

isodont adj. Describing the condition of having identical upper and lower teeth as typified by herbivores. Compare ANISODONT.

isognathous adj. Having jaws of approximately the same width.

isotonic adj. Describing solutions which have the same *osmotic pressure. Compare HYPERTONIC; HYPOTONIC.

isthmus n. A narrow or constricted piece of tissue or part of an organ such as the narrow part of a tooth cavity.

-itis Suffix denoting inflammation of an organ or tissue e.g. **pulpitis** (inflammation of the dental pulp).

ivory n. A hard, white, opaque form of *dentine which forms the tusks of elephants, walruses, and other large mammals. It resembles the structure of bone and consists mainly of calcium and phosphate with radially distributed *collagen fibril bundles. Ivory forms in layers to create a pattern of concentric rings.

ivory matrix retainer See MATRIX RETAINER.

jacket crown *See* CROWN.

jacquette (jaquette) scaler *n.* A periodontal hand instrument used for root debridement and the removal of subgingival calculus. *See also* SCALER.

Jakarta Declaration A declaration defined by the *World Health Organization in 1997 outlining priorities in health promotion. These include promoting social responsibility for health, increasing investment in health development, expanding partnerships for health promotion, increasing the empowerment of the individual, and securing an infrastructure for health promotion.

jaundice *n.* An accumulation of bilirubin (a chemical breakdown product of *haemoglobin) in the blood, resulting in a yellow complexion. It may be **obstructive**, when bile cannot flow from the liver due to disease or bile duct obstruction, or **haemolytic,** due to the premature breakdown of haemoglobin producing excess bilirubin. *Prilocaine local anaesthetic should be avoided in patients with haemolytic jaundice.

jaw *n.* A common name referring to either the *maxilla (upper jaw) or *mandible (lower jaw).

jaw relation *See* RELATION.

jaw thrust A manoeuvre to open an airway in an unconscious or anaesthetized patient. The mandible is pushed forwards by applying an upward finger pressure bilaterally behind the angle of the mandible with the hands placed on either side of the head. When the mandible is displaced forward, it pulls the tongue forward and prevents it from blocking the entrance to the trachea.

jeweller's rouge *See* FERRIC OXIDE.

Jiffy tube *n.* A disposable cellulose acetate or plastic tube with a straight or curved end of reduced dimension used to introduce materials into a root canal.

Johnson twin wire arch [J. E. Johnson (1888–1969), American orthodontist] *n.* An orthodontic appliance consisting of two thin stainless steel archwires attached to the teeth by orthodontic bands. It is used to correct tooth misalignment within a tooth arch.

joint *n.* The junction point at which two or more bones are connected. **Fibrous joints** connect bones without allowing any movement (e.g. the skull bones). **Cartilaginous joints** have a layer of *cartilage separating the bones and allow limited movement (e.g. the ribs). A **synovial joint (diarthrosis)** is a freely moveable joint in which the bony surfaces are covered by articular *cartilage with a space between the articulating bones (synovial cavity) containing *synovial fluid, allowing greater flexibility of movement (e.g. the temporomandibular joint).

Jourdain's disease [A. L. B. Jourdain (1734–1816), French physician] An early, now obsolete, name used to describe acute *gingivitis or *periodontitis.

junctional epithelium *n. See* EPITHELIAL ATTACHMENT.

jurisprudence *n.* The science or philosophy of law. **Dental jurisprudence** is the application of dental science to the civil and criminal law; it describes the legal limitations and regulations related to the practice of dentistry.

justification *n.* The first stage in reducing the dose of ionizing radiation to the patient and a legal requirement in the UK prior to taking any radiograph. The risks of the ionizing exposure have to be outweighed by the benefits to the patient; the radiograph must affect the diagnosis or management of the patient.

juvenile periodontitis A name formerly used to describe localized aggressive *periodontitis which is characterized by generalized inflammatory changes in the *periodontium, with interproximal attachment loss affecting molars and incisors around the time of puberty. *See also* CLASSIFICATION OF CONDITIONS OF THE PERIODONTIUM.

juxtaoral organ *See* CHIEVITZ'S ORGAN.

kaffir D *n*. The alpha form of *gypsum (calcium sulphate hemihydrate; $(CaSO_4)2H_2O$) made by heating gypsum under pressure to 120–150°C. It is frequently coloured yellow. It has greater compressive and tensile strength in comparison with plaster of Paris, due to its regular crystalline structure. It is used extensively as a model material. When used as a denture mould, it minimizes the dimensional changes which occur during the polymerization of acrylic resin. *See also* STONE.

kaolin *n*. A silicate mineral with the chemical composition $Al_2Si_2O_5(OH)_4$ used in the manufacture of *porcelain teeth.

Kaposi's sarcoma [M. Kaposi (1837–1902), Austrian dermatologist] A malignant tumour of lymphatic endothelium caused by human herpes virus 8. It is very common in AIDS patients but is also seen in transplant patients. It is characterized by painless pink, purple, or dark brown spots or nodules on the surface of the skin or oral cavity, which may grow to 1 cm in diameter. The most common affected site is the palate, but lymph nodes, respiratory tract, and gastrointestinal tract may be affected. Cases associated with HIV respond to HAART (highly active antiretroviral therapy) but some are treated by cryotherapy or radiation.

Kawasaki disease An uncommon illness in children that is characterized by fever of at least 5 days' duration, generalized rash, bilateral conjunctivitis, *strawberry tongue, reddening of the oropharyngeal mucosa, cervical *lymph gland involvement, and red, dry cracked lips. It can lead to swelling of the coronary arteries, which may result in inflammation of the heart muscle (myocarditis) and *aneurysms. Kawasaki disease is treated with gammaglobulin and high doses of aspirin.

((ⓕ)) SEE WEB LINKS

- Medicinenet page that describes in more detail the signs, symptoms, and treatment of the disease.

Kazanjian's operation [V. H. Kazanjian (1879–1974), American oral surgeon] A surgical procedure to deepen the vestibular sulcus of an edentulous ridge for an improved prosthetic foundation.

keloid *n*. An abnormal overgrowth of fibrous scar tissue following accidental trauma or surgery to the skin. It tends to return after excision. The ear lobes and neck are more susceptible to keloid scar formation than the facial tissues.

Kelsey Fry, Sir William (1899–1963) Sir William Kelsey Fry was formative in pioneering the development of maxillofacial surgery. He established a postgraduate teaching centre at East Grinstead, Sussex, during the Second World War and played a key role in establishing the Postgraduate Dental School at the Eastman Dental Hospital. With Sir Terrance Ward, he co-authored *The Dental Treatment of Maxillofacial Injuries*, one of the foremost textbooks in the field. In recognition of his services to his country and his profession he was awarded the CBE in 1948 and was knighted in 1951. He was dean of the Faculty of Dental Surgery of the Royal College of Surgeons of England during the period 1950–53. He became a fellow of the Royal College of Surgeons of England in 1953 and in 1955 was made a DSc of McGill University.

Kennedy classification [E. Kennedy (1883–1952), American dentist] A method of describing partially *edentulous arches or partial dentures based on the location of the edentulous areas within the arch.

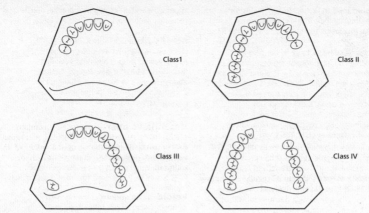

Kennedy Denture Classification

The Kennedy classification of dental arches

Class	Description
I	The edentulous area is bilateral and posterior to the remaining natural teeth.
II	The edentulous area is unilateral and posterior to the remaining natural teeth.
III	The edentulous area is between the anterior and posterior natural teeth and may be either unilateral or bilateral.
IV	A single edentulous area which crosses the midline and is anterior to the remaining natural teeth.

keratin *n.* (*v.* **keratinize**) An insoluble protein which is a major constituent of nails, hair, and the outermost layers of the skin. Keratin is present on the surface of the attached gingivae and gives it its pale pink colour when healthy.

keratinocyte *n.* A specialized *epidermal cell that synthesizes keratin.

keratocyst *n.* See CYST.

keratosis *n.* A condition of excess *keratin in epithelial tissue. **Frictional keratosis** is characterized by white patches on the buccal mucosa associated with chronic trauma such as cheek biting, sharp cusps, an overextended denture, or an ill-fitting orthodontic appliance. It can also occur on the attached *gingivae due to excessive or incorrect use of a toothbrush. **Chronic senile keratosis** can occur on the lips of elderly people and may lead to *malignant change. **Smoker's keratosis (nicotinic stomatitis)**, affecting particularly the palate, can be the result of excessive cigarette, cigar, or pipe smoking. *See also* STOMATITIS.

Keyes technique A treatment approach to the management of chronic periodontitis described by P. Keyes in 1978. It was also known as the 'salt out' technique and involved the conventional therapy of periodontitis-affected tissues (oral hygiene instruction and root planing) followed by the placement of a paste of sodium bicarbonate into the diseased pocket. The pocket flora was monitored using phase contrast microscopy.

kidney *n.* One of a pair of organs primarily responsible for the excretion of nitrogenous waste through the production of urine. The kidneys have secondary functions including the production of hormones and the regulation of electrolytes, acid-base balance and blood pressure.

((⊕)) SEE WEB LINKS

• The website of World Anaesthesia online which gives an overview of the physiology of the kidney

kinaesthesia *n.* (*US* kinesthesia) The sense of awareness that enables the brain to locate the position and be aware of the movement of muscles in different parts of the body. The study

of human motion (**kinaesiology**) is important in understanding mandibular movement.
See also PROPRIOCEPTOR.

Knoop hardness test A method of measuring the hardness of a material using a microscope (developed by F. Knoop in 1939), in which a pyramidal diamond point is used to make an indentation into the test material. It produces a much smaller indentation than the *Vickers hardness test because of the lower indentation pressure. The **Knoop Hardness Number (HK, KHN)** is a measure of the load divided by the size of the indentation.

Koplick's spots (Filatov's spots) [H. Koplick (1858–1927), American physician] Small red spots with white centres that appear on the oral *mucosa in the early stages of *measles.

Korff's fibres [K. von Korff (b. 1867), German anatomist] Precollagenous fibres of the dental pulp. They pass between the odontoblasts in developing dentine and undergo a collagenous change, eventually becoming incorporated into the dentine matrix.
The cellular origin of Korff's fibres is controversial.

Kurer anchor system A preformed parallel-sided, threaded, endodontic stainless metal post system, first described by P. F. Kurer in 1968, used to support an artificial *crown.

k

labial *adj.* Relating to the lips. The labial surface of a tooth is the surface adjacent to the lips. *See also* TOOTH SURFACES.

labial bar *n. See* BAR.

labial bow *n.* A component of a removable *orthodontic appliance consisting of an *archwire, usually made of stainless steel or nickel titanium, which extends across the anterior teeth to guide orthodontic tooth movement and to provide anterior retention. Acrylic resin may be added to provide additional retention.

labial commissure The corner of the mouth where the *lips meet at the outer edges of the mouth.

labial frenulum (fraenum) *See* FRENULUM.

labial glands *n.* A large number of small secretory glands resembling salivary glands in structure located between the mucosa and muscles of the lips. They are small and circular in form and have ducts opening into the mouth on the surface of the mucosa.

labial mucosa The *epithelial surface lining on the inner aspect of the *lips within the oral cavity. *See also* MUCOSA.

labioplasty *n. See* CHEILOPLASTY.

labiotenaculum *n.* An instrument used for holding the lips during a surgical procedure.

labioversion *n.* Deviation of an anterior tooth toward the lips from the normal line of occlusion.

labrale inferior *n.* A point where the boundary of the lower lip and the skin is intersected in the median sagittal plane; it is the lowest point of the lower lip.

labrale superior *n.* A point where the boundary of the upper lip and the skin is intersected in the median sagittal plane; it is the uppermost point of the upper lip.

labrette (labret) *n.* An ornamental device, usually a stud, ring, or bar, inserted into a perforation in the lip. A **lowbret** is located as low

as possible in the lower lip. A **Madonna** is a labrette placed in the upper lip. *See also* ORAL PIERCING.

lacebacks *pl. n.* Metal ligatures tied from the molars to the canines under the main archwire of an orthodontic appliance. They help to maintain the arch length and prevent the lower incisors from proclining as the canines upright. They can be used on one side only (unilaterally) to help centreline correction.

lacrimal *adj.* Relating to tears. The **lacrimal glands** are *exocrine glands which secrete fluid across the surface of the eye and drain via the lacrimal ducts into the nasal cavity. They are situated in the lacrimal fossae in the upper lateral part of each eye socket.

lacrimation *n.* Relating to the production of tears.

lactic acid *n.* The chemical produced by bacterial action on *carbohydrate food residues in the mouth. It can result in acid *demineralization of the teeth leading to *caries. Because of its high acidity (low pH) it is an important food preservative. During strenuous exercise pyruvic acid is converted to lactic acid, which may accumulate in the muscles and cause cramp.

Lactobacillus *n.* A genus of *Gram-positive anaerobic or *facultatively anaerobic bacteria (e.g. *Lactobacillus acidophilus*) capable of converting *lactose and other simple sugars (*monosaccharides) into *lactic acid. *Lactobacilli* have long been regarded as the main microbiological agent of dental caries; however, studies have shown that lactobacilli colonized carious lesions after their initial formation and that they were not prevalent in dental plaque during lesion formation. *Lactobacilli* multiply in an acid environment and their numbers in saliva are therefore related to sugar consumption and have been used as a *caries test.

Further Reading: Ireland, R. *Clinical Textbook of Dental Hygiene and Therapy* Chapter 4: dental caries and pulpitis. Blackwell Munksgaard. 2006:75–81.

lactose *n.* A complex sugar (*disaccharide) with one unit each of *glucose and *galactose, found in milk. It is broken down by the enzyme **lactase** to glucose and galactose.

lacuna *n.* A small cavity such as is found in compact *bone. *See also* HOWSHIP'S LACUNA.

lambda *n.* An anatomical landmark at the junction of the sagittal and lamboid sutures of the parietal and occipital bones.

lamella *n.* A thin layer or membrane such as the concentric layers of calcified matrix found around a *Haversian canal in *bone. *See also* ENAMEL.

lamina *n.* A thin membrane or layer of tissue. The **lamina dura** is a dense thin layer of cortical bone forming the wall of the *alveolus next to the tooth; radiographically it appears as a white line next to the dark line of the *periodontal ligament. The loss of lamina dura on a radiograph may be an indication of associated disease. The **lamina propria** is a highly vascular loose *connective tissue layer underneath the mucosal *epithelium.

lance *v.* To open by cutting or piercing, usually with a scalpel or *lancet. It is undertaken to establish drainage, such as when lancing an *abscess (boil).

lancet *n.* A surgical knife with a sharp point and a broad double-edged blade used for puncturing and making small incisions.

lancinating *adj.* Describing a sharp stabbing or cutting pain.

Langer curette *n. See* CURETTE.

Langerhans cell histiocytosis [P. Langerhans (1847–88), German physician and anatomist] A spectrum of disease characterized by accumulations of histiocytes and eosinophils. A localized form occurs in adults (eosinophilic granuloma) and may affect the jaws, causing bone destruction and loosening of teeth. Lesions occurring in children are more extensive and aggressive.

Langerhans cells [P. Langerhans (1847–88), German physician and anatomist] 1. The cells of the *pancreas that produce insulin. 2. Antigen-presenting dendritic cells (*macrophages) found in epithelium and epidermis.

laniary *adj.* Tearing or lacerating; of or relating to a pointed conical tooth such as a canine.

Larsen syndrome [L. J. Larsen (1914–), American orthopaedic surgeon] A rare autosomal dominant genetic condition characterized by cleft palate, flattened nasal bridge and facial features, prominent forehead, multiple congenital dislocations, and deformities of the hands and feet.

laryngopharynx (hypopharynx) *n.* The third part of the pharynx extending from the oropharyngeal isthmus and the hyoid bone to the lower border of the cricoid cartilage.

laryngoscope *n.* An instrument consisting of a handle, curved blade, and a light used to examine the upper respiratory tract and the larynx or to aid the insertion of a tube into the trachea (endotracheal tube).

laryngospasm *n.* Spasmodic contraction of the larynx. It sometimes occurs during the induction phase of general anaesthesia.

larynx *n.* (*adj.* **laryngeal**) A cartilaginous organ located above the *trachea and below the *oropharynx. It serves as part of the air passage from the pharynx to the lungs and as a *sphincter preventing food from entering the airway; it has a pair of vocal folds responsible for voice production (*phonation).

laser *n.* A device which produces a high-energy light source. The word laser is an acronym for 'light amplification by stimulated emission of radiation'. Lasers are used for surgery because of the ability to use them in small areas without causing damage to surrounding structures. **Argon lasers** emit a blue-green light and are used for polymerizing resin composite. **Carbon dioxide (CO_2) lasers** use carbon dioxide gas, which is readily absorbed by soft tissues because of the high cellular water content, causing surface cell vaporization to a depth of about 0.1mm. They operate at a wave band of 10600nm. Because the beam from a CO_2 laser is invisible, a second laser beam, based on the elements helium and neon, adds a visible red beam, so that the laser beam can be accurately focused. CO_2 lasers are used for gingival surgery, *fraenectomy, *biopsies, and the removal of benign or malignant soft tissue lesions. **Erbium:yttrium aluminium-garnet (erbium: YAG) lasers** have also been used for periapical surgery and the removal of hard tissue such as tooth enamel and dentine as an alternative method of cavity preparation, but access can be difficult and the cutting speed is slow; excessive heat generation can cause pulpal damage. **Neodymium:YAG lasers** penetrate more deeply than CO_2 lasers and utilize a jet of cool water or air to minimize possible heat damage; they operate at a wave band of 1064nm; these lasers may be used for soft tissue surgery but they can cause excessive damage to thin tissues. **Holmium:yttrium aluminium-garnet (holmium:**

YAG) lasers have been used experimentally for the removal of the cartilaginous disc in the *temporomandibular joint.

Further Reading: Sulieman M.An overview of the use of lasers in general dental practice: 2. Laser wavelengths, soft and hard tissue clinical applications. *Dent Update* 2005;32(5):286–8, 291–4, 296.

latent *adj.* Describing a condition that is present but not yet active or causing symptoms.

latent period 1. The very short interval between the time that a nerve impulse reaches a muscle fibre and the time the fibre starts to contract. 2. An alternative description for *incubation period.

lateral *adj.* Situated or occurring at the side of an organ or tissue.

lateral cephalogram An extra-oral radiograph which provides a standardized reproducible image of the lateral skull. It is a widely used diagnostic tool in orthodontics as it allows the antero-posterior and vertical relationships of the teeth, jaws, and soft tissues to be assessed. It is taken using a *cephalostat.

lateral deviation 1. An asymmetry of the face when viewed from the front. 2. A movement of the mandible to one side on opening or during forward thrusting due to a condition of the *temporomandibular joint, *muscles of mastication, or the teeth.

lateral excursion The sideways movement of the mandible from a centric position.

lateral nasal processes *n.* Soft tissue protrusions formed from the *fronto-nasal process at about 5 weeks of intrauterine life.

lateral oblique radiograph *n.* See OBLIQUE LATERAL RADIOGRAPH.

lateral repositioned flap (graft) See FLAP.

latero- A prefix denoting at the side of or towards the side.

lateroalveolism *n.* A condition in which the *alveolar process is shifted laterally on the base of the jaw. *Compare* MESIOALVEOLISM.

laterogenia *n.* A condition in which the chin prominence is shifted to one side in relation to the normal mandible.

lateromaxillism *n.* A condition in which the base of the *maxilla has shifted laterally but is of normal size and width. The most common cause is trauma.

laterotrusion *n.* The sideways movement of the mandible produced by the *muscles of mastication.

latex *n.* A milky fluid derived from the rubber tree and used for the manufacture of gloves, tubes, etc.

latex allergy A *hypersensitivity to natural latex characterized by skin irritation and inflammation (*dermatitis), itchy eyes, nasal irritation; in severe cases it can result in *anaphylaxis. Latex products include gloves, *dental dam, prophylactic polishing cups, and the bungs in local anaesthetic cartridges. Latex allergy has become more common and presents a significant hazard in dentistry. *See also* LATEX DERMATITIS.

latex dermatitis A skin inflammation in response to a *hypersensitivity to latex. **Irritant contact dermatitis** is a common non-allergic reaction to chemicals present in latex products, especially gloves; this is reduced by the use of powder-free gloves. **Allergic contact dermatitis** is an allergic reaction to specific proteins present in the natural latex.

Further Reading: Vozza I., Ranghi G., Quaranta A. Allergy and desensitization to latex. Clinical study on 50 dentistry subjects. *Minerva Stomatol* 2005;54(4):237–45.

lathe *n.* A machine tool with a rotating shaft to which may be attached various cutting instruments, grinding stones, and polishing wheels. It is used for grinding and polishing dental appliances.

lathe-cut amalgam alloy See AMALGAM.

lavage *n.* Washing out or irrigating a body cavity with water or a medicated solution.

lead apron A protective patient covering equivalent to 0.25mm lead used when taking dental *radiographs. It is only required when the primary x-ray beam is aimed directly at the reproductive organs i.e. for a vertex occlusal radiograph. There is a recommendation to offer the use of a lead apron in pregnancies for its psychological benefit.

lead line A grey or bluish line present at the gingival margin due to the deposition of lead sulphide; it is a sign of lead poisoning. It is also known as **Burton's line** [H. Burton (1799–1849), English physician].

Le Cron carver See CARVER.

Ledermix® *n.* The trade name for a water-soluble paste containing a synthetic corticosteroid (triamcinolone acetonide) and a

broad-spectrum antibiotic
(demethylchlortetracyline) used in the initial
treatment of irreversible pulpitis. It has
anti-inflammatory and bacteriostatic properties
but also suppresses pulpal defences, resulting
in the rapid increase in any bacteria not affected
by the antibiotic it contains. The paste has
been reported to cause discoloration of the
crowns of immature teeth.

Further Reading: Kim S. T., Abbott P. V., McGinley P. The
effects of Ledermix paste on discolouration of immature
teeth. *Int Endod J* 2000;33(3):233–7.

ledge *n.* A shelf-like projection at the junction
of two solid materials. It can be unintentionally
created at the margin of an amalgam, resin
composite, or cast restoration, frequently
resulting in the formation of a stagnation area or a
potential cause of soft tissue irritation; with
respect to the restoration the ledge can be either
positive or negative.

leeway space (E space) The difference in
combined width between the primary canine, first
molar, and second molar, and their permanent
successors (the permanent canine and
premolars). In Caucasians it is greater in the
primary dentition by about 1–1.5mm in the
maxilla and 2–2.5mm in the mandible.

Le Fort classification [L. C. Le Fort (1829–93),
French surgeon] A classification of fractures of
the maxilla and orbit. **Type I** is a horizontal
transmaxillary fracture running above the apices
of the teeth extending back to and including the
pterygoid plates; the maxillary antrum is involved
between the maxillary floor and the orbital floor.
Type II is a pyramidal fracture extending through
the nasal bones and including the anterior orbit.
Type III is also a pyramidal fracture but extends

to include the posterior orbit and the pyramidal
processes of the maxilla and zygoma.

((∰)) SEE WEB LINKS
• United States Army Institute of Surgical Research
web page giving an overview of neck and facial
injuries.

lentulo *n.* A flexible spiral wire instrument used
in a dental handpiece to introduce paste filling
materials into inaccessible areas such as root
canals.

leptostaphyline *adj. See* CHAMESTAPHYLINE.

lesion *n.* An area of tissue damage due to
disease or trauma resulting in impaired function.
Primary lesions include abscesses, ulcers, and
tumours; **secondary lesions**, such as crusts and
scars, are usually derived from primary lesions.

lethal dose (LD) An indication of the amount
of radiation, toxic drug, or compound that causes
death in humans or animals. The most common
indicator (LD_{50}) is the dose that will kill 50% of
subjects in a specified period of time.

leucocyte *n.* A white blood cell produced by
the *bone marrow and *lymph nodes. They are
subdivided into *granulocytes (neutrophils,
basophils, and eosinophils) and agranulocytes
(*lymphocytes and *monocytes). Leucocytes are
involved in *antibody production as part of the
body's defence mechanism.

leucocytosis *n.* An increase in the number of
*leucocytes.

leucopenia *n.* A reduction in the number of
*leucocytes.

leukaemia *n.* Any of a group of malignant
diseases in which there is an increase of abnormal

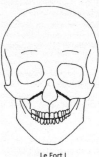
Le Fort I

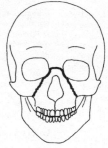
Le Fort II

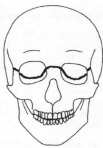
Le Fort III

Le Fort classification

*leucocytes in the blood. The increase in abnormal white blood cells suppresses the production of normal white cells, red cells, and *platelets, increasing the susceptibility to infection. **Acute leukaemia** is characterized by pallor, fatigue, and shortness of breath; there may also be spontaneous bleeding from the nose or oral mucosa, joint pain, and lymph node enlargement. In **chronic leukaemia** there is an increase in the number of leucocytes with different degrees of maturation. Chronic leukaemia may present as **chronic myeloid leukaemia**, which is due to a translocation between a part of chromosome 9 and a part of chromosome 22, or **chronic lymphatic leukaemia**, which is characterized by an increase in the number of circulating B-lymphocytes. Of oral significance in chronic leukaemia are symptoms of numbness or tingling sensation in the mouth together with swollen (oedematous) interdental gingivae which appear red and painful. Treatment for the condition by immune suppressive therapy can result in *gingival hyperplasia.

leukoedema, oral *n.* A variation of normal oral mucosa characterized by an asymptomatic bilateral diffuse, whitish-grey translucency of the mucosa. It is most common in the black population and is caused by intracellular oedema of the prickle cell layer of the epithelium. The clinical appearance should be differentiated from *leukoplakia, *lichen planus, and *keratosis. No treatment is necessary.

leukoplakia (leucoplakia) *n.* A potentially pre-malignant condition presenting as thickened white patches that develop on the sides of the tongue, floor of the mouth, gingivae, palate, and buccal mucous membrane. The patches cannot be removed by rubbing and they usually have no obvious cause, although lesions on the buccal mucosa are found more frequently where there is a history of *betel quid (paan) chewing. **Homogenous leukoplakia** is characterized by white lesions with a uniform flat appearance with a smooth, wrinkled, or corrugated surface with a consistent texture throughout; it has a low risk of malignancy. **Non-homogenous leukoplakia** is characterized by white or white and red lesions which may be flat, nodular, verruciform, *exophytic, or speckled; it has a high risk of malignancy. Treatment of leukoplakia is by removal of any local irritants and possible surgical removal of the lesion. **Hairy leukoplakia** is a white lesion present on the lateral surface of the dorsum of the tongue and more rarely on the buccal mucosa, occurring in patients with *HIV infection or suppressed immune systems. It is thought to be caused by a member of the

*herpes virus family. Treatment is usually unnecessary unless the lesion is causing pain, in which case the anti-herpes drug *aciclovir may be prescribed. 📷

levan *n.* Any one of a group of *polysaccharides formed from sucrose solutions (such as may be found in plaque) by the action of certain bacteria e.g. *Streptococcus mutans* and *Bacillus subtilis*. *See also* DEXTRAN.

levarterenol *n. See* NORADRENALINE.

levelling *n.* The orthodontic process of reducing the occlusal plane of the teeth in the antero-posterior plane (*curve of Spee).

Levene's test (in statistics) A test to assess the equality of *variance in different samples, first described by H. Levene in 1960. Many statistical procedures assume the variances of a population from which different samples are taken are equal; Levene's test examines this assumption.

lichenoid *adj.* Describing lesions that clinically resemble *lichen planus. Oral hypoglycaemic drugs and beta blockers can induce the formation of lichenoid lesions, as can hypersensitivity reactions to amalgam restorations.

lichen planus *n.* An oral condition characterized by bilateral, reticular, white, interlacing lines or striations present on the buccal mucosa, tongue, and occasionally on the lips. The gingivae may appear fiery red and the mucosa may be erythematous and show areas of *erosion or ulceration (desquamative *gingivitis). Skin lesions may also be present on the wrists or shins. The condition is usually asymptomatic and is more common in middle-aged women than men. The cause is unknown but lesions are the result of a cell-mediated immune reaction. If the condition is painful, treatment with topical corticosteroids may give symptomatic relief. Lesions that clinically resemble lichen planus (*lichenoid) may be caused by drugs (e.g. antihypertensive drugs for high blood pressure and oral hypoglycaemic drugs for diabetes) or reactions to dental materials such as amalgam. 📷

lidocaine *n. See* LIGNOCAINE.

ligament *n.* A tough band of white fibrous connective tissue that connects bones or supports organs.

ligation *n.* The means of attaching an orthodontic *archwire to an orthodontic *bracket, usually by means of *elastomeric modules or wire *ligatures. **Self ligation** is a term used to describe an orthodontic bracket which has a rotating or sliding mechanism to ligate an archwire. This type of bracket is an alternative to ligating using elastomeric modules.

ligature *n.* (*v.* ligate) 1. A wire used to secure the *archwire into the archwire slot of a *bracket on a fixed *orthodontic appliance; unlike *elastomeric modules, they can be tightened to maximize the contact between the wire and the bracket. 2. A cord or thread tied around a tooth to hold a *dental dam in place. 3. A cord, wire, or thread used to tie a blood vessel.

light curing *See* CURING LIGHT.

light-emitting diode (LED) A small semiconductor device that emits light as current flows through it. It is used in dentistry for *polymerizing resins; the narrow band width of 460–480nm enables it to work effectively with *resin composite materials containing *camphorquinone. *See also* CURING LIGHT.

lightening strip *See* SEPARATING STRIP.

lignocaine (lidocaine) *n.* An amide derivative of xylidine used as a local *anaesthetic agent. Used in sufficient quantities without *adrenaline (epinephrine) or with adrenaline as a vasoconstrictor (usually in a concentration of 1:80,000 or 1:100,000) it will produce pulpal analgesia of 1–1.5 hours' duration. It is metabolized by the liver. It can also be used as a topical anaesthetic agent. Trade names: **Xylocaine, Lidocaine.**

likelihood *n.* (in statistics) The probability of getting a set of observations given the parameters of a model fitted to those observations. It enables the estimation of unknown parameters based on known outcomes.

limitation of radiation dose The dose equivalent to all individuals which should not exceed the limits recommended by the International Commission for Radiological Protection.

linea alba buccalis *n.* A thickened whitish line on the buccal mucosa at the level of the occlusal plane extending from the corners of the mouth to the posterior teeth. It is usually associated with the frictional activity of the teeth and may be accentuated by cheek biting or *parafunction. The appearance is caused by a *keratosis of the epithelial tissue which cannot be rubbed off. It is asymptomatic and is usually present bilaterally. Linea alba buccalis is frequently associated with a crenated tongue

which may be a sign of *bruxism. The condition does not require treatment.

line angle The angle made by the junction of two surfaces. It is described by the names of the two surfaces.

linen strip *See* ABRASIVE.

liner *See* LINING.

lingual *adj.* Related to or situated close to the *tongue e.g. lingual *bar, lingual *plate. The lingual surface of a tooth is the surface adjacent to the tongue. *See also* TOOTH SURFACES.

lingual fraenum *See* FRENULUM.

lingual split technique A surgical technique for removing mandibular third molars where the lingual plate is fractured using a *chisel.

lingual tonsil *See* TONSIL.

lingula *n.* A small projection of bone forming the anterior border of the mandibular foramen. It forms the inferior attachment of the sphenomandibular ligament.

linguoversion *n.* The state of being inclined towards the tongue.

lining (cavity liner, lining) *n.* A material placed inside a prepared cavity prior to the placement of a restoration. Linings are used for protective, therapeutic, or structural reasons. Deep cavities may benefit from a lining material providing thermal protection, particularly for metallic restorations, although an additional *sublining may be necessary. A therapeutic lining material may be placed to stimulate the odontoblasts to lay down reparative dentine, to encourage remineralization, or to discourage bacterial activity. Structural linings reduce the volume of restorative material required and restore the internal form of the cavity; this can be advantageous for cast metal restorations by removing undercut areas and reducing the bulk of the restorative material. Lining materials include *calcium hydroxide, *resin modified glass ionomer cements, *zinc-oxide eugenol, *zinc phosphate, and *glass ionomer.

lip *n.* 1. The upper or lower fleshy folds of tissue surrounding the opening to the oral cavity. The musculature of the lips is made up of a sphincter muscle (orbicularis oris) and a number of dilator muscles. **Competent lips** meet together at rest without any undue strain on the lip musculature; if there is a space between the lips when at rest they are said to be **incompetent. Lip biting** can be the result of a conscious habit or due to a malocclusion of one or more anterior teeth.

The **high lip line** is the maximum height that the upper lip is raised in normal function. The **low lip line** is the lowest position of the lower lip during smiling or voluntary movement. 2. The top edge of a vessel or container.

lipid *n.* Any of a group of naturally occurring fats or fat-like substances characterized by being insoluble in water but soluble in solvents such as chloroform or alcohol. Lipids are an important dietary constituent.

lipo- (lip-) prefix denoting fat.

lipoid *adj.* Describing a resemblance to fat.

lipoma *n.* A common *benign tumour characterized by the presence of fat cells.

lipoprotein *n.* A compound of *protein that carries fats and fat-like substances, such as *cholesterol, in the blood.

lip pits Malformations of the lip characterized by unilateral or bilateral depressions. They may be hereditary or associated with cleft lip or palate with pits in the lower lip (**Van der Woude syndrome**).

lip retractor An instrument used to retract the lips to improve visibility for the purposes of taking intra-oral photographs or undertaking intra-oral procedures. They are usually made of plastic with curved rounded edges.

lithotripsy *n.* The process of using an externally applied, high-intensity acoustic pulse to disintegrate renal or salivary calculi.

litmus *n.* A water-soluble mixture of dyes, often absorbed onto a piece of filter paper, used to test for acidity. Blue litmus paper turns red under *acid conditions and red litmus paper turns blue under alkaline conditions.

liver *n.* The largest organ of the body, located in the upper right part of the abdominal cavity under the lowest ribs of the thorax (**right hypochondrium**). It has many functions, including secreting bile, neutralizing poisons, synthesizing proteins, and storing glycogen and certain vitamins and minerals.

local analgesic *n.* See ANALGESIC.

Local Dental Committee (LDC) A UK statutory body primarily representing general dental practitioners based in a *Primary Care Trust (PCT). The PCT has an obligation to consult with representative bodies such as the LDC on issues relating to the provision of primary care dentistry.

lockjaw *n.* A lay term for *tetanus; so called because of the *trismus that may be a symptom of the condition.

loculation *n.* The division of a fluid-filled cavity into a number of smaller cavities (loculi) by fibrous septa.

locum tenens A healthcare provider such as a dentist or doctor who stands in temporarily for a colleague who is absent or ill, and fulfils their duties in the practice or clinic. Often shortened to **locum**.

loglinear analysis *n.* (in statistics) A statistical procedure that is an extension of the *chi-square test. It analyses situations in which there are more than two categorical *variables; it enables the assessment of relationships between these variables.

logo- (log-) A prefix denoting speech or words.

logopaedics (*US* logopedics) *n.* The scientific study of defects and disabilities of speech and the methods used to correct them.

-logy (-ology) Suffix denoting field of study e.g. **cytology** (study of cells).

longitudinal study An epidemiological study that records data over an extended period of time or is repeated at certain intervals in order to analyse changes over time.

long junctional epithelium See EPITHELIAL ATTACHMENT.

loph *n.* An enamel ridge connecting cusps on the surface of a molar tooth.

lophodont *adj.* Describing teeth in which the occlusal surface shows a well-marked pattern of elongated ridges between the cusps. It is most pronounced in elephants and many rodents. *Compare* BUNODONT.

loss of attachment See ATTACHMENT.

lost wax process A casting technique in which a model made of wax is enclosed in a plaster *investment mould. The mould is then heated and the wax melted out through a vent and molten metal, such as gold or chromium cobalt, is poured or centrifuged in to replace it.

loupe, binocular *n.* Magnifying lenses for both eyes contained within an optical frame and worn like spectacles. 📷

lowbret *n.* See LABRETTE.

lower face height *n.* See FACE HEIGHT.

low-fusing alloy An alloy containing mainly lead, tin, and bismuth which melts in the temperature range 47°–170°C (117°–338°F) used for making casts and *dies.

lozenge (troche) *n.* A medicated tablet containing sugar. Lozenges dissolve slowly in the mouth so that the medication comes into prolonged contact with the mucous membranes of the mouth and throat.

Ludwig's angina [W. F. von Ludwig (1770–1865), German surgeon] A bacterial infection resulting in a severe *cellulitis and fascial space involvement of the sublingual and submandibular tissue spaces bilaterally. It can lead to swelling in the neck, elevation of the tongue, and potential airway obstruction. The source of the infection can be an infected tooth pulp usually from the lower second or third molars.

Further Reading: Bonilla E. D., Ayala H. S., Moguel M. J. L. Report of 16 cases of Ludwig's angina: 5-year review. *Pract Odontol* 1991;12(4):23–4, 2.

Luer fitting [H. W. Luer (1868–1943), German instrument maker] A standardized system for making leak-free connections between a male-taper fitting and its mating female part on medical and laboratory instruments.

lumen *n.* 1. The space within a tubular structure such as a blood vessel or salivary gland duct. 2. The international (SI) unit of luminous flux or quantity of light; a lumen equals the amount of light that is spread over a square foot of surface by one candle power (candela) when all parts of the surface are exactly one foot from the light source.

lupus erythematosus (LE) A chronic inflammatory autoimmune disease affecting the skin and mucous membranes as well as other organs. There are a spectrum of presentations from **chronic discoid LE**, which affects the skin and mucous membranes only, to **systemic LE (SLE)**, which affects the whole body and is characterized by renal disease, arthritis, and circulating auto-antibodies. The disease is much more common in females than males. Typically there is a red scaly rash on the face, usually extending across the bridge of the nose and zygoma (**butterfly rash**) and oral lesions include mucosal white patches and erosions. Treatment is by corticosteroids or immunosuppressant drugs.

lupus vulgaris An uncommon tuberculous infection of the skin characterized by nodular lesions on the face with dark red patches on the nose or cheek. It often starts in childhood and can lead to ulceration and scarring if left untreated. Treatment is with antituberculous drugs.

luting agent A material that bonds, seals, or cements objects together, such as the thin layer of *cement between a tooth preparation and an artificial crown. A luting cement should have low solubility, low viscosity, and high fracture resistance; examples are *zinc phosphate, *glass ionomer, and resin-based adhesives.

Further Reading: Burke F. J. T. Trends in indirect dentistry: 3. Luting materials. *Dent Update* 2005;32:251–60.

luxation *n.* The *dislocation or displacement of a tooth or joint. A tooth may be displaced laterally, labially, palatally, or lingually. A luxated tooth needs to be repositioned as soon as possible and then held in position with a splint for 2–3 weeks; loss of vitality is common if root formation of the tooth is complete. External or internal resorption or root canal obliteration may also occur.

luxatome (luxator) *n.* An instrument used to produce the partial dislocation or displacement of a tooth or tooth root prior to its extraction. The blade of the instrument is inserted between the tooth root and the *alveolar bone.

lymph *n.* The thin, opalescent fluid similar to blood *plasma contained within the vessels of the lymphatic system and filtered by the *lymph nodes. The cellular content is mainly *lymphocytes. **Lymph nodes** are small swellings composed of lymphoid tissue situated at intervals throughout the *lymphatic system. They act as filters preventing foreign particles entering the bloodstream.

lymphadenopathy *n.* Any disease that affects a *lymph node or nodes. Often used as a description of enlarged or tender lymph nodes identified during diagnostic investigation.

lymphangioma *n.* A benign tumour of the lymph vessels. It may consist of small capillary-sized lymph vessels, but more commonly cavernous lymphatic spaces are present. It is usually found on the tongue but may also occur on the buccal mucosa or palate.

lymphatic system A network of vessels and *lymph nodes carrying lymph fluid from the tissues to the bloodstream. It helps to maintain and protect the fluid environment of the body. The lymphatic drainage of the neck is arranged into deep and superficial chains; the deep jugular chain receives primary lymph drainage from the deeper structures in the head and neck including the tongue, larynx, soft palate, tonsils, and thyroid gland; the superficial nodes, including the facial,

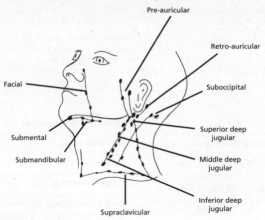

Lymph drainage and nodes of the head and neck

submental, and submandibular, receive drainage from the anterior part of the mouth and face and drain secondarily to the superior deep jugular nodes. All of these lymphatics eventually drain into the venous system.

SEE WEB LINKS

- Memorial University, Canada, web page that provides an outline of lymphatic drainage of the head and neck.

lymphocyte *n.* A type of white blood cell (*leucocyte) found in the blood, *lymph nodes, and certain organs. They may be divided into **T-lymphocytes** (T-cells), which develop in an organ called the thymus and are responsible for cell-mediated *immunity, and **B-lymphocytes**, which develop in the bone marrow and are responsible for the production of *antibodies (immunoglobulins).

lymphoid tissue A tissue responsible for the production of *antibodies and *lymphocytes. It is found in discrete organs (*lymph nodes, *tonsils, thymus, and *spleen) and as diffuse groups of cells.

lymphoma *n.* A *malignant *neoplasm of leucocytes which usually arises in lymph nodes. **Non-Hodgkins lymphoma** is a neoplasm of lymphoid tissue which may be derived from B-cells or T-cells. *See also* HODGKIN'S DISEASE.

lysergic acid diethylamide (LSD) A hallucinogenic drug which was formerly used for the treatment of psychological disorders but is now a drug of abuse. The physical effects include dilated pupils, higher body temperature, increased heart rate and blood pressure, sweating, loss of appetite, sleeplessness, dry mouth (*xerostomia), and tremors. The dry mouth, usually combined with poor oral hygiene, can result in a higher incidence of caries and periodontal disease.

lysis *n.* Cell disintegration due to rupture of the cell membrane or the breakdown of the cell wall.

-lysis A suffix denoting 1. Remission of symptoms. 2. Cellular disintegration.

lysogen *n.* A bacterial cell harbouring the genome of a *bacteriophage integrated into the bacterial cell's chromosomal DNA. Lysogens are latent forms of bacteriophages. A lysogenized phage genome is often referred to as a **prophage**. Prophages sometimes encode genes for toxins that are expressed by their bacterial host cell. Examples include diphtheria toxin, scarlet fever toxin, *Staphylococcus aureus* Panton-Valentine leukocidin, and enterotoxin A.

lysosome *n.* A membrane-bound sac inside a cell which has enzymes that can break down cellular components that need to be destroyed.

lysozyme *n.* An antibacterial enzyme occurring in saliva, mucus, and tears that has the ability to dissolve, or lyse, the structure of certain bacteria by breaking down their polysaccharide walls. Most of the bacteria affected by lysozyme are not *pathogenic.

maceration *n.* The softening of a substance or tissue caused by soaking in a liquid or due to excessive moisture e.g. skin under a wet dressing.

Macfarlane scaler *See* SCALER.

Mackenzie's syndrome [S. Mackenzie (1844–1909), English physician] A unilateral paralysis of the soft palate, pharynx, larynx, and vocal folds due to a lesion affecting one half of the brain stem.

macro- (macr-) A prefix denoting large size or enlargement.

macroalveolism *n.* A condition in which the *alveolar process of the mandible or maxilla is excessively large in all dimensions. *Compare* MICROALVEOLISM.

macrocheilia *n.* A congenital condition in which the lips are abnormally large.

macrodontia (megadontia) *n.* A developmental defect in which the teeth are larger than normal for a particular tooth type.

macrofilled resin composite *See* RESIN COMPOSITE.

macrogenia *n.* A condition in which the height, projection, and width of the *chin prominence is too large in relation to the rest of the facial skeleton. *Compare* MICROGENIA.

macroglossia *n.* An enlarged tongue which may be developmental or due to *thyroid deficiency (cretinism), a tumour, or obstruction of the *lymph drainage.

macrognathia *n.* A condition in which one or both jaws are unusually large.

macrophage *n.* A large scavenger cell present in connective tissue, major organs, and tissues that ingests bacteria, degenerated cells, and foreign bodies.

macrostomia *n.* The condition of having an abnormally large mouth.

macula *n.* (*pl.* **maculae**) A small anatomical area or spot that is distinguishable from the surrounding tissue.

Madonna *n. See* LABRETTE.

Magill's forceps *See* FORCEPS.

magnetic resonance imaging (MRI) A diagnostic procedure that uses a magnetic field to provide three-dimensional images of internal body structures based on the magnetic fields of hydrogen atoms in the body. It does not produce potentially damaging ionizing radiation. However, it can interfere with cardiac pacemakers. There is currently insufficient evidence for the efficacy of MRI for diagnosing temporomandibular joint disorders.

main effect (in statistics) The effect of a predictor *variable (or independent variable) on an outcome variable. The main effect is examined in an *analysis of variance (ANOVA).

maintainer *n. See* SPACE MAINTAINER.

maintenance phase The period following active treatment during which there is periodical review and assessment. Long-term maintenance is an important aspect of periodontal treatment.

malaise *n.* A general feeling of being unwell, sick, or nauseous which may indicate the presence of disease.

malalignment *n.* 1. A condition in which one or more teeth are situated outside the line of the dental arch. 2. A condition in which the two ends of a fractured bone are poorly located in relation to each other.

malar bone *n. See* ZYGOMATIC BONE.

Malassez, rest cells of [L. C. Malassez (1842–1909), French physiologist] Cells thought to be the remnants of *Hertwig's epithelial root sheath which remain after root development is complete. They are found near the *cementum of most teeth, mainly around the apical and cervical area.

malignant *n.* Any disease or condition which becomes life-threatening if untreated. It is characterized by progressive and uncontrolled growth. *Compare* BENIGN.

malleability *n.* The physical property of a material, such as gold, signifying its capability of permanent deformation, especially by hammering or rolling.

mallet *n.* An instrument used for hammering. An **automatic mallet** is used for the condensation of cohesive gold *foil. The first mechanical gold mallet is attributed to William G. Bonwill in 1867.

malnutrition *n.* An imbalance between food ingested and food required to maintain health. It may result from a poor diet which is deficient in one or more essential nutrients or the inability to utilize the nutrients ingested.

malocclusion *n.* A deviation of the teeth or a malrelationship of the dental arches outside the accepted range of normal. It may be the result of an abnormal jaw size, malformed teeth, missing teeth, *supernumerary teeth, retained, *impacted or unerupted teeth, *macrodontia, *microdontia, developmental abnormalities such as *cleft lip or palate, or environmental factors such as *digit sucking and trauma. *See also* INCISOR RELATIONSHIP; MOLAR RELATIONSHIP; SKELETAL PATTERN.

malposition *n.* An abnormal position of a tissue, structure (such as a tooth), or organ of the body.

malrelation *n.* An abnormal relationship of two connected parts or structures such as the *malocclusion of the teeth.

maltase *n.* An *enzyme present in *saliva and pancreatic juice that converts the disaccharide *maltose into *glucose during digestion.

maltose *n.* A *disaccharide consisting of two molecules of *glucose. It is broken down by the enzyme *maltase.

mamelon *n.* One of three rounded prominences on the incisal edge of a recently erupted incisor. Normal chewing and biting usually wear down mamelons to leave a smooth incisal edge; they are therefore not usually seen in the adult dentition. 📷

mandible *n.* (*adj.* **mandibular**) The bone of the lower jaw which accommodates the lower dentition in the alveolar process. It is formed from the mandibular process of the *stomodeum as a

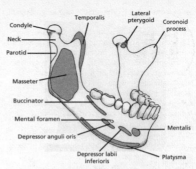

Mandible—external surface (muscle attachments in grey)

band of dense fibrous tissue known as *Meckel's cartilage. When fully developed, it has a horseshoe-shaped **body** which extends backwards and upwards to form the **ramus**. The ramus has two extensions, the posterior **condylar process**, which forms part of the temporomandibular joint, and the anterior **coronoid process** to which the temporal muscle is attached. On the external surface of the body of the mandible, the **mental foramen** is located between the first and second premolar teeth, midway between the upper and lower borders of the body and through which pass the mental nerve and blood vessels. Posterior to the mental foramen is the **external oblique line** which provides attachment for the buccinator muscle. Anteriorly near the midline there is a triangular prominence known as the **mental protuberance**. On the inner (lingual) surface of the mandible at the lower border near the midline is an oval depression (**digastric fossa**) to which the digastric muscle is attached. The **mylohyoid**

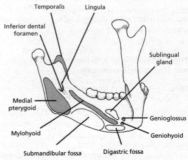

Mandible—internal surface (muscle attachments in grey)

ridge is an oblique ridge on the lingual surface of the mandible which extends anteriorly from the level of the roots of the third molar and is the bony attachment for the mylohyoid muscles which form part of the floor of the mouth. The **mylohyoid line**, to which the mylohyoid muscle is attached, extends from the third molar diagonally downwards and forwards on the lingual surface. Below this lies the **submandibular fossa** which accommodates the submandibular *salivary gland. At the centre of the inner surface of the ramus is the **mandibular foramen** through which pass the inferior alveolar (dental) nerve and blood vessels.

⊕ SEE WEB LINKS
- Yahoo Education page with further anatomical detail of the mandible.

mandibular advancement appliance (MAA) An appliance designed to posture the mandible forwards during sleep for patients with sleep-disordered breathing. The appliance aims to draw the tongue forwards through its muscular attachments and thereby increase the size of the pharyngeal airway; it may be prefabricated or custom-made, using soft or hard resin.

Further Reading: Johal A. A review of the use of mandibular advancement appliances in sleep disordered breathing. *Dent Update* 2008;35:230–35.

mandibular plane *n. See* CEPHALOMETRIC ANALYSIS.

mandibulectomy *n.* The surgical removal of part or all of the lower jaw. It is usually undertaken as part of the treatment for a malignant lesion.

mandibuloacral dysplasia (MAD) A rare *autosomal recessive disorder, characterized by postnatal growth retardation, craniofacial anomalies, dental crowding, skeletal malformations, and mottled skin pigmentation.

mandibulofacial dysostosis *see* TREACHER COLLINS SYNDROME.

mandrel *n.* A rotary instrument used in a dental handpiece for grinding, smoothing, or polishing. It has a screw (Huey's) or split stud (Moore's) at one end to secure a disc, wheel, stone, or cup.

manikin *n.* A replica of part or all of the human body used for teaching or instructional purposes.

manipulation time That part of the working time during which a material can be manipulated without adversely affecting its properties.

mannosidosis (α-mannosidosis) *n.* A very rare congenital deficiency of α-mannosidase, an *enzyme which breaks down the sugar mannose. It is characterized by learning disabilities and a susceptibility to infection, together with changes in facial features such as a prominent forehead, a flattened nasal bridge, a small nose, and a broad mouth.

⊕ SEE WEB LINKS
- The Society for Mucopolysaccharide diseases website, which provides information on the causes and treatment of mannosidosis.

Mann–Whitney test (Wilkoxson rank-sum test, Wilcoxon-Mann-Whitney test) A non-parametric test used in statistics to examine the differences between two independent samples. It examines whether the populations from which two samples are taken have the same location. It was initially developed by F. Wilcoxon in 1945 and extended by Mann and Whitney in 1947.

marble bone disease *See* OSTEOPETROSIS.

margin *n.* An edge or border. The **alveolar margin** forms the peripheral edge of bone around the tooth socket. The **cavity margin** is where the prepared surface of the cavity meets the external surface of the tooth. The **enamel margin** of a cavity is that part of the margin of a cavity preparation which lies on enamel. The **free gingival margin** is the edge of the gingival tissue adjacent to the crown of a natural tooth and forms the outer edge of the gingival crevice (sulcus) which in health is normally about 2mm deep. The **gingival margin** of a cavity is that part of the margin of a tooth preparation closest to the tooth root apex.

marginal bleeding index *see* GINGIVAL BLEEDING INDEX.

marginal ridge An enamel elevation on the crown of a tooth which forms the mesial or distal border of the *occlusal surface.

margin trimmer An angulated chisel-like hand instrument used to bevel the gingival margin of a tooth cavity preparation.

marsupialization *n.* An operative technique for the removal of a cyst in which an incision is made into the cyst and the cyst lining is sutured to the oral mucosa, thus creating a pouch which is open to the oral environment. The wound is kept open with either a *pack or a *stent until healing is complete.

Maryland bridge *See* BRIDGE.

mastication *n*. The process of chewing food. It occurs in three phases: incision of the food, chewing of the bolus, and finally the act of swallowing. It involves the opening, closing, left lateral, right lateral, and antero-posterior movement of the mandible controlled by the *muscles of mastication. The amplitude of the jaw movement increases with an increase in the size or hardness of the food being chewed and decreases as the masticatory sequence progresses.

mastoid process *n*. A protuberance of the petrous part of the temporal bone found immediately behind and below the external part of the ear. It contains air cells and can become infected as part of a generalized sinus infection. The sternocleidomastoid muscle is attached to the mastoid process.

matched sample (in statistics) A sample group that is the same in terms of specific factors (e.g. sex, age).

materia alba *n*. A soft non-mineralized whitish deposit found on the tooth surface around the gingival margins, usually associated with poor oral hygiene. It consists of food debris, micro-organisms, and dead tissue cells. Unlike dental plaque, it can be washed off with water.

matrix *n*. 1. (in histology) The substance of a tissue or organ such as dentine. 2. A mechanical or artificial wall or mould used to support a plastic material; it may be in the form of a strip (*see* MATRIX BAND) or a mould approximating the external surface of the tooth (**sectional matrix**). 3. The female part of a *precision attachment. 4. (in statistics) A mathematical table containing a collection of numbers arranged in rows and columns.

matrix band A thin band of metal, *mylar®, or acetate used to provide a temporary wall when inserting a plastic restorative material. It may also provide the desired tooth contour and optimal surface finish to a restorative material. A **metal matrix band** is used when *amalgam is condensed into a cavity with a missing proximal wall. An *acetate or **mylar® matrix band** or **strip**, which permits the transmission of light, may be used to provide an artificial wall when placing chemically cured or light activated *resin composites. A **circumferential metal, mylar®** or **acetate band** may be used when much of the external tooth surface is missing. A *wedge is recommended when using matrix bands for posterior restorations to avoid a gingival overhang of restorative material. There are a large number of commercial designs of matrix system developed for use with resin composite

restorations; these are either sectional e.g. V-ring®, Composi-Tight silver plus®, Contact matrix®, or circumferential e.g. Greater Curve Tofflemire Band®.

matrix retainer A mechanical device designed to hold a matrix band in position on the tooth. There are many different designs in current use. The **ivory retainer** has claws which engage in holes strategically placed in the band to allow for teeth of different circumference; it can be used for posterior teeth with only one missing proximal wall. The **Siqveland retainer** is self-adjusting to provide a narrower circumference at the gingival area of a cavity preparation and can be used for preparations with more than one missing proximal wall. It is available in two sizes to take either narrow or broad bands. **Tofflemire retainers** utilize pre-shaped annular bands held by screw tension; a knurled nut is rotated to tighten the band round the tooth; the band can be removed before the retainer is released separately; Tofflemire bands can also be used for preparations with more than one missing wall.

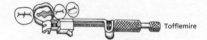
Tofflemire

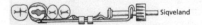
Siqveland

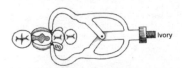
Ivory

Types of matrix retainer

A **circumferential retainer** can be tightened to give a band with a narrower circumference in the gingival area and wider circumference at the occlusal. **Contact ring matrix retainers** (trade names: BiTine, Contact matrix, Composi-Tight) have been developed for use with sectional matrices to provide tooth wedging and reduce the need for interproximal wedging.

maturation *n*. The process of arriving at complete development. It can be applied to a material such as *enamel or to a structure such as a tooth.

maxilla *n.* (*pl.* **maxillae**; *adj.* **maxillary**) One of two bones which are mirror images of each other and which together form the upper jaw and contain the upper teeth. It is a hollow structure containing a large air-filled space, the *maxillary sinus (antrum). It forms the boundaries of the roof of the mouth, the floor of the nose, and the floor of the orbit. It has four processes. The **frontal process** projects upwards and forms the lateral wall of the nose and meets with the frontal bone of the skull; the **zygomatic process** meets the *zygomatic (cheek) bone; the horizontal **palatine process** forms the major part of the hard palate; and the curved **alveolar process** projects downwards and provides the supporting *alveolar bone structure for the maxillary teeth. The **maxillary tuberosity** is the most distal extension of the alveolar process. Through the **infra-orbital foramen**, located on the anterior surface below the lower border of the orbit, pass the infraorbital nerve and blood vessels. In the midline immediately behind the upper incisor teeth is the **incisive foramen**, through which pass the nasopalatine nerve and artery. During the development of the maxilla, ossification begins around the 8th week of intrauterine life at the area of the developing primary canines. Growth, which takes place by a process of remodelling and sutural growth, carries the maxilla forwards and downwards.

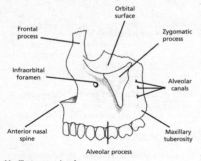

Maxilla—external surface

Labels: Orbital surface; Frontal process; Zygomatic process; Infraorbital foramen; Alveolar canals; Anterior nasal spine; Maxillary tuberosity; Alveolar process

maxillary plane *n.* See CEPHALOMETRIC ANALYSIS.

maxillary sinus (antrum) The largest of the paranasal sinuses occupying the body of the maxilla; if large, it may extend into the zygomatic bone. On its roof it is separated from the orbital cavity by a thin orbital plate through which run the infra-orbital vessels and nerve. The sinus floor is closely related to the apices of the permanent molar teeth and is a potential hazard during tooth

extraction, as a tooth may be inadvertently pushed into the sinus. The anterior wall of the sinus is bounded by the facial surface of the maxilla and the posterior wall is related to the pterygo-palatine fossa. The middle and anterior alveolar (dental) nerves run in canals in the lateral and anterior walls of the sinus. The opening into the sinus is high up on the nasal wall close to the roof and communicates with the middle meatus of the nasal cavity; this location makes the gravitational drainage of pus and fluids from the sinus difficult. The medial (nasal) wall of the sinus, composed mainly of *cartilage, is bounded by the nasal surface of the body of the maxilla and by parts of the palatine, lacrimal, ethmoid, and inferior turbinate bones. The sinus is lined with ciliated *mucoperiosteum.

maxillectomy *n.* The surgical removal of part or all of the upper jaw. It is usually undertaken as part of the treatment for a malignant lesion.

maxillofacial *adj.* Pertaining to the maxilla and face. **Maxillofacial surgery** is a recognized area of specialization in dentistry.

maxillotomy *n.* Surgical sectioning of the maxilla to allow for repositioning.

maximum permissible dose (MPD) Defined by the International Commission on Radiological Protection (ICRP) as the greatest dose of radiation which, in the light of present knowledge, is not expected to cause detectable bodily injury to a person at any time during their lifetime.

McCall's festoons Semilunar-shaped enlargements of the marginal gingivae primarily on the labial surfaces of the anterior and premolar teeth, described by John Oppie McCall in 1922. They were believed to be caused by *occlusal traumatism but this has not been confirmed by later studies.

McCune–Albright syndrome See DYSPLASIA.

mean (arithmetic mean) *n.* The average of a group of observations calculated by adding their values together and dividing by the number in the group. The **median** is the midpoint in a series of numbers such that half the data values are above the median and half are below it; when there is an even number of observations, the median is the average of the two scores that are on each side of what would be the middle value. The **mode** is the value that has the largest number of observations, namely the most frequent value or values. The mode is not necessarily unique, unlike the mean value.

measles (rubeola) A highly infectious viral disease that mainly affects children. It has an incubation period of 4–12 days and is characterized by cold-like symptoms, fever, and a blotchy pink rash which appears around the face and ears. Oral lesions are characterized by small red spots with white centres (*Koplick's spots) on the buccal mucosa, although these are often transient. Patients are infectious until 3–5 days after the appearance of the rash. Effective immunity is provided by vaccination. *See also* GERMAN MEASLES.

meatus *n*. (in anatomy) A passage or opening. The **auditory meatus** is the passage leading from the pinna of the outer ear to the eardrum. There are four paired structures within the nasal cavity; these are the **superior nasal meatus**, the **middle nasal meatus**, the **inferior nasal meatus**, and a **common nasal meatus**. The middle meatus contains an *antrum, the ethmoidal bulla, and the ethmoidal infundibulum.

Meckel's cartilage [J. F. Meckel the younger (1781–1833), German anatomist] A dense band of cartilaginous tissue which forms at about 6 weeks of intrauterine life and provides a framework for the development of the *mandible.

medial *adj*. 1. Relating to or denoting the parts of the body that are closest to the *median plane of the body. 2. Relating to or situated in the central region of a tissue, organ, or the body.

median *n*. 1. (in anatomy) Situated in the centre or the midline which divides the body into two halves 2. (in statistics) *See* MEAN.

Medicaid A US federal assistance programme that provides payment for medical care for certain low-income individuals and families. It is an entitlement programme that is jointly funded by the states and federal government, and is managed by the states. *See also* MEDICARE.

(⊕) SEE WEB LINKS
• Centers for Medicare and Medicaid services overview.

Medical Devices Directive A directive issued by the European Economic Commission (EEC) which covers the manufacture, placing on the market, and putting into service of medical devices. These include such items as manufactured orthodontic *brackets and *implants. The directive does not cover custom-made appliances such as dentures and bridges, which are manufactured in accordance with the written prescription of a duly qualified medical or dental practitioner and are intended for the sole use of a particular patient.

(⊕) SEE WEB LINKS
• Medical Devices Directive page on the Medicines and Healthcare Products Regulatory Agency website.

medical history A record of a patient's previous medical conditions, treatment, inoculations, allergies, and *medication. It may be stored in a paper or electronic format.

medical record *See* MEDICAL HISTORY.

medical status An assessment of a patient's current medical condition including medication. It may be used in the assessment of a patient's suitability for treatment, such as using the American Society of Anesthesiologists (ASA) medical status scale prior to sedation for dental treatment.

medicament *n*. A drug or preparation used for the prevention of disease or that promotes recovery from an injury, ailment, or disease.

Medicare A US federal insurance programme that provides certain in-patient hospital and physician services for all persons aged 65 and older, and eligible individuals with a disability. *See also* MEDICAID.

medication *n*. 1. A substance introduced into the body for the purposes of treatment. 2. The treatment of a patient using drugs.

medicine *n*. 1. The science or practice of the diagnosis, treatment, and prevention of disease. 2. The practice of the non-surgical treatment of disease. 3. Any drug or preparation administered (particularly by mouth) for the treatment or prevention of disease.

Medicines Information Service A part of the UK National Health Service that provides information and advice for medical and dental healthcare professionals on drug therapy related to medicine and dentistry.

mediotrusion *n*. Thrusting of the mandibular condyle towards the midline during movement of the mandible.

medium opening activator (MOA) A one-piece functional *orthodontic appliance used to reduce a deep *overbite. The upper and lower sections are joined by two rigid acrylic resin posts and only the lower anterior teeth are covered with acrylic allowing the lower molars freedom to erupt.

MEDLARS Acronym for Medical Literature Analysis and Retrieval System, a computerized index system of the US National Library of Medicine. *See also* MEDLINE.

MEDLINE (from MEDLARS on-line) The bibliographic database of the United States National Library of Medicine (NLM), covering journals in the fields of medicine, dentistry, nursing, veterinary medicine, healthcare administration, and the pre-clinical sciences dating back to 1949.

(⊕) SEE WEB LINKS

- US National Library of Medicine MEDLINE access page.

mega- A prefix denoting large size or abnormal enlargement or distension.

megadontia *n. See* MACRODONTIA.

megaloglossia *n.* A form of *macroglossia due to enlargement (*hypertrophy) of the tongue muscle.

meiosis *n.* (*adj.* **meiotic**) A type of cell division (reduction division) that produces four daughter cells, each having half the number of chromosomes of the original cell. *Compare* MITOSIS.

melanin *n.* A pigment produced by melanocytes in the basal layer of the skin and mucous membranes and transferred to the basal *keratinocytes. The amount of melanin produced is variable and differences are present between dark and fair skinned races. Pigment may be seen in the oral mucosa particularly the gingivae.

melanin incontinence Spillage of melanin from the basal *keratinocytes into the underlying connective tissue. It is commonly found in inflammatory lesions.

melanin pigmentation A change in the amount of *melanin produced. It may be developmental (*see* MELANOCYTIC NAEVUS; PEUTZ-JEGHERS SYNDROME; CAFÉ AU LAIT SPOTS) or acquired as the result of systemic disease (*see* ADDISON'S DISEASE), malignancy (*see* MELANOMA), or a simple local disorder (*see* MELANOTIC MACULE). Pigmentation of the soft palate is associated with smoking and bronchiogenic carcinoma. Certain drugs may also cause oral pigmentation.

melanocytic naevus A developmental lesion composed of melanocytes. They are common on the skin, where they are referred to as moles, but rare in the oral cavity.

melanoma *n.* A highly malignant tumour of pigment-producing cells (**melanocytes**). They usually occur on the skin due to excessive sunlight, but can also occur on the *mucosa,

particularly the palate. They are usually dark in colour but may also be pigment-free. Treatment is by surgical excision.

melanoplakia *n.* Pigmented patches of melanin on the surface of the tongue and in the mucous membrane (*mucosa) lining the cheeks.

melanotic macule (freckle) A localized increase in *melanin in the basal cell layer of the skin or mucous membranes.

melanotic neuro-ectodermal tumour of infancy A rare pigmented tumour which most often affects the maxilla in infants. It causes enlargement of the maxilla and is treated by excision.

melatonin *n.* A hormone produced by the pineal gland and present in the saliva. It is a powerful *antioxidant and protects cells against inflammatory processes. Salivary melatonin may play an important role in maintaining periodontal health.

Further Reading: Cutando A., Galindo P., Gomez-Moreno G., Arana C., Bolanos J., Acuna-Castroviejo D., Wang H. L. Relationship between salivary melatonin and severity of periodontal disease. *J Periodontol* 2006;77:1533–8.

melitis *n.* Inflammation of the cheek.

melitoptyalism *n.* A condition in which the secretion of saliva contains glucose.

Melkersson–Rosenthal syndrome [E. G. Melkersson (1898–1932), Swedish physician; C. Rosenthal (1892–1937), German neurologist] A rare neurological disorder characterized by recurring facial paralysis, swelling of the face and lips (usually the upper lip), enlargement of the glottis, and the development of enlargement (*hypertrophy) of the tongue, together with folds and furrows. The onset is in childhood or early adolescence. The lips may become hard, cracked, and fissured with a reddish-brown discoloration. Some cases are associated with *Crohn's disease and sarcoid. Treatment is symptomatic.

membrane *n.* (*adj.* **membranous**) A thin layer of tissue covering the whole or part of an organ or structure. The **basement membrane** is a thin, transparent, acellular layer of tissue beneath the epithelium and anchoring it to the underlying connective tissue. **Cell membrane** *see* CELL. **Mucous membrane** *see* MUCOSA. **Periodontal membrane** *see* PERIODONTAL LIGAMENT. The **synovial membrane** forms the inner surface of synovial *joints and secretes *synovial fluid into the joint cavity.

meniscectomy *n.* The surgical removal of the interarticular disc such as from the *temporomandibular joint.

meniscus *n.* (in anatomy) A crescent-shaped structure such as the fibrocartilaginous disc in the *temporomandibular joint.

menopause (climacteric) *n.* A hormonal change in women when the ovaries cease to produce an egg cell every four weeks. It usually takes place between the ages of 45 and 55. The hormonal change is known to cause oral changes which can include altered taste, a burning sensation in the mouth, greater sensitivity to hot and cold foods and beverages, and a decreased salivary flow that can lead to *xerostomia and gingival inflammation.

mental *adj.* (in dentistry) Relating to the *chin.

Mental Capacity Act (MCA) 2005 An act of the UK parliament which provides a legal framework for people whose capacity is impaired. It is meant to ensure that they participate as much as possible in any decisions made on their behalf, and that these are made in their best interests. It also allows people to plan ahead for a time in the future when they might lack the capacity, for any number of reasons, to make decisions for themselves. The MCA is supported by a detailed code of practice ('the code') which sets out best practice for professionals when treating patients who lack capacity. Dental care professionals have a duty to have regard to the code when necessary and failure to comply with it can also be used as evidence in court or tribunal proceedings. The MCA is underpinned by five principles that should guide dental care professionals and others involved in treating or caring for those whose capacity is impaired: a person must be assumed to have capacity unless it is established that he lacks capacity; a person is not to be treated as unable to make a decision unless all practicable steps to help him to do so have been taken without success; a person is not to be treated as unable to make a decision merely because he makes an unwise decision; an act done, or decision made, under the act for or on behalf of the person who lacks capacity must be done, or made, in his best interests. Before the act is done, or the decision is made, regard must be had as to whether the purpose for which it is needed can effectively be achieved in a way which is less restrictive of the person's rights and freedom of action. The act has been substantially amended by the *Mental Health Act 2007.

mental foramen *n. See* MANDIBLE.

Mental Health Act 2007 An act of the UK parliament to amend the Mental Health Act 1983, the Domestic Violence, Crime and Victims Act 2004, and the *Mental Capacity Act 2005 in relation to mentally disordered persons.

(🌐) **SEE WEB LINKS**
● The Department of Health web pages on mental health; they provide an overview and summary of the main provisions of the act.

mental protuberance *See* MANDIBLE.

mental spine *See* TUBERCLE.

menton *n. See* CEPHALOMETRIC ANALYSIS.

mepivacaine hydrochloride *n.* An *amide local anaesthetic agent having a similar action to *lignocaine but producing less vasodilatation. The formulation usually contains a *vasoconstrictor to prolong *analgesia, although the vasoconstrictor may be omitted when it is essential to retain a good blood supply to the operative site, such as when patients who have had radiotherapy to the head and neck and require tooth extraction. Known side-effects are dizziness, drowsiness, and blurred vision. Trade names: **Isocaine, Polocaine**.

mercaptan *n.* An ingredient in the base component of polysulphide *impression material. Mercaptan groups are the functional groups (sulphur and hydrogen atoms) in the base component and give the material its rather unpleasant smell.

mercurial line A very rare condition characterized by a grey or bluish line present at the *gingival margin caused by the deposition of *mercury.

mercurial stomatitis *n. See* STOMATITIS.

mercury *n.* A metallic element which is liquid at room temperature. It is combined with *amalgam alloy as a permanent restorative material. It is a hazardous substance which can be absorbed through the skin, by ingestion, or by inhaling vapour. **Chronic mercury poisoning** is difficult to identify because it is characterized by the common symptoms of tiredness, fatigue, and lethargy; more severe symptoms include irritability, excessive salivation, metallic taste, slurred speech, and gingival inflammation, which may include a gingival *mercurial line. Deaths from **acute mercury poisoning** of healthcare professionals in dental practice have been reported. Because of the mercury content in waste amalgam, it should be stored in a sealed container with a mercury suppressant.

mercury spillage kit Materials and equipment used to retrieve spilt mercury and minimize the potential health risk. A brush is used to localize the spillage and as much free mercury as possible is aspirated into a closed syringe and placed in a waste container. Flowers of sulphur and calcium oxide are then mixed to a paste with water and painted on and around the remaining spillage; when dry the mixture is transferred to a suitable sealed waste container.

meridian system Part of traditional Chinese medicine which describes a network of energy pathways consisting of 12 meridians that run through the body nourishing and vitalizing the organs and tissues. The theory is that any impediment in this circulation can be removed by inserting needles into specifically defined points on the meridian system and thereby remove pain (which may be of dental origin), and treat certain disorders. *See also* ACUPUNCTURE.

mesenchyme *n.* (*adj.* **mesenchymal**) Embryonic connective tissue that develops mainly from the middle layer (*mesoderm) of the embryo. It later becomes differentiated into blood vessels, smooth muscles, and skeletal and connective tissue. It is in this layer that the embryonic tooth buds begin to develop.

mesial *adj.* 1. Medial; nearer to the midline. 2. (in dentistry) Nearer to the midline in the dental arch or jaw. *See also* TOOTH SURFACES. **Mesial drift** is the gradual migration of teeth toward the midline or anteriorly in the dental arch; it occurs naturally with age due to the abrasion of the interproximal tooth surfaces and may occur more quickly when a tooth is lost and no appliance is inserted to maintain the space.

mesio- A prefix signifying mesial or towards the midline e.g. mesio-incisal, mesio-buccal, mesio-occlusal-distal (MOD).

mesioalveolism *n.* A condition in which the *alveolar process is shifted mesially on the base of the jaw. *Compare* LATEROALVEOLISM.

mesiocclusion *n.* A form of *malocclusion in which the mandibular teeth occlude mesially to the normal position of the maxillary teeth. *Compare* DISTOCCLUSION.

mesiodens *n.* A supernumerary tooth either erupted or unerupted found between the two maxillary central incisors. The cause is currently not well understood.

mesiognathic *adj.* Describing the malposition of one or both jaws in a more forward position than normal.

mesioversion *n.* 1. Indicating a tooth is closer than normal to or inclined towards the midline. 2. Indicating that the maxilla or mandible is anterior to its normal position.

mesocephalic *adj. See* CEPHALIC INDEX.

mesoderm *n.* (*adj.* **mesodermal**) The middle germ layer of the primitive embryo, between the *ectoderm and the *endoderm. It gives rise to cartilage, muscle, bone, blood, kidneys, gonads and their ducts, and connective tissue. It has an outer (**somatic**) layer and an inner (**splanchnic**) layer, separated by a cavity which becomes the body cavity. *See also* MESENCHYME.

mesodont *adj.* Describing teeth of moderate size.

mesodontia *pl. n.* Medium-sized teeth.

mesognathic *adj.* Having the jaws slightly projecting. *Compare* PROGNATHISM. *See also* GNATHIC INDEX.

mesoprosopic *adj.* Describing a face of moderate width.

mesostaphyline *adj. See* CHAMESTAPHYLINE.

mesostyle *n.* A minor cusp or fold of enamel on the buccal aspect of the occlusal surface of a maxillary molar or premolar situated between the *parastyle and the *metastyle present in some mammalian or primate species.

Messing root canal gun A modified amalgam carrier designed by J. J. Messing, an English endodontist, used when placing a root canal sealant restoration such as amalgam or *mineral trioxide aggregate (MTA) in a retrograde root filling procedure. It has a narrow orifice and a plunger with a thumb ring and a barrel that may be straight or curved.

meta-analysis *n.* A statistical practice of combining the data of a number of comparable research studies and synthesizing the pooled results to produce a more accurate single estimate or evaluation.

Further Reading: Understanding the statistical pooling of data, in *Evidence based dentistry for effective practice*, ed. J. Clarkson et al. Martin Dunitz, 2003.

metabolism *n.* (*adj.* **metabolic**) The chemical and physiological processes by which the body builds and maintains itself and by which it breaks down food and nutrients to enable its continued growth and functioning.

metacone *n.* The disto-buccal cusp of a mammalian upper molar tooth.

metaconid *n.* The disto-buccal cusp of a mammalian lower molar tooth.

metamerism *n.* The effect of producing a change of colour by viewing under different lighting conditions. It can affect colour selection for porcelain restorations.

metaplasia *n.* A reversible condition characterized by the replacement of one mature cell type with another mature cell type. It can be caused by chronic exposure to toxins, chronic inflammation, or physical irritants; for example, metaplasia is frequently seen in the respiratory tract of smokers.

metastasis *n.* (*adj.* **metastatic**) The spread of a malignant tumour to a distant part of the body. It usually occurs via the bloodstream, through the lymphatic system, or across body cavities.

metastyle (**distostyle**) *n.* A minor cusp or fold of enamel on the buccal aspect of the occlusal surface of a maxillary molar or premolar distal to the *mesostyle and disto-buccal to the *metacone present in some mammalian or primate species. A **metastylid** is a minor cusp or fold of enamel in the same location on a mandibular molar or premolar tooth.

methadone *n.* A long-acting synthetic opiate used in the treatment of opiate addiction. Because it is also an analgesic and sometimes used in the management of chronic pain, the seeking of dental treatment may be delayed until disease is advanced. Methadone can produce dry mouth (*xerostomia) which, combined with a usually high sugar intake, can result in extensive *caries. Because of the high acidity and a lifestyle involving gastric reflux and vomiting, there is an increased risk of tooth erosion.

Further Reading: Graham C. H., Meechan J. G. Dental management of patients taking methadone. *Dent Update* 2005;32(8):477–8, 481–2, 485.
Nathwani N. S., Gallagher J. E. Methadone: dental risks and preventive action. *Dent Update* 2008;35:542–8.

methaemoglobinaemia *n.* A condition of the blood in which the iron atoms of the blood pigment haemoglobin have been oxidized from the ferrous to the ferric form. This form of haemoglobin (**methaemoglobin**) cannot transport oxygen and carbon dioxide round the body. In health ongoing exposure of red blood cells to oxidizing agents results in low levels (<1%) of methaemoglobin production, which is maintained at this low level by the reduction enzyme system. Exposure to high levels of oxidizing agents beyond the capacity of the reduction enzyme system will result in greater quantities of methaemoglobin production. Once

levels rise above 30% symptoms will result. It is characterized by fatigue, headache, *cyanosis, and dizziness. It is a toxic effect sometimes associated with excessive dosage of *prilocaine analgesic such as *EMLA. Treatment is with methylene blue.

methamphetamine *n.* A psycho-stimulant drug popular for its recreational use. Medical uses include the treatment of *attention deficit hyperactivity disorder (ADHD), narcolepsy, and extreme obesity. It enters the brain triggering release of noradrenaline, dopamine, and serotonin. Methamphetamine addicts may develop a condition known as **meth mouth** in which there is extensive caries and periodontal disease, probably due to reduced salivary flow, poor oral hygiene, frequent consumption of carbonated drinks (because of an increased thirst), and tooth clenching and grinding (*bruxism).

meth mouth *n. See* METHAMPHETAMINE.

methylene blue *n.* A chemical compound used to stain residual proteinaceous material in the root canal during *endodontic procedures.

methyl methacrylate *n.* A monomer used in the production of *polymethylmethacrylate resin used primarily as a denture base material and for surgical prostheses. Residual methyl methacrylate in a prosthesis can cause contact *dermatitis characterized by generalized redness and itchiness of the tissues with which it is in contact.

metopion *n.* The craniometric point midway between the frontal eminences on the forehead.

metronidazole *n.* An antibacterial drug used in the treatment of infections caused by susceptible anaerobic organisms such as *necrotizing ulcerative periodontal disease and *pericoronitis. In dentistry it is administered orally. Side-effects include digestive upsets and an unpleasant taste. It should not be taken at the same time as alcohol because it inhibits its breakdown, leading to an accumulation of acetaldehyde; in addition, alcohol should be avoided for 2 days beyond the end of the course of treatment as it interacts with the metabolites of metronidazole. Trade names: **Flagyl, Metrozol.** It is also available as a sustained release, local delivery gel. The gel is injected into the periodontal pocket where it forms crystals which slowly release the antibiotic: the drug tends to be washed from the pocket in the gingival crevicular (sulcular) fluid. Trade name: **Elyzol.**

miconazole *n.* An imidazole antifungal agent commonly applied topically to the skin or mucous membranes. Side-effects include itching, skin rash, nausea, and vomiting. Trade name: **Daktarin**.

microabrasion *n*. The process of applying an abrasive material, such as aluminium oxide, to the tooth surface to remove superficial stains and discoloration. The abrasive material may be mixed with hydrochloric acid.

Further Reading: Wong F. S. L., Winter G. B. Effectiveness of microabrasion technique for improvement of dental aesthetics. *Br Dent J* 2002;193:155–8.

microalveolism *n*. A condition in which the *alveolar process of the mandible or maxilla is excessively small in all dimensions. *Compare* MACROALVEOLISM.

microbe *n*. *See* MICRO-ORGANISM.

microbiologist *n*. A scientist or clinician who specializes in the field of *microbiology.

microbiology *n*. The study of *micro-organisms, including *prokaryotes such as bacteria, and *eukaryotes such as fungi and protozoa. Most micro-organisms are single-celled (unicellular). Viruses and prions, although not considered living, are also included within microbiology. Microbiology consists of many branches including *bacteriology, *virology, and *mycology. *See also* ORAL FLORA.

microcheilia *n*. Abnormally small size of lips.

microdontia *n*. The condition of having abnormally small teeth. It may apply to one, several, or all the teeth in an individual.

micro-filled resin composite *See* RESIN COMPOSITE.

microgenia *n*. A condition in which the height, projection, and width of the *chin prominence is too small in relation to the rest of the facial skeleton. *Compare* MACROGENIA.

microglossia *n*. Abnormally small size of the tongue.

micrognathia *n*. A condition in which one or both jaws are congenitally unusually small.

microleakage *n*. The seepage of fluids, micro-organisms, debris, and breakdown products along the junction between a restoration and the walls of the cavity preparation. Microleakage around *amalgam restorations is minimized over time because of the accumulation of corrosion products at the tooth–amalgam interface.

micromotor *n*. A miniature electric motor which can be linked directly to a contra-angle or straight dental *handpiece. The rotational speed achieved is approximately 0–35,000 rpm.

micron (μ) *n*. One thousandth of a millimetre.

micro-organism *n*. An organism, often referred to as a microbe, that is invisible to the naked eye (i.e. microscopic). Micro-organisms include *bacteria, *fungi, protozoa, and *archaea. Micro-organisms that cause disease are termed pathogenic.

microstomia *n*. The condition of having an abnormally small mouth.

midazolam *n*. A water-soluble *benzodiazepine drug used in dentistry for intravenous, oral, and intranasal conscious *sedation. It is at least twice as potent as *diazepam and more likely to cause amnesia. Its *anxiolytic properties make it suitable for patients with severe dental anxiety or phobia. The most serious side-effect is respiratory depression. Trade name: **Hypnovel**.

midline *n*. A line drawn down the middle of the body or a structure.

migration *n*. 1. The movement of teeth from their normal position in the dental arch. It can be caused by the loss of an adjacent tooth, the loss of an opposing tooth, traumatic tooth relationships, inflammation or disease of the supporting structures, or oral habits such as *digit sucking. *See also* DRIFTING. 2. The movement of the *junctional epithelium onto the root surface with the development of chronic periodontitis and resultant loss of attachment.

Mikulicz's disease [J. von Mikulicz-Radecki (1850–1905), Polish surgeon] A name formerly used to describe bilateral parotid *salivary gland and *lacrimal gland enlargement. It occurs mainly in adults over 50 years of age and is usually asymptomatic. Mikulicz's syndrome was used to describe similar lesions associated with other diseases such as *Sjögren's syndrome, but this terminology is not common in modern clinical practice.

milk teeth *n*. The lay term used to describe the *primary (deciduous) dentition.

Miller's elevator *See* ELEVATOR.

mineralization *n*. The bioprecipitation of an inorganic material. *Calcium and phosphate ions are deposited during the mineralization of *enamel, *dentine, and *cementum. Plaque may be mineralized to form *calculus by the incorporation of inorganic ions.

minerals *n.* Inorganic substances required for the structural composition and proper functioning of the hard and soft tissues of the body. Of oral significance are *calcium and *iron. A deficiency of calcium can result in enamel or dentine *hypoplasia and defective bone formation; a deficiency of iron can result in *glossitis or *angular cheilitis.

mineral trioxide aggregate (MTA) An endodontic cement composed of tricalcium silicate, dicalcium silicate, tricalcium aluminate, tetracalcium aluminoferrite, calcium sulphate, and bismuth oxide used as a *retrograde root filling material in root end preparations, for *pulpotomies, *pulp capping, or for root perforations. It is an antimicrobial, alkaline powder mixed with water to make a grainy paste with a pH of 11.5–12.5.

Further Reading: Bortoluzzi E. A., Broon N. J., Bramante C. M., Garcia R. B., de Moraes I. G., Bernardineli N. Sealing ability of MTA and radiopaque Portland cement with or without calcium chloride for root-end filling. *J Endod* 2006;32(9):897–900.

minocycline *n.* A *tetracycline broad-spectrum antibiotic which may be used for the treatment of periodontal infections in conjunction with mechanical therapy. It is also used in the treatment of respiratory and genital mycoplasma infections, chronic bronchitis, and acne. It is administered by mouth or *topically as a gel. Side-effects include dizziness, paraesthesia, pigmentation of the skin (which may be permanent) and rarely the oral mucosa, loss of appetite, and skin rashes. It is not recommended during pregnancy because of the potential to cause discoloration of the developing foetal dentition. Trade names: **Minocin, Dyancin, Dentomycin.**

Misuse of Drugs Act 1971 (in the UK) An act of parliament restricting the use of dangerous drugs. These controlled drugs are divided up into classes A, B, and C, according to how much harm they can cause when misused. The act specifies certain requirements for writing prescriptions for these drugs.

Mitchell's trimmer *n. See* TRIMMER.

mitosis *n.* (*adj.* **mitotic**) The process of nuclear division in a cell that produces two daughter cells that are genetically identical to each other and to the parent cell. *Compare* MEIOSIS.

mixed dentition *n. See* DENTITION.

mixed design (in statistics) An experimental design incorporating two or more independent *variables with at least one being manipulated using different participants (or other entries being measured) and at least one being manipulated using the same participants (or entries).

mixing time That part of the *working time required to achieve a satisfactory mix of all the constituents of a material. If either the mixing time or the *manipulation time are prolonged, it may negatively affect the properties of the material.

mobility, tooth *n. See* TOOTH MOBILITY.

mode *n.* (in statistics) *See* MEAN.

model *n.* A positive reproduction or *cast made from an *impression of an object. It is used as a diagnostic or status record or as a base for the construction of a prosthetic or *orthodontic appliance. A **model trimmer** is an instrument with an abrasive wheel used to shape and remove excess stone or plaster from a cast.

modelling *n.* A psychological technique by which behaviour may be taught or learnt by imitating behaviour exhibited by another individual (the model). The technique is most effective if the model is of a similar age, gender, and ethnic origin. Photographs or drawings may be used to replace the live model.

modified dental anxiety scale (MDAS) A self-reported psychometric anxiety questionnaire used to objectively evaluate the level of a patient's anxiety. It is a 5 item questionnaire with a maximum score of 25. A score of 19 or above indicates a highly dentally anxious patient and possibly a dental phobic. *See also* DENTAL ANXIETY SCALE.

Further Reading: Humphris G. M., Morrison T., Lindsay S. J. E. The Modified Dental Anxiety Scale: validation and United Kingdom norms. *Community Den Health* 1995;12:143–50.

modified gingival index *See* GINGIVAL INDEX.

modified Widman flap *See* FLAP.

modiolus *n.* Subcutaneous muscular structure around the mouth held together by fibrous tissue, which is the meeting point of muscles involved in the movement of the mouth and facial expression. It is contributed to by the orbicularis oris, buccinator, levator anguli oris, depressor anguli oris, zygomaticus major, zygomaticus minor, and risorius muscles.

moisture control The means of minimizing blood, water, or saliva contamination during an intra-oral restorative procedure. *Dental dam (rubber dam) is the most effective method but may be supplemented by absorbent materials such as cotton wool, sponge, or gauze.

molar glands *n.* A small group of secretory glands situated between the masseter and buccinator muscles and beneath the *mucosa around the distal extremity of the duct of the *parotid gland. Their ducts open into the mouth opposite the last molar tooth.

molariform *adj.* Having the form of a molar tooth.

molar incisor hypomineralization (MIH) Enamel *hypomineralization of probably systemic origin that affects one or more of the first permanent molars and is often associated with affected permanent incisors.

molar, permanent mandibular first *n.* The tooth located in the permanent *dentition of the *mandible between the second premolar tooth and the second molar. It has no primary tooth predecessor and erupts immediately posterior to the second primary molar. The crown is longer mesio-distally than bucco-lingually and longer buccally than lingually. There are four large cusps (mesio-buccal, mesio-lingual, disto-buccal, and disto-lingual) and one small distal cusp. The four large cusps are separated by a cruciate pattern of grooves (fissures) with a central pit (*fossa). The lingual fissure may extend onto the lingual surface and the buccal fissure may extend onto the buccal surface and may end up in a small pit which is often a sight of a carious lesion. The distal fissure divides, one arm extending over the buccal surface and the other dividing the distal and disto-lingual cusps and possibly extending onto the distal surface. The mesial cusps are connected by a mesial marginal ridge, and the distal and disto-lingual cusps are connected by a distal marginal ridge. The four walls of the crown are all convex, particularly the buccal. There are two roots, one mesial and one distal united by a common undivided part below the crown. Both roots are broad and flattened on the mesial and distal surfaces. The mesial root is inclined distally and has a marked vertical groove on its distal surface. The smaller distal root has a narrower vertical groove on its mesial surface and may show little distal curvature. The pulp chamber has four pulp horns

directed towards the four large cusps. There are normally two root canals in the mesial root and one in the distal root but this is subject to considerable variation with the distal root sometimes having two root canals. *Calcification of the tooth begins at or shortly before birth and the crown is normally complete by 2½–3 years of age. The tooth erupts at about 6–7 years and the calcification of the root is complete at about 9–10 years.

molar, permanent mandibular second *n.* The tooth located in the permanent *dentition of the *mandible between the first and the third molar teeth. It has no primary tooth predecessor. The crown is similar in shape to the first permanent mandibular molar, although it usually only has four cusps (mesio-buccal, mesio-lingual, disto-buccal, and disto-lingual). The disto-buccal cusp is larger than in the first molar and located more distally. There are four grooves (fissures) separating the four cusps in a cruciate pattern. The buccal fissure usually extends onto the buccal surface. There are two roots which usually curve distally and may be fused for part of their length; they are normally shorter and weaker than those of the first molar. The pulp chamber has four pulp horns directed towards the four cusps. The root canal structure is very variable and is similar to the mandibular first molar. *Calcification of the tooth begins at 2½–3 years after birth and the crown is normally complete by 7–8 years of age. The tooth erupts at about 11–13 years and the calcification of the root is complete at about 14–15 years.

molar, permanent mandibular third (wisdom tooth) *n.* The tooth located in the permanent *dentition of the *mandible between the posterior to the second molar tooth. It has no primary tooth predecessor and it is usually the smallest of the three lower molar teeth. The crown shows considerable variation and may present with either four or five cusps. The distal surface is markedly convex. The roots may be similar to those of the second molar but fusion of the roots sometimes leads to the formation of a simple cone-shaped root. There are usually only two root canals, a mesial and a distal. *Calcification of the tooth begins at 8–10 years after birth and the crown is normally complete by 12–16 years of age. The tooth erupts at about 17–21 years and the calcification of the root is complete at about 18–25 years.

molar, permanent maxillary first *n.* The tooth located in the permanent *dentition of the *maxilla between the second premolar tooth and the second molar. The occlusal surface of the crown is diamond-shaped with the longest

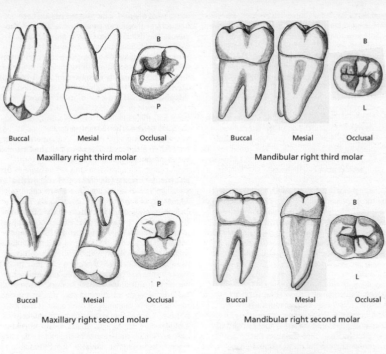

Buccal	Mesial	Occlusal

Maxillary right third molar

Buccal	Mesial	Occlusal

Mandibular right third molar

Buccal	Mesial	Occlusal

Maxillary right second molar

Buccal	Mesial	Occlusal

Mandibular right second molar

Buccal	Mesial	Occlusal

Maxillary right first molar

Buccal	Mesial	Occlusal

Mandibular right first molar

Permanent molars

diagonal extending from the mesio-buccal corner to the disto-lingual corner. It has four cusps (mesio-buccal, mesio-palatal, disto-buccal, and disto-palatal) separated by an H-shaped configuration of grooves (fissures). Mesial and distal marginal ridges connect the mesial and distal cusps respectively. An oblique ridge joins the mesio-palatal and disto-buccal cusps to divide the occlusal surface into a larger mesial

and smaller distal area both containing pits (fossae). A buccal fissure from the mesial pit extends onto the buccal surface. A fissure runs from the small distal pit parallel to the oblique ridge and turns on to the palatal surface of the crown. A fifth cusp, or small elevation (the *tubercle of Carabelli), is sometimes found on the palatal surface about midway between the apex and the cervical margin. The buccal, palatal, and distal surfaces of the crown are convex, whereas the mesial surface is almost flat. There are three roots (mesio-buccal, disto-buccal, and palatal) which remain united towards the crown. The buccal roots are flattened on their mesial and distal surfaces and are shorter than the much longer and straighter palatal root which diverges widely from the other two roots. The pulp chamber has four horns extending into the base of each of the four cusps. There are normally three root canals but in many cases there may be four or more. *Calcification of the tooth begins at or shortly after birth and the crown is normally complete by 2½–3 years of age. The tooth erupts at about 6–7 years and the calcification of the root is complete at about 9–10 years.

molar, permanent maxillary second *n.*
The tooth located in the permanent *dentition of the *maxilla between the first and third molar teeth. The form of the crown is similar to that of the first maxillary molar although it shows more variation and is smaller. The mesio-distal diameter is reduced and the diamond shape is usually more pronounced. Both the disto-palatal and disto-buccal cusps are reduced and sometimes the disto-palatal cusp is replaced by two smaller cusps or absent completely to give a tricuspid, triangular-shaped tooth where the distal margin of the crown is replaced by the oblique ridge joining the mesio-palatal and disto-buccal cusps. In a third variation the crown is compressed across the mesio-palatal disto-buccal diameter to give the crown the shape of a long oval, the long diameter of which runs from mesio-buccal to disto-palatal. It is very rare for a fifth cusp (the *tubercle of Carabelli) to be present on the palatal surface as in the upper first molar. The root pattern is usually similar to the first molar although the divergence is less pronounced. Sometimes the palatal root may be united with one of the buccal roots, usually the mesio-buccal. The pulp chamber and root canals are similar to the first molar but can show considerable variation. *Calcification of the tooth begins at 2½–3 years after birth and the crown is normally complete by 7–8 years of age. The tooth erupts at about 12–13 years and the calcification of the root is complete at about 14–16 years.

molar, permanent maxillary third (wisdom tooth) *n.* The tooth located in the permanent *dentition of the *maxilla distal to the second molar tooth. It is similar in form but smaller than the second molar tooth and is the most variable in the human dentition. Although it may have four cusps, it is most commonly present as a tricuspid tooth with the disto-palatal cusp and distal fossa being missing. A further reduction in size of the crown may present as a peg-shaped

tooth with a small cone-shaped crown. Sometimes there may be one or more accessory cusps. The distal surface of the crown is usually more convex than that of the first and second molars. There may be up to three roots but, more often, the roots are fused along most or all of their length and frequently show irregular curvature. There are many variations in the size and shape of the pulp chamber and the number of root canals. *Calcification of the tooth begins at 7–9 years after birth and the crown is normally complete by 12–16 years of age. The tooth erupts at about 17–21 years, but this is very variable and sometimes it may fail to erupt at all. The calcification of the root is complete at about 18–25+ years.

molar, primary (deciduous) mandibular first *n.* The tooth located in the primary *dentition of the *mandible distal to the primary canine tooth. It is succeeded by the mandibular first premolar. It has a crown elongated and oval in a mesio-distal direction and has four cusps (mesio-buccal, disto-buccal, mesio-lingual, disto-lingual), the largest of which is the mesio-lingual. A mesio-distal groove (fissure) separates the buccal from the lingual cusps and terminates at the mesial and distal marginal ridges. The lingual half of the tooth is narrower than the buccal and the mesio-lingual angle of the crown is markedly obtuse. A transverse enamel ridge frequently connects the mesio-lingual and mesio-buccal cusps to create mesial and distal pits (fossae). The buccal surface of the crown is very bulbous towards the cervical margin where there may be a distinct tubercle in the mesio-cervical part. It has a mesial and a distal root which diverge markedly to make room for the tooth germ of the mandibular first *premolar. The root apices may converge towards each other, further embracing the permanent tooth germ, which can result in its unintentional removal if extraction is attempted when the roots are fully formed. *Calcification of the tooth begins at about 5 months of foetal life. The tooth erupts at about 12 months after birth and the calcification of the root is complete at about 2½ years.

molar, primary (deciduous) mandibular second *n.* The tooth located in the primary *dentition of the *mandible distal to the primary first molar tooth. It is succeeded by the mandibular second premolar. The form of the crown is similar to but smaller than that of the first permanent mandibular molar. It has four cusps but the central pit (fossa) is significantly more extensive. The mesial and distal surfaces are strongly convex and there is a pronounced bulge on the buccal surface. It has a mesial and a distal root which diverge markedly to make room for the tooth germ of the mandibular second *premolar. The

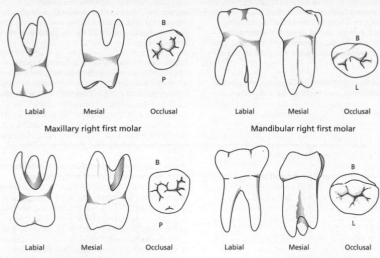

| Labial | Mesial | Occlusal | Labial | Mesial | Occlusal |

Maxillary right first molar   Mandibular right first molar

| Labial | Mesial | Occlusal | Labial | Mesial | Occlusal |

Maxillary right second molar   Mandibular right second molar

Primary (deciduous) molars

mesial root may show some partial buccal and lingual division. The root apices may converge towards each other, further embracing the permanent tooth germ, which can result in its unintentional removal if extraction is attempted when the roots are fully formed. *Calcification of the tooth begins at about 6 months of foetal life. The tooth erupts at about 20 months after birth and the calcification of the root is complete at about 3 years.

molar, primary (deciduous) maxillary first *n.* The tooth located in the primary *dentition of the *mandible distal to the primary canine tooth. It is succeeded by the maxillary first premolar. The occlusal surface of the crown is irregularly quadrilateral with the buccal side longer than the lingual and an obtuse mesio-palatal angle. The occlusal surface is divided into buccal and palatal parts by a deep groove running mesio-distally terminating in poorly defined mesial and distal marginal ridges. The buccal surface is markedly bulged and may be accentuated in the mesial half to create a tubercle (the *tubercle of Zuckerhandl). It has three roots, mesio-buccal, disto-buccal, and palatal, which are markedly divergent to make room for the tooth germ of the maxillary first *premolar. The palatal

root is the largest and longest and is almost circular in cross-section. The other two roots are flattened in a mesio-distal direction. The palatal and disto-buccal roots are sometimes fused. *Calcification of the tooth begins at about 5 months of foetal life. The tooth erupts at about 14 months after birth and the calcification of the root is complete at about 2½ years.

molar, primary (deciduous) maxillary second *n.* The tooth located in the primary *dentition of the *mandible distal to the primary first molar tooth. It is succeeded by the maxillary second premolar. The crown is very similar to although smaller than the permanent maxillary first molar. It does, however, have a more bulbous buccal surface in its cervical region but no *tubercle as with the first primary molar. A tubercle of Carabelli may be found on the mesial half of the palatal surface. In some rare occasions the disto-palatal cusp may be reduced or missing. The mesio-palatal cusp is the largest and is connected by an oblique ridge to the disto-buccal cusp to give a large mesial pit (fossa) and a small distal pit. It has three roots, mesio-buccal, disto-buccal, and palatal, which are divergent to make room for the

tooth germ of the maxillary second *premolar. Sometimes the palatal and disto-buccal roots are fused. *Calcification of the tooth begins at about 6 months of foetal life. The tooth erupts at about 24 months after birth and the calcification of the root is complete at about 3 years.

molar relationship The positioning of the mandibular molar teeth in relation to the maxillary molar teeth when the teeth are in maximum contact. Angle's classification is commonly used to describe the molars in occlusion. [Edward Angle (1835–1930), American orthodontist].

monilia *n.* A genus of fungi first introduced in the 18th century that originally included fungi isolated from vegetation and subsequently yeasts recovered from cases of oral and vaginal thrush.

Class	Relationship	
I	The mesio-buccal cusp of the upperfirst molar lies in the buccal groove of the lower first molar	
II	The mesio-buccal cusp of the upper first molar lies anterior to the buccal groove of the lower first molar	
III	The mesio-buccal cusp of the upper first molar lies posterior to the buccal groove of the lower first molar	

Mandibular and maxillary molar relationships

Several yeast species recovered from humans including *Candida albicans* were originally classified within the genus *Monilia* but are now classified within the genus *Candida*.

moniliasis *n.* An archaic former name for *candidiasis, an infection caused by *Candida albicans* or other *Candida* species.

monitoring badge See FILM BADGE.

monoamine oxidase inhibitor (MAOI) *n.* A class of antidepressants used in the treatment of depression. MAOIs work by inhibiting the activity of monoamine oxidase, thus preventing the breakdown of the brain's monoamine neurotransmitters. Side-effects include dry mouth, dizziness, and a feeling of being light-headed. Local *analgesic solutions containing *epinephrine should be used with caution in patients taking MAOIs because of the potential interaction with the vasoconstrictor.

monobloc *n.* A removable *activator-type *orthodontic appliance utilizing muscle forces to modify the growth of the jaws to correct a malocclusion. It is made from one block of acrylic resin. See also FUNCTIONAL APPLIANCE.

monocyte *n.* (*adj.* **monocytic**) A type of white blood cell with a kidney-shaped nucleus which is found in the bloodstream. They differentiate into macrophages once they enter the tissues and they ingest foreign particles such as bacteria and tissue debris. They can live for months or years.

monofluor-phosphate *n.* A chemical complex containing *fluoride. The sodium salt may be added to *toothpaste or as a topical application because of its caries inhibitory action.

monomer *n.* A molecule that can join with other molecules to form a large long chain molecule called a *polymer in a process known as *polymerization. In dentistry monomers are chemically combined to produce resin composite materials and denture base resins (*polymethylmethacrylate). Acrylic monomer is highly inflammable and skin contact or vapour inhalation is potentially hazardous.

monophyodont *adj.* Possessing only one generation of teeth. It is a characteristic of some mammals, including the manatee, seal, and walrus.

monosaccharide *n.* A simple sugar having the general formula $(CH_2O)_n$. They are classified according to the number of carbon atoms they possess. The most abundant monosaccharide is *glucose with six carbon atoms (a hexose).

Monson's curve See CURVE OF MONSON.

Moon's molars [H. Moon (1845–92), English surgeon] Small, domed first permanent molars sometimes seen in patients with congenital *syphilis.

Moorehead's retractor See RETRACTOR.

morbidity *n.* The state of being diseased. The **morbidity rate** is the number of cases of a disease occurring in a defined number of the population, usually stated as cases per 100,000 or per million. See also INCIDENCE; PREVALENCE.

morphine *n.* A highly potent opioid analgesic which acts directly on the nervous system to relieve severe and persistent pain. It has a high potential for addiction, and tolerance develops with regular use.

morphology *n.* The study of the form or shape of an organism or part of an organism. **Occlusal morphology** refers to the external form of the biting surface of a tooth. The **determinants of occlusal morphology** are the variable factors that determine the morphology of the restored crown of a tooth. **Vertical determinants** that affect the cusp height and fossa depth include the *condylar guidance, the anterior guidance, the plane of occlusion, the *curve of Spee, and the lateral translation movement. The **horizontal determinants** which influence the ridge and groove direction include the distance from the rotating condyle, the distance from the mid-sagittal plane, the lateral translation movement, and the intercondylar distance.

(((•))) SEE WEB LINKS
• An overview slide presentation from the Faculty of Dentistry, Chiang Mai University.

mortality rate The incidence of death in a population over a given period of time.

mortar *n.* An urn-shaped vessel in which materials may be crushed or ground with a *pestle. It was formerly used for mixing *amalgam alloy powder and *mercury (*trituration).

motile *adj.* Being able to move spontaneously and independently; usually applied to a cell or micro-organism.

motor nerve See NERVE.

motor neuron disease (MND) A progressive degenerative condition of the cells in the brain and the nerve-conducting pathways; of unknown cause. There is general muscle weakness and the tongue may be reduced in size and have limited movement. Patients may have difficulty in managing oral secretions and swallowing.

mottling *n. See* FLUOROSIS.

mould *n.* 1. The growth produced by certain types of fungi. 2. A form in which an object is cast or shaped. It is used to describe the shape of an artificial tooth. A **mould guide** is used to select the shape of an artificial tooth or teeth.

mouth breathing The state of inhaling or exhaling through the mouth, commonly seen in conditions which have caused a total or partial nasal blockage. The normal individual breathes through the nose at rest and simultaneously through the nose and mouth during vigorous aerobic exercise. Mouth breathing can produce excessive drying of the oral mucosa with a tendency to gingival enlargement or inflammation. Mouth breathing can also cause excessive *tongue thrusting and a resultant tooth *malocclusion. Untreated it can be the source of *temporomandibular joint problems.

mouth gag *n. See* GAG.

mouth guard A soft resilient intra-oral device, usually made of resin, worn to protect the teeth and associated supporting tissues from potential injury during participation in contact sports such as boxing, rugby, and hockey. 📷

mouth mirror A small circular reflector on a handle used in the examination of the teeth and oral tissues to provide indirect vision, to reflect light, or to retract soft tissues. Mouth mirrors are numbered according to size and may be magnifying, reflecting from the front surface, or reflecting from the back surface.

mouth prop [F. W. Hewitt (1857–1916), British anaesthetist] *n.* A device that is placed in a patient's mouth to keep it open during surgical work on the mouth or throat. **Hewitt's metal props** are in sets of three different sizes on a chain.

mouthrinse *n. See* MOUTHWASH.

mouthwash *n.* A medicated aqueous solution containing antiseptic, astringent, or deodorizing properties used for rinsing or gargling. **Fluoride mouthwashes** usually contain sodium fluoride added to reduce the incidence of dental caries at an approximate level of 0.05% (225 parts per million) for a daily rinse and 0.2% (900 ppm) for a weekly rinse. *Chlorhexidine gluconate mouthwash is used to treat the symptoms of *aphthous ulcers and to reduce gingival or periodontal inflammation; it has the disadvantage of potentially producing brown *extrinsic tooth staining. The use of stannous fluoride and chlorhexidine mouthwashes together may reduce the efficacy of both agents. Some mouthwashes have a significant alcohol content (15–30%) to aid the blending of oil-based products and increase the astringent properties; these should be avoided in patients with an alcohol dependency. **Zinc chloride mouthrinse** has been shown to reduce the rate of supragingival *calculus accumulation. **Homeopathic mouthwashes** are available that include such herbal agents as aloe vera, sodium carrageenan, *echinacea, and bee *propolis and are claimed to have antiseptic and anti-inflammatory properties although the current evidence base is poor. Rinsing with water after using a mouthrinse should be deferred for at least 30 minutes to prevent clearance of the rinse and a reduction in its effectiveness.

MRI *See* MAGNETIC RESONANCE IMAGING.

MRSA (Meticillin [originally spelled methicillin] resistant Staphylococcus aureus) *pl. n.* Derivatives of the common bacterium *Staphylococcus aureus* that are resistant to beta-lactam antibiotics including penicillin, meticillin, and cephalosporins. MRSA is endemic in hospitals in many countries around the world and is a common cause of nosocomial *infection. MRSA often exhibits resistance to a wide range of antibiotic groups apart from beta-lactams. Over the last decade community-acquired MRSAs have emerged as a significant cause of infection in the community in many countries. There are several distinct major subgroups of MRSA and a wide variety of variants. In the healthcare setting, patients with open wounds, indwelling devices, or a weakened immune system are significantly more at risk of infection. Healthcare staff who do not follow good cross-infection control and prevention practice can spread MRSA from patient to patient. *See also* STAPHYLOCOCCUS.

Further Reading: Dawson M. P., Smith A. J. Superbugs and the dentist: an update. *Dent Update* 2006;33(4):198–200, 202–4, 207–8.

mucilaginous *adj.* Resembling mucilage; moist and sticky or having a heavy gluey quality.

mucin *n.* A mucopolysaccharide which is the chief constituent of *mucus. It is a mixture of *glycoproteins soluble in water.

mucobuccal fold The line of flexure of the mucous membrane as it passes from the cheek to the mandibular or maxillary surface.

mucocoele (mucous cyst) *n.* A clinical term used to describe a bluish, soft, often fluffant swelling caused by either blockage or rupture of a *salivary gland duct. They are common on the lower lip and are caused by trauma. Histologically two types are recognized: mucous retention cysts in which the mucous is surrounded by ductal epithelium and mucous extravasation cysts. *See also* CYST.

mucoepidermoid carcinoma A *malignant *neoplasm of glandular tissue, particularly the ducts of the salivary glands. It contains both *mucous cells and *epidermal cells.

mucoepithelial dysplasia A rare hereditary multiepithelial disorder mainly characterized by chronic mucosal lesions of the mouth, nose, conjunctiva, vagina, anus, and bladder. Red, periorificial mucosal lesions involving these structures may be noted by 1 year of age and can persist throughout life.

mucogingival *adj.* Describing the portion of the oral mucosa that covers the alveolar process including the gingivae (keratinized tissue) and the adjacent alveolar mucosa. The **mucogingival junction** is a line of demarcation between the pale pink attached keratinized *gingiva and the darker red non-keratinized alveolar *mucosa. The **mucogingival complex** is a generic term used to describe anything that includes both the gingivae and the alveolar *mucosa; it includes the junctional epithelium, the periodontal ligament, and the attached gingivae.

mucolabial fold *n. See* FOLD.

mucoperiosteal flap A piece of tissue composed of mucous membrane and periosteum (*mucoperiosteum) such as from the hard palate or gingivae, raised during a surgical procedure.

mucoperiosteum *n.* A layer of *connective tissue covering bone which is a fusion of the *periosteum and the mucous membrane (*mucosa). It forms the mucosal lining of the maxillary sinuses and the hard palate.

mucopolysaccharide *n.* One of a group of complex *carbohydrates consisting of long unbranched *polysaccharides functioning as structural components in connective tissue. An example is *chondroitin sulphate, present in cartilage.

mucopolysaccharidosis *n.* Any one of a group of rare genetic disorders involving *polysaccharide metabolism in which the storage of complex carbohydrates is disordered e.g. *Hurler's syndrome.

mucosa (mucous membrane) *n.* A membrane lining the oral cavity. It consists of a surface layer of stratified squamous *epithelium and an underlying layer of highly vascular *connective tissue (*lamina propria). It is attached to underlying structures by connective tissue of varying thickness. The structure of the mucosa varies according to function. The **lining mucosa** covers the intra-oral surfaces of the cheeks and lips, the alveolar processes, soft palate, under-surface of the tongue, and the floor of the mouth; it is non-keratinized, loosely attached, and contains numerous salivary ducts. The **masticatory mucosa** covers the hard palate and the gingivae; it is *keratinized and firmly attached to the underlying bone and has no submucosa layer. **Specialized mucosa** which is keratinized covers the dorsum of the *tongue and contains taste buds.

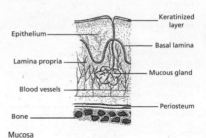

Mucosa

mucositis *n.* Inflammation of the *mucosa (mucous membrane). It is seen as a side-effect of *chemotherapy or *radiotherapy of the head and neck and is characterized by a burning sensation, areas of redness, and sometimes ulceration. **Chronic senile mucositis** is characterized by mucosal *atrophy and is seen primarily in elderly women.

mucostatic *adj.* 1. Pertaining to the normal relaxed condition of the mucosal tissues covering the jaws. A **mucostatic impression material** (e.g. plaster of Paris) causes minimum displacement of the mucosal tissues. 2. An agent or drug which arrests the secretion of *mucus.

mucous *n.* Relating to mucus.

mucous acinus *n.* A group of secretary cells in the *salivary glands from which *saliva is produced.

mucous extravasation cyst *n. See* CYST.

mucous membrane *n. See* MUCOSA.

mucous retention cyst *n. See* CYST.

mucus *n.* (*adj.* **mucous**) A viscous secretion of *mucosa which acts as a protective barrier and lubricant. It contains water, *mucin, white blood cells, inorganic salts, *enzymes, and exfoliated cells.

mulberry molars *See* MOON'S MOLARS.

mulling *n.* The final mixing and kneading stage in the process of *amalgam *trituration. Dentists used to mull amalgam in the palm of the hand; this added moisture and sodium chloride to the mix, which led to severe corroding of the amalgam and harmful consequences for the dentist because of mercury absorption.

multifactorial *adj.* Describing traits or diseases that are the result of the interaction between multiple genetic and environmental factors.

multiple endocrine neoplasia syndrome (MEN) A genetic syndrome with a spectrum of types. Type 3 is characterized by multiple mucosal neuromas and medullary *carcinoma of the thyroid gland.

multiple regression A statistical test in which an outcome is predicted by a linear combination of two or more *variables.

multiple sclerosis (MS) A chronic *autoimmune disease of the central nervous system affecting young adults. It is characterized by a progressive deterioration of neurological function and is subject to periods of remission and relapse. Of oral significance are possible signs of abnormal peri-oral hypersensitivity or anaesthesia, *trigeminal neuralgia, or facial paralysis. Treatment is based on physiotherapy and drug therapy to reduce muscular spasticity. The drug therapy can result in a dry mouth (*xerostomia) and gingival inflammation. At present there is no sound scientific evidence to link mercury from amalgam restorations with multiple sclerosis.

multituberculate (polybunodont) *adj.* Describing a tooth which bears numerous conical cusps; held by some to be the primitive condition of the mammalian teeth. *See also* TRITUBERCULAR THEORY.

multivariate *adj.* (in statistics) Describing two or more *variables.

multivariate analysis of variance (MANOVA) A group of statistical tests that applies the *analysis of variance to situations in which more than one outcome *variable is being measured.

mummification *n.* The application of a fixative agent to the dental *pulp to render it inert and to prevent decomposition. Many mummifying pastes contain *formocresol, *formaldehyde, or *paraformaldehyde. Parachlorophenol and camphor may be included for their antiseptic properties. Evidence of the *carcinogenicity and toxicity of formocresol, formaldehyde, paraformaldehyde, and mummifying agents which contain arsenic are a continued cause of serious concern. *See also* N2.

mumps (viral sialadenitis) *n.* A common contagious viral inflammation affecting school-age children. It is characterized 2–3 weeks after exposure by swelling of the *parotid glands which may or may not be bilateral. Frequently the parotid gland on one side of the face swells up days before the other. The infection may spread to other salivary glands, pancreas, brain, or testicles. The symptoms usually disappear within 3 days but the patient remains infectious until all the swelling has completely disappeared. Most cases are mild but complications include deafness and meningitis. Effective immunity is provided by *vaccination. *See also* PAROTITIS; SIALADENITIS.

muscle *n.* A tissue which by cellular contraction produces movement. There are three types of muscle. **Smooth muscle** (unstriated) is the simplest type of muscle and is found in such structures as the stomach, digestive tract, blood vessels, and ducts of glands. **Striated muscle** forms the bulk of the body and is under voluntary control; striated muscles are attached to the bones of the skeleton; they are composed of parallel bundles of multinucleate fibres, which reveal cross-banding when viewed under the microscope. **Cardiac muscle** (striated) forms the walls of the heart and contracts involuntarily.

muscles of facial expression The muscles surrounding the eyes, nose, and mouth which act as contractors and dilators of these openings. They are a large group of superficial muscles which have their insertion into the skin rather than bones. They aid speech and chewing and also modify the expression of the face by their action on the forehead, eyelids, cheeks, nostrils, and lips. They are derived from the second pharyngeal arch and are innervated by the facial nerve.

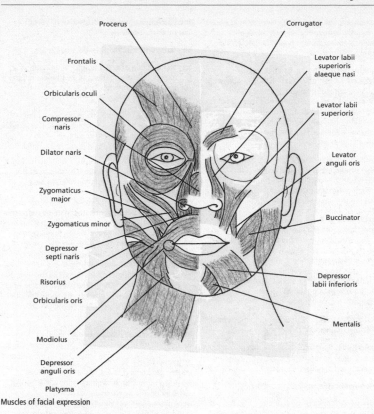

Muscles of facial expression

Labels (clockwise from top): Procerus, Corrugator, Levator labii superioris alaeque nasi, Levator labii superioris, Levator anguli oris, Buccinator, Depressor labii inferioris, Mentalis, Platysma, Depressor anguli oris, Modiolus, Orbicularis oris, Risorius, Depressor septi naris, Zygomaticus minor, Zygomaticus major, Dilator naris, Compressor naris, Orbicularis oculi, Frontalis

The functions of the muscles of mastication	
Muscles involved	Jaw action
Lateral pterygoid Digastric	Opening
Temporalis Masseter (superficial head)	Closing
Masseter (superficial head) Lateral pterygoid Medial pterygoid	Protrusion
Temporalis Masseter (deep head)	Retrusion
Temporalis on the same side Masseter Pterygoid muscles on the one side move the jaw to the opposite side	Chewing

muscles of mastication A group of muscles which act together to produce a coordinated movement of the *mandible during *chewing. They are innervated by the mandibular branch of the trigeminal nerve. The muscles consist of the temporalis, masseter, medial pterygoid, lateral pterygoid, and digastric. During mastication they act in conjunction with each other.

muscle trimming The shaping of impression material in the mouth, before reaching its final set, to determine the border of a denture by the manipulation of the lips and cheeks to conform the impression material to the shape of the *vestibule.

muscular dystrophy A group of genetic muscle disorders in which the affected muscles degenerate and are replaced by fatty tissue. Of dental significance is that the condition may result in a malocclusion because of the altered balance of the soft tissues. There may also be an open-mouth posture and muscle weakness of the circum-oral musculature, possibly associated with poor oral hygiene.

muscular triangle *n.* An anatomical description of a region of the neck also known as the **inferior carotid triangle**. It is bounded anteriorly by the median line of the neck from the hyoid bone to the sternum, posteriorly by the anterior border of the sternocleidomastoid muscle, and superiorly by the superior belly of the omohyoid muscle.

mutan *n.* A water-insoluble *polymer of *glucose produced by *Streptococcus mutans*. It may facilitate its establishment in dental *plaque since such polymers are necessary for the adherence of *S. mutans* to enamel.

myasthenia gravis (MG) A chronic autoimmune disease characterized by abnormal weakness and fatigue of specific muscles. The first to be affected are usually the facial muscles and the muscles associated with the eyes, mouth, and throat, which can lead to difficulty in swallowing (*dysphagia). Relief is obtained by rest and immunosuppressive drugs such as steroids.

mycologist *n.* A person who specializes in the field of *mycology.

mycology *n.* The branch of microbiology concerned with the study of fungi, which includes yeasts such as *Candida albicans*.

myeloblastoma *n. See* CHLOROMA.

myeloma (multiple myeloma, myelomatosis) *n.* A malignant neoplasm of plasma cells which produce antibodies. Lesions may affect many organs and if present in bone cause destruction and pain. It is incurable but can be stabilized by chemotherapy, steroids, and thalidomide.

mylar® *n.* A transparent polyester material used in the form of strips or bands as a *matrix during the placement of resin composite or glass ionomer restorations.

mylohyoid ridge *See* MANDIBLE.

myoblastoma *n.* A benign *neoplasm with large cells resembling immature muscle cells (myoblasts). It most frequently occurs in the tongue.

myocardial infarction *n.* Death of part of the heart muscle due to a blockage of the arteries supplying it (*coronary thrombosis). It is characterized by sudden severe chest pain which may radiate to the arms and throat.

myocardium *n.* The middle of the three layers forming the wall of the heart. It is composed of cardiac muscle.

myofascial pain dysfunction syndrome (MPDS) Pain associated with inflammation or irritation of muscles or the fascia surrounding muscles. It usually involves the *muscles of mastication as well as the neck and shoulder muscles. It is characterized by painful or sensitive areas (trigger points) in the muscle or the junction of the muscle and fascia. Diagnosis and treatment are difficult because there can be many causes including anxiety, trauma, systemic conditions, and muscle strain.

myofunctional appliance *See* ORTHODONTIC APPLIANCE.

myxoedema *n.* The clinical condition caused by an under-activity of the *thyroid gland in adult life. It is characterized by dry hair and skin, thinning of the eyebrows, slowness of speech, and mental dullness. Treatment is by the administration of *thyroxine.

myxoma *n.* A locally invasive but benign *odontogenic tumour characterized by odontogenic connective tissue. It presents as a multilocular radiolucency commonly at the angle of the mandible. Treatment is by excision.

m

N2 *n.* A single-visit endodontic technique that uses *formaldehyde as a mummification agent. 5% formaldehyde is added to a zinc oxide root canal sealer. It is also known as the **Sargenti technique**. Serious concerns have been raised concerning this technique since formaldehyde is known to cause permanent tissue damage if not confined to the pulp chamber or root canal system.

Further Reading: Orr D. L. Paresthesia of the second division of the trigeminal nerve secondary to endodontic manipulation with N2. *Journal of Head and Face Pain* 1987;27 (1):21.
Scully C., Ng Y. -L., Gulabivala K. Systemic complications due to endodontic manipulations. *Endodontic Topics* 2003;4 (1):60–68.

Nabers furcation probe *See* PROBE.

naevus (*pl.* **naevi)** *n.* A clearly defined pigmented area of skin or mucous membrane usually present at birth (**birth mark**). The **strawberry naevus** is a *haemangioma which appears as a raised red nodule on the face; it grows rapidly during the first month of life and disappears between the ages of 5 and 10 years. The **capillary naevus** (haemangioma) is permanent and purplish in colour, and usually occurs on the upper part of the body. **White sponge naevus (Cannon's disease)** is a rare hereditary condition characterized by benign white asymptomatic plaques with a shaggy or spongy wrinkled surface affecting the bucaal mucosa and/or floor of the mouth. **Melanocytic naevi** (moles) are characterized by accumulations of melanocytes and usually arise around puberty.

Further Reading: Ram S., Siar C. H. Cannon's disease: clinical and diagnostic implications: a case report. *Dent Update* 2004;31:557–9.

Nance appliance A fixed orthodontic appliance, first described by H. N. Nance in 1947, used either to rotate molar teeth, stabilize them, or prevent them from drifting mesially. It consists of fixed bands on molars either side of the arch with a connecting palatal archwire, in the centre of which is a button of acrylic resin which fits against the palatal surface. *See also* SPACE MAINTAINER.

Nance's analysis of arch length A method of assessing the arch length for the permanent dentition first defined by H. N. Nance in 1947. It is the difference in length of the space occupied by the primary canine and two primary molars and the space occupied by the permanent canine and two premolars on each side of the arch.

narcosis *n.* A state of unconsciousness induced by a drug.

narcotic *n.* A drug that induces insensibility and relieves pain.

naris (*pl.* **nares)** *n.* A nostril.

nasal *adj.* Relating to the nose. The **nasal bridge** is the upper bony part of the nose. The **nasal cavity** consists of two large irregular air-filled spaces (**nasal vestibule**) separated by a quadrilateral vertical septum (**nasal septum**) with membranous, cartilaginous, and bony parts situated either side of the midline and extending from the cranial base to the roof of the mouth; it communicates anteriorly with the nostrils (anterior nares) and posteriorly with the *nasopharynx. The nasal cavity is lined with mucous membrane containing olfactory receptors. The **anterior nasal spine** is a pointed forwards projection from the centre of the nasal part of the frontal bone; the tip (acanthion) is used as a *cephalometric landmark. The **posterior nasal spine** is the sharp posterior extremity of the nasal crest at the rear of the palate.

nasion *n. See* CEPHALOMETRIC ANALYSIS.

Nasmyth's membrane (primary enamel cuticle) [A. Nasmyth (1758–1840), anatomist and Scottish dental surgeon] The temporary remnants of the *reduced enamel epithelium covering the crown of the tooth after eruption.

nasolabial angle The angle formed by the labial surface of the upper lip and the lower border of the nose. It is a measure of protrusion of the upper anterior teeth.

nasolabial (nasoalveolar) cyst *n. See* CYST.

nasolacrimal duct A tubular duct that conveys tears from the *lacrimal gland to the nose.

nasopalatine canal Also known as the **incisive canal.** One of two canals running downward, anteriorly, and medially from the nasal floor close to the midline to meet at a common opening, the incisive fossa (anterior palatine foramen) on the anterior surface of the maxilla. A developmental nasopalatine *cyst can arise from the nasopalatine epithelium.

nasopharyngeal carcinoma *See* CARCINOMA.

nasopharynx *n.* (*adj.* nasopharyngeal) The part of the *pharynx that lies above the junction of the hard and soft palates. It connects the *nasal cavity to the *oropharynx.

natal teeth Teeth present at birth. They may be present due to the premature eruption of primary teeth or they may be *supernumerary teeth. The most commonly affected teeth are the mandibular incisors. They can cause discomfort to the nursing mother and may necessitate extraction. *See also* NEONATAL TEETH.

National Clinical Assessment Service (NCAS) A body that promotes patient safety by providing confidential advice and support to the *National Health Service (NHS) in situations where the performance of doctors and dentists is giving cause for concern. Managers or practitioners themselves can contact NCAS for advice. Advice may lead to formal assessment of clinical performance or to other forms of help. A performance assessment aims to clarify concerns and make recommendations which will support managers and practitioners in resolving the concerns.

 SEE WEB LINKS
• The National Clinical Assessment Service website.

National Examining Board for Dental Nurses (NEBDN) A body established in the UK in 1943 to advance the education of dental nurses for the benefit of the public. It provides examinations for the National Certificate for Dental Nurses and post-qualification nursing certificates in dental sedation, orthodontics, dental anaesthetics, oral health education, special care, and radiography.

SEE WEB LINKS
• The National Examining Board for Dental Nurses website.

National Health Service (NHS) (in Britain) A publicly funded healthcare system established in 1948. It provides comprehensive therapeutic and preventive medical, dental, and surgical care including the prescription and dispensing of medicines, spectacles, and medical appliances. NHS dental care is provided through the hospital service, the salaried dental service, and by *general dental practitioners practising within the *general dental services. As a result of major changes to NHS dentistry (introduced in April 2006), *Primary Care Trusts (PCTs) are responsible for commissioning dental services; this covers routine care and specialized care services. Dental practices are legally permitted to provide a mixture of NHS and private care. The NHS dental services provided by general dental practitioners depend on local oral health needs and the contract agreed with the PCT.

SEE WEB LINKS
• The National Health Service web pages about the NHS.

National Health Service (Primary Care) Act 1997 (in Britain) An act of parliament to provide for new arrangements in relation to the provision within the National Health Service of medical, dental, pharmaceutical, and other services. It provided the legislation for pilot schemes of the *Personal Dental Service replaced in 2006 by a new contract for NHS dental practitioners.

SEE WEB LINKS
• The National Health Service (Primary Care) Act 1997 on the Office of Public Sector Information website.

National Institute for Health and Clinical Excellence (NICE) An independent organization responsible for providing national guidance on promoting good health and preventing and treating ill health. It produces guidance on public health, health technologies, and clinical practice. Guidance is developed using the expertise of the *National Health Service (NHS) and the wider healthcare community including NHS staff, healthcare professionals, patients and carers, industry, and the academic world. NICE has issued guidelines on a number of issues relevant to dentistry such as dental examination recall (clinical guideline 19). It also undertakes technology appraisals and issues guidance on interventional procedures e.g. the extraction of wisdom teeth.

SEE WEB LINKS
• The National Institute for Health and Clinical Excellence website.

National Institutes of Health (NIH) An agency within the United States Public Health Service comprising several institutes and constituent divisions, including the National

Library of Medicine and the National Institute for Dental Research. It is a part of the US Department of Health and Human Services, and is the primary Federal agency for conducting and supporting medical research.

• The National Institutes of Health website.

National Patient Safety Agency (NPSA)
A Special Health Authority, covering England, created in July 2001 to coordinate the efforts of the entire country to report, and to learn from, mistakes and problems that affect patient safety.

SEE WEB LINKS

• The National Patient Safety Agency website.

National Performance Frameworks
A system established in the UK to assess how well each part of the *National Health Service delivers quality services. They address issues such as the outcome of healthcare provided, access to healthcare facilities, the efficiency of the services provided, and the experiences of the patient or carer.

National Service Framework
A UK advisory body concerned with the organization of services within the *National Health Service and advising on the standard that these services are expected to meet.

National Training Number (NTN)
A number issued to doctors or dentists who have competed and been accepted for a training programme which may lead to the award of a **Certificate of Completion of Specialist Training** (CCST).

National Vocational Qualification (NVQ)
A framework of work-related, competence-based qualifications in the UK based on national occupational standards. They reflect the skills and knowledge needed to do a job effectively, and show that a candidate is competent in the area of work the NVQ represents. Dental nurses are eligible to be entered onto the *General Dental Council register if they have achieved the relevant NVQ at level 3 and have the appropriate clinical experience. *See also* VOCATIONAL RELATED QUALIFICATION.

nausea *n.* The feeling of sickness or a tendency to vomit.

nebulizer *n.* A device that turns liquid medication into a fine mist so that it can be inhaled into the airways and lungs.

neck *n.* 1. That part of a tooth where the crown joins the root. 2. The narrower area below the condylar process of the ramus of the mandible.

neckstrap *n.* An extra-oral component part of *headgear used in *orthodontic therapy. It is attached to the outer bow of the *facebow and exerts a distal and extrusive force on the molars or maxilla. It can be used for patients with a reduced *vertical dimension. *See also* HEADCAP.

necrosis *n.* The death of some or all the cells in a tissue or organ. It may be caused by disease, physical trauma, or chemical trauma (**chemonecrosis**), *radiation, or interruption of the blood supply. **Exanthematous necrosis** is a severe, often gangrenous inflammation involving the gingivae, maxilla, mandible, and associated soft tissues. It primarily affects children and is of unknown cause. *See also* NOMA. **Ischaemic necrosis**, due to loss of blood supply, can occur in the periodontal membrane usually as a result of occlusal traumatism or excessive forces being applied to a tooth during orthodontic therapy. Necrosis of bone tissue (**osteonecrosis**) may be caused by trauma, poor blood supply (ischaemia), infection, drugs, malignant neoplasia, or ionizing radiation. **Osteonecrosis of the jaw** (ONJ) is a known risk in patients being treated for osteoporosis with oral *bisphosphonate therapy. **Radionecrosis** is an unwanted side-effect of radiation therapy: it can affect the bone (*osteoradionecrosis), skin, muscles, and organs. It is characterized by *hyperaemia, inflammation of blood vessels (endarteritis), *thrombosis, cellular loss, reduced vascularity, and progressive *fibrosis; blood vessels become scarred and narrow, depriving the tissues of oxygen and other nutrients.

Further Reading: Arrain Y., Masud T. Recent recommendations on bisphosphonates-associated osteonecrosis of the jaw. *Dent Update* 2008;35:238–42.

necrotizing fasciitis A rare life-threatening bacterial infection of the layer of *fascia beneath the skin. It can arise as a complication of an infection of dental origin, particularly related to mandibular second and third molars. Prompt treatment is required with excision of the involved tissue and the administration of intravenous antibiotics.

necrotizing sialometaplasia An inflammatory benign self-limiting disease of the minor salivary glands, usually caused by a restricted blood supply (ischaemia). It is characterized by necrotic ulceration which is usually painless and may be mistaken clinically as a malignant disease. Predisposing factors include traumatic injury, denture-wearing, smoking, heavy alcohol consumption, and dental local anaesthetic injection. In most cases the hard palate is involved but other sites such as the lower lip, retromolar area, tongue, and parotid glands may also be involved. Treatment is by conservative management such as the use of an antiseptic mouthwash.

necrotizing stomatitis *See* STOMATITIS.

necrotizing ulcerative gingivitis *See* GINGIVITIS, NECROTIZING.

necrotizing ulcerative periodontitis *See* PERIODONTITIS, ACUTE ULCERATING.

need *n.* A condition referring to something that a person or people must have, such as a need for dental care. **Normative need** is the need of an individual or groups of individuals as defined by an expert or health professional. **Perceived need** is a patient's own assessment of what they want. **Expressed need** is perceived need converted into action and expressed as a demand. **Comparative need** is an assessment of the problems which emerge by comparison with others who are not in need, such as the comparison of oral healthcare facilities in different geographical areas in order to determine which areas are most deprived. **Unmet need** represents the shortfall or deficiency in meeting the need of an individual or group.

needle *n.* A sharp-pointed metal instrument used for penetrating tissue. A **biopsy needle** is hollow and is used for the removal of a tissue sample for examination. A **Gilmore needle** (dental standard BS 29917 & 6039) is used for measuring the working and setting time of a material such as dental cement or *plaster of Paris. **Hypodermic needles** are hollow and used for injecting substances such as local anaesthetic into tissues or for aspirating fluid from a cavity. **Local anaesthetic needles** are manufactured in varying lengths from about 35mm for nerve block injections to about 6mm for *intraligamentary injections; they are also made in varying gauges from 25 gauge for block injections to provide some needle rigidity to finer 27 or 30 gauge for intraligamentary analgesia. The finer gauge needles are, however, unreliable when checking for blood aspiration. A **suture needle** is a straight, curved, or J-shaped pointed needle used for sewing tissues; it may be round, cutting, or reverse cutting. Cutting needles have three cutting edges, one on either side and one on the inside curve. A 16–22mm curved cutting or reverse cutting needle held in a needle holder is used for most intra-oral surgery. The needle may be equipped with an eye for the *suture material or may have the suture material fused into it (a so-called **atraumatic needle**).

needle holder *n.* Forceps used to hold a suture *needle as it is passed through tissue.

needle-stick injury An accidental puncture injury, usually to the hands or fingers as a result of handling a sterile or contaminated needle. It can result in transmitted infections such as *hepatitis or *AIDS. A strict protocol should be observed when the injury involves a contaminated needle.

negligence *n.* The failure by a health professional to provide a patient with the degree of care and vigilance that the circumstances demand. **Clinical negligence** occurs when a dental professional's clinical management or performance falls below the standard expected of a reasonably competent dental professional acting in a manner considered acceptable by a responsible body of dental practitioners. To establish a claim for clinical negligence, the patient has to prove that the failure by the dental professional actually caused the injuries complained of.

Neisseria [A. L. S. Neisser (1855–1916), German physician] *n.* A genus of *Gram-negative, aerobic to facultatively *anaerobic, non-motile bacterial *diplococci. Several species of *Neisseria* are normal inhabitants of the mouth and respiratory tract. The genus also includes a number of *pathogenic species including *N. gonorrhoeae*, the causative agent of gonorrhoea, and *N. meningitidis*, one of the most common causes of bacterial meningitis.

neomycin *n.* An aminoglycoside *antibiotic used to treat mainly *Gram-negative bacterial infections of the skin. It is used in many topical medications such as creams, ointments, and eye drops. It may be combined with *bacitracin and known by the trade name **Cicatrin**.

neonatal *adj.* Pertaining to the first 4 weeks after birth. A **neonatal line** is produced by altered dentine or enamel, which marks the disruption in its formation at birth. It is only seen in primary teeth or first permanent molars; it can provide an important forensic landmark. **Neonatal teeth** may erupt during the period immediately after birth and continuing through the first 28 days of life. *See also* NATAL TEETH.

neoplasia *n.* The formation of abnormal cells due to genetic changes.

neoplasm *n.* (*adj.* **neoplastic**) A new or abnormal growth of tissue which is uncoordinated with that of the normal tissues; any *benign or *malignant tumour.

nerve *n.* A cordlike structure that transmits impulses either from the brain or spinal cord to muscles and glands (**motor nerves**), or in the opposite direction from the sense organs to the brain and spinal cord (**sensory nerves**). The nerve cell (**neurone**) consists of a nucleated cell body with projections (*dendrites) that receive stimuli. The nerve fibre (**axon**) is an extension of the neurone. There is a point of contact between one neurone and another (*synapse). The conduction of a stimulus along a nerve fibre is dependent upon changes in the electrophysiological status of the nerve membrane.

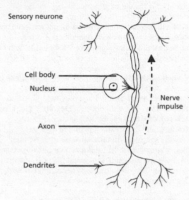

Sensory neurone

Cell body
Nucleus
Nerve impulse
Axon
Dendrites

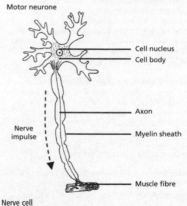

Motor neurone

Cell nucleus
Cell body
Axon
Nerve impulse
Myelin sheath
Muscle fibre

Nerve cell

((()) SEE WEB LINKS

• Eastern Kentucky University web pages that describe neurons and the nervous system.

nerve block A method of obtaining *analgesia in a defined region of the body by temporarily blocking the passage of pain impulses in the sensory *nerve of supply. A local analgesic, such as lignocaine, is injected into the tissues in close proximity to the nerve to produce a localized area of anaesthesia.

nervous system A network of specialized cells and tissues which carry information in the form of impulses to and from all parts of the body to provide sensory input or bodily action. The brain and spinal cord make up the **central nervous system**. The remaining **peripheral nervous system** includes the *sympathetic and *parasympathetic nervous systems.

Neumann's sheath [E. F. C. Neumann (1834–1918), German pathologist] The thin layer of dentine immediately surrounding each dentinal tubule.

neuralgia n. Pain associated with a nerve or nerves. **Post-herpetic neuralgia** is an intense debilitating pain following infection with *herpes zoster (shingles). The pain may be continuous and occurs in the distribution of the nerve that was affected by the herpes virus. **Trigeminal neuralgia (tic douloureux)** is characterized by severe paroxysms of pain, affecting areas of the face in the region of distribution of the trigeminal nerve and can be associated with involuntary contraction of the facial muscles; it is frequently initiated by a very minor stimulus (**trigger zone**) which causes sufferers to be very protective of the trigger zone. Treatment is usually by anticonvulsant drugs, although in severe cases neurosurgical treatment may be necessary. *See also* FACIAL PAIN.

Further Reading: Zakrzewska J. M., Lopez B. C. Trigeminal neuralgia. *Clin Evid* 2006;(15):1827–35.

neurapraxia n. A temporary loss of nerve function resulting in tingling, numbness, and weakness, usually due to trauma or nerve compression. It is followed by rapid and complete recovery.

neurilemmoma (schwannoma) n. A benign *neoplasm derived from the Schwann cells of the nerve sheath. Clinically it is similar to a *neurofibroma.

neuritis n. An inflammatory disease of peripheral nerves. It can cause pain over the associated nerves, disturbed sensation, paralysis, wasting, or loss of reflexes.

neurocranium n. Part of the skull enclosing the brain.

neurofibroma n. A benign *neoplasm derived from the cells of the nerve sheath. It is characterized by **Schwann cells** and fibroblasts.

They may occur at any site but in the oral cavity present as *sessile swellings.

neuroglia (glia) *n.* The specialized connective tissue of the central nervous system. It has various supportive and nutritive functions.

neuro-linguistic programming (NLP) A field of psychology that examines the way different people think and communicate with each other. NLP suggests that a person can communicate visually, auditorially, or *kinaesthetically.

Further Reading: Kay E. J., Tinsley S. *Communication and the dental team.* London: Stephen Hancocks Ltd, 2004, 60–75.

neuroma *n.* An overgrowth of nerve tissue usually associated with injury to a nerve such as following tooth extraction. They may also occur in multiple endocrine neoplasia syndrome.

neurone *n.* A nerve cell which forms the basic functional unit of the nervous system. *See also* NERVE.

neurosis *n.* (*pl.* **neuroses**) An emotional maladjustment with the predominant symptom of *anxiety together with possible impairment of thinking or judgement. It may be characterized by phobias, obsessions, compulsions, or sexual dysfunction. Neurosis is now more generally referred to as **anxiety disorder**.

neurotransmitter *n.* A specialized chemical substance (e.g. acetylcholine, dopamine, norepinephrine, serotonin) that sends a message from one nerve ending across gaps (*synapses) to other nerve endings.

neutral zone *n.* The potential space bounded by the lips and the cheeks on the one side and the tongue on the other; natural teeth situated in this area are subject to equal and opposite forces from the surrounding musculature. Artificial teeth are placed in the neutral zone to give maximum *stability.

neutropenia *n.* A decrease in the number of *neutrophils in the circulating blood. It can be caused by a wide variety of diseases and results in an increased susceptibility to infection. **Cyclic neutropenia** was first described by Leale in 1910; it is a rare condition of unknown aetiology that exhibits neutropenic episodes on a cyclical basis. Dental and oral symptoms include *aphthous ulcers and aggressive *periodontitis at a young age. *See also* CLASSIFICATION OF CONDITIONS OF THE PERIODONTIUM.

neutrophil *n.* A polymorphonuclear granular *leucocyte (*granulocyte) which provides an important role in defence against infection.

nevus *n. See* NAEVUS.

new variant CJD *See* CREUTZFELDT–JAKOB DISEASE.

NHS (National Health Service) Direct A 24-hour telephone and internet helpline established in the UK in 1997 providing advice about health, illness, and healthcare services on medical and dental issues. Since 2004 it has provided an NHS Direct digital TV service.

(((∰))) SEE WEB LINKS
• NHS Direct website.

nib *n.* The part of a condensing instrument that comes into contact with the material being condensed. The end (face) of it may be smooth or serrated.

nickel-chrome alloy *n.* A base metal alloy which may also include molybdenum and beryllium, used as an alternative to gold in the fabrication of metal-ceramic restorations and in the construction of removable partial denture frameworks. It has the advantage over gold in being cheaper, providing greater rigidity, and being stronger in thin section. The disadvantages include the potential biological hazards, difficult handling, and uncontrolled chromium oxide formation.

nickel-titanium alloy (NiTi) An alloy of titanium typically containing 50–55% nickel. Because of its strength and ability to deform without fracture it is used in orthodontics for brackets and wires and in endodontics, where nickel-titanium alloy files are used to clean and shape the root canals during root canal therapy.

nicorandil *n.* An oral medication used for the treatment and prevention of *angina by activation of potassium channels causing arterial and venous vasodilatation effects. It can result in severe oral ulceration which may occur many years after the start of treatment, especially with high doses, and which may be resistant to treatment. Trade name: **Ikorel.**

nicotine *n.* A substance derived from the leaves of the nightshade family of plants. In low concentrations it acts as a stimulant and is responsible for the addictive quality of cigarette *smoking. Pharmacologically this addictive quality is similar to that of heroine. Nicotine plays an indirect role in carcinogenesis by impeding the process of *apoptosis. Tobacco smoking and chewing are directly associated with the aetiology of oral squamous cell carcinomas. Nicotine has also been shown to be associated with the progression of *periodontitis.

nicotinic stomatitis *See* STOMATITIS.

nidus *n.* 1. A focus of infection as a result of favourable local conditions for bacterial growth. 2. The nucleus of a crystal.

nifedipine *n.* A dihydropyridine *calcium channel blocker used to control high blood pressure and *angina. Side-effects include fibrous enlargement (*hyperplasia, *fibromatosis) of the gingival tissues, disturbed taste and *erythema multiforme. The gingival hyperplasia is similar in clinical appearance to that produced by *phenytoin-associated gingival enlargement.

Further Reading: Gibson R. M., Meechan J. G. The effects of antihypertensive medication on dental treatment. *Dent Update* 2007;34:70–78.

night-grinding *See* BRUXISM.

night guard A removable acrylic resin appliance designed to cover the occlusal and incisal surfaces of the teeth to protect them from the destructive forces of *bruxism or night grinding.

Nikolskiy's sign [P. V. Nikolskiy (1858–1940), Russian dermatologist] *n.* A phenomenon of skin fragility used as a diagnostic criterion, first described by Valsiliyevich Nikolskiy in 1894. In 1957 **Sir William Lutz** described **Nikolskiy's phenomenon** as the condition in which gentle pressure applied to the mucosa may lead to the formation of a blister (*bulla) in certain oral diseases such as *pemphigus vulgaris.

Further Reading: Juneja M. Nikolskiy's sign revisited. *J Oral Sci* 2008;50:213–14.

nitrile rubber A synthetic rubber copolymer of acrylonitrile and butadiene used as an alternative to *latex for the manufacture of surgical gloves. Butadiene adds softness and flexibility and contributes to the elasticity of the glove. Nitrile is protein-free and is therefore less likely to cause the irritation and allergic reactions sometimes experienced with latex; however, many of the chemicals used in the manufacture of nitrile gloves are the same as those used for manufacturing latex gloves, and therefore allergic contact *dermatitis may still occur. Nitrile gloves are resistant to puncturing, tearing, and abrasion and are frequently coloured blue to make pin holes more visible. A high modulus of elasticity can lead to hand fatigue over time.

nitroglycerin *n. See* GLYCERYL TRINITRATE.

nitrous oxide Also known as dinitrogen oxide (N_2O). A colourless non-inflammable gas used in dentistry for its sedative, *anaesthetic, and *analgesic properties. It was first produced by Joseph Priestley, an English chemist, in 1772, and first used for a dental extraction by Horace Wells, an American dentist, in 1844. When inhaled alone it can produce euphoric effects, which has led to the common name of **laughing gas**. It is administered by inhalation in conjunction with oxygen as a method of *conscious sedation (relative analgesia) or when mixed with potent anaesthetic vapours such as isoflurane to produce general *anaesthesia. **Nitrous oxide cylinders** have a French blue shoulder; colour coding applies to the shoulder (curved part at the top of the cylinder) only and is harmonized within Europe under the *International Standards Organization (ISO 32); in the US colour coding is not regulated by law.

NK cell (natural killer cell) *n.* A type of lymphocyte that forms part of the natural immune system, capable of killing virus infected and cancerous cells. Their function is regulated by activating and inhibitory receptors.

NMES (non-milk extrinsic sugars) *n. See* SUGAR.

nociception *n.* The process of detection and signalling the presence of a noxious stimulus, including high-intensity mechanical, thermal, or chemical stimuli. **Nociceptors** are specialized sensory receptors that provide information about tissue damage; this information is processed by the central nervous system and experienced as pain. Nociceptors are classified according to the stimulus that activates them (mechanical, thermal, or polymodal).

node *n.* A swelling or knob of tissue. *Lymph nodes form part of the lymphatic drainage system.

nodule *n.* A small swelling or knot of tissue which can be easily felt. It may be present in the *epidermis, *dermis, or *subcutaneous tissue.

noma *n. See* CANCRUM ORIS.

nomenclature *n.* A system of names or naming as applied to the subjects or study in any art, science, or profession.

nominal variable *n. See* VARIABLE.

non-accidental injury *n. See* CHILD ABUSE.

non-milk extrinsic sugars (NMES) *n. See* SUGAR.

nonparametric statistics *n.* A branch of statistics used on data that are significantly skewed. The data distribution cannot be characterized by a few parameters. *Compare* PARAMETRIC STATISTICS.

n

non-steroidal anti-inflammatory drugs (NSAIDs) A group of drugs that interfere with biochemical mediators of inflammation, especially those associated with pain. By blocking the cyclo-oxygenase pathway, they interfere with prostaglandin synthesis in the peripheries. They act as anti-inflammatory agents as well as *analgesics and have a central *antipyretic action. This group of drugs includes *aspirin, *ibuprofen, mefenamic acid, and diclofenac. The use of NSAIDs in the treatment of chronic periodontitis remains controversial.

Further Reading: Milner N., Dickenson A., Thomas A. The use of NSAIDs in dentistry: a case study of gastrointestinal complications. *Dent Update* 2006;33(8):487-8, 491.

non-vital *adj.* Describing a tooth in which the pulp has undergone degenerative change (*necrosis) and does not respond to thermal or electrical stimulation. *Compare* VITAL.

non-working side The side away from which the mandible is moving (the working side) during lateral movement. It may be applied to natural or artificial teeth. *See also* BALANCING.

Noonan's syndrome [J. A. Noonan (1921–), US paediatrician] A genetic disorder affecting both males and females, with a family history reported in 50% of cases. It is characterized by heart defects, a webbed neck, chest deformity, learning disabilities, and short stature. Dental signs include *cysts and tumours in the mandible, congenital absence and delayed eruption of teeth, and severe periodontal disease.

Further Reading: Mendez H. M. M., Opitz J. M. Noonan syndrome: a review. *Am J Med Genet* 1985;21:493–506.

noradrenaline (norepinephrine, levarterenol) *n.* A hormone secreted by the medulla of the *adrenal gland and also released as a neurotransmitter by sympathetic nerve endings. It produces a wide range of actions, including an increase in blood pressure produced by constriction of small blood vessels. It is closely related to *adrenaline.

normoalveolism *n.* A condition in which the *alveolar process is normal in height, width, and position in relation to the respective jaw base.

normogenia *n.* A condition in which the chin prominence is adequate in height, projection, and width in relation to the mandible.

normomaxillism *n.* A condition in which the base of the maxilla is normal in length, width, and position.

nose *n.* The organ of the sense of smell (*olfaction), which also acts as an air passage to warm, moisten, and filter air on its passage to the lungs. The **external nose** is triangular in shape with two external openings (**nostrils**) and consists of cartilage covered by skin. It leads to the *nasal cavity which is divided into two chambers by the nasal septum. The nose can be divided into the root, dorsum, apex, and ala.

nosocomial infection *See* INFECTION.

nosode *n.* A homeopathic remedy prepared from diseased tissue or the product of disease.

notation *n. See* TOOTH NOTATION.

notch *n.* A depression or indentation. The **buccal notch** is found on a denture flange to accommodate the buccal *fraenum; the **labial notch** accommodates the labial fraenum. The **mandibular notch** is situated on the border of the ramus of the *mandible between the condyle and coronoid process. The **supraorbital notch** is a small depression (sometimes a foramen) on the supraorbital margin of the frontal bone through which pass the supraorbital nerve and vessels.

Novocaine *n.* The trade name for *procaine hydrochloride. Often used as a lay term for all types of dental local anaesthesia.

NSAIDs *See* NON-STEROIDAL ANTI-INFLAMMATORY DRUGS.

nucleotide *n.* One of the structural components, or building blocks, of *deoxyribonucleic acid (DNA) and **ribonucleic acid** (RNA). A nucleotide consists of a base (one of four chemicals: adenine, thymine, guanine, and cytosine) plus a molecule of sugar and one of phosphoric acid.

nudger appliance An *orthodontic appliance designed to achieve distal movement of the molar teeth. It incorporates palatal finger springs to retract the upper first permanent molars and is used in conjunction with bands on these teeth linked with *headgear.

Nuffield Report A document produced as a result of the Nuffield inquiry on the education and training of personnel auxiliary to dentistry, published in the UK in 1993 and named after the chairman of the inquiry, Lord Nuffield. It focused on a redefinition of the dental team through which dental care would be delivered and also examined whether and how far the role of auxiliaries could be expanded. It was concerned specifically with the education and training of auxiliary dental personnel now known as *dental care professionals (DCPs).

Further Reading: *Education and training of personnel auxiliary to dentistry.* London: Nuffield Foundation, 1993.

Baltutis L, Morgan M. The changing role of dental auxiliaries: A literature review. *Australian Dent J* 2008;43:354–8.

Nuhn's gland [A. Nuhn (1814–89), German anatomist] One of the small anterior sublingual *salivary glands situated either side of the *frenulum in the floor of the mouth.

null hypothesis (in statistics) The prediction that an observed difference is due to chance alone and not due to a specific cause; this hypothesis is tested by statistical analysis, and accepted or rejected. If the null hypothesis is proved to be true then the findings from the study are the result of chance or random factors.

number needed to treat (NNT) The number of people who must be exposed to a specific intervention to see one occurrence of a specific outcome.

nursing caries *n. See* CARIES.

nutrition *n.* The process by which essential food elements (e.g. carbohydrates, fats, proteins, vitamins, and mineral elements) in the diet are assimilated.

nystatin *n.* An antifungal drug of the polyene group which is active against *Candida albicans* and some other fungi. It is not absorbed by the gastrointestinal tract and has a topical effect only. It is used in the treatment of oral candidal infections in suspension form and should be used for 10–14 days.

n

objective structured clinical examination (OSCE) A method of assessment in which the candidate is required to attend a series of stations and undertake a clinical exercise at each station within a defined period of time.

obligate *adj.* Restricted to a particular set of environmental conditions without which an organism cannot survive e.g. an obligate anaerobe can only grow under anaerobic conditions.

oblique lateral radiograph An extra-oral radiograph that can be taken using a dental x-ray set which will allow visualization of the posterior teeth, angle, ramus, and condyle of the mandible and posterior maxilla. *See also* BIMOLAR RADIOGRAPH.

observational study *n.* Where the study is non-experimental and current behaviour is observed without intervention. No attempt is made to affect the outcome.

obtund *v.* To diminish or blunt sensitivity or pain.

obtundent *n.* An agent or drug that has the property of reducing or relieving pain.

obturation *n.* 1. The act of closing, obstructing, or occluding. 2. The process of filling the root canal system with an inert material following complete extirpation of the pulpal tissue. Research currently indicates that obturation beyond the radiographic apex of the root results in a poorer prognosis.

obturator *n.* A prosthesis used to close or cover a defect in the palate and restore the occlusion. The defect may be consequent upon the removal of a tumour or be congenital, as in a *cleft palate. An obturator is usually made of resin or a rubberized material and may be hollow to reduce the weight.

Further Reading: Walter J. Obturators for acquired palatal defects. *Dent Update* 2005;32(5):277–80, 283–4.

occipital bone *n.* The bone forming the back and part of the base of the cranium.

occipital triangle An anatomical description of a region of the neck. It is bounded posteriorly by the trapezius muscle, anteriorly by the sternocleidomastoid muscle, and inferiorly by the omohyoid muscle.

occiput *n.* The most posterior part of the skull.

occlude *v.* To close or shut. In dentistry it describes bringing the opposing jaws together to bring the teeth into contact.

occluding paper *n.* Inked paper or ribbon (usually blue or red) placed between natural or artificial teeth to record tooth contacts. *See also* WAX.

occlusal *adj.* Relating to the chewing or grinding surfaces of the molar or premolar teeth. *See also* TOOTH SURFACES.

occlusal adjustment The selective grinding of the occluding (contacting) surfaces of the teeth in order to remove premature contacts or occlusal interferences and to establish maximum masticatory efficiency. It is also undertaken to eliminate *occlusal trauma and abnormal muscle tension, to aid the stabilization of orthodontic therapy, to aid periodontal therapy, and following complex restorative treatment. It has been used to eliminate *temporomandibular joint problems, although the evidence to support this is controversial. *See also* BALANCED OCCLUSION.

Further Reading: Fricton J. Current evidence providing clarity in management of temporomandibular disorders: summary of a systematic review of randomized clinical trials for intra-oral appliances and occlusal therapies. *J Evid Based Dent Pract* 2006;6(1):48–52.
Milosevic A. Occlusion: 2. Occlusal splints, analysis and adjustment. *Dent Update* 2003;30(8):416–22.

occlusal analysis The study of the relationship of the occlusal surfaces of opposing teeth. It may be undertaken in the mouth or by the use of articulated study casts.

occlusal classification *See* INCISOR RELATIONSHIP; MOLAR RELATIONSHIP.

occlusal contact The point at which the occluding surfaces of one or more opposing posterior teeth meet. A **deflective occlusal contact** is a condition in which the tooth contacts divert the mandible from a normal path of closure; it may occur in the natural or artificial dentition. An **interceptive occlusal contact** is an interference with the normal movement of the mandible on initial tooth contact.

occlusal contouring The modification of the occlusal tooth *morphology to achieve a harmonious *occlusion and to protect the periodontal tissues.

occlusal curvature *See* CURVE OF MONSON; CURVE OF SPEE.

occlusal embrasure *See* EMBRASURE.

occlusal equilibration *See* EQUILIBRATION.

occlusal form *See* FORM.

occlusal guard *See* OCCLUSAL SPLINT.

occlusal indicator wax *See* WAX.

occlusal interference A condition that occurs when any tooth contact inhibits the remaining occluding tooth surfaces from achieving stable and harmonious contacts.

occlusal morphology *See* MORPHOLOGY.

occlusal neurosis *See* BRUXISM.

occlusal pattern The shape or form of the occlusal surface of a tooth or teeth which may or may not conform to that of the natural anatomical form.

occlusal plane An imaginary surface that theoretically touches the tips of the cusps of the posterior teeth and the incisal tips of the anterior teeth.

occlusal radiograph An intra-oral radiograph placed with the film between occluded teeth. It may be taken to show the upper anterior teeth (**standard upper occlusal**) or posterior teeth (**upper oblique occlusal**) or the mandibular teeth (**lower true occlusal**, **lower 45° occlusal** or **lower oblique occlusal**) ▣

occlusal record A means of recording the relationship between the occlusal surfaces of the maxillary and mandibular teeth. It allows the accurate articulation of laboratory plaster casts. It is usually created from a syringable *impression material or a *wax that is initially softened and hardens at mouth temperature.

Further Reading: Shargill I., Ashley M. Good night, squashbite: a 'how to' paper on better wax occlusal records. *Dent Update* 2006;33:626–31.

occlusal rest A rigid, usually metal, extension of a removable partial denture which rests on the occlusal surface of a posterior tooth for the support of a prosthesis. The occlusal rest is usually accommodated in a shallow prepared depression on the occlusal surface (**occlusal rest seat**) which allows the normal occlusal morphology of the tooth to be maintained.

occlusal rim The wax occlusal extension of a denture base used to establish jaw and tooth relationships during the construction of a complete or partial denture. Also known as **bite block**, **bite rim**, *bite plate, or **occlusal record block**.

occlusal splint (**occlusal guard**) A fabricated appliance, usually made from laboratory-processed acrylic resin, designed to cover the occlusal tooth surfaces and modify the occlusal contacts with the opposing dentition. The occlusal surface of the splint is flat without indentations so that the mandible is not guided into any predetermined position. An occlusal splint can have many functions, including to prevent tooth surface loss, to manage mandibular dysfunction, to create space to restore worn anterior teeth, to provide pre-restorative stabilization, and to protect the teeth and new restorations from destructive *parafunction.

Further Reading: Capp N. J. Part 3: Occlusion and splint therapy. *Br Dent J* 1999;186:217–22.
DuPont J. S. Jr, Brown C. E. Occlusal splints from the beginning to the present. *Cranio*. 2006;24(2):141–5.

occlusal table The total occlusal or grinding surface of the molars and premolars, including the *cusps, marginal *ridges, fossae, and grooves.

occlusal traumatism Abnormal occlusal contacts resulting in damage to the periodontium (periodontal *traumatism) or other supporting structures. Occlusal trauma has been investigated in relation to the progression of *periodontal disease. Studies do not support the role of occlusal trauma in the healthy, plaque-free dentition; there is evidence to suggest that occlusal trauma may be a risk factor for disease progression in the periodontium with established periodontitis. Diagnostic features include tooth mobility, tooth migration, discomfort on chewing or tooth percussion, muscle tenderness, excessive occlusal wear facets, chipped teeth, *fremitus, and radiographically visible widening of the periodontal ligament space.

occlusal vertical dimension (**OVD**) The vertical dimension, usually recorded from two fixed anatomical points, when the teeth (natural or artificial) or *occlusal rims are in contact. An increase in occlusal vertical dimension may occur as a result of a modification to the occlusal rims, tooth form or position, or denture rebasing or relining. A decrease in occlusal vertical dimension may result from attrition or drifting of the teeth, or the resorption of the alveolar ridges in edentulous patients.

occlusion *n*. 1. The relation of the upper and lower teeth when they are in contact. 2. The act of closing or the state of being closed. **Balanced occlusion** is the harmonious relationship between the upper and lower teeth of a natural or artificial dentition within the normal functional range of mandibular movement. It may be achieved entirely intra-orally or with the aid of an *articulator. **Centric occlusion** is the relationship of the mandible to the maxilla when the teeth are in maximum occlusal contact, irrespective of the position or alignment of the mandibular condyle. **Functional occlusion** refers to tooth contacts made within the functional range of the opposing teeth and is independent of aesthetics. **Lingualized occlusion** is where the maxillary teeth on a denture are placed buccally to the crest of the ridge so that occlusion only occurs between the palatal cusps of the upper teeth and the central fossae of the lower teeth, except for the first premolars where the situation is reversed. This occlusion has one upper tooth only contacting with its lower counterpart and not contacting any other tooth.

Further Reading: Davies S. Conformative, re-organized or unorganized. *Dent Update* 2004;31:334–45.
Davies S., Gray R. M. J. Occlusion: what is occlusion? *Br Dent J* 2001;191:235–41.

occupational disease A disease to which workers in specific occupations are particularly prone e.g. workers in contact with acid fumes can show evidence of acid tooth *erosion. Historically *mercury was used in the making of hats and the workers ingested the fumes; this resulted in mercury poisoning with kidney and brain damage (mad hatter syndrome).

odds *n*. A way of expressing the chance of an event, calculated by dividing the number of individuals in a sample who experienced the event by the number for whom it did not occur. For example, if in a sample of 100, 20 people were infected and 80 were infection free, the odds of being infected are 20/80 or 0.25.

odds ratio (OR) The odds of having the target condition or disease in the experimental group relative to the odds in favour of having the disease or condition in the *control group. The value of an odds ratio can be less than, equal to, or greater than 1. An odds ratio less than 1 indicates an inverse or negative association. The effects being measured may be adverse such as death, or desirable such as smoking cessation.

odontalgia *n*. (*adj*. **odontalgic**) Pain in a tooth or teeth (toothache). **Phantom odontalgia** is pain interpreted as toothache referred from an area or socket where a tooth has been extracted.

odontectomy *n*. The removal (usually surgically) of a tooth or tooth root.

odonterism *n*. Chattering of the teeth.

odontiasis *n*. *See* TEETHING.

odontoameloblastoma *n*. A very rare *odontogenic neoplasm containing dentine and enamel in the form of an odontome (*odontoma) with an epithelioid component that is similar to an *ameloblastoma in its locally aggressive behaviour.

odontoblast *n*. A dentine-forming cell. They are mesodermal in origin and are formed from cells at the periphery of the *dental papilla at about 17–18 weeks in utero. Odontoblasts are columnar cells that initially secrete a collagenous unmineralized matrix to form predentine; as they retreat towards the dental pulp they leave an elongated process (**odontoblast process**). Functionally active odontoblasts have long cell bodies, which contain a well-developed granular endoplasmic reticulum, many mitochondria, a Golgi apparatus, a nucleus, and several secretory vesicles; they secrete dentine throughout life. *See also* DENTINE.

odontocele *n*. A *cyst in the *alveolus of a tooth: a dentoalveolar cyst.

odontoclast *n*. A cell responsible for the resorption of *dentine and cementum. They are usually associated with the normal physiological resorption of the roots of the primary (deciduous) dentition prior to *exfoliation. Occasionally there may be pathological odontoclastic resorption of the roots of a permanent tooth.

odontoclastoma (pink spot) *n*. Internal tooth resorption which begins centrally within the tooth and is characterized by a pink discoloration of the crown. The resorbed tooth tissue is replaced by hyperplastic vascular tissue. *See also* ROOT RESORPTION.

Further Reading: Tripathi A. M., Pandey R. K. Odontoclastoma. *J Indian Soc Pedod Prev Dent* 2006;24(Suppl):S18–S19.

odontocnesis *n*. An itching sensation in the gingival tissue.

odontodynia *n*. *See* TOOTHACHE.

odontodysplasia (ghost teeth, odontogenesis imperfecta) *n.* A localized developmental disturbance of tooth formation causing multiple defects in the epithelial and mesenchymal tissues of tooth development characterized by abnormal tooth *morphology. The affected teeth have a rough discoloured surface with deficient dentine and enamel formation. The condition tends to affect several adjacent teeth, more commonly in the maxilla, but does not usually cross the midline. There may be evidence of mineralization in the pulp. The cause is unknown. *See also* AMELOGENESIS; DENTINOGENESIS.

Further Reading: Hamdan M. A., Sawair F. A., Rajab L. D., Hamdan A. M., Al-Omari I. K. Regional odontodysplasia: a review of the literature and report of a case. *Int J Paediatr Dent* 2004;14(5):363–70.

odontogenesis (odontogeny) *n.* The process of tooth formation and development.

odontogenesis imperfecta *n. See* ODONTODYSPLASIA.

odontogenic *adj.* Of or relating to the formation and development of teeth or tooth tissue.

odontogenic cyst *See* CYST.

odontogenic tumour Any one of a group of *lesions derived from the tooth-forming apparatus. They are only found in the jaws. *See also* AMELOBLASTOMA; AMELOBLASTIC FIBROMA; CEMENTOBLASTOMA; MYXOMA; ODONTOMA.

(⊕) SEE WEB LINKS

• A description of mandibular cysts and odontogenic tumours on the emedicine website.

odontogeny *n. See* ODONTOGENESIS.

odontoid *adj.* Shaped like a tooth.

odontology *n.* The scientific study of the structure and diseases of teeth. *See also* DENTISTRY.

odontolysis *n.* Tooth resorption. *See also* ROOT RESORPTION.

odontoma (odontome) *n.* A relatively common *benign *odontogenic malformation (*hamartoma) composed of dental hard tissues. Two types are recognized: a **complex odontoma** consists of a disorganized mixture of enamel, dentine, and cementum; a **compound odontoma** contains a more organized mixture of dental tissues often arranged to form miniature tooth-like structures surrounded by a fibrous sac. They often present in young patients and may cause a delay in or an abnormal path of eruption

of permanent teeth. Treatment is by surgical removal.

odontome *n. See* ODONTOMA.

odontometry *n.* The application of measurements and statistics in the study of the face, jaws, and teeth.

odontonomy *n.* The nomenclature of dental structures and tissues.

odontophobia *n.* An intense, abnormal, or illogical fear of teeth, usually applied to dentistry in general.

odontoplasty (enameloplasty, prophylactic odontotomy) *n.* The selective recontouring or reshaping of the morphological anomalies of the tooth surface, such as occlusal fissures, by removal of small amounts of enamel to change the surface, length, or shape of a tooth. This procedure has been adopted to reduce *plaque retention but has been largely replaced by the more conservative approach of using *fissure sealants.

odontoprisis *n.* The grinding together of the teeth. *See* BRUXISM.

odontorrhagia *n.* Profuse bleeding from the socket after the extraction of a tooth.

odontoscope *n.* 1. A device which contains a plane or magnifying dental mirror used for the examination of the teeth and oral tissues. 2. An optical device, similar to closed circuit television, that projects an image of the oral cavity onto a monitor to make multiple viewing possible.

odontoscopy *n.* The use of an *odontoscope for the examination of the oral cavity. It is used for the intimate examination of tooth structures such as to study the markings of the cutting edges of the tooth surfaces, used like fingerprints, as a method of forensic identification.

odontoseisis *n.* Looseness of a tooth or teeth.

odontotomy *n.* The act or procedure of cutting into the crown of a tooth. *Odontoplasty (prophylactic odontotomy) may be undertaken to improve plaque control.

odynophobia *n.* A morbid fear of pain.

oedema (*US* edema; *adj.* **oedematous,** *US* **edematous)** *n.* An accumulation of fluid in the body tissues which occurs during inflammation. **Angioneurotic oedema** is characterized by painless spontaneous swelling of the lips, cheeks, tongue, eyelids, soft palate, *pharynx, and *glottis due to increased permeability of the capillaries, often as a result of *allergy to food or drugs.

oesophagus (*US* **esophagus**) *n.* A muscular tube that extends from the *pharynx to the stomach, forming part of the digestive tract. It is about 25–30cm long and is the narrowest part of the gastrointestinal tract; it is lined with stratified squamous (non-keratinizing) *epithelium, becoming columnar at the stomach. Mucous glands are present in the mucosa and submucosa.

oil of cloves An essential oil from the clove plant. It contains the active ingredient *eugenol which has *analgesic properties and is included in some temporary tooth dressing materials. It can be irritant if applied topically to mucous membranes.

ointment *n.* A greasy substance which may or may not contain medication for use as a lubricant or as a topical application to the skin or mucous membrane.

olfaction *n.* (*adj.* **olfactory**) 1. The sense of smell. 2. The process of smelling. Specialized receptors are present in the mucous membrane (**olfactory epithelium**) lining the posterior part of the nasal cavity; these are stimulated by odorants (volatile chemical compounds) which send electrical signals via the olfactory nerve to the olfactory cortex of the brain.

oligodontia *n.* A condition in which one or more teeth are congenitally missing (partial *anodontia).

-ology *See* -LOGY.

-oma Suffix denoting a tumour e.g. **lymphoma** (of the lymph nodes).

omoclavicular triangle (subclavian triangle) *n.* An anatomical description of a triangular area of the neck bounded inferiorly by the clavicle, superiorly by the inferior belly of the omohyoid muscle, and anteriorly by the sternocleidomastoid muscle.

oncocyte *n.* An epithelial cell characterized by markedly pink cytoplasm containing numerous abnormal mitochondria. Their numbers increase with age in salivary glands; they are also found in certain salivary gland tumours.

oncocytoma *n.* A benign *neoplasm composed of *oncocytes.

oncogene *n.* A gene that has the potential to cause cancer.

oncogenic *adj.* Describing a substance, organism, or environment which is known to be a causal factor in the production of a tumour.

oncology *n.* The scientific study of tumours.

one-tailed test (in statistics) A test of a directional hypothesis. A **two-tailed test** is a test of a non-directional hypothesis.

onlay *n.* 1. A laboratory-processed restoration made of metal, porcelain, or resin composite that replaces one or more cusps and adjoining *occlusal surfaces of a tooth. 2. The *occlusal rest part of a removable partial denture that is extended to cover the entire occlusal surface of the tooth.

onplant (temporary anchorage device, orthodontic mini-implant) *n.* A *hydroxyapatite-coated thin titanium disc which sits on and is *osseointegrated with the palatal cortical bone beneath the *periosteum, and used as a means of *anchorage during orthodontic treatment. It is placed surgically and about 10 weeks later, after osseointegration has taken place, it is surgically exposed. It is removed on completion of orthodontic treatment under local anaesthetic. Onplants have advantages over implants in that they are less invasive, can be removed on completion of treatment, and are less expensive.

Further Reading: Skeggs R. M., Benson P. E., Dyer F. Reinforcement of anchorage during orthodontic brace treatment with implants or other surgical methods. *Cochrane Database of Systematic Reviews* 2007, Issue 3. Art. No.: CD005098. DOI: 10.1002/14651858.CD005098.pub2
Kalha A. S. Is anchorage reinforcement with implants effective in orthodontics? *Evidence-Based Dentistry* 2008;9:13–14.

onychophagia *n.* Habitual nail biting.

opacifier *n.* A material used to reduce the transparency or transluscency of a material. Metal oxides are used to opacify dental porcelains e.g. titanium oxide used to mask the metallic hue in porcelain fused to metal systems.

opalescent dentine *n.* Dentine which gives an unusually opalescent or translucent appearance to the teeth, usually associated with *dentinogenesis imperfecta.

opaque *adj.* Describing a material that does not transmit light but either absorbs it or reflects it from its surface. The degree of opacity is dependent upon the type of light source and the composition of the material.

open bite *See* BITE.

open contact *n.* A region in which there is a failure of adjacent teeth to make contact with each other. It can be due to a developmental anomaly, abnormal tooth position, missing teeth, oral disease, habits such as pencil sucking, or an overdevelopment of the fraenal attachments. It can result in *food trapping and lead to *periodontal disease or *caries.

operative dentistry The specialist area of dentistry concerned with the functional, restorative, and aesthetic problems associated with the teeth.

operculectomy *n.* The surgical removal of the flap of mucosal tissue (*operculum) that partially or completely covers an unerupted or partially erupted tooth. It may be undertaken for the treatment of *pericoronitis, often associated with a partially erupted mandibular third molar.

operculitis *n. See* PERICORONITIS.

operculum *n.* The flap of mucosal tissue that partially or completely covers an unerupted or partially erupted tooth.

ophthalmic *adj.* Relating to the eye.

opisthion *n.* The midpoint on the posterior border of the *foramen magnum. It is used as a *craniometric landmark.

opisthogenia *n.* Defective development of the jaws following *ankylosis of the jaw.

opportunistic disease *n.* A disease that occurs due to an impairment of the patient's immune system such as by an infection, another disease, or by drugs.

opsialgia *n.* Facial *neuralgia.

optimization *n.* The process of keeping all radiation exposures as low as reasonably practicable (ALARP), taking into account both social and economic factors.

Orabase® *n.* The brand name of a topical dental paste containing an adrenocorticoid (hydrocortisone acetate). It is used for the temporary relief of symptoms associated with oral inflammation such as *aphthous ulcers.

oral *adj.* 1. Pertaining to the mouth. 2. Taken by mouth (e.g. medicines).

oral and maxillofacial pathology A specialized area within dentistry concerned with the causes, pathogenesis, and diagnosis of oral diseases including the mucosa, jaws, and salivary glands. The histological changes in the tissues are studied by microscopy and a report issued indicating the changes and diagnosis.

oral cancer A *malignant neoplasm of any structure or tissue within the oral cavity. Most oral cancers are squamous cell *carcinomas which commonly involve the lips, lateral border of the tongue, floor of the mouth, and retromolar area (posterior to the third molars). The clinical features of oral cancer can include long-standing asymptomatic ulceration, firmness or hardness on palpation, and, in advanced cases, hard cervical *lymph nodes with loss of weight and pale complexion. Some cancers may appear as velvety red patches (*erythroplakia) or may arise from pre-existing raised white patches (*leukoplakia). Causative agents include *carcinogens in tobacco (smoking and smokeless tobacco including paan), and sunlight on the lips. *Alcohol itself is not carcinogenic but it potentiates the effects of carcinogens by increasing the permeability of the oral mucosa. Oral squamous cell carcinoma infiltrates local tissues and spreads via the lymphatics to the cervical lymph nodes, where it may escape into the tissues of the neck. Oral cancer *screening is an important part of routine dental examinations. Early diagnosis by *biopsy is essential for a good outcome *prognosis. Treatment is by surgical excision which may be accompanied by *radiotherapy. The prognosis tends to be generally worse when tumours arise in the more posterior parts of the oral cavity and oropharynx, when they are large, or have spread to the cervical lymph nodes and tissues of the neck. The incidence of oral cancer is rising particularly in the young and this may be related to an increase in alcohol consumption.

Further Reading: Scully C., Newman L., Bagan J. V. The role of the dental team in preventing and diagnosing cancer: 2. Oral cancer risk factors. *Dent Update* 2005;32(5):261–2, 264–6, 269–70.

Kujan O., Glenny A. M., Oliver R. J., Thakker N., Sloan P. Screening programmes for the early detection and prevention of oral cancer. *Cochrane Database of Systematic Reviews* 2006, Issue 3. Art.No.CD004150.DOI:10.1002/14651858.CD004150. pub2

oral cavity *n. See* CAVITY, ORAL.

oral flora Micro-organisms that normally inhabit the oral cavity, of which bacteria are the predominant group. The oral cavity is sterile at birth, but quickly becomes colonized by *bacteria (both aerobic and facultative anaerobic organisms). With the eruption of the teeth, the microbial flora becomes more complex. More than 700 bacterial species have been identified in the healthy oral cavity, many of which are site- and subject-specific. Most sites possess a *biofilm containing 20–30 different predominant species that alter in the presence of disease such as *caries or *periodontal disease. The bacteria in oral biofilms cluster together to form microcolonies which provide an anaerobic environment at the centre and a more aerobic environment at the periphery, resulting in a diversity of species. Oral bacteria can be classified primarily into Gram-positive and Gram-negative micro-organisms, and secondarily as being either *anaerobic or facultatively anaerobic, according to their oxygen requirements. Bacteria which are commonly isolated from the healthy oral flora include *Streptococcus mutans, Streptococcus salivarius, Streptococcus mitis, Staphylococcus aureus, Streptococcus intermedius, Actinomyces israelli*, and *Lactobacillus acidophilus*.

Further Reading: Aas J. A., Paster B. J., Stokes L. N., Olsen I., Dewhirst F. E. Defining the normal bacterial flora of the oral cavity. *J Clin Microbiol* 2005;43(11):5721–32.

oral health education (OHE) The process of providing individuals with personally relevant information about their oral health based on scientific principles and evidence. It involves motivating, teaching, and training both individuals and small groups. Successful oral health education is influenced by attitudes, beliefs, and values.

Further Reading: Levine R. S. The scientific basis of dental health education. A Health Education Council Policy Document. *Br Dent J* 1985;158(6):223–6.

oral health index (OHI) A statistical measure that quantifies a number of aspects of an individual's oral health status and assigns them a numerical value.

Further Reading: Burke F. J., Busby M., McHugh S., Delargy S., Mullins A., Matthews R. Evaluation of an oral health scoring system by dentists in general dental practice. *Br Dent J* 2003;194(4):215–18.

oral health promotion (OHP) The process of oral health education that encompasses involvement in planning and evaluating strategies, identifying and networking with appropriate agencies and individuals, and working with health educators to maximize their effectiveness. It can also include political lobbying and influencing policy makers in the healthcare domain.

Further Reading: Petersen P. E., Kwan S. Evaluation of community-based oral health promotion and oral disease prevention – WHO recommendations for improved evidence in public health practice. *Community Dent Health* 2004;21 (4 Suppl):319–29.

oral hygiene The practice of personal maintenance and cleanliness of the hard and soft tissues of the oral cavity. **Oral hygiene instruction** involves instruction on the use of a variety of oral hygiene aids including toothbrushes, toothpaste (*dentifrice), dental floss, dental tape, interdental brushes, wood points, and disclosing agents, and

why these may be of benefit. *See also* PLAQUE CONTROL.

oral hygiene index *See* GREENE–VERMILLION INDEX.

oral irrigator An oral hygiene device for delivering under pressure fluid such as water, sometimes together with antibacterial solutions and other *medicaments, for the purpose of flushing out loose debris and *plaque in areas of the mouth that are difficult to access (e.g. beneath fixed bridgework). It may also be used for subgingival irrigation of periodontal pockets. The device may be electrically or manually powered.

oral jewellery Objects attached to the teeth for the purposes of adornment and serving no functional value. Although it has been used for many years, it has recently become more popular; it usually takes the form of crystal embellishments bonded to the labial surfaces of anterior teeth using *resin composite. It may also include non-functional colour-contrasting inlays in crowns or prosthetic appliances. *See also* ORAL PIERCING.

oral medicine A specialty concerned with the oral healthcare of patients with chronic recurrent and medically related disorders of the mouth and with their diagnosis and non-surgical management.

oral microbiology The scientific study of micro-organisms of the oral cavity and their interactions with each other and the host. It is a clinical specialty undertaken by laboratory-based personnel who provide reports and advice based on the interpretation of microbiological data.

oral mucosa *See* MUCOSA.

oral pantomograph *See* DENTAL PANORAMIC TOMOGRAM.

oral pathology The study of the disease processes of the structures within and associated with the oral cavity, with the aim of understanding their nature and causes and dealing with their management.

oral piercing The penetration of the oral soft tissues, such as the lips (*labrette), tongue, cheeks, fraenum, or uvula, followed by the insertion of a metal ring, stud, or bar. It is becoming increasingly popular and is usually carried out for cosmetic, religious, cultural, or sexual reasons. It may be undertaken by placing a needle of the same shape and size as the device being inserted into the tissues inside a plastic sheath and puncturing the soft tissue. The needle is then removed, leaving the sheath in situ until a temporary device is placed. The temporary device must be longer than the permanent replacement to allow for post-operative swelling. A permanent device may be inserted at the time of perforation or after 3–6 weeks. Complications include haemorrhage, nerve damage, pain, swelling, infection, and trauma to both the hard and soft tissues.

(((🌐))) SEE WEB LINKS

• A comprehensive overview of oral piercing on the American Dental Association website.

oral rehabilitation The procedure of reconstructing a dentition which has been damaged by disease, wear, or trauma aimed at improving function or aesthetics.

oral surgery A specialized area of dentistry that deals with the diagnosis and treatment of oral conditions of the jaws and structures associated with the mouth that require surgical intervention.

oral ulceration A break or defect through the full thickness of the oral epithelium, exposing the underlying connective tissue to saliva and micro-organisms. The surface of the ulcer is covered by a white-grey slough composed of *fibrin and neutrophils and the base is replaced by *granulation tissue (endothelial cells and fibroblasts) infiltrated by lymphocytes and plasma cells. The margins appear red and inflamed. **Traumatic oral ulceration** may be caused by sharp tooth edges, orthodontic appliances, ill-fitting dentures, or habits such as lip or cheek biting (**factious ulceration**). The shape, size, and position of the ulcer, which is accompanied by redness and inflammation of the surrounding connective tissue, is related to the suspected cause. Once the cause is removed, healing usually takes place within a few days. **Chemical ulceration** is relatively uncommon but may be caused by drugs such as *aspirin tablets being placed on the oral mucosa; injudicious use of *phosphoric acid used in the *acid-etch technique can result in ulceration of the lips or gingival tissues. **Neoplastic ulceration** is normally painless and diagnosed by *biopsy (*see also* ORAL CANCER). The ingestion of excessively hot foods or liquids can result in **thermal ulceration**; healing usually occurs quickly and without the formation of scar tissue. Oral ulceration is also a feature of *aphthous ulcers, *oral cancer, some viral infections such as *herpes, bacterial infections including tuberculosis and syphilis, certain autoimmune blistering conditions such as *pemphigus vulgaris and pemphigoid, and gastrointestinal diseases such as Crohn's disease.

oral vestibule *See* VESTIBULE.

orbitale *n.* The lowest point on the lower edge of the orbit that may be felt under the skin which is used as a reference point in *cephalometric analysis. It is the point at which the tip of the *orbital marker on a *facebow is placed.

orbital marker The projection on a *facebow that marks the position of the *orbitale. It is used as a marker for the orientation of plaster casts on an *articulator.

ordinal data Data that are classified into more than two discrete categories which have a natural order and can be ranked, for example, heavy smokers, light smokers, and non-smokers.

ordinal variable *n. See* VARIABLE.

organ *n.* A part of the body composed of more than one tissue which has a specific function. *See also* ENAMEL ORGAN.

origin *n.* 1. The point of attachment of a muscle that remains relatively fixed during contraction of the muscle. *Compare* INSERTION. 2. The point at which a nerve or blood vessel branches from a main nerve or blood vessel.

oroantral fistula An abnormal pathway that connects the oral cavity with the *maxillary antrum. It can be created unintentionally following the extraction of an upper posterior tooth with roots that penetrate the antrum. It is usually treated by surgical closure if healing is not spontaneous.

orodigitalfacial dysostosis (OFD syndrome) A rare condition in which there is abnormal development of the jaws, tongue, lip, palate, and malformation of the bones of the skull. There may also be malformation of the fingers and learning disabilities.

orofacial granulomatosis (OFG) A diffuse swelling of the lips, and/or cheeks, and face characterized by *granulomas in the tissues. It is associated with allergy to various foodstufs as well as Crohn's disease and sarcoid. *See also* MELKERSSON–ROSENTHAL SYNDROME.

orofacial pain Pain involving the facial and oral regions which may be of dental or non-dental origin. Pain from the dento-alveolar complex may be pulpal, dentinal, or periodontal in origin or may also arise from thermal sensitivity, *cracked tooth syndrome, or maxillary *sinusitis. Orofacial pain may arise from the musculo-ligamentous or soft tissues such as idiopathic orofacial pain, temperomandibular dysfunction, salivary gland disease, oral lesions, *candidiasis, or malignancy. Orofacial pain of neurological or vascular origin may be associated with *burning mouth syndrome, *trigeminal neuralgia, cluster headache, post-herpetic neuralgia, cranial arteritis, or glossopharyngeal neuralgia. *See also* FACIAL PAIN.

Further Reading: Zakrzawska J. M. Diagnosis and management of non-dental orofacial pain. *Dent Update* 2007;34:134–9.

oronasal *adj.* Pertaining to the mouth and nose. An **oronasal fistula** is an abnormal communication between the mouth and nasal cavity; this may cause problems with fluids and solids passing from the mouth to the nose and if large may result in speech defects. Most can be treated by surgical closure.

oropharynx *n.* (*adj.* **oropharyngeal**) The part of the *pharynx that lies between the junction of the hard and soft *palates above, the *hyoid bone below, and the arch of the soft palate anteriorly. It contains the *tonsils.

orthodentine *n.* Dentine containing tubes through which nutrients pass from the pulp tissue; these tubes are seen in mammalian teeth.

orthodontic appliance An appliance used to move teeth as part of orthodontic therapy. Movement of the teeth may be achieved by intra-oral or extra-oral *traction. **Fixed appliances** are attached directly to the teeth. The components of fixed appliances, namely *bands or *brackets, adhere to the tooth surface and archwires attached to them apply a force to the teeth and are capable of changing the mesio-distal angle of the teeth (tipping), changing the bucco-lingual inclination of the teeth (*torquing), rotating or bodily moving teeth. They utilize *archwires and *auxiliaries (e.g. ligatures, elastics, springs, separators). Fixed appliances have an advantage over removable appliances in that they can be used for multiple tooth movement and they make it possible to exercise precise control over force distribution to individual teeth. Examples are the *edgewise, *Begg, and *tip-edge appliances. **Removable appliances** are capable of being removed by the patient for cleaning. They can be used as active appliances by utilizing springs, wires, bows, screws, elastics, or the acrylic resin baseplate. A **functional appliance** (**myofunctional appliance**) is used to correct jaw disharmonies by modifying the growth of the jaws in an actively growing patient by utilizing the forces generated within the masticatory and facial muscles. They act on both upper and lower teeth at the same time and may be either fixed or removable. Changes induced by functional appliances are thought to be due to changes in the dento-alveolar complex, skeletal changes, or changes in the *glenoid fossa of the *temporomandibular joint. There are many different appliance types used to treat specific malocclusions; these include the *Andresen, *Bimler, *Frankel, *monobloc, and *twin block appliances. A **lingual orthodontic appliance** is a fixed orthodontic appliance placed on the lingual or palatal tooth surface. A **vacuum-formed appliance** is usually made of clear plastic, using a 'suck-down' machine that forces the plastic to adapt to the contours of the model; it is often used as a retainer following active treatment but may also be used for minor tooth movements.

orthodontic nurse *See* DENTAL NURSE.

orthodontics *pl. n.* (*adj.* **orthodontic**) *n.* The specialist branch of dentistry concerned with the growth and development of the face and jaws and the treatment of irregularities of the teeth.

orthodontic specialist list A list, first established in 1998, held by the General Dental Council in the UK of orthodontists who have undergone an approved period of postgraduate training that has led to the attainment of a relevant qualification. The list is published annually in paper and electronic formats.

orthodontic specialist practitioner A dental practitioner who has received specialist postgraduate education and is able to provide advice on the need for orthodontic therapy and any intervention required in a developing *malocclusion. They can also provide treatment for patients with moderate or severe malocclusions who may need treatment by means of removable, functional, or upper or lower fixed *orthodontic appliances.

orthodontic therapist *See* THERAPIST, DENTAL.

orthodontic tube *See* TUBE.

orthodontist *n.* A dental specialist who has undertaken appropriate postgraduate training in the special area of orthodontics.

orthognathic *adj.* Describing a condition of the upper jaw in which it is in an approximately vertical relationship. **Orthognathic surgery** is the surgical correction of severe *malocclusion in which development of one or both jaws is abnormal. The skeletal discrepancy can occur in an antero-posterior, vertical, or transverse plane of space or any combination of all three. Treatment is usually undertaken in conjunction with orthodontic therapy; additionally, restorative treatment may be involved if there are missing, damaged, or malformed teeth.

orthograde root filling See ROOT FILLING.

orthopantomograph *n.* See DENTAL PANORAMIC TOMOGRAM.

orthopnoea *n.* A breathing difficulty that occurs when lying flat. It is a symptom of *heart failure. It can also occur in individuals with *asthma or chronic bronchitis.

orthostaphyline *adj.* See CHAMESTAPHYLINE.

osmosis *n.* The diffusion of a *solvent from a less concentrated solution to a more concentrated solution through a semipermeable membrane. This tends to result in an equalization of the concentration of the two solutions. In living organisms, the distribution of water (the solvent) through cell membranes (the semipermeable membrane) is an important process. The **osmotic pressure** is the pressure generated by water moving by osmosis through a semipermeable membrane; the more concentrated the solution, the greater is the osmotic pressure.

osphresis *n.* **(***adj.* **osphretic)** The sense of smell.

osseointegration *n.* A direct structural, functional, and biological adhesion between living bone and the surface of a load-carrying *titanium implant without a foreign-body reaction. The dental implant is retained rigidly within the bone without any functional mobility because of the absence of a *periodontal membrane between the bone and the implant.

osseous dysplasia See DYSPLASIA.

ossification (osteogenesis) *n.* The process of bone formation by the action of bone forming cells (*osteoblasts). Bone may form by the conversion of cartilage into bone (**endochondral ossification**), such as occurs in the long bones, or by development from tissue or membrane (**intramembranous ossification**) as in the formation of the bones of the skull.

ossifying fibroma See FIBROMA.

ostectomy (osteoectomy) *n.* The surgical removal of alveolar bone around a tooth root to improve the bone contour and eliminate an intra-bony periodontal pocket.

osteitis *n.* Inflammation of the bone due to infection, trauma, or metabolic disorder.

Localized osteitis of the alveolar process following tooth extraction is usually referred to as *alveolitis or dry socket. **Condensing osteitis** is characterized by unusually dense bone, sometimes associated with non-vital teeth or at the site of extraction of non-vital teeth. **Osteitis deformans** is a condition of unknown cause in which there are repeated episodes of bone resorption followed by periods of repair resulting in weakened dense-deformed bones. Radiographically the bone has a cotton wool appearance. It is characterized clinically by enlarged cranial bones and frequently enlargement of the mandible or maxillae. The teeth may show *hypercementosis resulting in difficulties with extraction and, due to the dense bone and reduced blood supply, they are predisposed to infection. The condition is also known as **Paget's disease** [Sir James Paget (1814–99), English surgeon].

osteo- Prefix denoting bone.

osteoarthritis *n.* A chronic degenerative disease of the joints resulting in painful and restrictive movement. The condition very rarely affects the temporomandibular joint.

osteoblast *n.* A cuboidal-shaped cell responsible for the formation of bone.

osteoblastoma *n.* A rare usually *benign primary *neoplasm of the bone, characterized histologically by the formation of immature bone (*osteoid) and fibrovascular connective tissue. It can produce pain of several months' duration. The cause is unknown.

osteocementum *n.* A hard bone-like layer of secondary *cementum deposited after root formation is complete. It is typically laid down in incremental layers because of intermittent deposition on the root surface. See also HYPERCEMENTOSIS.

osteoclast *n.* A large multinucleate cell responsible for the resorption of bone. Their activity allows tooth movement through bone to take place during orthodontic therapy.

osteoclastoma *n.* A *benign tumour of bone characterized by numerous multinucleate giant cells that resemble osteoclasts. It occurs near the end of long bones and is rarely if at all seen in the jaw bones. Occasionally it may become malignant.

osteochondroma *n.* A rare benign lesion of osseous and cartilaginous origin. It is characterized by growing hyaline *cartilage at the periphery of the tumour, which ossifies upon cessation of growth. It rarely occurs in the facial bones but has been reported occurring in the mandibular condyle.

osteocyte *n.* A bone cell: an *osteoblast that has ceased bone-forming activity and has become embedded in the bone matrix.

osteodistraction *n.* The gradual and controlled displacement of a surgical fracture. It is used in oral and maxillofacial surgery such as in the correction of alveolar bone defects. The gap (distraction zone) created by the bone displacement fills with immature non-calcified bone which subsequently matures during the fixation period.

osteoectomy *n. See* OSTECTOMY.

osteogenesis (ossification) *n.* The formation of bone by the action of special cells (*osteoblasts). A meshwork of *collagen is first laid down, followed by a cementing polysaccharide. The cement is finally impregnated with tiny crystals of calcium. On completion of bone formation, the osteoblasts become trapped within the matrix as *osteocytes. Osteogenesis may be encouraged as part of a planned surgical procedure (*distraction osteogenesis).

osteogenesis imperfecta (fragilitas ossium) *n.* A congenital genetic, often inherited, condition characterized by unusually brittle and fragile bones. It is caused by mutations in the genes that code for Type 1 collagen and at least seven recognized forms of the disorder occur, representing a range of severities. It may also be associated with *dentinogenesis imperfecta and deformed teeth.

osteoid *n.* A protein mixture (mucopolysaccharide-protein complex) secreted by *osteoblasts which later becomes calcified to form *bone.

osteoma (*pl.* **osteomata)** *n.* A *benign overgrowth of bone (*exostosis) caused by excessive osteoblast activity. When occurring on long bones they can be painful. In the jaws they may occur as part of Gardner's syndrome.

Further Reading: Goodger N. M., Jones J. Giant osteomata of the mandible. *Dent Update* 2004;31:224–29.

osteomalacia *n.* A condition of the skeleton, usually due to a deficiency of *vitamin D, and characterized by softening of the bones because of reduced mineralization. When it occurs in children it is called *rickets.

osteomyelitis *n.* Inflammation of the bone due to infection. **Acute osteomyelitis** occurs most commonly in children when bacteria from another infected site enter the bone from the bloodstream and is characterized by severe pain, tenderness, and redness over the involved bone. **Chronic osteomyelitis** may develop from acute osteomyelitis or following surgery involving bone tissue. It is characterized by pus accumulation and the formation of islands of necrotic bone (*sequestra). Pain and swelling are always present, although less severe than in the acute condition. Radiologically the sequestra appear as radiopaque surrounded by areas of radiolucency. Predisposing factors include trauma, radiotherapy, and systemic conditions such as *diabetes, *AIDS and *osteoporosis, malnutrition, and immunosuppression. Alcohol and tobacco use are frequently associated with osteomyelitis. It is seen rarely in the jaws but may occur following oral surgery or a traumatic tooth extraction due to the contiguous spread of infection from pulpal or periapical tissues; when it does occur, it is more common in the mandible than the maxilla because of the greater bone density and reduced blood supply. It is treated by prolonged antibiotic therapy. **Garre's osteomyelitis** [C. Garre (1857–1928), Swiss surgeon] is a type of chronic sclerosing osteomyelitis that primarily affects children and adolescents; this rare condition is usually associated with either chronic periocoronitis or chronic periapical periodontitis, which results in a proliferative response of the periosteum. It is characterized by swelling and usually affects the body and ramus of the mandible.

osteonecrosis *n. See* NECROSIS.

osteopathy *n.* The study of the inter-relationship between the structure of the body and the way in which it functions. It offers a form of diagnosis and therapy for many problems affecting the neuro-musculo-skeletal systems. Treatment can include palpation, manipulation, and massage.

osteopenia *n.* A reduction in bone mineral density characterized by increased bone radiolucency. It is not as severe as, but may develop into, *osteoporosis. Metabolic or eating disorders such as *anorexia nervosa can contribute to this condition due to the deficiency of vitamins and minerals.

(()) SEE WEB LINKS

• An overview of osteopenia on the WebMD website.

osteopetrosis (Albers–Schönberg disease, marble bone disease) *n.* A congenital abnormality characterized by abnormally dense and brittle bones which have a tendency to fracture. It may be associated with delayed tooth eruption, and *osteomyelitis or *necrosis following dental infection.

osteoplasty *n.* The surgical reshaping of bone, such as the reshaping of the *alveolar process to produce a contour favourable for a healthy *periodontium without the loss of bone support for the tooth roots.

osteoporosis *n.* A systemic disorder resulting in brittle bones which have a tendency to fracture. It usually occurs in the elderly and in women it often follows the menopause. Evidence of osteoporosis in the jaws may be seen radiographically by a loss of alveolar bone height not directly related to periodontal disease. Prevention relies on regular exercise, adequate diet, and avoidance of smoking and excessive alcohol consumption.

osteoradionecrosis (ORN) *n.* A condition where osteomyelitis develops at a site of radiation injury; it can be spontaneous but most commonly results from tissue injury such as denture-related injury, ulcers, periodontal procedures, or tooth extraction. Pain may be severe and there may be a raised body temperature (pyrexia). It is the result of a reduction in bone vascularity and damage to the bone cells (*osteocytes) due to radiation damage which reduce their potential for repair. The mandible is more commonly affected than the maxilla because of its natural reduced vascularity. The overlying mucosa often appears pale due to radiation damage.

osteosarcoma *n.* A malignant *neoplasm of bone. It is most common in the long bones and relatively rare in the jaws.

osteosclerosis *n.* An abnormal increase in the density of bone. It can occur as a result of poor blood supply, chronic infection, or a tumour. It may also occur as a sign of excessive ingestion of fluoride either occurring naturally or introduced artificially into the water supply.

osteotome *n.* An instrument used for cutting or dividing bone. The blades may be curved, straight, or interchangeable.

osteotomy *n.* The surgical process of cutting a bone into two sections followed by realignment. The mandible may be advanced or retracted by splitting it bilaterally in the region of the molar teeth (**sagittal split osteotomy**); this procedure is usually undertaken as part of orthognathic therapy.

(⊕) SEE WEB LINKS
- A review of orthognathic surgery of the mandible on the University of Oulu website.

Ottawa Charter A document on health promotion defined by the *World Health Organization in 1986. It identified the key areas of health promotion to be: building a healthy public policy, creating supporting environments, developing personal skills, strengthening community action, and reorienting health services towards prevention and health promotion.

(⊕) SEE WEB LINKS
- A detailed description of the Ottawa Charter on the World Health Organization website.

outlier *n.* (in statistics) Any value that is markedly smaller or larger than other values in a data set.

outline form *n. See* FORM.

out of hours service *See* EMERGENCY DENTAL SERVICE.

out-patient *n.* A person who receives treatment, examination, or observation in a hospital but is not admitted to a bed in a hospital ward. *Compare* IN-PATIENT; DAY-PATIENT.

overbite *n.* The vertical overlap of the incisor teeth. It is described as **average**, when the upper incisors overlap the lower incisors by a third of their height, **reduced** when the upper incisors overlap the lower incisors by less than a third of their height, or **increased** when the upper incisors overlap the lower incisors by more than a third of their height. An overbite can also be described as **complete** where there is contact between the lower incisors and either the upper incisors or the junction of the teeth with the palate, or **incomplete** where the lower incisors make no contact with the opposing upper incisors or the palatal mucosa when the buccal segment teeth are in *occlusion. *Compare* OVERJET.

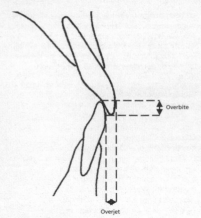

Overbite and overjet

Further Reading: Naini F. B., Gill D. S., Sharma A., Tredwin C. The aetiology, diagnosis and management of deep overbite. *Dent Update* 2006;33(6):326–8, 330–32, 334–6.

overclosure *n.* A form of malocclusion in which the jaws are in an abnormally close relationship. It is caused by a loss of occlusal *vertical dimension usually due to tooth loss or *attrition in the natural dentition.

overcontour *n.* An overbuilding of the crown of a tooth as part of a restorative process. Overcontouring can cause a loss of the normal self-cleansing morphology of the tooth, resulting in potential periodontal problems.

overcrowding *n.* A condition in which there is insufficient room in the dental arch to accommodate all the teeth present.

overdenture *n.* A complete or partial denture provided with additional retention or support by being placed over or attached to existing retained teeth, tooth roots, or *implants. Overdentures may be tooth (or implant) supported or tooth (or implant) and tissue supported. Benefits of overdentures can include prevention of *alveolar bone loss by retention of teeth or tooth roots, improved speech, management of tooth wear, improved jaw alignment, and improved masticatory efficiency. Retention (resistance to vertical displacement) and stability (resistance to lateral or rotational displacement) are enhanced in comparison with conventional complete or partial dentures. A high standard of oral hygiene must be maintained to minimize the risk of caries on the root faces.

overeruption *n.* The condition of having a tooth extruded from its socket such that the occlusal surface of the tooth extends beyond the normal *occlusal plane. It is particularly likely to occur when a tooth is unopposed; the contact area between the over-erupted tooth and the adjacent teeth is lost. This creates an increased clinical risk of dental caries and periodontal disease on the exposed root surface of the over-erupted tooth.

Further Reading: Craddock H. L., Franklin P. Overeruption – another challenge? *Dent Update* 2005;32(10):605–8, 610.

overextension *n.* The extension of the periphery of a prosthetic or *orthodontic appliance such that it excessively compresses the mucosal tissues or impinges on the muscular attachments.

overhang *n.* 1. An excess of restorative material projecting beyond the cavity margin. 2. An overcontoured crown margin projecting beyond the crown preparation margin. An overhang creates a site for dental plaque accumulation and an increased risk for the development of *gingivitis and *periodontitis.

overjet *n.* The horizontal distance between the labial surface of the tips of the upper incisors and the labial surface of the lower incisors. *Compare* OVERBITE. A **reverse overjet** occurs when the mandibular incisor edges occlude anterior to the mandibular incisor edges.

overlap (horizontal) *n. See* OVERJET.

overlap (vertical) *n. See* OVERBITE.

overlay *n. See* ONLAY.

Overseas Registration Examination (ORE) *See* INTERNATIONAL QUALIFYING EXAMINATION.

Owen's contour lines *See* CONTOUR LINES OF OWEN.

oximetry *n.* The determination of the oxygen saturation of the blood by measuring the amount of light transmitted through an area of skin. *See also* PULSE OXIMETER.

oxygen *n.* An odourless, colourless gas that makes up 20% of the atmosphere. It combines with glucose to provide energy for metabolic processes. It is transported in the blood by combining with *haemoglobin in red blood cells to form oxyhaemoglobin. The amount of oxygen in the tissues is termed the **oxygen tension** and is measured in kilopascals (kPa). Oxygen is administered with the sedative drug nitrous oxide, using specialized equipment, to achieve conscious *sedation (relative analgesia) by inhalation. **Oxygen cylinders** have a white shoulder (previously black in the UK); colour coding applies to the shoulder (curved part at the top of the cylinder) only and is harmonized within Europe under the *International Standards Organization (ISO 32); in the US colour coding is not regulated by law.

oxygen inhibition layer A thin (approximately 1–3µ) layer of non-polymerized resin on the surface of a resin composite material produced as a result of the action of atmospheric oxygen. The oxygen inhibition layer consists of mainly uncured monomers. Viscous glycerine-based gels are designed to prevent the formation of an oxygen inhibition layer on the surface of resin materials when they are polymerized. Trade name: **DeOx®**.

ozone *n.* An allotrope of oxygen (O_3) containing three oxygen atoms. It is a powerful oxidizing agent and has been advocated for the treatment of *caries because of its ability to kill the great majority of micro-organisms in carious lesions; however, the evidence is currently conflicting.

Further Reading: Baysan A., Lynch E. The use of ozone in dentistry and medicine. *Prim Dent Care* 2005;12(2):47–52.

ozostomia *n.* Having bad breath (*halitosis).

pachy- Prefix denoting thickening of a part or parts.

pachyglossia *n*. Abnormal thickness of the tongue.

pachygnathous *adj*. Describing a condition characterized by a large or thick jaw.

pachyonychia congenita *n*. A rare hereditary condition that can affect the nails, skin, mouth, hair, larynx, and eyes. It is characterized by oval benign white patches on the tongue and oral mucosa.

(⊕) SEE WEB LINKS
• Emedicine web page giving an overview of the condition.

pack *n*. A protective material used to fill a space, prevent wound contamination, or to prevent haemorrhage. A **periodontal pack** or dressing is used to protect the gingival tissues after periodontal surgery; periodontal packs may contain *eugenol (e.g. zinc oxide eugenol paste) or be eugenol-free (e.g. **COE-PAK™ dressing**, the brand name of a chemically cured glyoxide dressing material which does not contain asbestos). They are applied as a soft putty-like material that sets hard after a few minutes but remains pliable. The pack is normally left in situ for about one week after surgery.

pad, dental dam *n*. A piece of gauze or absorbent material placed between the *dental dam and the face as a means of facial protection.

pad, retromolar *n*. The mass of soft tissue located at the *distal end of the mandibular ridge behind the last molar tooth.

paediatric dentistry (*US* **pediatric dentistry**) *n*. The specialist branch of dentistry concerned with the oral healthcare of children and adolescents.

paedodontics (*US* **pedodontics**) *n. See* PAEDIATRIC DENTISTRY.

Paget's disease *n. See* OSTEITIS.

pain *n*. An unpleasant sensation produced in response to impulses from the peripheral nerves in damaged tissue transmitted along nerve pathways to the central nervous system. **Pain control** is achieved by the use of *analgesics either acting centrally on the central nervous system such as *aspirin, *ibuprofen, and *paracetamol, or locally using topical or injected analgesics such as *benzocaine and *lignocaine. **Referred pain** (synalgia) is pain produced by a causative agent in one area but manifested in another (e.g. pain from pulpitis referred from a maxillary tooth to a mandibular tooth). *See also* ODONTALGIA.

pairwise comparison (in statistics) The comparison of a pair of *means.

palatal *adj*. Relating to the palate. The palatal surface of a tooth is that surface adjacent to the palate. *See also* TOOTH SURFACES.

palatal bar *n. See* BAR.

palatal index (palatomaxillary index, palatine index) The ratio of the length of the hard palate (palatomaxillary length) to its width (palatomaxillary width) multiplied by 100. The measurement of the length is from the most anterior point on the maxillary anterior process in the midline (alveolar point) to the middle of a transverse line touching the posterior borders of the two maxillae; the measurement of the width is from the outer borders of the alveolar arch just above the middle of the second permanent molar tooth. It is used in anthropology to define the varying forms of the dental arch and palate.

palatal plate *See* PLATE.

palatal shelf A medially directed outgrowth of the embryonic *maxilla which fuses with its opposite number to form the secondary *palate. Failure of the secondary palate to develop correctly may result in a *cleft palate.

palate *n*. (*adj*. **palatal**) The bone and soft tissue that forms the roof of the mouth and separates the mouth from the nasal cavity. The **development of the palate** begins at about 5 to 6 weeks of intrauterine life, when the fronto-nasal process forms the medial and lateral nasal processes, the primary nasal septum, and the **primary palate** (the primary palate contains the maxillary incisor teeth). A *palatal shelf develops laterally behind the primary nasal septum from the two maxillary processes. The *secondary nasal septum grows from the roof of the primitive oral cavity, dividing the nasal cavity into two chambers. The palatal shelves contact each other to form the **secondary palate** separating the oral and nasal cavities. The secondary palate anteriorly becomes the **hard palate** which includes the palatal extensions of the maxillary and palatine bones covered by mucous membrane and posteriorly the **soft palate**, a flexible fold of mucous membrane that tapers at the back of the mouth to form a fleshy flap of tissue, the *uvula. Failure of the maxillary and nasal processes to fuse can result in a *cleft lip or palate.

palatine *adj.* Relating to the palate or palatal processes.

palatine bone The bone forming the posterior part of the hard palate (**horizontal plate**) and the lateral wall of the nose and the floor of the orbit (**vertical plate**). It has pyramidal, orbital, and sphenoidal processes.

palatine index *See* PALATAL INDEX.

palatomaxillary index *See* PALATAL INDEX.

palatoplasty *n.* The surgical repair of defects of the palate.

palatorrhaphy *n.* The surgical repair of a cleft palate using sutures.

palladium *n.* A metallic element (Pd) resistant to tarnish and corrosion; it is used in dental alloys with copper, cobalt, silver, or gold for inlays, bridgework, and orthodontic appliances. It is now less popular as an alloy because it is more expensive than gold.

palliative *n.* An agent or medicine which temporarily relieves without actually curing the disease.

pallor *n.* Abnormal paleness of the skin.

Palmer tooth notation *n.* *See* TOOTH NOTATION.

palm grip *n.* *See* GRIP.

palpation *n.* A method of examination by using the hands or fingers. It enables solid and fluid-filled swellings to be distinguished.

palpitation *n.* An uncomfortable awareness of the heart beat. Palpitation may be due to a normal heart beat made more prominent by anxiety, emotion, or exercise, or may be a symptom of heart disease, arrhythmias, neurosis, or overactivity of the circulation.

palsy *n.* *See* BELL'S PALSY.

panacea *n.* A medicine or remedy claimed to be a cure for all diseases.

pancreas *n.* A compound gland situated behind the stomach that releases enzymes concerned with digestion into the duodenum via the pancreatic duct. The gland contains isolated groups of cells (*islets of Langerhans) which secrete *insulin and *glucagon into the bloodstream.

pandemic *n.* An *epidemic that spreads through human populations over a very wide area, crossing international boundaries and usually affecting a large number of people.

Pankey, Lindsey Dewey, Snr

(1901–1989) He qualified in dentistry at the University of Louisville and entered dental practice in Kentucky. In 1943 he was elected President of the American Association of Dental Examiners. He is most well known for advocating a new philosophy in dentistry and for his work and publications on occlusal rehabilitation. He retired from dental practice in 1969. In 1971 he was elected an honorary fellow of the Academy of Prosthodontists and in 1972 the Pankey Institute was established in his name to continue his educational philosophy.

(((⊕))) SEE WEB LINKS

• The Pankey Institute website.

panoral *adj.* Pertaining to the whole mouth. A **panoral radiograph** includes all the teeth in both dental arches on one film. *See* DENTAL PANORAMIC TOMOGRAM.

panoramic radiograph *n.* *See* DENTAL PANORAMIC TOMOGRAM.

pantograph *n.* An instrument used to measure or record mandibular jaw movements during reconstructive restorative therapy. The jaw movements may be recorded on an articulator, on paper (**pantographic tracing**), or electronically by interfacing with a computer.

paper point *n.* A cone of absorbent paper available in assorted sizes and used by inserting

into a root canal to absorb fluids, transfer
*medicaments, or to take fluid samples for
culture.

papilla *n.* (*pl.* **papillae**) Any small nipple-
shaped protuberance. The **circumvallate papillae**
are situated on the dorsum of the *tongue
immediately in front of a V-shaped groove (sulcus
terminalis): they number 10–15 and are 1–2mm
diameter mushroom-shaped papillae surrounded
by a trough. The **dental papilla** is a condensation
of *mesenchymal cells formed during tooth
development and located beneath the inner
*enamel epithelium which eventually forms the
*pulp of the fully developed tooth. The **filiform
papillae** are situated on the dorsum of the tongue
and are numerous conical elevations which give
the tongue its rough texture. **Fungiform papillae**
contain *taste buds and can be seen as numerous
red dots at the tip and sides of the tongue. **Foliate
papilla** contain taste buds and are found
posteriorly along the lateral borders of the tongue.
The **incisive papilla** is a soft tissue elevation
situated palatal to the upper central incisors and
covering the incisive *foramen. The **interdental
papilla** fills the interproximal space between two
adjacent teeth. The **interproximal papilla** is a
conical projection of gingival tissue which fills the
interdental space up to the contact area when
viewed from the labial, buccal, lingual, or palatal
aspects; when viewed buccolingually the
interproximal papilla appears as a rounded cavity
below the contact area; this is known as the
interdental *col. The **parotid papilla** is a small soft
tissue projection on the buccal mucosa near the
maxillary second molar which guards the
entrance into the oral cavity of the *parotid duct.
The **retrocuspid papilla** is a small raised nodule
of gingival tissue with a broad or pedunculated
base on the lingual side of the mandibular
canines usually occurring bilaterally; it is a
normal anatomical feature which may regress
with age and requires no treatment.

**papillary marginal attached (PMA)
index** A numerical system for recording the
gingival health used primarily in children. It was
first described by I. Schour and M. Massler in
1947. The 'P' represents that part of the gingival
tissue occupying the interproximal space between
two teeth (papilla); the 'M' represents the free
gingival tissue collar on the labial, lingual, and
buccal aspects of the teeth (marginal gingiva) and
the 'A' represents the gingiva firmly attached to
the underlying bone (attached gingiva). The
severity of the inflammation is indicated on a
scale of 0–4. When first described, only the labial
gingivae of the lower six anterior teeth were
examined.

**papillary marginal gingival index
(PMGI)** A numerical system of scoring gingival
inflammation which is a combination of the
*papillary marginal attached index and the
*gingival index of Loe and Silness, first described
by M. De La Rosa and O. P. Sturzenberger in 1976.
The labial and lingual papillae and margins are
scored 0 for no inflammation, 1 for mild
inflammation, 2 for moderate inflammation, and
3 for severe inflammation. The individual score is
the number of inflammatory scores divided by the
number of sites examined.

papillary marginal (PM) index An index
based on gingival margin bleeding on gentle
probing as an early sign of periodontal disease. It
has been renamed the *sulcus bleeding index
(SBI).

**papillary marginal recession (PMR)
index** A periodontal index in which the
recession (R) component replaces the attached
gingiva (A) component of the *papillary marginal
attached (PMA) index.

papilloma *n.* (*adj.* **papillomatous**) A benign
wart-like *neoplasm of the *epithelium or
*mucosa. A **squamous cell papilloma** of the
mouth usually occurs on the tongue and the
inside surfaces of the cheeks or lips and is
probably of viral origin; it is an oral variant of the
common wart (*verruca vulgaris). Single lesions
are most common and are characterized by soft
pedunculated swellings which are either pink
when non-keratinized or white if heavily
*keratinized; they usually require no treatment
but, if indicated, treatment is by surgical
excision. 📷

(⊕) SEE WEB LINKS

• DermNet NZ web page giving details of squamous
cell papilloma of the mouth and throat.

papillomatosis *n.* A disorder presenting with
multiple papillomas forming a microscopically
undulating surface such as *Cowden's syndrome.

Papillon Lefévre syndrome (PLS) A very
rare genetic disorder also known as **focal
palmoplantar and gingival hyperkeratosis**, first
described by M. M. Papillon and Paul Lefévre in
1924, that usually becomes apparent in the first 5
years of life. It is characterized by the
development of dry scaly patches
(*hyperkeratosis) on the skin of the palms of the
hands and the soles of the feet, attached gingivae,
retromolar pads, and the palate, together with
severe inflammation and degeneration of the
periodontal structures. The intra-oral
hyperkeratosis is more generalized than that seen
in frictional *keratosis due to trauma such as

friction from excessively heavy toothbrushing. The primary (deciduous) teeth frequently become loose and fall out by about 5 years of age. Without treatment, most of the permanent teeth may also be lost by approximately the age of 17. Additional symptoms may include pus-producing skin infections, abnormalities of the nails, and excessive perspiration; fissuring on the hands and feet can cause pain. Treatment is by a multidisciplinary approach.

papule *n.* A pimple. It is a solid raised lesion with distinct borders and is usually less than 1cm ($^3/_8$ inch) in diameter. Papules may be domed, flat-topped, or umbilicated and are often associated with secondary features such as scales or crusts. Unlike a *vesicle, a papule does not contain fluid.

para- Prefix denoting 1. By the side of or close to, e.g. **paranasal** (near the nasal cavity). 2. Resembling, e.g. **paradysentery** (a mild form of dysentery). 3. Abnormal, e.g. **paralalia** (abnormal speech).

paracetamol (acetaminophen) *n.* An analgesic drug that also reduces fever; it is used to treat mild to moderate pain such as toothache. It has no significant anti-inflammatory property. Side-effects may include digestive upsets and overdosage can cause liver damage; this can be a significant problem for patients with severe dental pain which may therefore result in accidental overdose. Liver damage can occur with doses of 10–15g / day and death at 25g / day. Trade names: **Calpol, Panadol, Panaleve.**

parachlorophenol (PCP) *n.* An antibacterial agent effective against most *Gram-negative organisms. It has been used alone or camphorated ($^1/_3$ parachlorophenol, $^2/_3$ camphor) as a topical application to disinfect root canals. Its use has declined because of its cytotoxicity and potential for damage to adjacent tissues.

parachute chain A metal chain having a finger ring at one end and a clip at the other capable of being attached to an endodontic *file or *reamer to prevent it from being inhaled or swallowed. This technique is not considered to be as effective as *dental dam isolation.

paracone *n.* The mesio-buccal cusp of a mammalian upper molar tooth.

paraconid *n.* The mesio-buccal cusp of a mammalian lower molar tooth.

paradontal (paradental) *adj.* Describing a location next to or alongside a tooth.

paradontosis *n.* An outmoded term used to describe *periodontitis as a degenerative condition. It was often used in relation to juvenile periodontitis.

paraesthesia *n.* A tingling or **pins and needles** sensation due to disruption of nerve function. It is a normal sensation experienced as the effect of a local anaesthetic begins to wear off. It can also occur as a result of nerve damage following surgery, trauma, or malignant involvement of the nerves. It can be a symptom of adrenocortical hormone insufficiency, vitamin B_{12} deficiency, a side-effect of some medications, and some neurological conditions and pathology.

paraformaldehyde *n.* A polymer of formaldehyde formerly used as a *devitalization preparation in the *pulpotomy procedure for a primary tooth. It penetrates through dentine and is gradually released as *formaldehyde, which has a destructive effect on periodontal and bone tissues. The material is no longer advocated because of its associated toxicity and potential carcinogenicity. Trade name: **Toxavit.**

Further Reading: Özgöz M., Yagiz H., Çiçek Y., Tezel A. Gingival necrosis following the use of a paraformaldehyde-containing paste: a case report. *International Endodontic Journal* 2004;37(2):157–61.

parafunction *n.* A normal movement of the mandible at an abnormal frequency (e.g. tooth *grinding or *clenching). It can take many forms such as single episodes (clenching) or rhythmic contractions (grinding). It can lead to tooth *attrition and more rarely to *temporomandibular joint dysfunction. Significant parafunction occurs during sleep. Symptoms of parafunction include headache, migraine, facial pain, jaw or neck pain often associated with restriction of movement, sinus pain, or feeling of pressure. Therapeutic management is directed at the parafunction's four components of intensity, duration, frequency, and position.

Further Reading: Porter R., Poyser N., Briggs P., Kelleher M. Demolition experts: Management of the parafunctional patient: 1. Diagnosis and prevention. *Dent Update* 2007;34:198–207.

parakeratosis *n.* An increase in the formation of parakeratin on the surface of stratified squamous epithelium.

paralgesia *n.* A disorder or abnormality of the sense of pain.

parallax *n.* The apparent motion of an object in relation to its adjacent structures when viewed from two different positions because of a perspective shift. It is a method used in dental *radiography to determine the position of an object in relationship to its adjacent structures by taking two radiographs at slightly different angles by changing the position of the x-ray tube. The object furthest from the x-ray beam will appear to move in the same direction as the tube shift. It is useful in determining whether an unerupted tooth lies buccal or palatal to the line of the arch.

paralleling technique A method of taking an intra-oral *radiograph in which the film is held in a film holder parallel to the tooth and the x-ray beam is directed at 90° to the tooth and the film. A 20cm *focus to skin distance is required to ensure that the x-ray beam is parallel rather than divergent. It gives less geometric distortion than the *bisecting angle technique and allows the use of rectangular *collimation.

parallelism n. The condition of two or more surfaces or lines which if extended to infinity would never meet. In prosthetic or restorative dentistry it is a principle used to gain maximum retention between vertical tooth surfaces and a restoration or appliance.

parallelometer n. An instrument used to establish the extent to which two or more objects are parallel with each other or to achieve *parallelism between two or more objects. *See also* SURVEYOR.

paralysis n. (*adj.* **paralytic**) Loss or impairment of muscle function due to nerve damage, usually as a result of disease or trauma.

paramedic n. A person trained to assist medical professionals and to provide emergency medical treatment.

parametric statistics Statistics carried out on data which are suitable for arithmetic operations such as addition and subtraction. This enables precise numbers (parameters) such as *mean and *standard deviation to be defined. They are appropriate where the population is normally distributed. *Compare* NONPARAMETRIC STATISTICS.

paramolar n. A *supernumerary tooth, usually rudimentary, in the molar region. They are most common in the maxillary arch of the permanent dentition.

paranasal sinus n. *See* SINUS.

paraplegia n. (*adj.* **paraplegic**) Paralysis of both legs and affecting all parts below the site of injury or disease of the spinal cord.

parapremolar n. A *supernumerary tooth that forms in the premolar region and resembles a premolar tooth.

parasite n. (*adj.* **parasitic**) Any living organism that lives in or on another living organism (host): they include fungi, bacteria, and viruses.

parastyle n. A minor cusp or fold of enamel on the buccal aspect of the occlusal surface of a maxillary molar or premolar situated mesial to the *mesostyle and buccal to the *paracone present in some mammalian or primate species.

parasympathetic nervous system One of the two divisions of the autonomic nervous system. It has nerve fibres that leave the brain and the lower part of the spinal cord and which supply internal organs, glands, and tissues and regulate their involuntary activity. It frequently opposes the actions of the *sympathetic nervous system.

parathyroid glands Two pairs of small *endocrine glands situated behind the *thyroid gland (but outside its capsule) which control the distribution of calcium and phosphate in the body. Each pair is located one above the other (superior and inferior) and are about the size of peas. An increase in parathyroid hormone can cause demineralization of bone. A lack of parathyroid hormone can lead to delayed dental development and *enamel hypoplasia.

parenteral *adj.* Administered by any way other than through the mouth (e.g. by injection).

parietal bone n. One of a pair of irregularly shaped quadrilateral bones situated between the frontal and occipital bones which together form the sides of the cranium.

PAR index *See* PEER ASSESSMENT RATING INDEX.

Parkinson's disease (PD) [J. Parkinson (1755–1824), British physician] A degenerative neurological disorder usually associated with aging. It may occur before the age of 40 (**young-onset PD**) and very rarely before the age of 20 (**juvenile PD**). It is characterized by slow, staccato-like movement; postural instability; tremor of the arms and head even at rest; and speech and swallowing difficulties. The control of the airway during dental procedures can present difficulties. A decreased quantity or quality of saliva can lead to *xerostomia and root caries. Oral hygiene tends to be poor because of the reduced manual dexterity.

paronychia n. *See* WHITLOW.

parotid gland *See* SALIVARY GLAND.

parotitis n. Inflammation of the parotid gland. **Acute bacterial parotitis** is characterized by redness, pain, tenderness, and swelling over the affected gland, often with a discharge of pus from the opening of the parotid duct on the inside of the cheek. It may occur following radiotherapy or in patients with a compromised immune system; treatment is with antibiotics and pain relief. **Infectious parotitis** (*mumps) is caused by a viral infection of one or both parotid glands. **Chronic recurrent parotitis** is characterized by discomfort and repeated swelling of the parotid gland frequently after eating; it is associated with a decreased flow of saliva, often due to a narrowing of the parotid duct or blockage by a *salivary stone. Less common causes of parotitis are *actinomycosis and *Sjögren's syndrome.

Parrot's ulcer [J. M. J. Parrot (1839–83), French physician] *n.* Ulcerative lesions of the mucous membrane seen in *thrush or *stomatitis.

partial anodontia *See* ANODONTIA.

partial denture *See* DENTURE.

parulis *n.* An inflammatory nodule on the gingival margin at the site of the opening of a draining sinus tract (gumboil). *See also* ABSCESS.

Passavant's ridge [P. G. Passavant (1815–93), German surgeon] *n.* (Passavant's bar, Passavant's pad) A bulge which appears on the posterior wall of the *pharynx during swallowing due to the constriction of the upper part of the pharyngeal constrictor muscle.

passive *adj.* Describing an orthodontic appliance which has been adjusted so as to provide no effective force on a tooth, teeth, or jaw. *Compare* ACTIVE.

passive eruption The apparent continued eruption of a tooth which is due to regression of the gingivae and surrounding alveolar bone and not to the movement of the tooth.

paste *n.* A semi-fluid, frequently medicated mixture. **Filler paste** is a thin easily displaced mixture of materials used to fill the root canal system. **Polishing paste**, used to smooth restorations and polish tooth surfaces, contains an abrasive such as pumice or diamond grit. **Pressure-indicating paste** is a thin, opaque, easily displaced material used to disclose areas of premature contact under restorations or prosthetic appliances. **Prophylactic paste** contains a number of abrasive materials with fluoride added to inhibit the caries process; it is used to aid the removal of tooth surface deposits and staining.

patch test *n.* A method used to determine if a specific substance causes inflammation of the skin (contact *dermatitis). It is often used to test for an *allergen. The allergen to be tested is first diluted in an appropriate vehicle to minimize its irritant potential; it is then fixed to the skin and covered with tape, usually on the upper back or upper arm. The tests are generally left on the skin for 48 hours to allow sufficient penetration of allergen to provoke a reaction.

patent *adj.* Open or unobstructed; applied to a hollow tube such as a root canal or airway.

path *n.* A defined course that is usually followed. The **centric path of closure** is the path taken by the mandible during closure when the musculature is in balance. The **occlusal path** is the line of movement of an occlusal surface as it glides over an opposing surface. The **path of insertion** is the direction in which a prosthesis is inserted into the mouth or a cast restoration is inserted into a tooth.

pathodontia *n.* The study of dental diseases.

pathogen *n.* (*adj.* **pathogenic**) An infectious agent, usually a micro-organism, capable of causing disease. Normal microbial flora and the immune system can protect the host from infection by pathogens. However, pathogens can cause disease when natural defences are breached. Normal commensal flora can behave as opportunistic (also called opportunist) pathogens in severely immunocompromised hosts (e.g. oral candidiasis caused by *Candida albicans* in HIV-infected and AIDS patients).

pathogenesis *n.* The mechanism by which an etiological agent (e.g. micro-organism) causes disease or the development of a disease from its beginning to its manifestation of *signs or *symptoms.

pathognomonic *adj.* Describing a *sign or *symptom that is diagnostic for a particular disease and that is unique to, or characteristic of, a specific disease (e.g. pseudomembranes on tonsils, pharynx, and nasal cavity are pathognomonic for diphtheria). Individual pathognomonic signs are relatively uncommon.

pathology *n.* (*n.* **pathologist**) The branch of medicine concerned with the study of disease and disease processes.

pathosis *n.* A disease entity or pathologic condition; a patient is said to have a pathosis, not a *pathology.

patrix *n.* The male portion of a *precision attachment. *Compare* MATRIX.

pattern *n.* A form or shape used to make a mould such as for an inlay or partial denture. *See also* OCCLUSAL PATTERN; WAX PATTERN; TOOTH WEAR.

pearl (enamel) *n. See* ENAMEL PEARL.

pediatric dentistry *See* PAEDIATRIC DENTISTRY.

pedicle flap *See* FLAP.

pedodontics *n. See* PAEDIATRIC DENTISTRY.

pedunculated *adj.* Raised on the end of a narrow stalk-like process. *Compare* SESSILE.

peer assessment rating (PAR) index An index used to assess the outcome of orthodontic treatment based on an evaluation of the pre- and post-treatment study models. A score is assigned to various occlusal traits that make up a malocclusion; these are then weighted and summated to obtain a total that represents the extent of deviation from normal alignment and occlusion; a low score indicates a low level of irregularity. The difference between the pre- and post-treatment scores represents the degree of improvement.

Further Reading: Richmond S., Shaw W. C., Roberts C. T., Andrews M. The PAR Index (Peer Assessment Rating): methods to determine outcome of orthodontic treatment in terms of improvement and standards. *Eur J Orthod* 1992;14 (3):180–87.

peer review 1. The procedure by which academic journal articles are reviewed by other researchers before being accepted for publication. 2. The process by which the activity of a professional is reviewed by one or more other professionals, usually in the same geographical area and specialty.

peg-shaped tooth A developmental anomaly, usually of the maxillary lateral incisor, which causes it to resemble a small peg; it may be associated with a missing lateral incisor in the other maxillary quadrant. The crown of the third molar may sometimes fail to develop fully and can also resemble a small peg.

pelican *n.* A beak-shaped instrument of varying design (resembling a pelican) once used for extracting teeth. It was first described by Guy de Chauliac in 1363 and consisted of a main shaft about 4 inches long with a serrated semicircular bolster at either end; riveted to the centre of the shaft were two arms of different lengths ending in claws. Each claw was placed over the crown of the tooth to be extracted with the bolster against the outer gingival tissue to act as a fulcrum; the tooth was then levered out with a downwards pressure. It was superseded by the *tooth key in the early 18th century. *See also* UBERWULF.

pellet *n.* A small round mass of material. **Cotton pellets** or pledgets are balls of cotton wool used to absorb fluid. **Foil pellets** consist of loosely rolled up balls of 24 carat gold foil which are malleted into a cavity.

pellicle (acquired pellicle) *n.* A thin deposit of salivary and bacterial glycoproteins deposited on the surface of a tooth within minutes of being cleaned. If left undisturbed it acquires further bacteria to form a thicker *biofilm (*plaque).

pemphigoid *n.* A chronic and relatively benign *autoimmune disease, usually of the elderly, characterized by recurrent sub-epithelial blistering which persists for several days. Different subtypes are recognized: **bullous pemphigoid** is an autoimmune disease characterized by blisters on the skin and occasionally the oral cavity; **cictricial pemphigoid** affects the conjunctiva as well as the oral mucosa. Patients present with bullae (blisters) which burst to leave ulcers. **Mucous membrane pemphigoid** affects the oral cavity and other mucous membranes with limited skin involvement. The disease is caused by autoantibodies that react with a component of the basement membrane, resulting in separation. It is treated with corticosteroids or *immunosuppressant drugs.

pemphigus (pemphigus vulgaris) *n.* A rare *autoimmune disease characterized by successive outbreaks of blisters and erosions that fail to heal. It may affect the mouth or skin, or both, and is caused by antibodies which react with the structures which hold epithelial cells together (*desmosomes), resulting in their separation. It is treated with immunosuppressants but before the advent of steroids was frequently fatal, due to loss of fluids and secondary infection.

pen grip *n. See* GRIP.

-penia Suffix denoting lack or deficiency.

penicillin *n.* An antibiotic originally derived from cultures of *Penicillium notatum* by Alexander Fleming (1881–1955, Scottish physician) in 1929. Penicillin acts by interfering with the ability to synthesize the bacterial cell wall. It first became available for treating infections in 1941. Since then a number of naturally occurring penicillins have been developed. **Penicillin G (benzyl penicillin)** is active against Gram-positive bacteria and is administered by intramuscular injection to give a prolonged low concentration; it cannot be taken orally since it is inactivated by gastric acid. **Penicillin V (phenoxymethylpenicillin)** is administered orally and is effective against oral infections where a high tissue concentration is not required. There are many antibiotics derived from the penicillins such as amoxicillin, ampicillin, and flucloxacillin (semi-synthetic penicillins). *Allergy can occur and is characterized by skin rashes, swelling of the throat, and fever. Some bacteria are **penicillin-resistant** and can inhibit the effect of penicillin by the production of *penicillinase, an enzyme that destroys penicillin. A current threat is meticillin-resistant *Staphylococcus aureus* (*MRSA).

penicillinase *n.* An enzyme, also known as a beta-lactamase, produced by bacteria capable of hydrolysing the beta-lactam ring of the antibiotic penicillin and thus inactivating penicillin's antibacterial properties.

pentobarbital sodium *n.* A short acting barbiturate which depresses brain cell activity. Trade name: **Nembutal Sodium.**

peptide *n.* A compound consisting of two or more amino acids linked by bonds (**peptide bonds**) between the amino group (-NH) and the carboxyl group (-CO).

percentile *n.* A descriptive measure that represents the relative position or rank of each priority score (along a 100 percentile band) among the scores assigned by a particular study section. For example, the 20th percentile is the value that has 20% of the observations below it.

percussion *n.* The technique of tapping a part of the body with the fingers or an instrument as an aid to diagnosing the condition of the area beneath by the sound obtained. It is used in dentistry to determine the sensitivity of a tooth to pressure by noting the patient's response.

percutaneous *adj.* Through the skin; frequently applied to the route of administration of a drug.

perforation *n.* The creation of a hole in an organ or tissue. This may occur due to disease or during instrumentation such as the lateral perforation of a root during endodontic therapy.

performer *n.* (in the UK) A *dental professional contracted with a dentist (the *provider) to provide healthcare services within the new framework of general dental services (nGDS). Performers may include other dentists, dental hygienists, and dental therapists.

perfusion *n.* 1. The passage of fluid through a tissue, such as blood through the lungs so as to pick up oxygen and release carbon dioxide. 2. The deliberate injection of a fluid, possibly

containing a drug, into a tissue usually via a blood vessel.

peri- Prefix denoting near, around, or enclosing e.g. periapical (in the region of the apex); **pericardial** (around the heart); **peritonsillar** (around the tonsil).

periapex *n.* The region immediately surrounding the apex of a tooth root.

periapical *adj.* Surrounding the apical area of a tooth root. **Periapical abscess** See ABSCESS. A **periapical granuloma** (*apical granuloma) consists of a mass of inflammatory cells, fibroblasts, and collagen at the apex of a tooth root, usually caused by disease progression from the pulp of an associated tooth root; it is frequently asymptomatic although the soft tissue over the apex may be tender to pressure. If left untreated it can develop *cystic change. Radiographically it appears as a well-defined area of *radiolucency. **Periapical periodontitis** refers to inflammation of the periapical tissues; it may be either acute or chronic. **Acute periapical periodontitis** is associated with increased blood flow and the formation of *oedema in the periapical tissues, and the tooth is very tender to pressure; there are minimal radiographic changes, although widening of the periodontal ligament may be seen; it may resolve or develop into **chronic periapical periodontitis** (periapical granuloma). *See also* PERIODONTITIS. **Periapical tissue** consists of the periapical *alveolar bone and the periodontal membrane in the region of the apex of the tooth, which interfaces between the tooth root and the alveolar bone.

periapical cemental dysplasia A *benign, asymptomatic condition affecting the development of the periapical tissues. It has a variable radiographic appearance depending on the phase at which it is diagnosed. In the initial phase, bone is lost around the apex of the tooth and replaced by fibrous *connective tissue giving a radiolucent appearance similar to a periapical *cyst or *granuloma. In the second, cementoblastic stage, there is calcification of the *radiolucent area of fibrosis and in the third phase an excessive amount of calcified tissue is laid down in the periapical area to give a markedly *radiopaque appearance. There is no loss of tooth vitality. The cause is unknown, although it has been associated with chronic trauma. It is more common in females, specifically black women in their forties. The mandibular anterior teeth are most frequently affected, usually involving two or more teeth. No treatment is required. *See also* CEMENTOMA.

periapical radiograph An intra-oral radiograph that shows the crown and root of one

p

or more teeth including the periapical tissues and is of diagnostic value in endodontic therapy and detecting periapical pathology.

periauricular *adj.* Surrounding the external ear e.g. periauricular pain.

pericision (fiberotomy) *n.* An orthodontic surgical procedure in which the interdental and dento-gingival *periodontal fibres are cut above the level of the *alveolar bone. It is undertaken to attempt to reduce the rotational *relapse of a tooth following orthodontic treatment.

pericoronal flap *n. See* FLAP.

pericoronitis (operculitis) *n.* Inflammation of the tissue flap (*operculum) covering the crown of a partially erupted tooth, most commonly the third mandibular molar. Treatment consists of irrigation under the tissue flap with *chlorhexidine and removal of any traumatizing, non-functional opposing teeth, possibly followed by surgical removal of the tissue flap. Antibiotic therapy may be indicated if there is *trismus or a raised temperature. 📷

peridens *n.* A supernumerary tooth found elsewhere than in the midline of the dental arch.

peri-implantitis *n.* Inflammation around the area of a dental *implant which may include loss of bony support. It is characterized by swelling and redness of the tissues possibly associated with bleeding and increased *probing depth. The cause may be related to poor *oral hygiene, the state of the tissue surrounding the implant, implant design, surface roughness, alignment of implant components, external morphology, or excessive mechanical load. Treatment is dependent on the cause.

Further Reading: Sanchez-Garces M. A., Gay-Escoda C. Periimplantitis. *Med Oral Patol Oral Cir Bucal* 2004;9 Suppl:69–74; 83–9.

perikymata *pl. n.* Incremental growth lines approximately 30–40µ apart that appear on the surface of enamel as a series of curved grooves. They indicate the termination of the *enamel striae of Retzius on the labial surface of the tooth. They may disappear over time due to surface abrasion.

perimolysis (perimylolysis) *n.* Mechanical or chemical *erosion of tooth enamel. It is frequently associated with conditions involving chronic regurgitation of acidic gastric contents (such as *bulimia or *anorexia nervosa) which affects the palatal surfaces of the maxillary anterior teeth (particularly the central and lateral incisors) and the occlusal surfaces of the posterior teeth.

Periochip *n. See* CHLORHEXIDINE GLUCONATE.

periodontal *adj.* Relating to the *periodontium.

periodontal abscess *See* ABSCESS.

periodontal attachment The connective tissue attachment between the root of the tooth and the alveolar bone. *See also* PERIODONTAL LIGAMENT.

periodontal disease Any of a group of diseases of the gingivae and supporting tissues of the teeth. These include *plaque and non-plaque induced gingival diseases, chronic and acute *periodontitis, aggressive periodontitis, periodontitis as a manifestation of systemic disease, necrotizing periodontal diseases, periodontal *abscess, periodontitis associated with endodontic lesions, and developmental or acquired deformities and conditions. Plaque is the principal aetiological factor in nearly all forms of periodontal disease although the role of bacteria present is unclear; current hypotheses suggest that periodontal disease may be due to bacterial accumulation irrespective of its composition, the result of an infection with a single specific pathogen, or the result of infection with a relatively small number of interacting bacterial species. There are a number of currently identified risk factors for the progression of the disease such as poor plaque control, smoking, family history, and various medical conditions. Periodontal disease appears to be associated with a significant increase in the risk of future *cardiovascular disease.

Further Reading: Palmer R. M., Floyd P. D. *A clinical guide to periodontology.* British Dental Association, 2003.

periodontal disease index (PDI) A method of assessing the periodontal status, first defined by Ramfjord in 1967, and used to establish the need for treatment and to evaluate the results following treatment. It is a modification of the *periodontal disease index of Russell. Six teeth are examined and scored for gingivitis, calculus and plaque deposits, mobility, lack of tooth contact, and depth of gingival crevice (mobility and lack of tooth contact may be omitted). The PDI is the total of the scores for each tooth divided by the number of teeth examined: the higher the score, the more severe the periodontal disease.

Further Reading: Ramfjord S. P. The Periodontal Disease Index (PDI). *J Periodontol* 1967;38(6):Suppl:602–10.

(🌐) SEE WEB LINKS
- An overview of the periodontal disease index on the Medical Algorithms website.

periodontal disease index of Russell (PI) An assessment tool, named after A. L. Russell, a contemporary American dentist, that estimates the degree of periodontal disease present by measuring gingival inflammation and bone loss. It is used for measuring periodontal disease in population surveys. Each tooth is scored separately according to defined criteria; the higher the score, the more marked the periodontal disease. The population score equals the average for the individual scores in the population examined.

periodontal dressing *See* PACK.

periodontal examination An assessment of the condition of the *periodontium by visual examination, *probing pocket depths, *furcation recording, measuring *gingival recession, tooth *mobility, *occlusion, and restorative status, and by radiographic examination.

periodontal fibres The principle collagenous fibres of the *periodontal ligament running from the *cementum to the *alveolar bone; their orientation varies according to their location.

periodontal hoe *See* HOE.

periodontal index Any of a number of measurements which represent the disease status of the periodontal tissues as a numerical value. These include plaque and calculus indices (*See* GREENE–VERMILLION INDEX), the *gingival bleeding index, the *mobility index, and the *sulcus bleeding index.

periodontal instruments *n.* Instruments used for the maintenance of the gingivae and supporting structures of the teeth or the treatment of conditions relating to them. They include *scalers, *hoes, and surgical cutting instruments such as the *Blakes gingivectomy knife.

periodontal ligament A dense connective tissue layer about 0.2mm thick enveloping the roots of teeth, located between the *cementum and *alveolar bone and consisting mainly of *collagen fibres (**desmodontium**) and ground substance (proteoglycans and glycoproteins). The cell types considered to be part of the periodontal ligament are the *fibroblast, *cementoblast, *osteoblast, and *osteoclast. It contains blood vessels, lymph vessels, and nerves. The periodontal ligament forms from collagen fibres within the *dental follicle (*Hertwig's sheath); cellular remnants of

Periodontal disease index of Russell

Criteria for field studies	Additional radiographic criteria	Score
No gingivitis (neither overt inflammation in the investing tissues, nor loss of function due to destruction of supporting tissues).	Normal radiographic appearance.	0
Mild gingivitis (overt area of inflammation in the free gingivae, but this area does not circumscribe the tooth).		1
Gingivitis (inflammation completely circumscribes the tooth, but there is no apparent break in the epithelial attachment).		2
Not used in field study.	Early, notch-like resorption of the alveolar crest.	4
Gingivitis with pocket formation (the epithelial attachment is broken, and there is a pocket). There is no interference with normal masticatory function, the tooth is firm in its socket, and has not drifted.	Horizontal bone loss involving the entire alveolar crest, up to half of the length of the tooth root (distance from apex to cemento-enamel junction).	6
Advanced destruction with loss of masticatory function (tooth may be loose; tooth may have drifted; tooth may sound dull on percussion with a metallic instrument; the tooth may be depressible in its socket).	Advanced bone loss, involving more than half of the length of the tooth root, or a definite intrabony pocket with definite widening of the periodontal membranes. There may be root resorption, or rarefaction at the apex.	8

p

Dentine

Cementum

Periodontal ligament

Alveolar bone

Periodontal ligament

Hertwig's sheath remain between the collagen fibres into adult life. Its functions are to provide a support mechanism for the tooth, to maintain the vertical position of the tooth, to form, maintain, and repair the surrounding alveolar bone and cementum, to detect pressures on the tooth through proprioceptive sensors, and to provide nutrients to the cement-forming cells (cementoblasts). The fibres of the periodontal ligament are grouped together to provide tooth stability. With age, the width of the periodontal ligament decreases and there is a decrease in collagen and protein synthesis.

Further Reading: Berkovitz B. K. B. Periodontal ligament: structural and clinical correlates. *Dent Update* 2004;31:46-54.

periodontal ostectomy *See* OSTECTOMY.

periodontal pack *See* PACK.

periodontal pocket . A pathological deepening of the gingival *sulcus (crevice) produced by the destruction of the supporting tissues and the apical migration of the *epithelial attachment. The *junctional epithelium is located apical to the *cemento-enamel junction. The base of the pocket is limited by the epithelial attachment to the cementum of the root surface. It provides an ideal protected environment for the continued growth of subgingival bacteria which release toxins that can damage the surrounding tissue and *cementum. The pocket may be **supra-bony**, with the base of the pocket above the crest of the alveolar bone, or **infra-bony**, with the base apical to the *crest of the alveolar bone.

periodontal probe *See* PROBE.

periodontal screening and recording (PSR) *See* BASIC PERIODONTAL EXAMINATION.

periodontal surgery Surgical intervention in the treatment of periodontal conditions, aimed

primarily at regenerating lost periodontal tissue rather than resecting diseased tissue. The *excisional new attachment procedure (ENAP) is the surgical removal of the diseased pocket epithelium. **Periodontal flap surgery** involves incisions made in the gingiva around the necks of the teeth with the elevation of a *flap, including the underlying soft tissues, to expose the supporting alveolar bone; the flap provides access to the underlying tissues. The flap is sutured into position post-operatively and usually covered by a protective *pack. *Gingivectomy involves the excision and removal of some of the gingival tissue. **Gingival curettage** is a procedure that involves an attempt to scrape away the lining of the *periodontal pocket using a *curette.

periodontal traumatism *See* TRAUMATISM.

periodontics *n. See* PERIODONTOLOGY.

periodontitis *n.* Inflammation of the supporting tissues of the teeth, resulting in permanent tissue destruction.

periodontitis, acute necrotizing An acute inflammatory condition of the supporting tissues of the teeth resulting in permanent tissue destruction and characterized by a change in gingival contour, bleeding, pain, and the loss of the apex of the gingival papilla, producing a punched-out appearance. Tissue death (*necrosis) frequently produces a grey slough (**pseudomembrane**) on the gingival surface, accompanied by *halitosis. There may also be swollen lymph glands and *pyrexia. Destruction of the tissues may progress to necrosis of the *alveolar bone, which can become a detached fragment (*sequestrum). General predisposing factors include increased stress, malnutrition, fatigue, suppression of the immune system, and systemic diseases such as *leukaemia and *HIV. Local predisposing factors include poor oral hygiene, cigarette smoking, and pre-existing *gingivitis. Treatment is by the removal of surface deposits, oral hygiene instruction, the prescription of mouth rinses such as *hydrogen peroxide and *chlorhexidine, and possibly antibiotics if there are systemic symptoms. *See also* PERIODONTITIS, CHRONIC.

periodontitis, aggressive Inflammation of the supporting tissues of the teeth resulting in rapid permanent tissue destruction; it characteristically manifests itself before the age of 35. It is also known as **juvenile, pre-pubertal** or **early-onset periodontitis.** It may affect an isolated group of teeth or the whole dentition, and only affects a small group of the population. There is rapid periodontal attachment loss with destruction of the periodontal ligament and supporting alveolar bone in an otherwise healthy mouth. Delayed diagnosis can result in rapid and extensive tooth loss. There is often a familial tendency; bacteria associated with this condition are *Actinobacillus actinomycetemcomitans* and *Porphyromonas gingivalis.* Clinical features include a low level of gingival inflammation, usually in combination with low plaque levels and good oral hygiene, which can cause the diagnosis to be overlooked; radiographically, however, bone loss is evident. Treatment is by the removal of surface deposits, oral hygiene instruction, and addressing any predisposing risk factors. A 7 day course of adjunctive antibiotics such as *metronidazole and *amoxicillin can improve the short-term clinical outcomes. *See also* PERIODONTITIS, AGGRESSIVE; CLASSIFICATION OF PERIODONTAL DISEASE. 📷

periodontitis, chronic

Inflammation of the supporting tissues of the teeth characterized by apical migration of the *junctional epithelium, loss of *periodontal attachment, and loss of *alveolar bone. The **clinical features** include purplish-red swollen (oedematous) and shiny gingival tissue, detachment of the *interdental papillae, an increase in the gingival crevice (sulcus) beyond 3mm (*periodontal pocket), usually no pain or discomfort, and bleeding on gentle probing. There may also be exudation of pus on digital pressure or probing, tooth mobility, drifting of the teeth, tooth loss, and gingival recession. Subgingival calculus is frequently present and causes additional irritation. The **initiation of chronic periodontitis** is thought to be due to gene polymorphism, which causes a change in the behaviour of *cytokines, substances which influence the immune system. Histologically there is extensive destruction of *collagen tissue and there may be *fibrosis of the tissue outside the inflamed area. Many bacterial species have been identified, including *Porphyromonas gingivalis, Bacillus forsythius,* and *Treponema denticola,* although their role in the disease process is not clearly defined. **General risk factors** include smoking, which reduces the gingival blood circulation, diabetes, stress, leukaemia, and hormonal changes such as puberty, pregnancy, and the menopause. **Local risk factors** include the presence of calculus, malpositioned teeth, poorly constructed restorations, removable partial dentures, poor tooth *contact areas, and a deep *overbite causing direct gingival trauma. Treatment is by the removal of surface deposits, oral hygiene instruction, and addressing any predisposing risk factors. *See also* GINGIVITIS.

periodontitis, early-onset *See* PERIODONTITIS, AGGRESSIVE.

periodontitis, juvenile *See* PERIODONTITIS, AGGRESSIVE.

periodontitis, periapical *See* PERIAPICAL.

periodontitis, pre-pubertal *See* PERIODONTITIS, AGGRESSIVE.

periodontitis, refractory Destructive periodontal diseases in patients who, when monitored over a period of time, demonstrate further attachment loss at one or more sites, despite well-undertaken therapeutic and patient efforts to halt the progression of disease.

periodontium *n.* The tissues that surround and support the teeth. It includes the *gingiva, *periodontal ligament, *cementum, and supporting *alveolar bone.

periodontology *n.* The specialty in dentistry concerned with the supporting structures of the teeth and the prevention and treatment of *periodontal disease.

periodontoscopy *n.* The examination of the periodontal structures by means of an *odontoscope.

periodontosis *n.* An outmoded term used to describe periodontal destruction in terms of degeneration rather than infection; it was often used to describe juvenile *periodontitis. *See* PERIODONTITIS, AGGRESSIVE.

period prevalence *See* PREVALENCE RATE.

perioral *adj.* In the region of the mouth.

Periostat *n.* See DOXYCYCLINE.

periosteal elevator *n.* See ELEVATOR.

periosteum *n.* A layer of dense fibrous *connective tissue covering bone surfaces, excluding the articular surfaces. The outer layer consists of dense *collagenous tissue rich in blood vessels; the inner layer is less vascular and more cellular, containing *osteoblasts. The periosteum provides attachment for muscles, tendons, and ligaments.

periostitis *n.* Inflammation of the *periosteum which can result in jaw swelling and ulceration. It usually occurs in response to chronic irritation to the periosteum, often from foreign material. **Periostitis ossificans** is a non-suppurative type of *osteomyelitis occurring in the mandible of children and young adults. It most commonly arises from the periapical infection of a first molar. Radiographically it is characterized by an 'onion skin' appearance. Treatment is antibiotic therapy with associated tooth extraction.

Further Reading: Kannan S. K., Sandhya G., Selvarani R. Periostitis ossificans (Garré's osteomyelitis) radiographic study of two cases. *International Journal of Paediatric Dentistry* 2006;16(1);59.

periotome *n.* A hand instrument with detachable flexible blades that have cutting surfaces. It is used with a vertical sawing motion for severing the periodontal membrane prior to tooth extraction to minimize gingival trauma and to facilitate the extraction. It may also be used to reflect and protect the gingival margin during implant placement.

peripheral ossifying fibroma (peripheral cementifying fibroma) A reactive focal gingival overgrowth derived from cells of the *periodontal ligament. It is characterized by a painless, haemorrhagic, and often lobulated mass of gingiva or alveolar mucosa usually 1–2cm in size, which may have large areas of surface ulceration. Radiographically there may be scattered areas of radiopacity due to the presence of small deposits of bone, cementum, or dystrophic calcification. It is most common in young adults but may occur at any age, particularly in the presence of poor oral hygiene or local irritation. Treatment is by surgical excision with diligent root planing of the adjacent teeth to avoid recurrence.

peripheral seal 1. The fit around the outer margins of a denture that creates an effective contact between the denture and the soft tissues and improves retention. 2. The peripheral contact between a restoration and the prepared tooth

tissue; also sometimes referred to as a **border seal**.

periradicular *adj.* Pertaining to the region around the root of a tooth.

peristalsis *n.* An involuntary wavelike movement that progresses along some of the tubes of the body. It is characteristic of tubes possessing circular and longitudinal muscle such as the intestines and oesophagus. It is induced by distension of the tube walls. Behind the distension the circular muscle contracts and in front of the distension the circular muscle relaxes and the longitudinal muscle contracts to advance the contents of the tube. Peristalsis follows *deglutition (swallowing).

perlèche *n.* Dryness and cracking at the angles of the mouth. See ANGULAR CHEILITIS.

permanent dentition The 32 teeth of the second dentition which replace the primary dentition. Each quadrant has 8 teeth: 2 *incisors, 1 *canine, 2 *premolars, and 3 *molars. The incisors, canines, and premolars replace the teeth of the primary dentition. *Eruption starts at about 5 years of age and is normally completed by the age of 21.

permucosal *adj.* Via or through the *mucosa, such as the penetration of the mucous membrane by a needle or dental *implant.

peroral *adj.* Through the mouth; administered by mouth.

peroxide *n.* See HYDROGEN PEROXIDE.

Personal Dental Service (PDS) A system of primary dental healthcare delivery within the National Health Service in the UK established in 1997 under the NHS Primary Care Act. The PDS was in part replaced in 2006 by the new General Dental Services (nGDS) contract.

personal development plan (PDP) A process whereby educational needs are identified, objectives set, and educational activities are planned. It usually includes evidence to indicate that skills, knowledge, or understanding have been achieved.

personal protective equipment (PPE) Clothing and equipment used to help provide a barrier between the dental healthcare worker and any potentially infectious material. It includes the wearing of latex or non-latex *gloves, *gowns, *facemasks or protective glasses, and appropriate shoes.

Further Reading: Kohn W. G., Collins A. S., Cleveland J. L., Harte J. A., Eklund K. J., Malvitz, D. M. Centers for Disease Control and Prevention (CDC), 2003. Guidelines for infection control in dental health-care settings—2003. *Morbidity and*

Mortality Weekly Report. Recommendations and Reports, 52 (RR–17), 1–61.

pestle *n.* An instrument used for pounding or grinding substances in a *mortar. It was originally used in dentistry for *triturating mercury and alloy powder to produce amalgam alloy.

petechiae *pl. n.* Small localized areas of bleeding from the blood vessels just beneath the surface of the skin or *mucosa, characterized by small dark red spots. They are typical of some blood dyscrasias, vitamin C deficiency, and sub-acute bacterial *endocarditis.

Petri dish [J. R. Petri (1852–1921), German bacteriologist] *n.* A shallow, plastic or glass, flat-bottomed, cylindrical dish with vertical sides and a loose-fitting lid, used to contain sterile solid *agar or gelatin culture media, used in bacteriology or mycology. Sterile dishes are filled with molten liquid agar supplemented with various nutrients, essential salts, and amino acids and allowed to solidify prior to being used to culture bacteria or fungi.

Peutz–Jeghers syndrome [J. L. A. Peutz (1886–1957), Dutch physician; H. J. Jeghers (1904–90), US physician] A hereditary disorder characterized by polyps of the small intestine and purple or black *hamartomatous freckles (melanin spots) around the lips and on the oral mucous membrane; the spots commonly disappear during the teenage period. Approximately half of those affected develop malignant tumours.

pH A measure of the acidity or alkalinity of a solution. A pH of 7.0 is neutral; greater than 7.0 is more basic; less than 7.0 is more acidic (the resting pH of saliva varies between 6.8 and 6.9).

phagocyte *n.* (*adj.* **phagocytic**) A cell capable of ingesting bacteria, cells, and other substances, and which therefore forms part of the body's defence mechanism.

phagocytosis *n.* The process of engulfing bacteria and other substances by *phagocytes.

pharmacist *n.* A suitably qualified person licensed to prepare and dispense medicines.

pharmacodynamics *n.* The branch of pharmacology concerned with the course of action, effect, and breakdown of drugs within the body.

pharmacokinetics *n.* The branch of pharmacology that deals with the fate of pharmacological substances within the body including their distribution, absorption, metabolism, and elimination.

pharyngitis *n.* Inflammation of the *pharynx (behind the soft palate).

pharynx *n.* A hollow muscular tube, lined with mucous membrane, about 12cm long and extending from behind the nose to the beginning of the trachea and oesophagus. It is divided into *nasopharynx, *laryngopharynx, and *oropharynx.

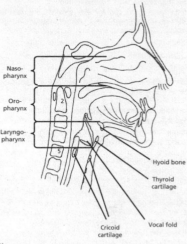

Pharynx

phenol *n.* An aromatic compound also known as **carbolic acid**. It has antiseptic properties but is toxic and a severe irritant to the skin. It is one of the main ingredients of commercial antiseptics such as trichlorophenol (TCP). **Phenol coefficient** is a test employed for determining the germicidal efficiency of disinfectants. *See also* PARACHLOROPHENOL.

phenoxymethylpenicillin *n. See* PENICILLIN.

phenytoin *n.* An anticonvulsant drug used in the treatment of *epilepsy and *trigeminal neuralgia. A common side-effect is gingival *hyperplasia (*fibromatosis) occurring in up to 50% of dentate patients. This begins with enlargement of the interdental papillae to produce triangular protruding tissue masses; these may fuse mesially and distally to partially obliterate the anatomical tooth crowns; it is most commonly seen on the labial surfaces of the anterior teeth. Trade names: **Dilantin**, **Epanutin**.

philtrum *n.* The vertical groove in the midline on the external surface of the upper lip. It is formed from the fusion of the nasal and maxillary processes during embryonic development. A failure of these processes to fully fuse results in a *cleft lip.

phlegm *n.* A non-medical term for *sputum.

phobia *n.* (*Suffix* **-phobia** denoting morbid fear or dread). An anxiety state characterized by an irrational fear of a specific object or situation; the fear response is excessive and disproportionate to the threat posed. The patient has little or no control over the phobia, which can significantly influence their behaviour. Management in the dental context includes the use of behaviour therapy, hypnotherapy, and conscious sedation.

phonation *n.* The production of vocal sounds, particularly speech.

phosphonecrosis (phossy jaw) *n.* A rare condition resulting in death (*necrosis) of the jaw bone, due to exposure to phosphorous. It is seen in workers exposed to yellow phosphorous fumes.

phosphoric acid *n.* A colourless, odourless, inorganic mineral acid (H_3PO_4). It is used in dentistry as an aqueous solution forming the liquid component of *zinc phosphate cement and as an etching liquid or gel when applied to dentine or enamel to remove calcium and provide a micro-mechanical bonding surface for restorative or preventive *resin restorations.

phosphorous tincture An alcohol-based *homeopathic *astringent used to control gingival haemorrhage in restorative procedures prior to impression taking.

phossy jaw *See* PHOSPHONECROSIS.

photoactivated disinfection (PAD) *See* PHOTODYNAMIC THEORY.

photodynamic therapy (PDT) The use of a solution of a light-sensitive dye or drug (photosensitizer) and a low-power *laser, such as a Helium Neon laser (trade name **Periowave**™), to produce the oxidative destruction of pathogenic bacteria. Also known as photoactivated disinfection (PAD). To be effective, sufficient time must be allowed for the low viscosity photosensitizer to migrate towards the bacteria before excitation with the light source. Dyes used include toluidine blue (tolonium chloride) and methylene blue. It has been used in the treatment of deep carious lesions, periodontitis, root canal infections, sites of *peri-implantitis, and in the treatment of pre-cancerous skin lesions of the face and scalp.

Further Reading: Garcez A. S., Ribeiro M. S., Tegos G. P., Nunez S. C., Jorge A. O., Hamblin M. R. Antimicrobial photodynamic therapy combined with conventional endodontic treatment to eliminate root canal biofilm infection. *Lasers Surg Med* 2007;39(1):59–66.

photo-initiator *n.* An agent which, when exposed to a specific waveband of light, starts a chain reaction in the formation of a resin polymer. Most commercial photo-initiators contain benzoyl groups such as *benzoyl peroxide and *camphorquinone, which are both used in some dental resins.

photon *n.* The quantum of electromagnetic energy, generally regarded as a discrete particle having zero mass, no electric charge, and an infinitely long lifetime. Specific ranges of photons provide curing energy for *bisphenol A-diglycidylether methacrylate (bis-GMA) resins of light cured *resin composite.

physiognomy *n.* 1. The physical appearance of one's face. 2. The assessment of someone's character or personality from their face and other external bodily features.

physiology *n.* The study of the mechanical, physical, and biochemical functions of living organisms and their parts.

pica *n.* The persistent eating of non-nutritive or harmful substances, such as paper or glass, or an abnormal appetite for some things that may be considered foods or food ingredients, such as flour, raw potato, and starch. The name comes from the Latin for magpie, a bird reputed to eat almost anything. The condition most commonly occurs in people with developmental and learning difficulties. The symptoms are related to the substances consumed. Oral features can include soft tissue trauma, nutritional deficiencies, and tooth wear.

Further Reading: Dougall A., Fiske J. Access to special care dentistry, part 6. Special care dentistry services for young people. *Br Dent J* 2008;205:235–49.

Ashcroft A., Milosevic A. The eating disorders: 1 Current scientific understanding and dental implications. *Dent Update* 2007;34:544–54.

Pickerill's lines [H. P. Pickerill (1879–1956), English surgeon] Imbrication lines on the enamel surface; also known as *perikymata.

pickling *v.* The process of cleaning metal surfaces by acid immersion. It is used to improve the bonding of porcelain to the metal surface by removing unwanted oxides on the metal surface. Pickling agents include phosphoric, nitric, hydrochloric, hydrofluoric, and sulphamic acids (sulfamic acid; trade name Neacid®). Commonly used acids for pickling gold alloys are 50% hydrofluoric acid and 30% hydrochloric acid.

pick-up impression *n. See* IMPRESSION.

p

pier *n.* An intermediate supporting or retaining abutment for a prosthetic appliance.

Pierre Robin sequence (Robin anomalad, Robin sequence) [P. Robin (1867–1950), French dentist] A congenital disease of unknown cause characterized by a very small lower jaw (*micrognathia), cleft soft palate, *natal teeth, and usually associated with a backward displacement of the tongue (*glossoptosis) which can result in respiratory difficulty.

piezograph *n.* A three-dimensional shape moulded in an impression material by the tongue, lips, and cheeks in edentulous areas of the mouth. It provides a functional recording of the *denture space.

pigmentation *n.* Discoloration of the body produced by the deposition of a pigment. It can be seen normally in oral mucous membrane of dark-complexioned individuals and pathologically in *Addison's disease. Amalgam remnants can become incorporated into the gingival tissues (*amalgam tattoo). Pigmentation can also be due to the ingestion of metals such as silver (*argyria).

pillars of fauces Two curved folds of tissue on either side of the pharyngeal opening extending from the *palate to the base of the *tongue. The anterior fold is known as the **palatoglossal arch** and the posterior as the **palatopharyngeal arch**.

pin *n.* 1. A thin metal rod used to provide fixation for bones in the treatment of fractures. 2. A thin metal rod used in dentistry as an aid to retention. Pins used to retain a restoration or core may be cemented, friction-retained by the elasticity of the dentine, or self-threaded utilizing a pre-drilled hole. **Dentine pin** *See* DENTINE. An **incisal guide pin** is a vertical metal rod which maintains the vertical dimension on an *articulator; it is attached to the upper part of the articulator and rests on the *incisal guide table.

pin dam A groove on the periphery of a removable partial denture *baseplate (narrower than that of a *post-dam) that is designed to increase the adaptation of the baseplate periphery to the mucosa.

Pindborg's tumour [J. J. Pindborg (1921–95), Danish oral pathologist] *n.* A calcifying epithelial *odontogenic tumour. It is a rare *benign *neoplasm, usually arising in the mandibular molar or premolar region.

pink disease *See* ACRODYNIA.

pink spot *See* ODONTOCLASTOMA.

pinlay *n.* A gold inlay or onlay which has its retention supplemented by a pin or pins embedded as part of the restoration.

pinledge *n.* A type of *pinlay retained by means of one or more parallel pins recessed into small grooves or ledges cut into the lingual or palatal surface of an anterior tooth.

pinna (auricle) *n.* The external part of the ear.

pit *n.* 1. A small depression on the enamel surface of a tooth. 2. A small depression on the surface of a restoration due to an air inclusion or resulting from non-uniform density.

pit and fissure sealant *n. See* SEALANT.

pitting *n.* The formation of small well-defined depressions on the surface of a material such as gold or amalgam. It is often associated with *corrosion.

pituitary gland A pea-sized *endocrine gland situated in a bony cavity at the base of the skull. It produces hormones essential for growth, metabolism, reproduction, and vascular control. Of dental significance, over-activity can result in *osteoporosis, thickening of the facial and cranial base bony structures, and *hypercementosis. Under-activity can cause delayed dental development, an anterior open *bite, and alteration in the dimensions of the facial skeleton.

placebo *n.* An inactive substance in the same form as an active drug, given for psychological effect or as a control in evaluating a medicine believed to be active. The **placebo effect** is the apparently beneficial result or positive reaction to a pharmacologically inactive or neutral substance by a recipient who believes it will be effective.

plane *n.* A flat surface that is defined by the position in space of three points. The **axial plane** is parallel to the long axis of an object. The **sagittal plane** is a vertical plane dividing the body into two halves which are equal in the mid-sagittal plane. The **transverse plane** (also known as horizontal or cross-sectional) divides the body into superior (upper) and inferior (lower) portions. *See also* FRANKFORT PLANE.

plantago *n.* A homeopathic tincture claimed to be effective at treating *dentine hypersensitivity and pulpal sensitivity but not currently supported by clinical evidence.

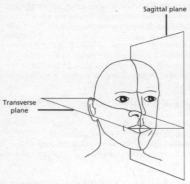

Sagittal plane

Transverse
plane

Sagittal and transverse planes

plaque *n.* 1. A *biofilm consisting of an organized bacterial community, *salivary mucins and proteins adhering to tooth surfaces, restorations, and prosthetic appliances. Plaque forms by attachment of bacteria to the outer surface of the *pellicle, predominantly in stagnation areas not having the benefit of the self-cleansing actions of the oral cavity. The bacterial composition of plaque is very dependent on the site location and local environment. If left undisturbed, initial colonization is predominantly by aerobic and facultative anaerobic *Gram-positive *Streptococci* and the thickness increases largely by bacterial cell division. With an increase in thickness there is a predominance of Gram-positive filaments such as *Actinomyces* and anaerobic Gram-negative bacteria which are suspected to be periodontal pathogens, although the role of bacteria in the initiation of disease is unclear. Three hypotheses put forward to explain the role of bacteria in periodontal disease are: the **non-specific plaque**

hypothesis that states that periodontal disease is due to bacterial accumulation, irrespective of its composition; the **specific plaque hypothesis** that states that periodontal disease is the result of an infection with a single specific pathogen; and the **multiple pathogen hypothesis** that states that periodontal disease is the result of interacting bacterial species. Plaque is normally invisible except when well established, when it appears milky white; it can be made visible using *disclosing agents. Mineralized deposits may be laid down in established plaque to form *calculus. 2. A raised patch on the skin. 3. A fatty deposit on the inner wall of an artery (*see* ATHEROMA). 4. A flat and often raised patch resulting from local damage e.g. on mucous membrane. 📷

Further Reading: Palmer R. M., Floyd P. D., Newton J. T., Hasan A. S. *A clinical guide to periodontology.* British Dental Association, 2003.
Roberts A. Bacteria in the mouth. *Dent Update* 2005;32:134–42.

plaque control The methods by which bacterial dental plaque is either removed or its formation inhibited. Control may be by supragingival or subgingival delivery systems. Control of the supragingival environment has a beneficial effect on the subgingival. Plaque control may also be either mechanical or chemical.

plaque-free zone A plaque-free area on the root surface coronal to the *junctional epithelium and apical to the tooth attached plaque, described by J. Waerhaug in 1952.

plaque index *n. See* GREENE–VERMILLION INDEX; QUIGLEY–HEIN PLAQUE INDEX.

plasma (blood plasma) *n.* The straw-coloured fluid component of blood. It contains many substances including *protein and the salts of sodium, potassium, and calcium.

Delivery systems for plaque control agents

Supragingival	Subgingival	
Local Delivery	Local Delivery	Systemic Delivery
Mouthrinse	Irrigator	Capsules/tablets
Dentifrice	*Fibres	Low-dose antimicrobials
Gel	*Gel	
Irrigator	*Acrylic strip	
Floss (medicated)		
Chewing gum		
Lozenges		
(sustained release)		

plasma cell (plasmocyte) An antibody-producing cell formed in the bone marrow, spleen, and lymph nodes.

plasma lamp (arc) A light source in which a current traverses a gas between two incandescent electrodes to generate an arc which produces light used to polymerize resins. It has a peak energy level of 900mW and a spectrum of 430–490nm, and therefore requires a much shorter curing time (1–2 seconds) than a conventional *halogen lamp (20–30 seconds).

plasma membrane The membrane that surrounds an entire cell, separates it from its environment, and which regulates the flow of substances to and from the cell. It consists of a double layer of phospholipids with embedded proteins.

plasmin *n.* The collective name for a group of protein-dissolving *enzymes capable of degrading *fibrin in the process of removing a blood clot.

plaster knife *n.* A metal knife with a stiff blade, usually with a wooden handle, used to trim plaster or stone models.

plaster of Paris *n.* A calcium sulphate hemihydrate ($CaSO_4$.0.5H_2O) derived by heating *gypsum (*calcination). It forms a solid mass with the addition of water and is used to make casts for prosthetic or orthodontic appliances.

plastic *n.* 1. A restorative material that is soft and malleable at the time of insertion and subsequently hardens, such as amalgam or composite resin. 2. A hand instrument used for contouring plastic restorative materials.

plasticizer *n.* A low molecular weight substance added to a polymer to reduce the forces of attraction between the polymer chains and make the polymer more flexible. Dibutyl phthalate is a plasticizer added to *polymethyl-methacrylate to make *soft linings for dentures.

plate *n.* A thin sheet of metal or resin forming part of an appliance. An **expansion plate** is an *orthodontic appliance with an acrylic palatal plate, split in an antero-posterior direction into two halves separated by a screw which can be progressively rotated to provide lateral pressure on the teeth. A **base plate** forms part of an orthodontic or prosthetic appliance which is contoured to fit the mucosa and to which are attached teeth, springs, or clasps. **Bite plate** *See* BITE. The **cortical plate** forms the superficial outer layer of bone. A **lingual plate** is a type of *connector used in a lower removable partial denture to join the right and left sides; it lies lingual to the alveolar ridge behind the anterior teeth and extends across the gingival margins to the cingulum of each tooth. A **palatal plate** is a type of *connector used to join the units of one side of a partial or complete denture with those located on the opposite side of the arch.

platelet (thrombocyte) *n.* A colourless anuclear disc-shaped cell 1–2μm in diameter present in the blood. Platelets have an important role in blood clotting.

platelet-derived growth factor (PDGF) A *glycoprotein carried in the granules of platelets and released during blood clotting; it regulates cell proliferation. It is a potent growth factor for cells of mesenchymal origin, including *fibroblasts and smooth muscle cells.

platinum (Pt) *n.* A silvery-white, soft metallic element. It is mixed with *gold, silver, *copper, or *zinc to produce alloys suitable for inlays, crowns, or bridges. It adds strength, stiffness, and durability to alloys. A thin layer of **platinum foil** is used as a matrix in the construction of the core of a porcelain crown to provide rigidity during fabrication and firing and allow separation of the porcelain from the *die.

platy- Prefix denoting broad or flat e.g. **platysma** (broad flat sheet of muscle in the neck); **platycephalic** (having a broad flat skull); **platyglossal** (having a broad flat tongue).

Plaut–Vincent gingivitis (angina) *See* GINGIVITIS, NECROTIZING.

pledget *n.* A small ball of cotton wool used to absorb fluids or transport liquid medicaments.

pleomorphic *adj.* Occurring in many distinct forms; in terms of cells, having variation in the size and shape of cells or their nuclei.

pleomorphic adenoma *See* ADENOMA.

pleurodont *adj.* Having teeth firmly attached (*ankylosed) by their sides to the inner surface of the jaw, as seen in some reptiles, rather than in sockets in the jaw bone.

plexus *n.* A network of blood vessels, nerves, or lymphatic vessels. The **plexus of Raschkow** is a network of nerves immediately beneath the odontoblast layer of the dentine, first described by J. Raschkow in 1835.

plica *n.* A fold of tissue. The **plica fimbriata** is a fringed fold of mucous membrane on the underside of the tongue either side of the lingual frenum and lateral to the lingual vein. The **plica sublingualis** is a ridge of soft tissue running outwards and posteriorly from each sublingual papilla that marks the upper edge of the sublingual *salivary gland and onto which most of the ducts of that gland open.

plicate *v.* (*n.* **plication**) To fold like a fan.

pliers *n.* A tool with small pincer-shaped jaws with two handles and a common pivot axle of varying designs, used for holding, bending, stretching, contouring, or cutting. **Adams pliers**, designed by C. Philip Adams, an English orthodontist, are used primarily for the adjustment of orthodontic appliances. **Adams universal pliers** have two short tapering rectangular beaks and are used to adjust headgear, facebows, and Adams cribs. **Adams spring-forming pliers** have a tapering rounded beak and a tapering rectangular beak and are used to adjust orthodontic springs and contour archwires.

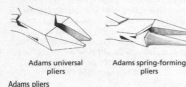

Adams universal pliers   Adams spring-forming pliers

Adams pliers

plugger *n.* See CONDENSER.

Plummer–Vinson syndrome [H. S. Plummer (1874–1936), American physician; P. P. Vinson (1890–1959), American surgeon] A rare form of chronic iron deficiency *anaemia, characterized by difficulty in swallowing due to small thin growths of tissue that block the *oesophagus. There may also be cracks at the corners of the mouth (*angular cheilitis), and a painful smooth red tongue.

plunger cusp *n.* A cusp whose movement during mastication forces food into interproximal areas.

pocket *n.* An abnormal space developing between the gingiva and the root of a tooth. The **pocket depth** is measured, usually in millimetres, from the gingival crest to the base of the pocket. A **false (pseudo-** or **gingival pocket)** is created when there is gingival enlargement due to inflammation, without an apical proliferation of the junctional epithelial attachment. **Pocket marking** accurately determines the pocket depth either as an aid to diagnosis or to provide a guideline for a *gingivectomy incision. See also PERIODONTAL POCKET.

pocket measuring probe An instrument used for determining the *probing depth of a *periodontal pocket. Its secondary function is to assess whether there is bleeding on probing used as a measure of inflammation. Probes in common use are the *basic periodontal examination (BPE)

probe, the *Williams 10mm probe, and, for inaccessible areas on the lingual aspect of lower molars, the Williams 15mm probe. The probe is inserted into the pocket using a pressure of 10–20gm, aligned with the long axis of the tooth until the base of the pocket is detected, and the depth recorded, usually in millimetres.

pogonion *n.* See CEPHALOMETRIC ANALYSIS.

poikilo- Prefix denoting variation, or irregularity.

poikilodentosis *n.* Enamel *hypoplasia (*mottling) due to excessive fluoride in the water supply.

point *n.* 1. A small spot or minute area. 2. The sharp end of an object or instrument. 3. A clearly defined approach to a surface, such as pus from an abscess. An **abrasive rotary point** is a small instrument inserted into a dental handpiece used for grinding, smoothing, or polishing. A **condenser point** is the small contact tip of an instrument used for condensing amalgam or gold foil. **Contact point** See CONTACT. **Gutta-percha point** See GUTTA-PERCHA. A **trigger point** is a specific spot on the body that will elicit pain if touched.

point angle *n.* The junction of three surfaces of a tooth crown or of cavity walls.

point prevalence *n.* See PREVALENCE RATE.

polishing *n.* The process of making a surface smooth. A **polishing cup** is the operative part of a rotary tool made of synthetic or natural rubber and mounted in a dental handpiece. A **polishing brush** is a rotary instrument made of synthetic or natural bristle mounted in a dental handpiece or on a lathe and used with a polishing paste. **Polishing paste** is a water-soluble mixture containing abrasive particles such as aluminium oxide paste used for polishing restorations or *pumice. 📷

poly- Prefix denoting many, multiple, excessive, generalized, or affecting many parts.

polyacrylic acid *n.* A colourless to pale yellow transparent polymer of acrylic acid which reacts with an ion-leachable glass in the presence of water to form *glass ionomer cement. Homopolymers (polymers formed from a single monomer) of polyacrylic acid can form *polycarboxylic acid. See also POLYALKENOIC ACID.

polyalkenoic acid *n.* A family of complex acids which includes *polyacrylic, polyitaconic, and polymaleic acid which react with an ion-leachable glass (usually calcium-alumino-silicate) in the presence of water to form a *glass ionomer cement (**polyalkenoates**).

polyamide *n.* A polymer resin that can occur naturally (e.g. wool, silk) or manufactured synthetically (e.g. nylon). Synthetic polyamide may be used as a substitute for *polymethylmethacrylate resin denture base material, particularly in cases of allergy. Trade name: **Valplast®**.

polybunodont *adj. See* MULTITUBERCULATE.

polycarboxylate cement *n.* A cement formed by the acid-base reaction of *zinc oxide (base component) with polycarboxylic acid (acidic component) in water. The zinc oxide is *sintered to reduce the reactivity and improve the manipulation. The viscosity of the liquid is controlled by the addition of tartaric acid. It is used as a luting cement and cavity liner.

polycarboxylic acid *n.* A *polymer generated from a series of straight-chain dicarboxylic acids which forms the acidic component in the acid-base reaction with zinc oxide in the formation of polycarboxylate cement.

polydontia *n. See* POLYODONTIA.

polyether *n.* A non-aqueous elastomeric impression material which polymerizes to form a cross-linked polymer when the monomer base (polyether), reactive group (ethyline imine), and catalyst (2,5 dichlorobenzene sulphonate) are mixed together. The material is used where an impression material of high dimensional *stability and accuracy is required.

polymer *n.* A chemical compound formed by combining many smaller molecules (*monomers) in a regular pattern in a process known as *polymerization.

polymerization *n.* A chemical reaction (also known as curing) in which the molecules of a simple substance (*monomer) are linked together to form large molecules (*polymers) whose molecular weight is a multiple of that of the monomer. **Addition polymerization** is a polymer formed by the reaction between two molecules to produce a larger molecule without the elimination of a smaller molecule e.g. water. If the two molecules are the same, a **homopolymer** is formed; if they are different, a **heteropolymer** is formed. **Condensation polymerization** is the reaction between two usually dissimilar molecules to form a larger molecule with the elimination of a smaller molecule (often water). **Polymerization shrinkage** is a potential problem, particularly with restorative polymers, which can result in cuspal fracture and is minimized by the addition of *fillers.

polymethylmethacrylate *n.* A polymer of methyl methacrylate. *See also* ACRYLIC RESIN.

polymorphous low-grade adenocarcinoma *n.* A malignant salivary gland *neoplasm that occurs almost exclusively on the palate.

polyodontia (polydontia) *n.* The condition of having *supernumerary teeth.

polyp *n.* A *pedunculated, usually *benign, growth from a mucous membrane. A **fibroepithelial polyp** is an overgrowth or firm nodule of fibrous tissue covered by epithelium usually formed in response to chronic irritation. A **pulp polyp**, sometimes known as **chronic hyperplastic pulpitis** or **proliferative pulpitis**, is a proliferation of vascular granulation tissue on the surface of an exposed pulp; pulpal tissue necrosis which would normally take place does not occur, partly due to the lack of significant intrapulpal pressure. Pulp polyps are often found in open carious lesions, particularly in children or as a result of pulpally involved tooth fracture or loss of a restoration.

polypeptide *n.* A molecule consisting of three or more amino acids linked together by covalent (peptide) bonds. *Protein molecules are polypeptides.

polyphagia *n.* Excessive or gluttonous appetite.

polypharmacy *n.* The prescription of more than one type of medicine.

polyphyodont *adj.* Pertaining to the development of generations of successional teeth, as found in most reptiles and fishes. The teeth usually have a brief functional lifespan and tend to be morphologically simple in structure.

polyprotodont *adj.* Referring to members of the marsupial order which have more than two lower incisors.

polysaccharide *n.* A complex carbohydrate formed from many monosaccharides joined together. They function as a storage form of energy e.g. glycogen in animals, and as structural elements e.g. mucopolysaccharides in animals and cellulose in plants.

polysialia *n.* Increased salivary flow (hypersalivation).

polystomatous *adj.* Having many mouths.

polysulphide *n.* A non-aqueous elastomeric impression material (*elastomer). It is prepared by mixing a base material (mercaptan) with either an inorganic catalyst (lead dioxide or lead peroxide) or an organic catalyst (benzoyl peroxide). It can be used in a dual impression technique combining heavy-bodied (high-viscosity) material with a high permanent set with a light-bodied (low-viscosity) material providing fine detail reproduction.

polytetrafluoroethylene (PTFE) *n.* An insoluble and chemically inert synthetic fluoropolymer. It is used for dental floss and tape because of the ease with which it slides between the teeth without fraying or shredding. It is also used as a liner when trying in intracoronally retained indirect restorations prior to cementation. Trade name: **Teflon®**.

polyvinylsiloxane *n. See* SILICONE IMPRESSION MATERIAL.

pontic *n.* A suspended member on a fixed partial denture. It replaces a natural tooth and restores its function and usually its aesthetics. A pontic may reproduce both the aesthetics and morphology of the natural tooth or it may be constructed on the posterior part of the mouth to allow a self-cleansing area between the pontic and the mucosal tissue covering the alveolar ridge (**sanitary, hygienic,** or **self-cleansing pontic**).

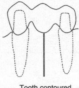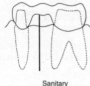

| Tooth contoured pontic | Sanitary pontic |

Pontic

Pont's index A method of predetermining the ideal dental arch width, first postulated by A. Pont in 1909. **Pont's premolar index** is the sum of the widths of the four maxillary incisors (taken from the distal contact points with the canines on either side) divided by the premolar arch width (taken from the first maxillary premolars of the left and right sides at the distal ends of their occlusal grooves), multiplied by 100. **Pont's molar index** is the sum of the widths of the four maxillary incisors divided by the molar arch width (taken from the maxillary left first permanent molar to the same of the right side at its mesial pit on the occlusal surface), multiplied by 100.

population *n.* (in statistics) Defines the total group with the characteristic which is being studied.

porcelain *n.* Dental porcelain consists mainly of silica (silicon dioxide, SiO_2), potassium, and sodium *feldspar. Some of the newer porcelains contain aluminium oxide (*alumina), zirconium oxide (zirconia), or magnesium aluminium oxide (spinelle) as the main components. Porcelain can

be classified according to fusion temperature: **high fusing** (1300°C), used for the manufacture of denture teeth; **medium fusing** (1101–1300°C), used for porcelain jacket crowns and inlays; **low fusing** (850–1100°C), used for metal ceramic and porcelain jacket crowns, inlays, and veneers; and **ultra-low fusing** (<850°C), used for titanium and titanium alloy crowns.

porion *n. See* CEPHALOMETRIC ANALYSIS.

porosity *n.* The presence of pores or small holes in a structure. In dental castings, porosity may occur due to the inability of gases to escape through the investment material or to localized shrinkage during solidification. Porosity can occur in *amalgam due to inadequate condensation.

porotic dentine *n. See* DENTINE.

Porphyromonas gingivalis *n.* A *Gram-negative, non-sporebearing anaerobic, rod-shaped bacterium associated with *periodontal disease.

> **(∰) SEE WEB LINKS**
> • The website of the *Porphyromonas gingivalis* Genome Project, with an overview of the bacterium.

port wine stain *See* HAEMANGIOMA.

position *n. See* RELATION.

positioner *n.* A resilient orthodontic appliance designed to move the teeth in a controlled and predetermined direction and used for finishing orthodontic cases. It is designed to achieve minor correction of sagittal plane arch relationship discrepancies. The appliance fills the *freeway space, and covers the clinical crowns of all the teeth and about 3mm of the buccal and lingual gingival mucosa. It is constructed over a predetermined ideal tooth configuration and fabricated from either plastic or a flexible material. *See also* INVISALIGN.

positron emission tomography (PET) An imaging technique that uses signals emitted by a short-lived radioactive tracer isotope to construct images of the distribution of the tracer in the body. The isotope is incorporated into a metabolically active molecule and is usually injected into the bloodstream where it travels to the target organ. As the radioisotope decays it undergoes positron emission. It is used as an alternative diagnostic technique to *computerized tomography (CT) or *magnetic resonance imaging (MRI) scanning for head and neck squamous cell carcinoma.

Further Reading: Valez T. L. Positron emission tomography: a promising diagnostic modality for head and neck pathology. *J Oral Maxillofac Surg* 2006;64:1272–7.

Posselt's envelope A sagittal view of maximum mandibular movement, first described by U. Posselt in 1952. Posselt also postulated that in the initial 20mm of opening and closing, the mandible only rotates and does not simultaneously move downward and forward.

post *n.* A metal, ceramic, or fibre-reinforced peg or dowel used to attach an artificial crown to the root of a natural tooth. A metal post may be either cast or preformed; preformed posts are either tapered or parallel-sided, and may have a thread for additional retention which enables them to be screwed into a prepared post hole. Examples of fibre-reinforced posts are carbon-fibre and glass-fibre. Posts are retained using a *luting cement. 📷

Further Reading: Bateman G., Tomson P. Trends in indirect dentistry: 2. post and core restorations. *Dent Update* 2005;32 (4):190–92, 194–6, 198.

postcristid *n.* An enamel ridge joining the *hypoconid and the *hypoconulid on the occlusal surface of a mandibular molar.

post crown Any artificial crown which can be attached to a tooth root by means of a *post, which may be preformed or cast metal. 📷

post-dam (post-palatal dam) *n.* A groove cut along the posterior palatal margin of a denture cast which produces a ridge on the finished denture and forms a more effective posterior seal to aid retention. It also acts to prevent food debris collecting between the palatal mucosa and the denture.

posterior *adj.* Describing a location behind or at the back of the body or an organ.

posterior nasal apertures *n.* See CHOANAE.

posterior open bite *n.* See BITE.

posterior triangle An anatomical term used to describe a region of the neck also known as the **lateral cervical triangle**. It is bounded anteriorly by the sternocleidomastoid muscle, posteriorly by the anterior border of the trapezius muscle, superiorly by the union of the sternoclaidomastoid and trapezius muscles, and inferiorly by the middle third of the clavicle. *See also* ANTERIOR TRIANGLE.

post hoc tests (in statistics) A set of comparisons between group means that were not thought of before data collection. The tests generally involve the comparison of *means from the different combinations of pairs of experimental conditions. They are used during the second stage of the *analysis of variance (ANOVA) or *multivariate analysis of variance (MANOVA) if the *null hypothesis is rejected.

post-operative complications *pl. n.* Unanticipated problems following surgery. They are, most commonly, bleeding, infection, or excessive pain.

post-operative haemorrhage *n.* Excessive bleeding following surgery. *See also* HAEMORRHAGE.

post-palatal seal *n. See* POST-DAM.

postprotocrista *n.* An enamel ridge joining the *metacone and the *protocone on the occlusal surface of a maxillary molar.

posture (balanced, neutral) *n.* The position of the operator when undertaking restorative dentistry in a seated position that is most ergonomic and provides the least muscular stress. A balanced posture is characterized by the upper arms being vertical and in contact with the rib cage, the forearms parallel to the floor, the body weight evenly balanced, and the seat height such that the heels rest comfortably on the floor.

Further Reading: Paul J. E. Four-handed dentistry. 1. Principles and techniques: a new look. *Dent Update* 1983;10(3):155–7, 159–60, 162–4.

((⬡)) **SEE WEB LINKS**
• An outline of the operating technique for four-handed (close support) dentistry.

potassium sulphate *n.* A chemical added in small quantities to gypsum products as an accelerator to increase the rate of reaction and shorten the setting time.

potentization *n.* The process of preparing a homeopathic remedy by repeated serial dilution with vigorous mixing (*succussion).

power *n.* (in statistics) The probability of detecting a meaningful difference, or effect, if one were to occur. Ideally, studies should have power levels of 0.80 or higher, which indicates an 80% chance or greater of finding an effect if one was really there.

practice effect Describes a participant's performance in an experiment being influenced, either positively or negatively, by repeating the task due to familiarity with the experimental situation or measures.

practice information leaflet (PIL) An information leaflet detailing the services provided to patients within a dental practice. It is a contractual requirement, under the National Health Service (NHS) regulations for practices treating patients under these regulations, to make such a leaflet available to their patients. The leaflet must contain details of the names and qualifications of all dental professionals providing NHS services (e.g dentists, hygienists, therapists), the services provided and their availability including emergency arrangements, the provision for patients with disabilities, the complaints procedures, and any foreign languages spoken.

Prader–Willi syndrome (PWS) Also known as **Prader–Labhart–Willi syndrome**. A rare genetic disorder linked to chromosome 15, and first described in 1956 by Andrea Prader, Inrich Willi, and Alexis Labhart. It is characterized by excessive hunger and an abnormally large intake of food (hyperphagia), oesophageal reflux, cognitive impairment, behaviour issues, reduced muscle tone (hypotonia), and hypogonadism. Oral conditions associated with PWS include enamel *hypoplasia, caries, a thick or reduced salivary flow, and excessive tooth wear in adults.

Further Reading: Dougall A., Fiske J. Access to special care dentistry, part 6. Special care dentistry services for young people. *Br Dent J* 2008;205:235–49.

pre-adjusted bracket *n. See* BRACKET.

precementum *n. See* CEMENTOID.

precision attachment *n.* Machined manufactured *connector with male and female components used to retain a removable bridge, partial, or complete denture (fixed or removable prosthesis); they may be either rigid or resilient. They are used to redirect the forces of occlusion so that the occlusal load distribution can be varied between the hard and soft tissues. One part is attached to a root, a tooth, or an implant and the other to the artificial prosthesis. **Intra-coronal**

attachments are housed within the contour of the tooth and provide either entirely frictional retention or frictional retention supplemented by mechanical means. The **Chayes attachment**, first described by Herman Chayes in 1906, is a T-shaped intracoronal attachment which provides retention mainly by the frictional surface area of contact between the two parts of the attachment. **Extra-coronal attachments** have part or all of their mechanism external to the contour of the tooth; they may project from an *abutment crown, may allow movement between two sections of a prosthesis, or be a combined unit with an extra-coronal hinge connected to an intra-coronal attachment. **Stud attachments** have a ball-shaped male component (patrix) soldered to a cast post and core and a female sleeve (matrix) cured into the fitting surface of the prosthesis; these attachments are used for retaining *overdentures; examples are Rothermann eccentric, Dalbo®-Rotex, and Zest anchor. **Bar attachments** may be parallel-sided for retaining partial dentures or can be round or ovoid for retaining complete dentures; they normally have a plastic or metal sleeve; straight bars allow for some rotation of the prosthesis around the bar creating some resiliency that permits the occlusal load to be distributed between the supporting teeth or implants and the soft tissues. Examples of bar attachments are the *Dolder, Ackerman, and Hadar attachments. **Magnetic attachments**, used specifically for overdentures, allow a degree of lateral movement which can be advantageous, providing the lateral movement is not too excessive; they can be produced in thin section and usually retain their magnetism for a clinically acceptable period of time.

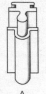 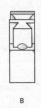

A

B

C

D

E

F

A   Intra-coronal (friction only)

B   Intra-coronal (mechanical supplementation)

C   Extra-coronal

D   Stud (Rothermann eccentric)

E   Stud (Dalbo®-Rotex)

F   Bar (Dolder)

Types of precision attachments

- A computer-aided learning programme on precision attachments from the University of Birmingham Dental School.

predentine *n. See* DENTINE.

preformed metal crown *See* CROWN.

pregnancy epulis *n. See* EPULIS.

pregnancy gingivitis *n. See* GINGIVITIS.

premalignant condition A generalized condition in which the patient has a higher risk of developing malignancy. Oral examples include *lichen planus, submucous fibrosis Plummer Vinson (Patterson Kelly) syndrome, and discoid *lupus erythematosus.

premalignant lesion A morphologically altered tissue which has a higher risk of turning malignant than normal tissue. In the oral cavity *leukoplakia and *erythroplakia are premalignant lesions.

premature contact *n. See* CONTACT.

premaxilla *n.* A bone on either side of the midline between the nose and the mouth, forming the anterior part of each half of the maxilla in the foetus. The premaxillae become united and form the incisal part of the upper jaw.

premedication *n.* Drugs administered to a patient prior to surgery to reduce anxiety and apprehension and aid sedation prior to anaesthesia.

premolar (bicuspid), mandibular first *n.* The tooth that replaces the primary first *molar located in the permanent *dentition of the *mandible between the canine and the second premolar tooth. The crown is roughly circular in outline, although slightly flattened mesio-lingually. It has one large buccal cusp and one much smaller lingual cusp whose apex is at a much lower level than the buccal cusp. The cusps are invariably connected by a central ridge running bucco-lingually, on either side of which is a pit (*fossa). The distal pit is normally larger than the mesial pit. Marginal ridges bound both pits and connect with the two cusps. Frequently a groove runs from the mesial pit over the mesial marginal ridge onto the mesio-lingual surface. The crown is inclined lingually, so that the apex of the buccal cusp lies directly over the vertical axis of the root. The mesial and distal surfaces are convex and slope towards the narrower lingual surface of the root. There is normally only one root with vertical grooves, on the flattened mesial and distal surfaces of which the mesial is more marked. There is

normally a single root with a pulp chamber having one pulp horn extending towards the apex of the buccal cusp and a single pulp canal, although this may be subject to considerable variation.
*Calcification of the tooth begins at about 1½–2 years after birth and the crown is normally complete by 5–6 years of age. The tooth erupts at about 10–12 years and the calcification of the root is complete at about 12–13 years.

premolar (bicuspid), mandibular second *n.* The tooth that replaces the primary second *molar located in the permanent *dentition of the *mandible between the first premolar tooth and the first molar. The crown is almost circular in outline and is larger than the crown of the first mandibular premolar but is subject to more variation. The two cusps are more equal in size and are united by a bucco-lingual ridge either side of which is a mesial and distal occlusal pit (*fossa). The lingual cusp may be divided into two smaller cusps, of which the mesial is normally the larger. The mesial and distal marginal ridges are well formed; they bound the occlusal pits and connect the two cusps. Often the disto-buccal ridge may be absent so that a mesio-distal groove (*fissure) connects the two pits. The mesial and distal surfaces are convex and slope towards the narrower lingual surface of the root. The lingual surface is wider than in the first premolar. There is a single root which, not uncommonly, curves distally towards the apex. It is oval in cross-section and flattened on the mesial and distal surfaces, often having vertical grooves. There is a single root canal with two pulp horns directed towards each cusp.
*Calcification of the tooth begins at about 2 years after birth and the crown is normally complete by 6–7 years of age. The tooth erupts at about 11–12 years and the calcification of the root is complete at about 13–14 years.

premolar (bicuspid), maxillary first *n.* The tooth that replaces the primary first *molar located in the permanent *dentition of the *maxilla between the *canine and the second premolar tooth. Viewed from the occlusal aspect, the crown is oval in shape, being broader buccally than palatally and narrower mesio-distally than bucco-palatally. The buccal, palatal, and distal surfaces of the crown are convex; the mesial surface is convex towards the occlusal surface but has a concavity towards the cervical margin (*canine fossa). The crown has a palatal cusp and a larger buccal cusp, the mesial slope of which is longer than the distal slope. The two cusps are separated by a well-defined central groove (*fissure) running mesio-distally and terminating in two small pits bounded by mesial and distal marginal ridges. A shallow extension of the central groove usually crosses the mesial marginal ridge to end on the mesial surface.

p

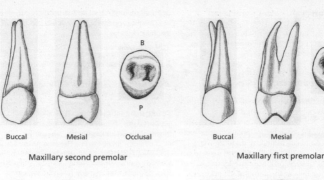

| Buccal | Mesial | Occlusal |

Maxillary second premolar

Maxillary first premolar

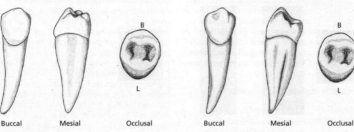

| Buccal | Mesial | Occlusal |

Mandibular second premolar

Mandibular first premolar

Premolars

There are normally two roots, located buccally and palatally, although occasionally there may only be one, within well-demarcated vertical grooves on the mesial and distal surfaces. The *pulp chamber is oval in cross-section, being longer bucco-palatally than mesio-distally. Two pulp horns extend into the buccal and palatal cusps. If there are two roots, there are normally two root canals, although this may be subject to considerable variation. *Calcification of the tooth begins at about 1½–2 years after birth and the crown is normally complete by 5–6 years of age. The tooth erupts at about 10–11 years and the calcification of the root is complete at about 12–13 years.

premolar (bicuspid), maxillary second *n.* The tooth that replaces the primary second *molar located in the permanent *dentition of the *maxilla between the first premolar and the first *molar tooth. The crown has a similar shape to the upper first molar but is slightly smaller and more oval and the two cusps are more equal in size. It has a mesio-distal central groove (*fissure) confined to the occlusal surface and less well defined than that of the upper first premolar. The buccal, palatal, mesial, and distal surfaces are all convex and, unlike the upper first premolar, there is no concavity on the

mesial surface. There is normally only one root with vertical grooves on the flattened mesial and distal surfaces. The *pulp chamber is similar in shape to the upper first premolar, with two pulp horns extending into the cusps. There are usually two root canals, although this may be subject to considerable variation. *Calcification of the tooth begins at about 2 years after birth and the crown is normally complete by 6–7 years of age. The tooth erupts at about 10–12 years and the calcification of the root is complete at about 12–14 years.

prenatal *adj.* Before birth.

preparation *n.* The process of modifying a tooth as part of a restorative procedure. This may include the removal of caries, previously placed restorative materials, unsupported enamel and dentine, or reshaping of the interior and exterior surfaces as required to allow a restorative procedure to be satisfactorily completed. *See also* CAVITY DESIGN. A **slice preparation** is a type of cavity preparation in which a slice of the proximal convexity of the tooth is removed to achieve a shoulderless and cleansable margin.

preprotocrista *n.* An enamel ridge joining the *protocone and the *paracone on the occlusal surface of a maxillary molar.

prescription *n.* An order in writing for dispensation of a medicine (in a legally prescribed format), signed by a person qualified by law to prescribe and made to a professional who is legally authorized to dispense.

presenility *n.* (*adj.* **presenile**) Premature ageing of either the mind or body.

prevalence rate A measure of the proportion of people in a population affected with a particular disease. **Point prevalence** is a measure of a condition or disease in a population at a given point in time; it is calculated by dividing the number of persons identified with the disease or condition at a specific point of time by the size of the total population at the same point of time. **Period prevalence** is the representation of the extent of a disease or condition in a population during a specific period of time; it is calculated by dividing the number of persons identified with the disease or condition during a specific period of time by the size of the population during the same period of time.

prevalence study *See* CROSS-SECTIONAL STUDY.

prevention *n.* The protection of an individual from disease. **Primary prevention** is aimed at keeping an individual or population healthy by prevention of the initiation of disease such as by *immunization, dietary advice, *plaque control programmes, and *fissure sealants. **Secondary prevention** aims to limit the progression and effect of a disease as soon as possible after onset. **Tertiary prevention** is concerned with limiting the extent of *disability once a disease has caused some functional limitation.

preventive dental unit (PDU) A designated area designed specifically for providing preventive dental advice and treatment for patients on an individual or group basis.

Further Reading: Oral health education, in *Advanced Dental Nursing*, ed. R. S. Ireland. Blackwell Munksgaard, 2004, 71–2.

preventive dentistry The branch of dentistry concerned with the prevention of dental disease. It includes such measures as dietary advice, *plaque control measures, *fluoride application, and the application of *fissure sealants.

preventive resin restoration The treatment of a small discrete *carious lesion within the pit and fissure system of a tooth with an adhesive resin restorative. The tooth is first cleaned with an abrasive solution and cavity access obtained with minimal enamel removal. Dentine caries is removed and the cavity restored

with a *resin composite using the *acid-etch technique. A protective pulpal *lining may be indicated.

Further Reading: Ripa L. W., Wolff M. S. Preventive resin restorations: indications, technique, and success. *Quintessence Int* 1992;23(5):307–15.

Prevotella intermedia A Gram-negative anaerobic pathogen (formerly *Bacteroides intermedius*) involved in periodontal infections. It has many of the virulence factors found with *P. gingivalis*. *P. intermedia* appears to be commonly associated with *gingivitis.

pre-wedging *n.* The procedure of inserting a *wedge between the interproximal surfaces of two adjacent teeth prior to cutting a cavity involving a proximal wall. The purpose is to achieve some tooth separation such that, after restoration, the teeth will return to their original position and a more positive tooth contact area will be achieved.

prilocaine *n.* An amide local analgesic agent. It produces less vasodilatation than *lignocaine. In high doses it can cause *methaemoglobinaemia and *cyanosis. It has a potent topical anaesthetic effect and is a constituent of *EMLA cream. Trade name: **Citanest**.

primary care *n.* Healthcare provided by a general medical or *dental practitioner, or other healthcare professional to whom patients have direct access and to whom they can normally self-refer. It is usually the first point of patient contact with a healthcare provider.

Primary Care Act 1997 An act passed by the UK parliament to provide for new arrangements in relation to the provision within the *National Health Service of medical, dental, pharmaceutical, and other services. It established pilot schemes for the *Personal Dental Service (PDS). The PDS was partially replaced in 2006 by the new General Dental Services (nGDS) contract.

Primary Care Trust (PCT) One of a group of freestanding statutory bodies within the *National Health Service responsible for working with dental providers to assess and meet the oral health needs of local communities and commission local healthcare.

primary (deciduous) dentition The first set of teeth which erupt into the mouth. Each mouth quadrant has 5 teeth—2 incisors anteriorly, 1 canine distal to the 2 incisors and 2 molars distal to the canine—to make a total dentition of 20 teeth. The incisors erupt at 6–9 months of age, followed by the first molars at 12–14 months, the canines at 16–18 months, and finally the second molars at 24–30 months. There can be considerable variation in eruption dates, although eruption of the central incisors after the lateral incisors usually indicates some pathology. The primary teeth differ from the permanent teeth in that they have shorter crowns, narrower occlusal surfaces, broader and flatter contact areas, thinner enamel and dentine, longer pulp horns, curved roots (to accommodate the developing permanent successor) with open apices, and are lighter in colour. Primary teeth are normally replaced by teeth of the succeeding *permanent dentition but, where a permanent tooth fails to erupt, the primary tooth may be retained into adult life. *See also* ERUPTION.

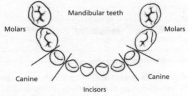

Primary (deciduous) dentition

primary dental care team *n.* *See* DENTAL CARE PROFESSIONAL.

primary enamel cuticle *See* NASMYTH'S MEMBRANE.

primary epithelial band A thickening of the ectodermal *epithelium underneath the oral *ectoderm at about the 6th week of intrauterine life. It differentiates into the *vestibular band, which eventually forms the lips and cheeks, and the *dental lamina from which the tooth germs develop.

primary intention, healing by *See* WOUND.

primary nasal septum A vertical soft tissue process formed from the *fronto-nasal process at about the 6th week of intrauterine life. It

eventually contacts the palatal shelves anteriorly to divide the nasal cavities.

primary palate *See* PALATE.

primary prevention *See* PREVENTION.

primate space (anthropoid space) A naturally occurring spacing between the teeth of the primary dentition. In the maxillary arch, it is located between the lateral incisors and canines, whereas in the mandibular arch the space is between the canines and first molars. It also occurs between the canine and first premolar teeth in adult primates.

primer *n.* A chemical used to treat the surface of enamel or dentine to improve bonding prior to the insertion of a restorative material. Primers, e.g. phosphoric acid, are usually applied in conjunction with an adhesive. Primers are also referred to as *conditioners. Primers may be water-based, *acetone-based, or alcohol-based.

prion *n.* An abnormal form of a constituent protein (PrP) of brain cells (prion is an acronym for proteinaceous infectious particle). Prions are composed solely of protein and can be infectious. They cause several diseases in a variety of mammals, including scrapie in sheep and bovine spongiform encephalopathy (BSE) in cattle, and are thought to be a causal agent of variant *Creutzfeldt–Jakob disease in humans (vCJD). Prions are very stable and present potential problems with cross-infection control because of their resistance to inactivation or destruction by standard thermal, chemical, and other means used for destroying micro-organisms in a dental healthcare environment. Prion disease is characterized by the destruction of brain and neural tissue, which is currently untreatable and eventually fatal.

Further Reading: Azarpazhooh A., Leake J. L. Prions in dentistry – what are they, should we be concerned, and what can we do? *Tex Dent J* 2006;123(5):421–8.

private dentistry Dental healthcare not funded by a state or governmental body. It is usually funded by direct payments from the patient on a fee-per-item basis, by fixed regular monthly payments, or by dental insurance policies. Dentists in Wales providing private dental care must register with the Healthcare Inspectorate Wales (HIW) under the Care Standards Act 2000 (modified by the Private Dentistry (Wales) Regulations 2008).

(((⊕))) SEE WEB LINKS

- Website of the Healthcare Inspectorate Wales.
- The Office of Fair Trading guide to private dentistry.

p

probability (p) value (in statistics) The chances of obtaining a certain pattern of results if there really is no relationship between the variables and the result could therefore have been caused by chance. For example, a p-value of 0.01 (p = 0.01) means there is a 1 in 100 chance the result occurred by chance. If the p value is less than 0.05 (<0.05) then the result is not due to chance and is statistically significant. The lower the p-value the more rigorous the criteria for concluding significance.

probe *n.* A thin flexible instrument designed to be inserted into a cavity or wound for the purposes of exploration. A probe with a sharp point used to investigate tooth surface defects is also called an *explorer. **BPE probe** *See* BASIC PERIODONTAL EXAMINATION. An **endodontic probe**, used to locate fine root canals, has an elongated working tip set at an angle to the handle. There are a number of designs of finely calibrated **periodontal probe** used for measuring the depth and topography of gingival and periodontal pockets. A **Goldman-Fox periodontal probe** is an angled tapering probe with a flat surface. A **Marquis® periodontal probe** has 3mm alternately coloured bands that mark 3, 6, 9, and 12mm, and is used for assessing the extent of oral soft tissue disease. The **Michigan-O periodontal probe** is a thin round cone-shaped probe, with circumferential markings at 3, 6, and 8mm, used for assessing oral disease; it is also available with Williams markings at 1, 2, 3, 5, 7, 8, 9, and 10mm. A **Nabers furcation probe**, named after Claude L. Nabers, a contemporary American periodontologist, is a hand instrument with a large curved tip used in assessing the extent of periodontal involvement between molar roots; it has circumferential markings at 2, 4, 6, and 8mm, made more visible by two black bands between the 2 and 4mm and the 6 and 8mm markings. The tip of the probe is moved towards the suspected location of the *furcation and then curved into the furcation area. Because of the difficulty in controlling pressure with manual probes, types of **automated probe** such as the **true pressure sensitive (TPS)®** probes have been developed to give more consistent, accurate, and reliable recordings; this probe consists of a tip connected to a special spring mechanism, which controls the pressure extended to the probe tip. According to the manufacturer, the force indicator lines coincide at approximately 20gm force. The **Florida periodontal probe** is an automated probe with a computerized device which combines a constant measured probing force with accurate periodontal pocket depth measurement. The **Williams periodontal probe**, developed by C. H. M. Williams in 1936, is a round, conical-shaped probe used for measuring periodontal pocket depths; it has circumferential markings at

1, 2, 3, 5, 7, 9, and 10mm; a 15mm extended version is available for probing inaccessible or deep pockets. *See also* POCKET MEASURING PROBE.

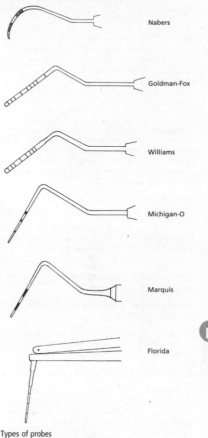

Nabers

Goldman-Fox

Williams

Michigan-O

Marquis

Florida

Types of probes

probing, circumferential The process of measuring the periodontal pocket depth of a tooth at a number of different locations around the circumference of the tooth.

probing depth The distance measured from the base of the pocket to the most apical point on the gingival margin. It dictates the patient's ability to maintain optimal plaque control. Probing depths in excess of 3mm are an indication for periodontal therapy.

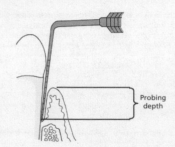

Probing depth

Probing depth

procaine *n.* An ester local *analgesic agent. Its use has now been replaced by *lignocaine but it may have an application for patients allergic to *amide local analgesic agents. It is no longer available in the United States in an injectable form. Trade name: **Novocain**.

process *n.* (in anatomy) A marked prominence or protuberance of bone such as the *alveolar process.

procheilia *n.* The condition in which one *lip protrudes further forward than its normal position.

procheilon *n.* The central prominence on the upper margin of the upper *lip.

proclination *n.* A sloping of the anterior teeth in a labial direction.

prodromal *adj.* Relating to the period of time between the first appearance of *symptoms of a disease and the development of a rash or fever.

professional ethics *n. See* ETHICS.

professional indemnity *n.* Legal protection against liability for professional *negligence or damages. Professional indemnity is a formal requirement by the *General Dental Council (GDC) in the UK and lack of it can lay the individual open to a charge of professional misconduct.

progeria (Hutchinson–Gilford syndrome) A rare collagen abnormality characterized by premature ageing in early childhood. The face is disproportionally small with a *retrognathic mandible, and beak-like nose. The average patient survives to the early teens.

proglossis *n.* The anterior portion or tip of the tongue.

prognathism *n.* (*adj.* **prognathic**) A condition of facial disharmony in which one jaw is markedly larger or projects further forward than the other. *See also* GNATHIC INDEX.

prognosis *n.* An assessment of the future course and probable outcome of a disease.

prokaryotes *pl. n.* (*adj.* **prokaryotic**) A group of organisms that do not have a cell nucleus or membrane-bound organelles. Most prokaryotes are unicellular and their DNA exists as a single chromosome that is not bounded by a nuclear membrane as occurs in *eukaryotes. Prokaryotes do not differentiate into multicellular forms and lack structural diversity. Prokaryotes are divided into two domains called *bacteria and *archaea, both of which have evolved differently. Bacteria are ubiquitous throughout the world and are essential for the recycling of nutrients. Some bacterial species cause disease in humans and animals. Archaea were originally described in extreme environments including very hot, very cold, highly acidic, highly alkaline, or highly salty environments; however, they are now also known to be ubiquitous. Whereas many bacterial species cause disease in humans and animals, currently there is little unequivocal evidence of archaeal pathogens.

prolabium *n.* The central area of the upper lip beneath the centre of the nose.

pronasion *n.* The point of the angle between the septum of the nose and the surface of the upper lip.

prop *n. See* MOUTH PROP.

prophylactic odontotomy *n. See* ODONTOPLASTY.

prophylactic paste *n. See* PASTE.

prophylaxis *n.* The use of any means to prevent disease. **Dental prophylaxis** involves the removal of *calculus, both sub- and supra-gingival, and *plaque from the surfaces of the teeth using hand or mechanical instrumentation accompanied by appropriate *oral hygiene instruction. **Antibiotic prophylaxis** is used to protect an individual from an anticipated bacterial invasion. *See also* ANTIBIOTIC. Fluoridation is a prophylactic measure used to prevent dental caries.

propofol *n.* A water-insoluble phenolic compound used as a general *anaesthetic intravenous induction agent. It may also be used as an intravenous *sedative agent for adult patients undergoing dental treatment. Trade name: **Diprivan**.

propolis *n.* A resinous material gathered by bees. It is a complex material containing 55% resinous compounds and balsam, 30% beeswax, 10% ethereal and aromatic oils, and 5% bee pollen. It has some antimicrobial action against fungi and some bacteria and viruses. It is used as a *homeopathic tincture in the treatment of *symptoms from oral ulceration, *pericoronitis, *alveolitis, and for the mummification of pulp tissue and as an adjunct to periodontal treatment; however, the evidence base for its efficacy is limited. It is an ingredient of some herbal *mouthwashes and toothpastes. Propolis is known to cause hypersensitivity and *anaphylaxis, and cases of allergic cheilitis and oral ulceration have been reported.

Further Reading: Gebaraa F. C., Pustiglioi A. N., de Lima L. A., Mayer M. P. Propolis extract as an adjunct to periodontal treatment. *Oral Health Prev Dent* 2003;1(1):29–35.

propranolol *n.* A beta blocker drug used to control abnormal heart rhythm, angina, and high blood pressure. It is administered by mouth or injection. Trade name: **Inderal.**

proprietary name (in pharmacy) The protected brand name or trademark registered with an appropriate patent office under which a manufacturer markets its product. It is written with an initial capital letter and is generally followed by the symbol®.

proprioceptor *n.* (*adj.* proprioceptive) A special nerve ending located in muscles, tendons, or joints that provides information about body movement and position. **Proprioception** is the unconscious perception of movement, body position, posture, balance, motion, and spatial orientation arising from stimuli within the body itself. *See also* KINAESTHESIA.

prosop- (prosopo-) Prefix denoting the face e.g. **prosopodynia** (pain in the face); **prosopoplegia** (facial paralysis); **prosoposchisis** (congenital facial cleft).

prospective study A study designed to follow one or more groups (cohorts) of participants forward in time, rather than retrospectively. It can determine the relationship over a defined period of time between a condition such as lung cancer, and a characteristic, such as smoking, shared by some members of the study group, noting the rate at which lung cancer occurs in the smokers and in the non-smokers. *Compare* RETROSPECTIVE STUDY.

prosthesis *n.* (*adj.* prosthetic) An artificial appliance used as a replacement for a body part or to correct a *congenital abnormality. In dentistry this includes partial and complete *dentures, *bridges (fixed prostheses), and

*orthodontic appliances. A **provisional prosthesis** is an interim prosthesis worn for a limited period of time, either to allow time to construct the permanent prosthesis or to allow for tissues to heal.

prosthetics *n. See* PROSTHODONTICS.

prosthion *n.* A craniometric point that is the most anterior point in the midline on the *alveolar process of the maxilla.

prosthodontics *n.* That branch of dentistry concerned with the functional and aesthetic rehabilitation of the masticatory system by artificial replacement of missing teeth and associated tissues. It may be subdivided into fixed prosthodontics (fixed bridgework), removable prosthodontics (*dentures and removable bridgework), and maxillofacial prosthetics.

prosthodontist *n.* A specialist in the practice of *prosthodontics.

protective clothing *n. See* PERSONAL PROTECTIVE EQUIPMENT.

protein *n.* A large complex molecule made up of one or more chains of *amino acids joined by *peptide bonds. Proteins are the principal constituents of cellular material and serve as enzymes, hormones, structural elements, and antibodies; they are synthesized in the body from their constituent amino acids.

proteolysis *n.* The breakdown of *proteins into their constituent *amino acids.

prothrombin *n.* A substance found in circulating blood (clotting factor II) that interacts with calcium salts to form **thrombin**, necessary for *blood coagulation.

protocone *n.* The mesio-palatal cusp of a mammalian maxillary molar tooth.

protoconid *n.* The mesio-lingual cusp of a mammalian mandibular molar tooth.

protocristid *n.* An enamel ridge joining the *metaconid and the *protoconid on the occlusal surface of a mandibular molar.

protostyle *n.* A minor cusp or fold of enamel on the palatal aspect of the occlusal surface of a maxillary molar or premolar situated mesio-palatal to the *protocone present in some mammalian or primate species. The **postprotostyle** is situated distal to the protostyle. A **protostylid** is a minor cusp or fold of enamel situated mesio-buccal to the *protoconid on a mandibular molar or premolar tooth.

protraction *n*. The condition in which the teeth of either jaw are located anterior to their normal position.

protrusion *n*. A forward projection of the teeth or jaws. **Bimaxillary protrusion** is associated with the maxillary and mandibular teeth, alveolar processes, or jaws.

protuberance *n*. An outward bulge, eminence, or knob of tissue.

provider *n*. 1. A healthcare institution. 2. A dental healthcare professional who holds a contract with the *Primary Care Trust in the UK. *See also* PERFORMER.

proving *n*. The testing of a homeopathic remedy by empiric means. The purpose is to gather symptoms experienced by a healthy person taking small doses of a homeopathic remedy.

provisional prosthesis *See* PROSTHESIS.

provisional restoration *See* RESTORATION.

provisional splint *See* SPLINT.

proximal *adj*. Situated towards the centre of the body. The area where the surfaces of two adjacent teeth in the same arch touch is the **proximal contact area**. The **proximal surface** describes either the *mesial or the *distal surface of a tooth.

pseudomembrane *n*. A loosely adherent grey layer of exudate and *necrotic *epithelium containing *leucocytes and bacteria. It is most commonly seen in *necrotizing gingivitis.

pseudo-pocket *n*. *See* POCKET.

pseudoprognathism *n*. The projection of the mandible forwards due to occlusal disharmonies that force it anteriorly. It can also occur as a result of decreased vertical dimension, such as the loss of the natural dentition without any prosthetic replacement causing a forward posturing of the mandible.

psychiatry *n*. (*adj*. **psychiatric**) The study of mental disorders and their diagnosis, management, and prevention.

psychology *n*. The scientific study of behaviour and its related mental processes.

psychomotor *adj*. Relating to muscular activity associated with mental activity. It is applied to conditions where cerebral disturbances affect muscular activity.

psychosis *n*. (*adj*. **psychotic**) A severe mental disorder, with or without organic damage, which may be chronic or transient, characterized by derangement of personality and loss of contact with reality, causing a deterioration of normal social functioning.

psychosomatic *adj*. Pertaining to the manifestation of physical symptoms resulting from a mental state and also to the reciprocal impact of disease on psychological functioning.

pterion *n*. An anatomical landmark at the junction of the sphenoid, frontal, parietal, and temporal bones.

pterygoid venous plexus The collection of veins occupying the *infratemporal fossa. It surrounds the maxillary artery and receives numerous branches that carry blood from the face and surrounding region to the facial and maxillary veins. It is connected to the **cavernous sinus** and the **pharyngeal venous plexus**. It is an important region because of the potential to spread dental infection; it can also be inadvertently penetrated when administering a block injection of the posterior superior alveolar nerve, potentially resulting in a *haematoma.

pterygomandibular raphe A tendinous band of the *buccopharyngeal fascia, attached by one extremity to the *hamulus of the medial pterygoid plate, and by the other to the posterior end of the mylohyoid line of the *mandible. It is formed by the union of the tendinous ends of the superior constrictor of the pharynx and buccinator muscles.

pterygomandibular space The space between the medial area of the mandible and the medial pterygoid muscle. It is a target area for administering block local anaesthesia of the inferior alveolar nerve. Infection in this area can spread to the parapharyngeal space.

ptyal- (ptyalo-) Prefix denoting saliva e.g. **ptyalorrhoea** (excessive flow of saliva); **ptyalolith** (a salivary *calculus).

ptyalectasis *n*. *See* SIALECTASIS.

ptyalin *n*. The enzyme amylase present in *saliva which breaks down starch into maltose and dextrin.

ptyalism (sialorrhoea) *n*. The excessive production of saliva. It is a symptom of a number of conditions including nervous disorders, infection, and *mercury poisoning.

ptyalith *n*. A stone (*calculus) in a salivary gland or duct.

ptychodont *adj*. Describing the crowns of molar teeth found in some animals (e.g. sharks) in which the enamel forms folds on the sides or occlusal surfaces. The enamel is fluted and folded upon itself longitudinally and laterally. Teeth lacking enamel folds are known as **aptychodont**.

puberty *n.* The time at which the secondary sex characteristics begin to develop and the reproductive organs become functional. It is brought about by an increase in sex hormone activity, due to stimulation of the ovaries and testes by pituitary hormones. It normally occurs from about the age of 10 in girls and 12 in boys. Girls going through puberty may experience swollen, sensitive, and bleeding gingivae, especially during their menstruation cycle. Sometimes ulcers may also appear in and around the mouth. **Precocious puberty** occurs at or before the age of 7 in girls and 9 in boys. Because of the early growth spurt this may lead to disruption in the normal tooth development pattern.

public health dentistry *See* DENTAL PUBLIC HEALTH.

pulp *n.* (in dentistry) A highly vascular connective tissue occupying the centre of the tooth. In addition to blood vessels, it contains nerves, *fibroblasts, *macrophages, and intercellular substances; it is surrounded by dentine, on the surface of which lies a layer of *odontoblasts capable of laying down dentine. The **pulp morphology** is dictated by the shape of the tooth and consists of a coronal portion in the crown of the tooth (**pulp chamber**) and root canals extending the length of the roots; small extensions (**pulp cornua, pulp horns**) project into the cusps of the tooth. The functions of the pulp include providing nutrients for the odontoblasts, acting as a sensory organ in response to external or internal stimuli, mobilizing defence cells (*histiocytes) when bacteria are present, and possibly contributing to the eruptive process of the tooth due to cellular proliferation causing increased pressure. The pulp may become inflamed (*pulpitis) as a result of the presence of bacteria or due to trauma. Pulpal age changes result in a reduction in volume due to continued secondary dentine formation, reduced cellular content and nerve supply, and an increase in collagen formation; calcific deposits (pulp stones or *denticles) may also be found.

pulpalgia *n.* Pain arising from the dental pulp. *See also* PULPITIS.

pulp cap *n.* An intervention to provide protection to the pulp. A **direct pulp cap** is a procedure in which a drug or medicament (e.g. calcium hydroxide or *mineral trioxide aggregate) is placed directly on the surface of an exposed pulp for the purpose of stimulating repair of the damaged or inflamed tissue. An **indirect pulp cap** involves placing a material, usually calcium hydroxide, on a thin residual layer of carious dentine remaining over the pulp to provide protection from external irritants.

Further Reading: Ricketts D. The management of the deep carious lesion and the vital pulp dentine complex. *Br Dent J* 2001;191:606–10.

pulp devitalization A procedure that destroys the vitality of the pulp. Chemicals such as *paraformaldehyde have been used for pulp devitalization but their use is no longer recommended because of their potentially toxic effect on adjacent tissues.

pulpectomy (pulp extirpation) *n.* The complete removal of the pulp tissue from the *pulp chamber and root canal system. It is a treatment option for irreversible *pulpitis. Pulpectomy may be undertaken in the *primary dentition to maintain the tooth free of infection, to biomechanically cleanse and obturate the root canals, to promote physiologic root resorption, and to maintain the space for the permanent successor tooth. *See also* PULPOTOMY.

pulp exposure The presence of a direct communication between the pulp tissue and the oral cavity. It can be a **traumatic exposure**, due to tooth fracture or injudicious cavity preparation, or a **carious exposure** following the spread of caries into the pulp chamber.

pulpitis *n.* Inflammation of the dental pulp. **Acute pulpitis** is characterized by a constant throbbing pain in the affected tooth (often made more severe by reclining), no pain on biting unless the inflammation has spread beyond the confines of the pulp tissue, and the inability to obtain relief from the pain. The pain is associated with the increased pulpal pressure caused by the influx of inflammatory cells, increased vascularity (*hyperaemia), and the inability of the pulp chamber to expand. Bacterial invasion may follow the inflammatory response. **Chronic pulpitis** may be the result of a persistent low-grade irritation or may follow acute pulpitis. It is characterized by a mild intermittent pain of varying intensity over a prolonged period which is difficult for the patient to localize. Pain is usually induced by thermal stimulation or sweet foods. There is a bacterial invasion with an increase in *plasma cells and *lymphocytes and an influx of *macrophages. Chronic pulpitis can resolve itself, progress to acute pulpitis, or result in pulp *necrosis following the accumulation of dead bacteria and necrotic debris. In an exposed pulp, the pulpal tissue may extrude through the communication into the oral cavity (**hyperplastic pulpitis**) to form a pulp *polyp; this is more common in primary teeth.

pulpotomy (partial pulpectomy) *n.* The removal of vital pulp from the crown of the tooth only. It is most commonly carried out on primary teeth where there is *pulp exposure but the tooth is asymptomatic or shows signs of reversible *pulpitis. The procedure involves the removal of residual caries, the removal of the coronal pulp as far as the base of the *pulp chamber, and the placement of a medicament such as *ferric sulphate or mineral trioxide aggregate (MTA) on the remaining pulp tissue for a short period of time; MTA is a biocompatible material when placed on the pulpal surface. The use of *formocresol as a pulpal medicament has raised concerns over its potential carcinogenicity and toxicity. The tooth is finally restored after the placement of an appropriate lining. A successful pulpotomy is indicated by an absence of tooth mobility, pain, tenderness to percussion, and pathological radiolucency.

Further Reading: Aeinechi M., Dadvand S., Fayazi S., Bayat-Movahed S. Randomized controlled trial of mineral trioxide aggregate and formocresol for pulpotomy in primary molar teeth. *Int Endod J* 2007;40:261–7.

(((●))) **SEE WEB LINKS**

• UK National Clinical Guidelines in Paediatric Dentistry on the British Society of Paediatric Dentistry website.

pulp polyp *See* POLYP.

pulp stone *See* DENTICLE.

pulp test The application of an external stimulus (electrical or thermal) to the surface of the tooth to determine the degree of *vitality of the pulp tissue. The electrical stimulus is provided by an instrument (**pulp tester**) which produces a high or low frequency current. Some recent tests have involved assessment of blood flow, and of these laser Doppler flowmetry has been the most widely used and beneficial to patients, particularly after traumatic injury.

Further Reading: Pitt Ford T. R., Patel S. Technical equipment for assessment of dental pulp status *Endodontic Topics* 2004;7(1):2.

pulse *n.* The expansion and contraction of an artery caused by contraction and subsequent relaxation of the heart muscle. It is most easily measured at the wrist (radial artery) or at the neck (carotid artery). The average **pulse rate** for a resting adult is 60–80 per minute.

pulse oximeter *n.* A non-invasive monitoring device for electro-mechanically monitoring arterial oxygen saturation. During the administration of conscious sedation it enables the operator to detect the early signs of *hypoxia. Its use is mandatory for intravenous, oral, and intranasal conscious sedation. It consists of a probe with a light emitting diode and photosensor, a digital display, an audible alarm, and a battery backup. It may in addition provide a graphic display of the pulse pressure. It works on the principle that the oxygenated blood is a brighter colour of red than the deoxygenated blood.

pumice *n.* A highly porous volcanic rock used as an *abrasive. It is produced with a variable grit size for use in polishing resin materials and as a *prophylactic paste for removing deposits or stain on natural teeth.

punch biopsy *n. See* BIOPSY.

purpura *n.* Purple spots (*petechiae) and patches caused by leakage of blood into the tissues under the skin or *mucosa.
Thrombocytopenic purpura is a rare condition occurring mainly in adults caused by a deficiency in blood *platelets and is characterized orally by spontaneous haemorrhage from any area of the mucous membrane.

purulent *adj.* Forming, consisting of, or containing *pus.

pus *n.* A thick yellowish liquid containing dead white blood cells (*leucocytes), necrotic tissue, and living and dead bacteria. It may drain from infected tissue or be retained within the tissue to form an *abscess.

push scaler *See* SCALER.

pustule *n.* (*adj.* **pustular**) A small *vesicle or blister on the skin containing *pus.

putrefaction *n.* The decomposition of proteins, particularly by anaerobic micro-organisms; the result is usually the formation of amines such as putrescine and cadaverine, which have a putrid smell.

p-value *See* PROBABILITY VALUE.

pyaemia *n.* Blood poisoning (*septicaemia) caused by pus-forming (pyogenic) bacteria released from an abscess; multiple abscesses may form as a result. *Compare* SEPTICAEMIA; TOXAEMIA.

pyogenic *adj.* *Pus-producing.

pyogenic granuloma *See* GRANULOMA.

pyorrhoea *n.* A lay or antiquated term used to describe *periodontal disease.

pyosis *n.* The formation and discharge of pus.

pyostomatitis vegetans *n.* A rare disorder affecting the oral mucosa and skin, associated with inflammatory bowel disease. It is characterized by oral ulceration, erosions, and papillary projections.

pyrexia (fever) *n.* An increase in body temperature above the normal oral temperature of 37°C (98.6°F) or rectal temperature of 37.2°C (99°F). This value is higher in children and lower in the elderly. It is usually caused by bacterial or viral infection and is generally associated with shivering, headache, nausea, constipation, or diarrhoea. Pyrexia may be intermittent with a rise and fall in body temperature returning to normal during the day.

qat (quat, khat) *n.* A green-leafed shrub (Catha edulis) whose leaves are chewed with the subsequent release of psychoactive agents. It is usually placed in the mucobuccal fold for several hours and is often accompanied by smoking *tobacco. It is reported to be associated with *periodontitis, *leukoplakia, and *oral cancer.

Further Reading: El-Wajeh Y. A. M., Thornhill M. H. Qat and its health effects. *Br Dent J* 2009;206:17–21.

quadhelix appliance *n.* A fixed slow-expansion *orthodontic appliance. It is attached to the teeth by *bands cemented to a molar tooth (usually the first molar) on each side of the arch. The spring between the molars is W-shaped and fabricated in 1mm stainless steel wire. In addition to expansion, the appliance can be used to de-rotate rotated molar teeth.

quadrant *n.* (in statistics) One half of each dental arch. The four quadrants are referred to as upper right, upper left, lower left, and lower right, with the dividing line being the midpoint of the arch.

qualitative research Gathers information that might aim to understand the reasons why a behaviour occurs. Qualitative research uses methods such as observation, in-depth interviewing, and focus groups. *Compare* QUANTITATIVE RESEARCH.

Quantiflex® machine The trade name for a machine used for delivering a continuous flow of nitrous oxide and oxygen to achieve and maintain conscious sedation.

quantitative research Information that can be expressed in numerical terms, counted, or compared on a scale. Quantitative research uses methods such as experimentation, observation, and surveys. *Compare* QUALITATIVE RESEARCH.

quarantine *n.* The period during which a person (or animal) is kept in isolation to prevent the spread of a *contagious disease.

quartile *n.* A statistical term describing one of four divisions of observations that have been grouped into four equal-sized sets based on their rank. For example, the first quartile is the point in a given distribution at which 25% of the observations fall below that point and 75% of the observations fall above it.

quartz *n.* *See* SILICA.

quartz-tungsten-halogen light *n.* The light source in many resin composite *curing lights. *See also* CURING LIGHT.

quaternary ammonium compounds *n.* Salts containing four alkyl or aryl groups attached to a nitrogen ion. They are *antiseptics and *surfactants such as benzalkonium chloride and cetylpyridinium chloride, used for their antiseptic properties as ingredients in *mouthwashes.

Quigley-Hein plaque index An index that evaluates the plaque revealed on the buccal and lingual non-restored surfaces of the teeth on a scale of 0 to 5, defined by G. A. Quigley and J. W. Hein in 1962 and modified by S. Turesky, N. D. Gilmore, and I. Glickman in 1970. All teeth except the third molars are assessed. An index for the entire mouth is determined by dividing the total score by the number of surfaces examined.

Quigley–Hain plaque index	
0	No plaque
1	Isolated flecks of plaque at the gingival margin
2	A continuous band of plaque up to 1mm at the gingival margin
3	Plaque greater than 1mm in width and covering up to one third of the tooth surface
4	Plaque covering from one thirds to two thirds of the tooth surface
5	Plaque covering more than two thirds of the tooth surface

quinsy *n.* A peritonsillar *abscess. *Pus accumulates in the space between the tonsil and the pharyngeal wall causing severe pain, *trismus, and difficulty in swallowing. Treatment is with antibiotics.

racemose *adj.* Resembling a bunch of grapes. It is used to describe a number of small sacs that form the secretory part of a compound gland e.g. a salivary gland.

rad *n.* An acronym for Radiation Absorbed Dose. One rad is equal to an absorbed dose of 0.01 joules per kilogram or 0.01 Gray.

radial pulse *See* PULSE.

radiation *n.* *See* IONIZING RADIATION.

radiation caries *See* CARIES.

radiation dermatitis *See* DERMATITIS.

radiation, diagnostic *Ionizing radiation used to establish the cause of a condition or disease. Examples used in dentistry are *computerized tomography (CT) and *x-rays.

radiation monitoring badge *See* FILM BADGE.

radiation mucositis *See* MUCOSITIS.

radiation necrosis *See* NECROSIS.

radiation protection The control of exposure to ionizing radiation. Protection against external radiation such as x-rays includes protective barriers (e.g. thyroid patient collars), ensuring an adequate distance from the radiation source is maintained, and keeping exposure times to a minimum. Radiation may be monitored by the operator wearing a personal *film badge.

radiation protection adviser (RPA) A person in the UK appointed in writing and approved under the *Ionizing Radiation Regulations 1999 (IRR99) to advise on matters relating to the taking of radiographs such as the testing of equipment, staff training, risk assessment, and quality assurance programmes.

radiation protection supervisor (RPS) A person in the UK responsible for implementing the local rules relating to the use of ionizing radiation equipment. The person may be an appropriately trained *dentist or a *dental care professional (DCP).

radiation therapy *n.* *See* RADIOTHERAPY.

radicular *adj.* Pertaining to the root of a tooth.

radicular cyst *n.* *See* CYST.

radiograph *n.* An image obtained by passing x-rays through the body onto a radiation-sensitive or light-sensitive film emulsion or digital imaging receptor. A useful diagnostic image is produced because the body absorbs different amounts of radiation depending on the atomic number of the tissue. Bone has a high atomic number and therefore absorbs more radiation than soft tissues, which have a lower atomic number. Dental radiographic films may be placed inside the mouth (**intra-oral**) or outside the mouth (**extra-oral**). Intra-oral radiographs include *bitewing, *periapical, and *occlusal radiographs. Extra-oral radiographs include *cephalometric radiographs (lateral cephalogram), *dental panoramic tomograms, and *oblique lateral radiographs.

radiographer *n.* A professional trained in taking radiographic images of parts of the body.

radiography *n.* The making of images on a photographic emulsion as a result of the action of *ionizing radiation.

radiography, digital

n. The result of an interaction of an x-ray beam with a digital sensor (which may be a charged couple device (CCD) or complementary metal oxide semiconductor (CMOS) receptor), which gives an instant image (**direct digital imaging**) or a photostimulable phosphor plate that requires processing in a laser reading device (**indirect digital imaging**). **Direct digital receptors** are either solid state CCDs or complementary metal oxide detectors; these provide an almost instant image. These sensors are available in a limited number of sizes and are more bulky than conventional film. Although wireless systems are available, most are connected to the personal computer through a cable, which can cause problems with cross-infection control. **Indirect digital sensors** consist of photostimulable phosphor (PSP) storage plates which require to be placed in a reader after exposure, to produce the image. The PSP plates are more like conventional film and are available in many sizes, including occlusal film size, and are thinner than direct digital receptors. The sensors can be reused many times but require careful handling to avoid scratches. In digital radiography, the image is made up of **pixels**; each pixel (2D image) represents the volume or voxel of the patient (3D image). Depending upon the number of x-ray photons absorbed by each pixel of the sensor, the pixel will be allocated a shade of grey between 0 and 256, with black being 0 and white being 256. **Digital image manipulation** can be achieved by altering the numbers allocated to each pixel; contrast and brightness are the most frequently manipulated functions. Brightness is compared to film blackening of a conventional film. **Brightness manipulation** will increase or decrease the shade of grey allocated to each pixel by the same amount. If the brightness is continually increased, the image will eventually become white as each pixel will reach 256 on the grey scale. **Contrast** is the visual difference between black and white; increasing contrast will decrease the number of shades of grey that can be observed. Contrast manipulation multiplies the shades of grey in each pixel by the same amount either increasing or decreasing the contrast.

radiologist *n.* A specialist trained in the interpretation of diagnostic x-rays and other imaging techniques and performing specialized x-ray procedures.

radiology *n.* A specialist branch of medicine or dentistry involving the study of radiographs and other imaging technologies.

radiolucent *adj.* Having the property of being transparent to x-rays. Radiolucent materials appear dark on an x-ray. *Compare* RADIOPAQUE.

radionecrosis *n. See* NECROSIS.

radiopaque *adj.* (*n.* **radiopacity**) Having the property of absorbing x-rays. Radiopaque materials appear light on an x-ray. Materials such as barium are added to *resin composite restoratives and crown posts to make them radiopaque: this is important as the detection of caries underneath non-radiopaque restorative materials is virtually impossible. Resin

composites should at least be as radiopaque as tooth enamel. *Compare* RADIOLUCENT.

radiotherapy *n.* The treatment of disease by *ionizing radiation to destroy *malignant cells or prevent their development. It may be given internally by drinking liquid, by injection, or by the implantation of radioactive needles, wires, or pellets, or externally by a shaped radiation beam aimed from several angles to intersect at the site of the tumour so that it receives a much larger absorbed dose than the surrounding healthy tissue.

radisectomy *n. See* HEMISECTOMY.

Ramsay Hunt syndrome [J. R. Hunt (1872–1937), American neurologist] An infection of the facial nerve caused by the varicella zoster virus. It is characterized by facial paralysis, vesicles on the same side in the pharynx, external auditory canal, and on the face, and sometimes on the roof of the mouth or tongue. Treatment is with antiviral medications. *See also* BELL'S PALSY.

ramus *n.* (*pl.* **rami**) 1. A branch of a nerve fibre or blood vessel. 2. A thin projection of a bone such as the ramus of the *mandible.

randomization *n.* The process of making something random. This often applies to the random assignment of participants to different experimental conditions.

randomized controlled trial An investigation in which subjects are randomly assigned to two groups: one (the experimental group) receiving the intervention that is being tested, and the other (the comparison group or *control group) receiving no intervention.

random sample A sample of a population where each member of the population has an equal chance of being included in the sample. It can be **stratified** such that separate samples are drawn from each of many layers of the population, for example by age or sex.

range *n.* (in statistics) The difference between the highest and lowest values in a data set.

Ranke's angle [J. Ranke (1836–1916), German physician and anthropologist] The angle between the horizontal plane of the skull and a line through the centre of the maxillary alveolar process and the centre of the nasofrontal suture.

ranula *n.* A mucous cyst (*mucocoele) formed under the tongue due to the obstruction of one of the ducts from either the submandibular or sublingual salivary glands. It is characterized by a bluish, translucent, fluctuant swelling with possible elevation of the tongue. Ranulas are normally asymptomatic but, if large, may interfere with swallowing. Treatment is usually by excision, although sometimes by *marsupialization.

raphe *n.* A ridge or crease which marks the midline of an organ or structure.

rapid maxillary expansion (RME) A process of orthodontic tooth movement using a fixed hyrax *screw appliance. The screw is turned twice a day and is designed to 'split' the maxillary midline palatal suture and affect expansion of the upper arch by skeletal movement as opposed to dento-alveolar movement. **Surgically assisted rapid maxillary expansion (SARME)** is the surgical splitting of the midline palatal suture to assist in rapid palatal expansion.

rarefaction *n.* A decrease in density of a substance or tissue such as bone.

Raschkow's plexus [I. Raschkow (1811–72), German physician] A network of nerves below the odontoblast layer in the pulpodentinal border zone of the pulp.

rash *n.* An inflammatory skin lesion usually characterized by a general reddening of the skin or by discrete red spots. It may be a local skin reaction, such as in response to local irritation, or the outward sign of a disorder or infectious disease e.g. chickenpox and measles, affecting the whole body.

Rathke's pouch [M. H. Rathke (1793–1860), German anatomist] A depression in the floor of the embryonic mouth, anterior to the buccopharyngeal membrane, which eventually loses its connection with the pharynx and gives rise to the anterior lobe of the *pituitary gland.

ratio *n.* The proportional amount or magnitude of one quantity relative to another. The **water–powder ratio** is the relative amounts of water and powder in a mixture e.g. *gypsum or *alginate impression material.

reamer *n.* A thin tapered metal instrument with a spiral cutting edge used to enlarge, shape, and remove debris from an irregularly shaped canal, to produce a canal round in cross-section. Reamers are usually made of stainless steel with a triangular or square cross-section. They may be hand held or mounted in a dental handpiece. *See also* FILE; GATES–GLIDDEN DRILL.

reattachment *n.* The process whereby healthy supragingival *periodontal fibres become reattached to bone or *cementum following flap surgery to treat *periodontal disease or for other oral surgical procedures. This should not be confused with new *attachment. *See also* GUIDED TISSUE REGENERATION.

rebase *n.* The process of replacing most or all of the base of a denture without altering the occlusal relations of the teeth. It is undertaken to improve the shape of the fitting surface. It may be carried out using either a self-cure or heat-cure resin.

recall examination The process of reviewing or re-examining a patient to monitor oral health or any disease progression. It is an important aspect of preventive dentistry. The frequency of patient recall examination is influenced by the predisposition to disease, the current disease experience, the disease experience since the last examination, past dental history, the ability to maintain good oral hygiene and dietary habits, risk factors to other disease processes, patient expectations, and patient lifestyle changes. The National Institute of Health and Clinical Excellence (NICE) provides guidelines on recall examination intervals under guidance document CG19.

Further Reading: *Clinical examination and record keeping: good practice guidelines.* Faculty of General Dental Practitioners (UK), 2001.

(⊕) SEE WEB LINKS
• The National Institute of Health and Clinical Excellence guidelines on recall intervals.

receptionist *n.* A non-clinical member of the dental team, usually responsible for patient appointment management and office administration.

receptor *n.* 1. A specialized cell or group of cells capable of detecting environmental change and sending impulses to the central nervous system. Examples are sensory nerve endings and *proprioceptor fibres in the periodontal membrane which detect movement. 2. A specialized area of a cell membrane that can bind with a *hormone, drug, or other chemical to produce an intra-cellular change.

recertification *n.* The process of renewing membership of a professional register, which usually includes the requirement to have undertaken appropriate continuing professional education or development.

recession *n. See* GINGIVAL RECESSION.

reciprocal force *n.* A balancing force used in orthodontic therapy or partial denture construction to counteract another applied force. *See also* CLASP.

reciprocation *n.* The countering of the effect of one part of a removable partial denture

Active   Passive

Reciprocation

framework with another part of the framework. It may be **active reciprocation**, when there are two opposing and balanced retentive *clasp arms, or **passive reciprocation**, where the rigid part of the clasp arm is located opposite the retentive arm and on or above the height of the contour line or on a guiding plane. *See also* BRACING.

Further Reading: Davenport J. C., Basker R. M., Heath J. R., Ralph J. P., Glantz P. O., Hammond P. Bracing and reciprocation. *Br Dent J* 2001;190:10–14.

recontour *v.* The restoration of a tooth to its original anatomical form by appropriate instrumentation.

record *n.* Information preserved in written or electronic format. A **centric interocclusal record** is a record of the maxillae and mandible when in *centric relation. A **clinical record** is a paper-based or electronic form which contains the medical or dental history of a patient, including any radiographic or image data. A **facebow record** is a registration procedure to orientate the maxillary cast to the hinge axis of the articulator using a *facebow. A **plaque record** is a measure of the extent to which *plaque deposits are present on the tooth surfaces. A **protrusive record** is the registration of the mandible when it is located anterior to its centric *relation to the maxillae.

recrudescence *n.* A return of signs and symptoms in a patient following a period of quiescence, abatement, or improvement when recovery seemed to be taking place.

reduced enamel epithelium *See* ENAMEL EPITHELIUM.

refereed journal *n.* A professional journal or publication in which articles or research papers are reviewed by a panel of readers or referees who are experts in the field; they advise the editor as to the suitability of the article for publication.

reference nutrient intake (RNI) A *dietary reference value used to estimate the protein, vitamin, and mineral requirements of a defined healthy group of the population.

referred pain *See* PAIN.

refined carbohydrate *See* CARBOHYDRATE.

reflective practice The process of retrospectively examining one's own professional performance in order to clarify the reasons for one's actions and decisions, and to learn from them.

reflex *n.* An automatic or involuntary response to a stimulus such as the pharyngeal or *gag reflex. Consciousness is not necessarily involved.

refractory flask *n. See* FLASK.

refractory investment *n.* An investment material that can withstand the high temperatures used in soldering or casting of dental appliances and restorations. *See also* CRISTOBALITE.

refractory period *n.* The brief period following an action potential during which normal stimulation of a nerve will not cause another action potential.

refractory periodontitis *n. See* PERIODONTITIS, REFRACTORY.

regional block analgesia *n. See* ANALGESIA.

registration *n.* A record of the maxillary and mandibular jaw relationships made for transfer to dental casts which are then mounted on an *articulator. It is an important stage in the construction of *complete dentures, and partial dentures where the remaining teeth are insufficient to define the jaw relationship.

registration paste *n.* A material used to record the occlusal relationships of the natural or artificial maxillary and mandibular teeth or the relationship of the occlusal surfaces of wax registration blocks. The material is usually applied in a flowable form and allowed to set in the mouth to a rigid or semi-rigid state.

regression *n.* A statistical analysis tool that quantifies the relationship between a dependent *variable and one or more independent variables. **Stepwise regression** is a method of multiple regression in which variables are entered into the model based on a statistical criterion; after a new variable is entered into the model, the variables are all assessed to see whether any can be removed.

regulated waste (US) *n.* Refuse, often contaminated with infectious material, which must be disposed of according to specific regulations and guidelines. *See also* CLINICAL WASTE.

regurgitation *n.* The backward flow of digested or undigested food from the oesophagus or stomach. It is a symptom of *bulimia and can result in acid *erosion of the teeth.

rehabilitation *n.* The restoration of form and function following damage or disease. **Oral rehabilitation** is the restoration of the form, function, and aesthetics of the mouth and teeth.

reimplantation *n.* The replacement of a tooth (or teeth) that has been *avulsed from its alveolar socket due to accidental or non-accidental trauma. Reimplanted teeth require stabilization with a functional *splint, such as one made of resin composite, for about 7–10 days to allow periodontal ligament *reattachment to take place. The splint should allow some normal tooth movement within the socket to avoid *ankylosis. Factors affecting the success of reimplantation include the time from avulsion to reimplantation, the storage medium, the splinting time, and the viability of the pulp. Unwanted sequelae of reimplantation are root resorption or ankylosis.

reinforcement *n.* A technique used in psychological patient behaviour management in which a pattern of behaviour may be enhanced by reward (**positive reinforcement**) or by punishment (**negative reinforcement**).

Reiter's syndrome [H. Reiter (1881–1969), German physician] A condition characterized by inflammation of the urethra, arthritis, conjunctivitis, and oral ulceration; horny areas may develop on the skin. It is caused by an overreaction of the immune system to an infection. Treatment involves treating any triggering infection as well as treating the symptoms of the syndrome itself.

relapse *n.* 1. Any change from the final tooth position following the completion of orthodontic treatment. The change may be towards the original malocclusion or may be due to reasons unrelated to the treatment such as age changes. 2. A return of disease symptoms after apparent recovery or the worsening of an apparently improving condition.

relation *n.* The association or position of one object to another. **Centric jaw relation** is the most retruded physiologic relation of the mandible to the maxillae, to and from which individual lateral movements can be made. **Eccentric jaw relation** is any relation of the mandible to the maxillae other than centric relation. The **jaw rest relation** (position) is the postural relation of the mandible to the maxillae when the patient is in an upright position and the masticatory musculature is in a state of maximum relaxation.

relative analgesia *n. See* SEDATION.

relative risk (risk ratio) *n.* The ratio of risk in the intervention group to risk in the *control group. A risk ratio (RR) greater than 1.0 means that an individual is estimated to be at an increased risk.

reliability *n.* (in statistics) The consistency of a measuring instrument or set of measurements used to describe a test. An experiment is unreliable if repeated measurements give different results. **Internal consistency reliability** is estimated by using a single measurement instrument given to a group of people on one occasion to assess the reliability of the instrument. **Inter-rater reliability (inter-observer reliability)** is the extent to which two or more researchers (or observers) give consistent estimates of the same phenomenon. **Split-half reliability** is a reliability measure obtained by splitting items on a measure into two halves (randomly) and then obtaining a score from each half of the scale; by taking a correlation between the two scores a measure of reliability is obtained. The **test-retest reliability** is estimated by administering the same test to the same sample on two different occasions; this assumes there are no significant changes in the construct being measured between the two occasions.

relief *n.* The reduction or elimination of pressure from a specific area underneath or on the periphery of a denture base. A **relief area** is an area on a plaster model defined to relieve pressure on the tissues underneath a denture base; a space is created using a tin foil spacer adapted to the model surface and removed after processing. A **relief chamber** is a recess cut into the base of a denture to reduce or eliminate potential pressure on a specific area; it may be used on the palatal surface of a *complete denture with the intention of improving retention by creating negative pressure.

reline *n.* The procedure whereby the fitting surface of a *denture is resurfaced to improve the accuracy of fit on a jaw that has undergone bone resorption or soft tissue change since the denture was originally made. The procedure is frequently necessary where the denture has been fitted immediately after the extraction of the teeth (immediate denture) due to post-operative bone resorption.

remineralization *n.* The reintroduction of mineral salts into calcified tissues such as bone, enamel, dentine, and cementum. During enamel remineralization, mineral ions restore the deficient latticework structure of the *hydroxyapatite crystals. The *saliva is a supersaturated solution of calcium and phosphate ions normally in equilibrium with the tooth enamel, but if the *pH of the saliva changes either *demineralization or remineralization takes place according to the equation:

$$Ca_5(PO_4)OH \leftrightarrow 5Ca^{2+} + 3PO_4^{3-} + OH^-$$

The critical pH below which demineralization of enamel takes place is 5.2–5.5.

remission *n.* 1. A temporary loss or decrease in severity of symptoms. 2. The reduction in size of a *malignant tumour and its related symptoms.

removable prosthesis *See* PROSTHESIS.

repair *n.* The restoration of continuity after injury or damage. 1. (dentures) *See* DENTURE. 2. (cementum) The laying down of new cellular or acellular *cementum to repair cemental resorption and damage. 3. (restorations) *See* RESTORATION. 4. (tissue) Damaged or diseased tissue is repaired by the action of tissue-building cells such as *fibroblasts, *osteoblasts, and *odontoblasts.

reparative dentine *n. See* DENTINE.

replantation *n. See* REIMPLANTATION.

Reporting of Injuries, Diseases and Dangerous Occurrences Regulations 1995 (RIDDOR) A UK parliament statutory instrument that requires the reporting of work-related accidents, diseases, and dangerous occurrences. It applies to all work activities but not to all incidents. It includes events such as fatalities, major injuries to employees and patients, and certain specified diseases.

(((⊕))) **SEE WEB LINKS**

• The Office of Public Centre Information Statutory Instrument.
• Health and Safety Executive guidance details for RIDDOR.

reproximation (enamel stripping) *n.* The removal of small amounts of enamel from the mesial or distal surface of a tooth. It is carried out to create space, to correct tooth size discrepancies, to improve the contact area of the tooth, or to change the shape of the tooth.

rescue breathing *See* BREATHING, RESCUE.

resection *n. See* AMPUTATION.

reservoir bag A collapsible container from which gases such as oxygen and nitrous oxide are inhaled and into which gases may be exhaled during general *anaesthesia, inhalational sedation, or during artificial ventilation as part of *basic life support.

reservoir bite guard *See* BITE GUARD.

residual *n.* (in statistics) The difference between the value a model predicts and the value observed in the *data on which the model is based; it represents the error in a result.

residual volume The quantity of air remaining in the lungs after maximum expiratory effort.

resin *n.* Any of a class of solid or semi-solid organic products, usually *polymers of natural or synthetic origin; they are soluble in ether or acetone but insoluble in water. **Polymethylmethacrylate denture base resin** is formed by mixing beads made from polymethylmethacrylate and an *initiator (benzoyl peroxide) with liquid methyl methacrylate monomer and *polymerizing (curing) at room temperature (**self-curing, cold-cure, auto-curing**) or by the addition of heat (**heat-cure**). The impact strength may be increased by grafting a rubber-like butadiene-styrene polymer to the acrylic molecules. If polymerization is incomplete, the residual monomer can result in a soft tissue sensitivity reaction.

resin composite

n. An organic *resin matrix and an inorganic particulate *filler bonded to the resin matrix by a *coupling agent. The filler is added to the resin to reduce the high coefficient of thermal expansion, polymerization shrinkage, and water absorption, and to improve the mechanical properties: the properties and therefore the applications of resin composite depend on the physical and chemical properties of its individual components. The **resin matrix** is usually based on either Bis-GMA or *urethane dimethacrylate (UDMA), both being liquid monomers of high viscosity to which low viscosity resins such as tri-ethylene glycol dimethacrylate (*TEGDMA) and hydroxyethylmethacrylate (*HEMA) are added to lower the density and improve the resin cross-linking. Other chemicals which are added to the resin matrix are light or chemical curing activating agents, stabilizers to increase the shelf life, and pigments for aesthetics. The filler in early composites consisted of large *quartz particles (**macrofilled resin composites**) which tended to produce restorations of poor strength which were difficult to polish, and readily stained. To overcome the problems of aesthetics and poor polishability, **microfilled resin composites** were developed containing colloidal *silica with a smaller particle size. Unfortunately these resins have a lower filler loading (about 50% by volume) which reduces the long-term strength and wear resistance. Because of the disadvantages of both micro- and macrofilled composites, **hybrid resin composites** were developed which contain both larger quartz particles and smaller silica particles. A recent addition is **flowable resin composites** which have a low filler content (50–70% by volume) and will flow easily into cavities, although their wear resistance is low; the main indications include use in small cavities, *preventive resin restorations, class V cavities caused by non-carious tooth surface loss, and the restoration of primary teeth. Resin composites harden by polymerization; this may be achieved as a two paste **self-curing** process, in which a tertiary aromatic amine is added to one paste and a catalyst such as benzoyl peroxide is added to the other paste, or as a single paste **light activated** process in which the resin, filler, and *activator (camphorquinone) are all in the same paste. In the latter case, when the camphorquinone is exposed to light of a specific waveband (approximately 470 nanometres), free radicals are produced that initiate polymerization. Light curing has the advantage that polymerization is under the control of the operator and is fast, small

increments can be dispensed, and there is minimal wastage: however, in deep cavities curing may be incomplete because of the lack of light penetration. **Dual-cure composite**, a restorative material partially set by light and partially by a slower chemical reaction, has been developed to overcome the individual disadvantages of the other two curing methods. The advantages of resin composite restorative materials are that, in conjunction with a dentine adhesive, they can be placed with no or minimal tooth preparation, light curing permits immediate finishing and polishing, dentine bonding reduces marginal leakage, secondary caries, and tooth sensitivity, aesthetics is good, and it is possible to add to the material at a later date. The disadvantages are that polymerization shrinkage (typically 2–3%) can disrupt marginal adaptation and fracture cusps, dentine bonding can be problematical in deep cavities, water absorption can lead to marginal staining, there can be operator or patient *sensitivity to the resin, and poor radiographic definition can make diagnostic interpretation difficult. Resin composite may be modified by the addition of glass ionomer particles (*giomer, resin-modified glass ionomer *cement).

Further Reading: Bonsor S. J. Contemporary use of flowable resin composite materials. *Dent Update* 2008;35:600–06.
Contemporary dental materials, ed. V. B. Dhuru, 57–65. Oxford University Press, 2004.

((🌐)) **SEE WEB LINKS**
• The International Association of Dental Research poster research presentations on dental polymers, April 2009.

resin composite, fibre reinforced *n.*
Resin composite with added fibrous material to improve strength and rigidity. Examples of reinforcing materials are ultra high molecular weight polyethylene, glass fibre, carbon fibre, quartz fibre, and fibre pre-impregnated with light curing resin. A good bond between fibre and polymer matrix is required to ensure good mechanical properties and to prevent diffusion of liquids along the fibres. Uses for fibre reinforced resin include occlusal and periodontal splints, permanent or temporary bridges, reinforcement of large restorations, and anatomical posts.

Further Reading: Butterworth C., Ellakawa A. E., Shortall A. C. C. Fibre-reinforced composites in restorative dentistry. *Dent Update* 2003;30:300–06.

resin modified glass ionomer cement *n.*
See CEMENT.

res ipsa loquitur *adj.* A Latin phrase meaning 'the thing speaks for itself'. A rule of evidence whereby the negligence of an alleged wrongdoer can be inferred from the fact that the accident happened. If a judge accepts this argument the burden falls on the defendant to prove they were not professionally negligent.

resistance *n.* 1. A measure of the body's ability to withstand disease. 2. The degree to which a pathogenic organism remains unaffected by antibiotics or other drugs.

resistance form *n. See* FORM.

resorption *n.* The physiological or pathological loss of substance. **Bone resorption** occurs due to the activity of *osteoclasts; it allows tooth movement to take place during normal eruption, tooth migration, and *orthodontic therapy. **Horizontal bone resorption** is a typical feature of chronic *periodontitis in which the crestal margins of the *alveolar bone are resorbed. Alveolar bone resorption around an individual tooth (**vertical bone resorption**) may be associated with *occlusal traumatism and periodontal disease. Osteoclastic and cementoclastic activity can result in *root resorption.

respiration *n.* (*adj.* **respiratory**) The process of gaseous exchange between a cell and its environment, or between an animal and its environment. **External respiration**, where oxygen is taken up by the capillaries of the lungs and carbon dioxide is released from the blood, is controlled by the respiratory centre in the brain. The normal respiration rate in a resting adult is 14–20 breaths per minute and approximately 500ml of air is exhaled with each breath (**tidal volume**). During **internal respiration**, oxygen is released to the tissues and carbon dioxide is absorbed by the blood.

respiratory arrest Cessation of breathing. It may be due to airway obstruction, brain or spinal injury, drug overdosage, or disease or trauma to the lungs, muscles, or nerves necessary for breathing. Treatment includes removal of any airway blockage and establishing ventilatory support as quickly as possible.

respiratory distress Severe difficulty in achieving adequate oxygen in the lungs in spite of efforts to breathe; it is usually associated with an increased rate of breathing (*respiratory rate) and the use of muscles of the shoulder, girdle, and chest wall together with the diaphragm. It can occur in both obstructive and non-obstructive lung conditions.

respiratory rate (RR) The number of breaths per minute. It is normally between 6 and 12 but will increase with exercise and *respiratory distress.

respiratory system The organs and tissues associated with breathing. They include the nose, throat, larynx, trachea, bronchi, and lungs, which together form the **respiratory tract**, and the diaphragm and other muscles associated with breathing. The secondary functions of the respiratory system are voice production in the larynx and the sense of smell.

response *n.* The way in which the body reacts to a stimulus. For example, stimulating the soft palate can induce a *gag reflex.

rest *n. See* OCCLUSAL REST.

rest cells of Malassez *n. See* MALASSEZ, REST CELLS OF.

restoration *n.* A generic term used to describe any filling, inlay, crown, bridge, implant, or removable prosthesis which replaces lost tooth tissue and restores form, function, or aesthetics. A **direct restoration** is a restoration prepared for immediate placement in the mouth, such as an amalgam or resin composite, and does not require any external fabrication. An **indirect restoration** is a restoration fabricated outside the mouth. A **provisional restoration** is a temporary restoration intended to restore either aesthetics or function, or both, prior to the placement of a permanent restoration; it is often placed to allow inflammatory conditions of the pulp or adjacent soft tissues to resolve. Provisional or temporary restorative materials include zinc oxide/eugenol and zinc phosphate cements.

restorative dentistry *n.* The specialist branch of dentistry which is involved with the restoration of diseased, injured, or abnormal teeth to normal form, function, and aesthetics.

rest seat *n.* A shallow preparation on a tooth to accommodate a metallic extension of a *denture (*rest). It may be on the incisal or lingual surfaces of an anterior tooth or on the occlusal surface of a posterior tooth.

resuscitation *n.* The restoration to life or consciousness of an individual showing no signs of life; it includes such measures as artificial respiration and cardiac massage. *See also* ADVANCED LIFE SUPPORT; BASIC LIFE SUPPORT.

Resuscitation Council An organization in the UK which provides education and reference materials to healthcare professionals and the general public in the most effective methods of resuscitation.

⊕ SEE WEB LINKS
• The Resuscitation Council website.

retainer *n.* 1. That part of a *bridge (fixed prosthesis) that joins the *abutment tooth to the suspended portion of the bridge. 2. An orthodontic appliance used to maintain the position of the teeth and help reduce *relapse following orthodontic therapy; the retainer may be either removable, e.g. *Hawley retainer, or fixed. 3. A clasp, attachment, or similar device used to connect to an abutment tooth and stabilize the prosthesis. A **continuous bar retainer** is a metal bar situated along the lingual surfaces of the anterior teeth attached to a major connector used to stabilize a distally extended partial denture. A **direct retainer** is a clasp or attachment on a partial denture applied to an abutment tooth in order to retain the denture in its intended position. An **indirect retainer** is that part of a partial denture that acts to resist displacement of a free end denture base away from its tissue support; it acts on the opposite fulcrum line to a direct retainer. *See also* MATRIX RETAINER.

retarder *n.* A chemical added to a material to slow down the chemical reaction and thereby extend the working time; for example, retarders such as monobasic sodium phosphate may be added to irreversible *hydrocolloid, or acetate, borate, or tartrate to *plaster of Paris impression materials.

retching *n.* Repeated unproductive efforts to vomit. It may be induced by stimulation of the soft palate, such as by an overextended denture palate or when taking an impression or by stimulation of the posterior third of the tongue.

retention *n.* 1. Resistance to displacement of a *restoration in an occlusal direction; this may be aided by the use of adhesives, cements, or bonding agents. It supplements resistance *form. *Pins may be used to improve the retention of both direct and indirect restorations. 2. Resistance to displacement of a denture in a direction opposite to the path of insertion. **Direct retention** of a removable partial denture is obtained by the use of clasps, attachments, or retentive arms on the supporting abutment teeth. **Indirect retention** (**anti-rotation**) of a removable partial denture is obtained by the use of indirect *retainers. 3. The period following the completion of orthodontic appliance therapy during which the teeth are stabilized in the desired position with the use of a *retainer.

Further Reading: McNally M., Mullin M., Dhopatkar A., Rock W. P. Orthodontic retention: why when and how? *Dent Update* 2003;30(8):446–52.

retention cyst *See* CYST.

retention form *See* FORM.

retention index *See* GINGIVAL INDEX; GREENE–VERMILLION INDEX.

rete (epithelial) ridges *n.* Deep extensions of oral epithelial tissue into the underlying connective tissue; formerly known as **rete pegs**.

reticular fibres Fine branching fibres of collagen-like protein that form a supporting network (reticulum) within *connective tissue.

reticular formation An area of the brain stem consisting of a network of nerve pathways and nuclei connecting motor and sensory nerves. It is an important regulator of the *autonomic nervous system controlling such functions as respiration rate, heart rate, gastrointestinal activity, and sleeping.

reticulocyte *n.* An immature red blood cell. Reticulocytes normally constitute 1% of all red blood cells and are increased when the rate of red cell production increases. They develop and mature in the red bone marrow.

retraction *n.* 1. The drawing back of tissue to gain access to or expose a given part. 2. The distal movement of teeth usually achieved during orthodontic therapy. 3. The distal or retrusive movement of the jaw. *See also* GINGIVAL RETRACTION.

retraction cord *n. See* GINGIVAL RETRACTION.

retractor *n.* A surgical instrument used to draw aside tissues to expose the site of operation. There are many designs in common use in dentistry. **Cheek retractors** have a broad flange to allow distal retraction of the cheeks. An **Austin retractor** has a retraction blade with terminal tissue hooks set at right angles to the handle. A **Kilner retractor** is straight with a curved lip at either end. The **Minnesota retractor** has a broad blunt blade to retract the cheek or tongue; it may be modified to provide a curved lip (**Cawood–Minnesota retractor**). *See also* ELEVATOR.

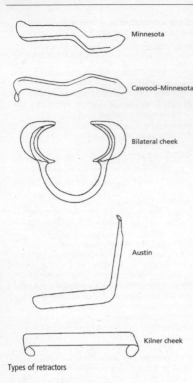

Minnesota

Cawood–Minnesota

Bilateral cheek

Austin

Kilner cheek

Types of retractors

retro- Prefix denoting at the back, behind, or reverse.

retroalveolism *n.* A condition in which the *alveolar process is normal in height and width but is positioned posteriorly on the respective jaw base. *Compare* ANTEALVEOLISM.

retrobuccal *adj.* Relating to the posterior part of the cheek, or behind the cheek.

retroclination *n.* The posterior angulation of the anterior teeth.

retrocuspid papilla See PAPILLA.

retrofill *v.* The process of obturating the apex of a tooth root canal by a direct surgical approach. *See also* ROOT FILLING.

retrogenia *n.* A condition in which the chin is placed too far back (distal) in relation to the rest of the facial skeleton. *Compare* ANTEGENIA.

retrognathic *adj.* Describing a mandible or maxilla that is retruded in its relationship with

other facial structures due to a discrepancy in size or abnormality of position. *See also* GNATHIC INDEX.

retrograde *adj.* Describing going backwards, or moving in the opposite direction to normal. Used to describe an apical *root filling or obturation undertaken using a direct surgical approach.

retrograde root filling See ROOT FILLING.

retromaxillism *n.* A condition in which the base of the maxilla is normal in length and width, but is positioned too far posteriorly. *Compare* ANTEMAXILLISM.

retromolar *adj.* Distal or posterior to the last molar tooth. **Retromolar pad** *see* PAD, RETROMOLAR. The **retromolar triangle** is a three-sided area posterior (distal) to the third molar tooth in the centre of which is a depression, the **retromolar fossa**. The retromolar fossa is bounded medially by the lowest part of the temporal crest and laterally by the external oblique ridge.

retrospective study A research study that investigates what happened when a certain treatment was given by looking backwards in time at treated individuals usually using healthcare records, interviews, or questionnaires. *Compare* PROSPECTIVE STUDY.

retruded arc of closure The arc of closure of the mandible with the condyles rotating about the *terminal hinge axis.

retruded axis position The position the mandibular condyle adopts during the terminal hinge movement of opening or closing. *See also* HINGE AXIS.

retruded contact position *n. See* CENTRIC RELATION.

retrusion *n.* Teeth or jaws situated posterior to their normal location.

reverse headgear *n. See* HEADGEAR.

reverse overjet *See* OVERJET.

Reye's syndrome [R. D. K. Reye (1912–77), Australian histopathologist] A rare but dangerous condition characterized by liver damage and encephalitis. *Aspirin has been implicated as a cause and should therefore not be prescribed to children under the age of 12.

rhagades *pl. n.* Cracks or scars of the skin, particularly around the mouth. They form from the healing fissures around the mouth of babies with congenital syphilis.

rhesus blood group system *See* BLOOD.

rheumatic fever A disease affecting mainly children and young adults, caused by infection of the upper respiratory tract by haemolytic *streptococci. It is characterized by upper respiratory tract infection, *fever, swelling of the cervical *lymph nodes, subcutaneous nodules, and inflammation of the heart muscle and valves. It may progress to **chronic rheumatic heart disease** and permanent heart damage.

rheumatoid arthritis A disease of the synovial lining of joints. It is characterized by painful, swollen, and stiff joints, which typically affects the joints of the wrists, elbows, knees, and ankles. It is a multi-system immunologically mediated disease occurring in genetically predisposed individuals and is three times more common in females than males. Oral manifestations include *xerostomia as part of secondary *Sjögren's syndrome and in some cases the temporomandibular joint (TMJ) may be affected, giving rise to pain, tenderness, and possibly swelling of the pre-auricular region with some limitation of mandibular movement. The TMJ signs and symptoms may periodically be subject to exacerbation and remission. There may also be erosion of the condylar head of the mandible, which can result in an anterior open bite or a loss of mandibular growth in children.

rheumatoid factor An autoantibody found in the serum of patients with rheumatoid arthritis.

rhin- (rhino-) Prefix denoting the nose e.g. rhinolith (a calculus or concretion in the nose).

rhinitis *n.* Inflammation of the *mucosa of the nose. It may be acute, viral, allergic, atrophic, or perennial (vasomotor).

rhinodymia *n.* Duplication of the nose on an otherwise normal face.

rhinophyma *n.* A large red swelling of the nose, most commonly seen in men. It is a complication of *rosacea. It is caused by enlargement of the *sebaceous glands and surrounding connective tissue. It is not related to alcohol consumption, although excessive intake of alcohol can aggravate the condition. Surgical treatment may be beneficial in severe cases.

rhinoplasty *n.* Reconstructive surgery of the nose, sometimes involving the use of implanted tissue.

rhinorrhoea *n.* A persistent watery mucous discharge from the nose, as in the common cold.

rhyparia *n.* An archaic name for *sordes.

riboflavin *n. See* VITAMIN B₂.

Richmond crown [C. M. Richmond (1835–1902), American dentist] A cast metal post retained crown with a porcelain facing constructed for an endodontically treated tooth.

rickets *n.* A childhood disease in which there is defective *mineralization of bone due to *vitamin D deficiency. The deficiency may be as a result of lack of exposure to sunlight, or dietary deficiency. Oral manifestations may include delayed mandibular development, delayed eruption, malposition of teeth, and enamel *hypoplasia.

RIDDOR *See* REPORTING OF INJURIES, DISEASES AND DANGEROUS OCCURRENCES REGULATIONS.

ridge *n.* A projecting or raised edge. **Alveolar ridge** *see* ALVEOLAR. The **marginal ridge** is an enamel elevation on the occlusal surface of a posterior tooth forming the boundary on the mesial or distal margins. **Mylohyoid ridge** *see* MANDIBLE. The **oblique ridge** is an enamel elevation which joins the distobuccal and mesiopalatal cusps on the occlusal surface of a maxillary molar.

ridge augmentation A surgical procedure to increase an edentulous area of an alveolar ridge which has resorbed. The augmentation may involve hard or soft tissue.

ridge lap *See* DENTURE.

Riga–Fede disease [A. Riga (1832–1919), Italian physician; F. Fede (1832–1913), Italian paediatrician] Ulceration on the under-surface of the tongue in infants with *natal or *neonatal teeth caused by the irritation from the teeth during sucking.

Riggs' disease [J. M. Riggs (1810–85), American dentist] An early name used to describe periodontal disease.

rim *n.* A well-defined outer edge. An **occlusal rim (record rim)** is a rim of wax mounted on a denture base and used to record the jaw relationships during denture construction.

Ringer's solution [S. Ringer (1835–1910), British physiologist] A clear colourless aqueous solution containing the chlorides of calcium, sodium, and potassium, which has the same osmotic pressure as blood plasma (isotonic). It is used in dentistry as a vehicle for local anaesthetic agents.

Risdon approach A surgical technique for the treatment of a fractured mandible, first described by F. Risdon in 1934, in which the submandibular area is approached extra-orally through an

r

incision below and behind the angle of the mandible.

risk difference (absolute risk reduction) The difference in size of risk between two groups. For example if one group has a 20% incidence of disease, and the other has a 15% incidence of the disease, the risk difference is 5%.

risk factor Anything that increases a person's chance of developing an illness, disease, or injury. Smoking is a risk factor for lung cancer and periodontal disease, and a high sugar intake is a risk factor for caries.

risk management Clinical and administrative activities undertaken to identify, evaluate, reduce, or eliminate the risk of injury, illness, or disease to patients, staff, and visitors.

risk ratio *n. See* RELATIVE RISK.

Roach clasp *n. See* CLASP.

Roach's attachment [F. E. Roach (1868–1960), American dentist] *n.* A type of attachment used for retaining a removable partial denture consisting of a ball and socket joint in which the socket is in a crown or inlay *retainer.

Robin sequence *See* PIERRE ROBIN SEQUENCE.

Rochette bridge *See* BRIDGE.

rod *n.* A cylindrical form of material. An **analysing rod** is the vertical arm of a model surveyor used to assess parallelism of different surfaces and to measure the extent of the cervical convergence of a tooth. **Enamel rod** *see* ENAMEL.

rodent ulcer *n. See* BASAL CELL CARCINOMA.

Roger Anderson pin fixation appliance [R. Anderson (1891–1971), American orthopaedic surgeon] An extra-oral appliance used in the fixation of mandibular fractures. Threaded steel pins are placed in the bone segments and joined by metal connecting rods.

roll *n. See* COTTON WOOL.

Romberg syndrome (Parry–Romberg syndrome) [C. H. Parry (1755–1822), British physician; M. H. Romberg (1795–1873), German neurologist] A rare craniofacial disorder characterized by hemifacial *atrophy of the subcutaneous muscles of the face associated with *trigeminal neuralgia. It is more common in females and appears around the first decade of life.

rongeur forceps *n. See* FORCEPS.

root *n.* 1. (in dentistry) That part of a tooth covered by *cementum and not covered by *enamel (**anatomical root**). An **accessory root** is a supplemental root differing in size, shape, and direction from the principal root. The **clinical root** is that portion of the root which is attached by the *periodontal ligament to the *alveolar bone. A **retained root** is a tooth root or part of a tooth root remaining in the alveolar bone or soft tissue following trauma, extraction, or extensive caries; it may be intentionally retained to prevent alveolar bone resorption or to use for the retention of a crown, bridge, or removable denture. 2. (in neurology) A nerve at its emergence from the spinal cord.

root canal *n.* That part of the tooth containing the *pulp between the pulp chamber and the root apex or apices. A **root canal instrument stop** is a device placed on a root canal instrument to provide a guide for instrumentation by measuring the depth of instrument penetration within the tooth.

root canal sealer *n. See* SEALER.

root canal therapy The process of removing an infected, inflamed, or necrotic pulp and filling the residual space with an inert material. Access must first be gained to the pulp chamber and root canal system; the pulp canals are then measured and the pulp tissue and any infected material removed; the canals are then shaped, irrigated, and cleaned of debris; the root canals are obturated with a *root filling material such as *gutta-percha and a sealant, and finally a coronal seal placed to prevent bacteria from the mouth entering the root canal system.

root debridement The process of removing soft or calcified deposits from the surface of a root using hand or ultrasonic instrumentation. The treatment is intended where there is evidence of periodontal disease with an increase in pocket depth. It may also involve the removal of diseased tissue within a pocket using a laser. *See also* ROOT PLANING.

root filling *n.* 1. The final stage of *root canal therapy in which the prepared canal is obturated with an inert filling material. 2. The inert material used to obturate a root canal; this is usually a core of gutta-percha with a thin coating of sealant cement. An alternative material to gutta-percha is a hydrophilic polymer resin which swells in a lateral dimension only when in contact with fluid in the root canal. Metals such as gold, tin, lead, copper, amalgam, and *silver have been used as root canal filling materials but are now only of historical interest. A **retrograde root filling** is a root filling material, such as *resin composite,

*amalgam, or *mineral trioxide aggregate (MTA), placed in a root canal from the apical end of the tooth root rather than the pulp chamber (**orthograde**) to provide an effective seal following an *apicectomy.

root fracture A complete or incomplete cleavage of the root in any direction. Treatment is influenced by the depth and direction (horizontal, vertical, or oblique) of the fracture, whether the pulp chamber is breached, and whether the fracture plane penetrates the external root surface. *See also* CRACKED TOOTH SYNDROME.

root planing A treatment procedure designed to remove deposits on the periodontally involved root surface, including the intentional removal of cementum or surface dentine that is rough, impregnated with calculus, or contaminated with toxins or micro-organisms; it was formerly considered necessary to remove cementum impregnated with bacterial endotoxins to facilitate periodontal healing following surgery, but this is now not accepted clinical practice. Root planing may be undertaken using manual or ultrasonic instrumentation.

root resection A surgical procedure to remove an untreatable or fractured root while retaining the remaining tooth structure in situ. It is undertaken in association with endodontic treatment either before, during, or shortly after the procedure. Resection may involve the removal of the apical portion of the root only (**root end resection**, *apicectomy).

root resorption *n.* The loss of hard dental tissue (cement or dentine) by *cementoclastic or *osteoclastic activity. It may be external or internal. **External root resorption (surface resorption)** can lead to a shortening of the root, when occurring in the apical area, or perforation of the pulp canal, when occurring on the lateral surface. External resorption may be caused by inflammation following trauma or infection, excessive forces applied to the tooth root during orthodontic therapy, or due to the eruptive pressure from an adjacent impacted tooth. It occurs in the primary dentition as a normal physiological process during *exfoliation. **Internal root resorption** can occur due to *osteoclastic activity, which removes the dentine creating an internal concavity which may be characterized externally by a pink discoloration (**pink spot**); it can occur anywhere in the root and may produce tenderness over the root apex or pulp sensitivity. Internal resorption may be caused by incomplete caries removal. *See also* ODONTOCLASTOMA.

Further Reading: Patel S., Pitt Ford T. Is the resorption external or internal? *Dent Update* 2007;34:218–29.

ropivacaine *n.* A long acting *amide local analgesic agent less cardiotoxic than bupivacaine. It may be formulated with or without *adrenaline.

rosacea *n.* A chronic inflammatory disease of the face that causes the skin to appear red like a flush or blush. It may progress to produce pimples without blackheads and red lines formed by prominent tiny blood vessels. It usually occurs in women in the mid-thirties and is of unknown cause. It responds to treatment with oral tetracycline. It is sometimes called acne rosacea, although it is a different condition from *acne; however, it can occur at the same time.

rosin *n.* A solid form of resin made by heating fresh liquid resin to vaporize some of the volatile liquid components. It is a constituent of some impression materials, varnishes, and chewing gum.

rouge *n. See* JEWELLER'S ROUGE.

-rrhagia Suffix denoting excessive or abnormal flow or discharge.

-rrhoea Suffix denoting an abnormal or excessive discharge or flow from an organ or part such as a discharge from the nose (*rhinorrhoea).

rubber dam *n. See* DENTAL DAM.

rubber polishing cup *n. See* POLISHING.

rubefacient *n.* An agent that causes reddening and warming of the skin. Rubefacients, such as methyl salicylate, are often used for the relief of muscle pain.

rubella *n. See* GERMAN MEASLES.

rubor *n.* Redness; one of the classical signs of tissue *inflammation.

ruga *n.* (*pl.* **rugae**) A fold, ridge, or crease, especially seen on the roof of the mouth (**palatal rugae**).

rule of ten A method of providing a guide as to whether an infiltration or a block injection of local *analgesic is appropriate for a child requiring treatment to a mandibular tooth. The primary tooth to be anaesthetized is assigned a number from 1 to 5 according to its location in the dental arch (central incisor = 1, second molar = 5). This number is added to the age of the child (in years), and if the number is 10 or less then an infiltration analgesic is most appropriate; if greater than 10, then an inferior dental nerve block is likely to be more effective.

rumination *n*. The voluntary process of regurgitation of partially digested food before rechewing it and swallowing it or spitting it out. The habit can cause severe acid *erosion of the teeth.

Rushton body [M. A. Rushton (1903–70), English pathologist] *n*. A transparent hyaline amorphous concretion found on histological examination in the epithelial lining of approximately 10% of odontogenic *cysts. The material is secreted by the reduced *enamel epithelium.

Ruspini, Bartholomew (1728–1813) Italian surgeon–dentist to King George IV, born in Romacoto, north-east of Milan. He studied surgery at the local hospital in Bergamo, and dentistry in Paris, then regarded as the leading city for dental education. He practised in Bath about 1758 before settling in London in 1766. In 1768 he published *A treatise on the teeth*, in which he described an anatomy of dental organs and stressed the importance of prevention and the detrimental effect of sugar and the dangers of using dentifrices containing mercury and caustics. He established the Royal Cumberland Freemason School in 1788 (now the Royal Masonic School for Girls) for the daughters of impoverished freemasons. The hereditary title of chevalier was conferred on him in recognition of his professional skill and generosity to persons in adversity or poverty.

Further Reading: Philanthropy and fame. *BDANews* 2007;20 (9):38.

Russell periodontal disease index *See* PERIODONTAL DISEASE INDEX OF RUSSELL.

Russell–Silver syndrome [A. Russell (20th century), British paediatrician; H.K. Silver (1918–), US paediatrician] A rare congenital growth disorder characterized by asymmetry of the body, short stature, a triangular face, and a small lower jaw with a pointed chin; the mouth tends to curve down.

Russell's sign An indication of bulimia in which calluses occur on the back of the hands or fingers, produced by inserting the hands into the throat against the teeth in an attempt to induce vomiting. First described by Gerald Russell in 1979.

r

sac *n.* A pouch or baglike structure. The dental sac encloses the *enamel organ.

saddle *n.* That part of a partial denture which is in contact with the alveolar mucosa. The saddle may have a natural tooth on either side of it (**bounded saddle**) or may have no natural tooth distally (**free-end saddle, distal extension saddle**).

safelight *n.* A special lamp emitting low-intensity red-orange light of long wavelength used in the darkroom to provide working visibility without affecting (fogging) the photosensitive emulsion of the radiographic film.

sagittal plane *adj.* Relating to a vertical plane or section dividing the body into right and left halves.

St John's wort (Hypericum perforatum) A homeopathic remedy for the treatment of depression and nerve damage. It is known to have an adverse effect by increasing the metabolism and elimination of other drugs that a patient may be taking.

salaried dental services A part of the National Health Service (NHS) dental service in the UK. It has replaced the Community Dental Service (CDS) and the Personal Dental Service (PDS).

salbutamol *n.* A short-acting beta 2 adrenergic receptor agonist used for the treatment of bronchospasm in conditions such as *asthma and chronic obstructive pulmonary disease. It is usually self-administered via an inhaler or a *nebulizer. Side-effects include dizziness, headache, tremor, and increased heart rate. Trade names: **Aerolin, Airomir, Asmasal, Ventolin, Albuterol.**

saline, physiological (normal saline) *n.* A solution containing 0.9% sodium chloride used mainly for irrigating wounds, as an ingredient of plasma substitutes, and as a diluent for drugs.

saliva *n.* (*adj.* **salivary**) The alkaline fluid secreted by the salivary glands and the oral mucous membrane. Saliva is 98% water but also contains mineral salts, *mucus (consisting mainly of mucopolysaccharides and *glycoproteins), antibacterial compounds, and enzymes such as *amylase and *lysozyme. The normal adult unstimulated salivary flow is 0.3–0.4ml per minute, of which about 60% is from the submandibular glands, 25% from the parotid glands, 7–8% from the sublingual glands, and the remainder from the minor salivary glands. Salivary flow increases in response to the chewing action of the jaws or to the thought, taste, sight, or smell of food; it decreases during sleep. The saliva produced by the parotid gland is thinner and less viscous than that produced by the other glands and contains no *mucin. Saliva has many functions, including the maintenance of the *pH in the oral cavity (by means of a *buffering action), facilitating *mastication and swallowing, protecting the teeth from acidic gastric reflux, removing oral debris, facilitating speech, direct antibacterial activity, and initiating the digestive process. Salivary flow may be reduced by radiotherapy, disease, drugs, hormonal disturbances, dehydration, or *atrophy. The treatment for reduced salivary flow (dry mouth or *xerostomia) is by drug administration such as pilocarpine, salivary stimulants (*sialagogues), contained in chewable pastilles or gum, or **artificial saliva** containing a lubricant. Saliva substitutes can be carboxymethyl cellulose-based (e.g. **Saliveze®, Salivart®**), mucin-based (e.g. sorbitol-based **saliva Orthana®**), or gel-based, containing enzymes normally present in saliva (trade name: **BioXtra®**). Sweets should be avoided as salivary stimulants because of the risk of causing dental caries.

Further Reading: Mandel I. D. The functions of saliva. *J Dent Res* 1987;66:623–7.

saliva ejector *n. See* ASPIRATION.

salivant *n.* An agent that increases the flow of *saliva.

salivary gland A gland that produces *saliva. There are three major pairs of salivary glands: the *parotid, submandibular, and sublingual glands. The **parotid gland** is one of a pair of salivary glands found in the subcutaneous tissue of the face, overlying the mandibular ramus and anterior and inferior to the external ear. The

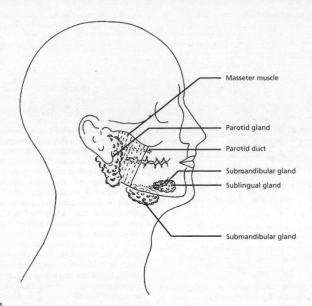

Masseter muscle

Parotid gland

Parotid duct

Submandibular gland

Sublingual gland

Submandibular gland

Salivary glands

parotid gland is the largest of the salivary glands and resembles a three-sided pyramid with the apex directed downwards; it empties into the oral cavity opposite the upper second molar tooth via the **parotid duct** (*Stensen's duct) marked by a small elevation of tissue (**parotid papilla**). The parotid gland produces *serous (as opposed to *mucous) saliva. The **submandibular glands** are a pair of round biconvex bodies located beneath the floor of the mouth, superior to the digastric muscles and both beneath and lingual to the body of the mandible. The inner surface is in contact with the stylohyoid, digastric, and styloglossus muscles posteriorly, and the hyoglossus and the posterior border of the mylohyoid muscle anteriorly. The submandibular duct (*Wharton's duct) is located on the upper part of the inner surface and passes along the inner surface of the sublingual gland to open into the floor of the oral cavity on a small papilla at the side of the lingual frenum. The submandibular glands produce a mixed serous and mucous secretion. The **sublingual glands** are located in a shallow depression close to the medial side of the mandible underneath the tongue in the floor of the mouth; they are covered superiorly by mucous membrane. There are several ducts which

sometimes unite with the submandibular duct before entering the oral cavity. The sublingual glands produce a predominantly mucous secretion. **Minor salivary glands** are situated in the cheeks, lips, tongue, and palate. Secretory glands (*Ebner's glands) are also situated at the base of the *circumvallate papillae on the dorsum of the tongue. The salivary glands are divided into lobules containing serous and mucous cells and surrounded by a connective tissue capsule. Diseases of the salivary glands include inflammation (sialoadenitis, *parotitis), *mumps and the autoimmune disorder, *Sjögren's syndrome. Tumours are usually *benign, such as pleomorphic *adenoma, but may be *malignant, such as mucoepidermoid *carcinoma.

Further Reading: Field E. A., Longman L. P., Fear S., Higham S., Rostron J., Willetts R. M., Ireland R. S. Oral signs and symptoms as predictors of salivary gland hypofunction in general dental practice. *Primary Dental Care* 2001;8(3):111–14.

salivary stone (sialolith, calculus) *n.* A small mass of calcified tissue which forms in a *salivary gland or one of the major salivary ducts. They may be asymptomatic but, when not, they are characterized by severe pain and glandular swelling due to the obstruction of the salivary flow. They occur most frequently in the submandibular salivary glands, possibly because of the viscosity of the secretion and the upward passage of the duct. Salivary stones can sometimes result in secondary infection. They may respond to massage or ultrasound (*lithotripsy), but surgical removal may be necessary.

salivation *n.* The secretion of *saliva by the salivary glands.

sample *n.* (in statistics) A selection of individual units from a population intended to yield some knowledge and truths about the population.

sandarac varnish *n.* A hard translucent resin obtained from the bark of a coniferous evergreen tree (*Tetraclinis articulata*). It has been used as a vehicle for the delivery of antimicrobial substances such as *chlorhexidine to tooth surfaces.

sarcoidosis *n.* A chronic *granulomatous disease of unknown cause in which many of the *lymph nodes are enlarged. Orofacial presentations are rare, although the *salivary glands may be involved, and submucosal lesions may also appear in the soft palate, floor of the mouth, gingivae, and cheeks. Most patients recover without intervention, although drugs may be used to relieve the symptoms and reduce inflammation; recovery is complete with minimal side-effects in most cases.

Further Reading: Poate T. W. J., Sharma R., Moutasim K. A., Escuier M. P., Warnakulasuriya S. Orofacial presentations of sarcoidosis—a case series and review of the literature. *Br Dent J* 2008;205:437–42.

sarcoma *n.* (*adj.* **sarcomatous**) Any *malignant tumour (cancer) of connective tissue such as cartilage, fat, bone, or muscle. Sarcomas are usually categorized according to their cell type such as **liposarcoma** (from fat tissue), *osteosarcoma (from bone tissue), and *leukaemia (from blood-forming tissue). *See also* KAPOSI'S SARCOMA.

Further Reading: Gahan R., Rout J., Webster K. Case report: oral manifestations and radiographic features of osteosarcoma. *Dent Update* 2007;34:52–54.

saturated *adj.* Describing a solution obtained when a *solvent (liquid) can dissolve no more of a *solute (usually a solid) at a particular temperature. Normally, a slight fall in temperature will cause some of the solute to crystallize out of solution;

when this fails to occur it is known as **supercooling**, and the solution is said to be *supersaturated.

scaler *n.* A hand instrument used principally to remove hard deposits such as *calculus from the surfaces of the teeth. A **jaquette (jacquette)** scaler is a hand instrument used for the removal of supragingival calculus; it has an angled blade with a straight, flat face and two cutting edges that come to a point. A **sickle scaler** has a triangular cross-section with two cutting edges and a sharp point, and is suitable for supragingival scaling; the shape makes it unsuitable for subgingival scaling because of the potential damage to the soft tissues. A **push (chisel) scaler** has a head angled at 45° and is applied from the labial aspect of mandibular anterior teeth to remove gross supragingival deposits from the approximal surfaces. **Sonic scalers** use air pressure to create mechanical vibrations that cause the instrument tip to vibrate at frequencies ranging from 2000 to 6000Hz. **Ultrasonic scalers** are water-cooled mechanical devices that produce a vibratory movement of the metal tip which causes microscopic bubbles to form in the water coolant (*cavitation). Electrical energy is converted to mechanical energy to create a tip oscillation of about 18,000–45,000 times per second at an amplitude of 0.006–0.1mm. The vibration of the tip dislodges the hard deposits, and the cavitation and the flushing effect of the water remove the plaque and may disrupt the bacterial cell walls. Ultrasonic scaler units may be magnetostrictive in which a pulsing magnetic field is applied to a metal 'stack' that flexes to move the vibrating tip in an elliptical pattern, or piezo-electric in which there is a linear pattern of vibration. The instrument is used with a light brushing motion with overlapping strokes; a variety of working tips are available. Ultrasonic scalers generate undesirable heat, requiring water for cooling the handpiece tip and adjacent tissues.

scaling *n.* The process of removing hard deposits, such as calculus, plaque, and stain from the surfaces of the teeth using *scalers. It can be undertaken with hand or ultrasonic instrumentation. Scaling may be apical to the gingival margin (**subgingival**) or coronal to the gingival margin (**supragingival**).

scalpel *n.* A small pointed surgical knife usually with a detachable disposable blade. The blade is available in a variety of shapes.

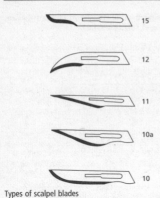

15

12

11

10a

10

Types of scalpel blades

scar *n.* A permanent mark left in the tissue after wound healing is complete. **Scar tissue** is thicker than the surrounding tissue, and also paler and denser because it has a reduced blood supply. It is limited in function, including movement, circulation, and sensation. An overgrowth of fibrous tissue following trauma to the skin results in a **keloid scar**. Keloid scars do not resolve spontaneously and tend to extend beyond the original wound. **Hypertrophic scars** consist of raised scar tissue and do not extend beyond the boundaries of the original wound and may reduce over time.

scarlet fever (scarlatina) *n.* A highly infectious disease caused by *Streptococcus pyogenes* (group A streptococcus) expressing *bacteriophage-encoded streptococcal pyrogenic *exotoxin type A (scarlet fever toxin). It is characterized by sore throat, fever, enlarged *lymph nodes in the neck, and a widespread scarlet rash; the tongue is initially covered by a thick white deposit before turning bright red (**strawberry tongue**). Antibiotic therapy reduces the risk of secondary infection.

Scarpa's foramina [A. Scarpa (1747–1832), Italian anatomist and surgeon] *n.* Two additional openings occasionally present in the midline of the hard palate which, if present, transmit the **nasopalatine nerves**, the left passing through the anterior foramen, and the right through the posterior foramen.

scatterplot *n.* (in statistics) A display of the values of one variable against a corresponding value of another variable. The value of one variable determines the position on the horizontal axis and the value of the other variable determines the position on the vertical axis.

scavenging device A piece of equipment that collects exhaled *nitrous oxide and removes it during the administration of inhalation sedation. The main component is the **scavenging nasal hood**. The device is recommended by the American Dental Association (ADA) to reduce the occupational exposure to the gas.

schisto- Prefix denoting a fissure or split.

schistoglossia *n.* A congenital fissure or cleft of the tongue. Congenital fissures are transverse, whereas those due to disease are usually longitudinal.

schizodontia *n. See* GEMINATION.

schizophrenia *n.* A severe disabling mental disorder that makes it difficult for a person to think clearly, relate to others, and function productively in society. It can lead to hallucinations, delusions, mood disturbances, and unusual speech or behaviour.

Schreger's lines (Hunter–Schreger bands) [C. H. T. Schreger (1768–1833), German anatomist] Broad light and dark bands visible under a light microscope that run obliquely from the amelodentinal junction through the inner two thirds of the thickness of the *enamel (mantel enamel). They are an optical phenomenon caused by the undulating and wavy pattern of the enamel rods. They are curved with the convexity facing apically.

scissors *pl. n.* An edge cutting tool having two crossed pivoting blades. **Scissors bite** *see* BITE. **Crown scissors (Beebee scissors)** have small broad curved or straight blades used to trim copper rings or metal strips. **Goldman-Fox scissors** have narrow fine-pointed blades for use in removing or trimming soft tissue in interproximal areas.

scleroderma *n.* A chronic autoimmune disorder, sometimes termed **systemic sclerosis**, of unknown cause. It is characterized by inflammation and fibrosis (excess collagen production) of viscera such as the lungs, heart, and gastrointestinal tract, and by either localized or generalized ivory-coloured fibrosis of the skin. Fibrosis of the facial skin can give rise to a mask-like expression and a reduction in the opening of the mouth (*microstomia). It can also affect the mucous membrane and periodontal tissues with degeneration of the periodontal fibres in the absence of inflammatory changes. Treatment includes systemic immunosuppressants but spontaneous resolution may occur.

s

sclerosis *n.* (*adj.* **sclerotic**) Tissue hardening usually after inflammation or due to ageing. Tracts of increased density can appear in dentine (**dentinal sclerosis**) under a carious lesion or in response to *abrasion, *attrition, or *erosion. **Pulp tissue sclerosis** occurs with age with the formation of fibrous tissue, a reduction in blood supply, and a reduction in pulp volume due to the laying down of secondary *dentine; pulp tissue sclerosis can also occur in response to chronic inflammation, infection, or trauma.

scorbutic *adj.* Describing the condition of being affected with *scurvy.

Scottish Intercollegiate Guidelines Network (SIGN) A network formed in 1993 to improve the quality of healthcare for patients in Scotland by reducing variation in practice and outcome, through the development and dissemination of national clinical guidelines containing recommendations for effective practice, based on current evidence.

(🌐) **SEE WEB LINKS**

• The Scottish Intercollegiate Guidelines Network website.

screening The process of testing a large number of asymptomatic or apparently healthy people to separate those who may have a specific disease and would benefit from further testing from those who probably do not. Screening is usually targeted at individuals who are most at risk of the disease, such as screening heavy smokers for oral cancer. Factors which need to be taken into account to determine the appropriateness of screening include the *epidemiology of the disease, efficacy and availability of treatment, safety, acceptability, cost, *sensitivity, and *specificity of the test. Screening for diseases that affect general health, such as diabetes and cardiovascular disease, may be undertaken within a primary dental care setting.

screen, intensifying *n.* A thin sheet of material consisting of fluorescent phosphor (usually rare earth phosphors), embedded in a plastic matrix which absorb the x-ray photons and convert the energy of the x-ray photon to light. One x-ray photon produces many light photons, thus decreasing the amount of x-rays required to produce an image and thereby reducing the dose to the patient. It is used in extra-oral radiography but not for digital imaging.

screen, oral *n.* An orthodontic appliance constructed to contact the tips of protruding maxillary teeth such that lip pressure tips the

incisors palatally. It is also used to inhibit mouth breathing and *digit sucking.

screw *n.* A threaded pin or post normally used as an attachment. A screw is used as part of an orthodontic *expansion plate to provide controlled separation of the plate; it is opened or closed by means of a key. The **hyrax screw** is an orthodontic screw designed for rapid palatal expansion. An **implant screw** is used as a means of primary retention of an implant or to cover an implant during the healing phase (**cover screw**). A **self-tapping screw** is a screw that cuts its own thread in bone, dentine, or enamel.

scrofula *n.* *See* TUBERCULOSIS.

scurvy *n.* A disease caused by *vitamin C (ascorbic acid) deficiency which results in a reduction in collagen formation. It is characterized by swollen bleeding gingivae and a rash of small bleeding spots around the hair follicles. There may also be weakness, poor wound healing, *anaemia, and haemorrhage under the *mucosa. The elderly living alone are particularly at risk.

seal *n.* Something that effectively closes or secures. An **anterior oral seal** is formed by lip contact or contact between the lower lip and the tongue or palatal mucosa. **Border seal** *see* PERIPHERAL SEAL. A **posterior palatal seal** is the seal at the posterior border of an upper denture obtained by producing extra pressure on the palatal mucosa, by creating a ridge or *post-dam in the denture. A **posterior oral seal** is created by the contact of the soft palate against the dorsum of the tongue during speech or swallowing.

sealant *n.* *See* FISSURE SEALANT.

sealer *n.* A material used to fill the space around *gutta-percha or silver points in a root canal. Most sealers contain materials such as zinc, barium, and bismuth salts to render them radiopaque. Root canal sealers require tissue compatibility, good dimensional *stability, and low solubility; they should also be readily removable if necessary. Sealers are available made from *zinc oxide eugenol, calcium hydroxide, resin, silicone, or *glass ionomer. Trade names: **Sealapex®**, **Tubliseal®**, **Apexit®**, **AH26®**.

sebaceous gland *n.* Any of the simple *exocrine glands of the skin that secrete an oily substance (*sebum) which reduces evaporation of sweat. They are present inside the oral cavity as yellowish-white spots (*Fordyce's spots), usually on the buccal or labial mucosa.

S

sebum *n.* An oily secretion from the *sebaceous glands that reduces the evaporation of water and has an antibacterial effect.

secodont *adj.* Describing a posterior tooth adapted for cutting, as in many of the carnivora.

second appropriate person A *dental care professional, required by the General Dental Council (GDC) in the UK, to assist a dentist who is acting as both operator and sedationist.

secondary care Healthcare provided by medical or dental specialists, usually in a hospital setting, but may also include some specialist services provided within the community.

secondary dentition *See* PERMANENT DENTITION.

secondary haemorrhage *See* HAEMORRHAGE.

secondary nasal septum A band of tissue formed around the 6th week of intrauterine life that grows behind the *primary nasal septum from the roof of the primitive oral cavity, dividing the *nasal cavity into two halves.

secondary palate *See* PALATE.

secondary prevention *See* PREVENTION.

second opinion *n.* An opinion about the appropriateness of proposed treatment by a practitioner other than the one originally making the recommendation.

Section 63 courses Educational programmes for dental practitioners funded by the National Health Service out of the medical and dental educational levy (MADEL).

sectional archwire *See* ARCHWIRE.

sectional impression *See* IMPRESSION.

sectorial teeth *See* CARNASSIAL.

sedation

n. The use of a drug or drugs to produce a restful state of mind, enabling dental treatment to be carried out. Drugs may be administered orally as a *premedication (e.g. the *benzodiazepines), intravenously (e.g. *midazolam, *propofol) or by inhalation (e.g. *nitrous oxide). **Conscious sedation** is defined in the UK by the General Dental Council as a technique in which the use of a drug or drugs produces a state of depression of the *central nervous system enabling treatment to be carried out, but where verbal contact with the patient is maintained throughout the period of sedation. The drugs and techniques used to provide conscious sedation for dental treatment should carry a margin of safety wide enough to render loss of consciousness unlikely; the level of sedation must be such that the patient remains conscious, retains protective reflexes, and is able to understand and respond to verbal commands. It has applications in dentistry for the management of patients with dental *anxiety and *phobia, medical conditions aggravated by stress, medical conditions producing involuntary movements (e.g. cerebral palsy, Parkinson's disease), and patients with learning difficulties who may become stressed during treatment. Conscious sedation is usually used in conjunction with local *analgesia. **Inhalational sedation**, also known as **relative analgesia** (RA), involves the administration of nitrous oxide and oxygen by titration. **Intranasal sedation** is gaining popularity, particularly for patients requiring special care dentistry. Both oral and intranasal sedation require the same monitoring and aftercare as intravenous sedation techniques. **Intravenous (IV) sedation** using titrated midazolam has the advantages over inhalational sedation of providing a more rapid onset, it does not have to be administered continuously throughout treatment, and mouth breathing does not influence the quality of sedation. However, intravenous sedation carries an increased risk of respiratory depression; *cannulation is invasive and may be difficult to achieve in some patients, and the patient will require an escort and post-operative care for the rest of the day. Drugs may be taken by mouth (**oral sedation**) in tablet or liquid form to reduce anxiety. However, it has the disadvantages of difficulty in assessing the correct dosage for individual patients and unreliable gastric absorption.

Further Reading: Paterson S. A., Tahmassebi J. F. Paediatric dentistry in the new millennium: 3. Use of inhalation sedation in paediatric dentistry. *Dent Update* 2003;30(7):350–56, 358.
Coulthard P. Conscious sedation guidance. *Evid Based Dent* 2006;7(4):90–91.
Craig D. C., Wildsmith J. A. W. Conscious sedation for dentistry: an update. *Br Dent J* 2007;203:629–31.

sedative *n.* A drug that has a calming effect, reducing anxiety (anxiolytic) and tension.

selective grinding *n. See* GRINDING.

selenodont *adj.* Describing teeth which are crescent-shaped in cross-section, e.g. as seen in sheep.

self-cleansing area An area of the teeth or gingival tissue which by its shape and contour is less likely to retain food debris or surface deposits during normal function; it should probably more accurately be described as a **readily cleansable area**.

self-curing resin *n. See* RESIN.

self-evaluation *n.* A critical appraisal of one's own actions or performance.

self-ligation *n.* A fixed appliance bracket system, which may be either active or passive. It is designed to reduce the friction in a fixed orthodontic appliance.

self-tapping implant *See* IMPLANT.

self-tapping screw *See* SCREW.

sella turcica *n.* A saddle-shaped depression in the sphenoid bone at the base of the skull which houses the *pituitary gland.

senescence *n.* (*adj.* **senescent**) The condition of ageing. **Dental senescence** is a condition in which the dental tissues show deterioration due to ageing (senility) or premature ageing.

sensitivity *n.* 1. A measure of the ability of a diagnostic or screening test to detect a condition or disease when it is truly present. *See also* SPECIFICITY. 2. **Dentine sensitivity** *see* DENTINE HYPERSENSITIVITY.

sensory nerve *n. See* NERVE.

separating medium *n.* 1. A material applied to a cast to facilitate separation from the resin denture base material after curing and to protect the resin from the moisture in the *gypsum, such as tinfoil, cellophane, or alginate. 2. A material applied to the fitting surface of an implant-retained denture during its construction to prevent material bonding to the denture base.

separating strip (lightening strip) *n.* A thin piece of metal or plastic used to prevent resin composite from bonding to the tooth adjacent to the one being restored.

separator *n.* 1. A device used to wedge teeth apart. It may be used to gain better access to the interproximal surface of a tooth for diagnostic purposes, to achieve a better interproximal contact area of a restoration, or to aid the finishing of a restoration. Care needs to be taken to avoid soft tissue damage. 2. A device used to separate waste amalgam from waste water using a range of techniques alone or in combination which include sedimentation, centrifugation, ion-exchange, or filtration.

sepsis *n.* The putrefactive destruction of tissues by disease causing bacteria or their toxins. **Oral sepsis** can provide a local source of infection which may spread to cause *systemic disease.

septicaemia *n.* A general term used to describe widespread tissue destruction due to the presence of *pathogenic organisms or *toxins in the bloodstream. *See also* TOXAEMIA.

septum *n.* A thin partition or dividing wall between two structures or tissue masses. The **interdental (interalveolar) septum** is an extension of alveolar bone between the roots of two adjacent teeth. The **nasal septum** divides the nasal cavity into left and right chambers. The **lingual septum** is a vertical fibrous partition in the midline of the tongue to which the intrinsic tongue muscles are attached.

sequela *n.* (*pl.* **sequelae**) Any pathological condition that results from an injury, disease, or treatment.

sequestrum *n.* (*pl.* **sequestra**) A fragment of dead (*necrotic) bone which has become separated from living (*vital) bone. Although rare, it can occur as a result of chronic *osteomyelitis of the jaws, more commonly in the mandible. It can be associated with the formation of pus. Treatment is usually by surgical removal of the piece of dead bone (**sequestectomy**). *See also* OSTEONECROSIS.

serial extraction *See* TOOTH EXTRACTION.

seroconvert *v.* To produce specific *antibodies in response to the presence of an *antigen e.g. a vaccine or a virus.

serology *n.* The branch of science dealing with the measurement and characterization of antibodies and other immunological substances in body fluids, particularly *serum.

serous *adj.* 1. Relating to or containing *serum. 2. Producing a fluid resembling serum.

serpiginous *adj.* Describing a chronic slowly progressing or creeping skin lesion, particularly one with a wavy border.

Serres glands [A. E. R. A. Serres (1786–1868), French physiologist] Epithelial remnants of the *dental lamina. They have the capacity to form small cysts (*Bohn's nodules). As early as 1817, Serres believed that gingival *crevicular fluid was secreted from this tissue.

serum (blood serum) *n.* The fluid component of blood excluding *fibrinogen and other coagulating substances.

S

serum hepatitis *n. See* HEPATITIS.

sessile *adj.* Describing being attached directly by its base. *Compare* PEDUNCULATED.

set-up *n.* 1. The arrangement of artificial teeth on a trial denture base. 2. Instruments placed on a tray in a predetermined order and location.

sevoflurane *n.* A fluorinated derivative of methyl isopropyl ether first synthesized in the 1970s. It is used in general anaesthesia and inhalational *sedation in combination with oxygen or nitrous oxide and oxygen.

sextant *n.* One of the three divisions of a dental arch; both arches are therefore divided up into six divisions. The anterior sextant of each arch includes the incisors and canines and the two posterior sextants include the premolars and molars.

shank *n.* The slender part of an instrument that connects the working end with the handle; it may be curved or straight. With rotary tools, such as burs and drills, it is the end that fits into the handpiece chuck.

sharpening tool An instrument used to restore the cutting edge of an instrument, usually a flat or cylindrical abrasive stone over which the cutting edge is drawn.

Sharpey's fibres [W. Sharpey (1802–80), English anatomist] The ends of the *collagen fibres within the *dental follicle which become embedded in the developing cementum and alveolar bone. The collagen fibres form the principal fibres of the *periodontal ligament.

sharps *pl. n.* Any object that can penetrate the skin, including needles, scalpels, endodontic files, and reamers. After use they are placed in a *sharps container and disposed of under clearly defined disposal regulations.

sharps container A yellow, rigid, leak-proof, puncture-resistant container that should comply with **BS 7320: 1990** Specification for sharps containers, **United Nations Standard 3291**, or their equivalent (regulated in America by the Occupational Safety and Health Administration (OSHA)).

(((●))) **SEE WEB LINKS**

• An overview of sharps management on the Community Practitioners and Health Visitors Association website.

sheath *n.* A connective tissue covering of structures such as nerves and muscles. The **epithelial root sheath** (*Hertwig's root sheath) is a continuation of the internal and external enamel epithelium which determines the root morphology.

shelf life *n.* 1. The length of time a material or product remains usable. 2. The length of time a material can be stored without deterioration in its properties.

shellac *n.* A resinous *polymer secreted by the lac insect, capable of being moulded by heat (thermoplastic) and contoured against a cast for use as a denture baseplate material.

shell crown *n. See* CROWN.

shimstock *n.* Very thin (8μ thickness) metal foil strip used to check for the presence of occlusal contacts when the teeth are in normal *occlusion.

Further Reading: Harper K. A., Setchell D. J. The use of shimstock to assess occlusal contacts: a laboratory study. *Int J Prosthodont* 2002;15(4):347–52.

shingles *n. See* HERPES.

shock *n.* The condition of acute circulatory failure in which the arterial blood pressure is insufficient to maintain an adequate supply of blood to the tissues. It is characterized by low blood pressure, cold sweaty pallid skin, weak rapid pulse, irregular breathing, dry mouth, dilated pupils, and reduced urinary flow. Shock has many causes including haemorrhage, burns, dehydration, severe allergic reaction (*anaphylactic shock), reduced activity of the heart, bacteria in the bloodstream (*bacteraemia), and drug overdosage, such as from insulin. **Galvanic shock** *see* GALVANISM.

shoulder *n.* The extra-coronal margin of a cavity preparation where the gingival floor meets the axial wall to form a ledge.

shrinkage *n.* A decrease in dimension. **Casting shrinkage** occurs when a molten metal such as gold alloy solidifies; it is compensated for by expansion of the *refractory casting material during setting and by thermal expansion prior to casting. **Polymerization shrinkage** can occur during the curing of a resin based material and can be a significant problem during the *polymerization of resin denture material or during the placement of a *resin composite restoration.

sial- (sialo-) Prefix denoting saliva or salivary gland.

sialadenitis (sialoadenitis) *n.* Inflammation of the salivary gland; it is often associated with pain, tenderness, redness, and gradual localized swelling of the affected area. **Acute bacterial sialadenitis** is characterized by swelling, pain, fever, and reddening of the overlying skin; it is commonly caused by bacteria entering the salivary ducts against the salivary flow since reduced salivary flow, such as in *Sjögren's syndrome, can be a predisposing factor. Treatment is by antibiotic therapy and gentle massage. **Chronic bacterial sialadenitis** most commonly affects the submandibular salivary gland and presents as a recurrent painful swelling particularly associated with eating and drinking; there may also be a purulent discharge producing a salty or unpleasant taste in the mouth. **Radiation sialadenitis** can occur as an unwanted side-effect following *radiotherapy, particularly when delivered to the head or neck; it can result in progressive fibrous replacement of the glandular tissue. **Viral sialadenitis** *see* MUMPS.

sialadenosis *n.* A condition characterized by bilateral swelling of the *salivary glands, usually the parotid. It is associated with hormonal disturbances, liver cirrhosis, and malnutrition, but may also be idiopathic.

sialagogue *n.* A substance that stimulates the flow of *saliva.

sialaporia *n.* A reduction or deficiency in the flow of saliva.

sialectasis (ptyalectasis) *n.* Dilation of a *salivary duct or ducts.

sialoangiectasis *n.* Dilation of a *salivary duct or ducts.

sialoangiitis *n.* Inflammation of a *salivary duct or ducts.

sialogenous *adj.* Producing saliva.

sialogram *n.* A radiograph taken of either the submandibular or the parotid glands following the introduction of a radiopaque contrast medium into the *salivary gland ducts, allowing visualization of the main and intra-glandular salivary ducts. It is used to diagnose *salivary calculi or strictures. 📷

sialography *n.* A technique for radiographic examination of the salivary glands. *See also* SIALOGRAM.

sialolith *n. See* SALIVARY STONE.

sialolithiasis *n.* The process of formation of a *salivary stone.

sialometaplasia *n. See* NECROTIZING SIALOMETAPLASIA.

sialorrhoea *n. See* PTYALISM.

sialoschesis *n.* The reduction in the flow, secretion, or amount of saliva.

sickle-cell trait The carrier condition of **sickle-cell disease** in which there is production of an abnormal type of haemoglobin. It is most common in people of African ancestry and can present potential problems when administering a general *anaesthetic.

sickle scaler *n. See* SCALER.

side-effect *n.* An unwanted effect produced by *medication in addition to its desired *therapeutic effect.

Sievert [R. M. Sievert (1896–1966), Swedish radiologist] *n.* The SI unit (*International System of Units) for measuring equivalent and effective radiation doses. *See also* DOSE.

sign *n.* A feature of a disease or condition as detected by the dental or medical professional during physical examination of a patient. It is therefore objective, as opposed to the patient's experience (*symptom), which is subjective.

sign test (in statistics) A test used to determine whether two related samples are different. It tests the hypothesis that there is no difference between the continuous distributions of two random *variables (e.g. X and Y).

silica (quartz) *n.* Silicon dioxide (SiO_2), which forms the main component in most dental ceramic materials providing a rigid crystalline three-dimensional structure. It can exist in the form of quartz, cristobalite, tridymite, or as a glass. Silica is particularly used in combination with aluminium oxide to produce alumino-silicate glasses such as glass ionomer *cement.

silicone impression material (polyvinylsiloxane) An organic–inorganic polymer in which some of the carbon atoms are replaced by silicon atoms. They may be divided into **condensation-cured silicones** (vinyl polydimethylsiloxanes) and **addition-cured silicones** (polydimethylsiloxanes). Crosslinking of condensation-cured silicones is achieved by the use of an activator paste containing tetraethyl silicate; the by-product of this reaction is alcohol which detrimentally affects the storage stability; impressions made with this material should therefore be cast immediately. The setting reaction of addition-cured silicones is via a platinum catalyst and a silanol. Because there is no by-product, addition-cured silicones have greater dimensional *stability. The wearing of latex gloves can cause the inhibition of the setting reaction of addition-cured silicone putty. Silicone *impression material is manufactured in a range of viscosities (light-, medium-, heavy-bodied, and putty) controlled by the amount of filler incorporated.

silk suture *n. See* SUTURE.

silver nitrate *n.* Nitrate of silver ($AgNO_3$), which is the light-sensitive ingredient of photographic film. In its ammoniacal form it was formerly used to disclose and arrest dental caries because of its ability to deposit black silver and its toxic effect on bacteria; however, it is a strong pulpal irritant.

silver point (cone) *n.* A radiopaque *endodontic filling material used in conjunction with an endodontic *sealer. They are not generally recommended as they fail to seal the root canal laterally or coronally and may cause tooth or gingival staining.

similars, the law of A homeopathic principle that states that the symptoms caused by a dose of a substance are the symptoms that can also be cured with an ultra-dilute dose of the same substance ('like cures like').

Simon's classification of malocclusion [P. W. Simon (1883–1957), German orthodontist] A classification of malocclusion, first described by Paul Simon in 1926, in which the teeth are related to the Frankfort, mid-sagittal, and orbital planes. Teeth too close to the Frankfort plane are in attraction, whereas those too distant are in distraction. Teeth too close to the mid-sagittal plane are in contraction, whereas those too far away are in distraction. Teeth too anterior to the orbital plane are in protraction, whereas those too posterior to the orbital plane are in retraction.

sinoatrial node *n.* The impulse generating tissue located on the wall of the right atrium of the heart near the entrance of the superior vena cava.

sintering *n.* The process of welding together powdered particles of a substance or mixture by heating to a temperature below the melting point of the components. A process used in the manufacture of dental *porcelain.

sinus *n.* 1. An air cavity within a bone. The **paranasal sinuses** are air-filled cavities surrounding and opening into the *nasal cavity. They are named after the bone in which they are situated i.e. frontal sinus, *maxillary sinus, ethmoid sinus, palatine sinus, and sphenoid sinus. 2. A channel containing venous blood. The **cavernous sinus** is one of a pair of large cavities in the sphenoid bone situated behind the eye sockets. It provides venous blood drainage from the brain, eye, nose, and upper part of the cheek. 3. A bulge in a tubular organ; for example, the carotid sinus.

sinusitis *n.* Inflammation of the mucous membrane of any sinus, especially of the maxillary and nasal sinuses. It is characterized by symptoms such as headache, pain around the eyes, toothache, jaw pain, nasal discharge, postnasal drip, coughing, swelling around the eyes, a stuffy nose, fatigue, bad breath, or a sore throat. It may be of bacterial, viral, fungal, allergic, or autoimmune origin. It can present as **acute sinusitis**, lasting up to about four weeks, or **chronic sinusitis**, lasting up to three months or more. *Asthma may be associated with recurrent sinusitis. Decongestants such as pseudoephedrine may be prescribed to reduce nasal swelling.

sinus lift A surgical procedure to raise the lining of the floor of the maxillary *antrum and allow bone from the tibia, iliac crest, or chin to be inserted into the space obtained. It produces an increase in the vertical height of the alveolar bone and is carried out in order to provide sufficient bone for the retention of a dental *implant.

Further Reading: Emmerich D., Att W., Stappert C. Sinus floor elevation using osteotomes: a systematic review and meta-analysis. *J Periodontol* 2005;76(8):1237–51.

sinus tract An infected tract leading from a focus of infection to the skin or a hollow organ. It is sometimes also called a *fistula. The tract is lined with epithelium. Although usually draining into the mouth, sinus tracts may lead from a focus of infection such as an infected tooth or periodontal disease to drain on the face or neck (**cutaneous sinus tract**). When a cutaneous sinus tract is present, the infected tooth is often asymptomatic, as the tract provides a pathway for inflammatory exudates, thereby relieving the pressure. Cutaneous dental sinus tracts may resemble a pimple, ulcer, or nodule.

Siqveland matrix retainer *n. See* MATRIX RETAINER.

Sjögren's syndrome [H. S. C. Sjögren (1899–1939), Swedish ophthalmologist] An autoimmune condition affecting the *exocrine glands, particularly salivary and lacrimal (tear) glands. It most commonly occurs in females and the middle-aged and is characterized in the **primary form (sicca syndrome)** by dry mouth (*xerostomia) and dryness of the eyes (xerophthalmia), and in the **secondary form** where the symptoms additionally include those of another autoimmune disorder, such as *rheumatoid arthritis or systemic *lupus erythematosus (SLE). Symptoms may also include intermittent swelling of the major salivary glands and an increased liability to acute suppurative *sialadenitis and *candidal infections. Treatment is aimed at minimizing the oral symptoms and managing any other associated autoimmune disease.

skeletal discrepancy *n.* The nature of a *malocclusion based on the malrelation of the skeletal structures to one another.

skeletal pattern The relationship of the structures of the face to each other. It is assessed with the patient seated in an upright position looking straight ahead, with the head positioned so that the *Frankfort plane is parallel to the floor and the teeth are in *occlusion. It can be assessed in antero-posterior, vertical, and transverse planes. The **antero-posterior plane** can be assessed with the tips of the index and middle fingers placed in the concavities between the upper lip and the base of the nose and the lower lip and the chin; the skeletal pattern is **class I** if the index finger is horizontal during the examination (the mandible is 2–3mm posterior to the maxilla), **class II** when the index finger slopes down (the mandible is retruded relative to the maxilla), and **class III** when the index finger slopes upwards (the mandible is protruded relative to the maxilla).

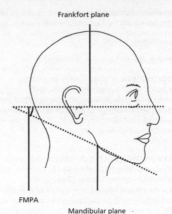

Skeletal pattern—vertical plane

The face height is divided into upper and lower parts. The lower face height (LFH) is of normal proportion when the distances from the glabella to the columella and the columella to the lower border of the chin are equal: the LFH is increased if the distance from the glabella to the columella is less than the distance from the columella to the lower border of the chin, and decreased if the distance from the glabella to the columella is greater than the distance from the columella to the lower border of the chin.

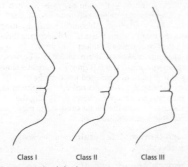

Antero-posterior skeletal pattern

Class I   Class II   Class III

The vertical plane is assessed from the side of the patient with the *Frankfort plane parallel to the floor and the teeth in occlusion. In a patient with an average Frankfort mandibular plane angle (FMPA), a finger placed on the lower border of the mandible and one placed on the Frankfort plane will produce an angle in which the long axes of the fingers will cross at the *occiput; with an increased FMPA the long axes will cross in front of the occiput, and with a reduced FMPA the long axes will cross behind the occiput.

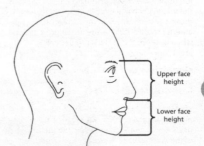

Skeletal pattern—face height

In the **transverse plane**, discrepancies may be either **unilateral** or **bilateral** depending on whether one or both sides respectively are affected. The transverse plane is in normal proportion if the width of the base of the nose is approximately the same as the inter-inner canthal width and the width of the mouth is the same as the distance between the medial sides of the irises.

S

skeletal relationship The orientation of the jaws to the bones of the skull. *See* SKELETAL PATTERN.

skeleton denture *See* DENTURE.

skew *n.* (in statistics) A measure of the symmetry of a frequency distribution. If frequent scores are clustered at the lower end of the distribution and the tail points towards the higher scores, this is a **positive skew**. Conversely, if the frequent scores cluster at the higher end of the distribution and the tail points to the lower scores, this is a **negative skew**.

skin *n.* The outer covering of the body made up of an outer layer, the *epidermis, and an inner layer, the *dermis. Its functions include protection of the body from trauma and infection, temperature regulation by means of hair and sweat glands, acting as an organ of excretion, and the prevention of dehydration. *See also* MUCOSA.

skull *n.* The entire bony framework of the head and face including the mandible. The skull has many functions including protecting the brain from injury and supporting the facial structures. It is made up of the *cranium and the mandible and consists of 22 bones (28 including the ossicles).

Apart from the mandible, the bones are joined together by sutures to form a rigid though elastic complex.

slaking *v.* A method of mixing zinc phosphate *cement by adding the powder to the liquid in small increments and waiting about 15 seconds between increments. This has the effect of prolonging the working time by reducing the accelerating effect of the *exothermic reaction.

slapped cheek disease *n. See* ERYTHEMA INFECTIOSUM.

SLOB rule An acronym (Same Lingual Opposite Buccal) describing a parallax radiographic technique used to identify the position of *ectopic teeth (usually maxillary canines). It compares the object movement with the x-ray tube head movement. If the tube head moves mesially, the image of a lingual object will also move mesially on the film, i.e. in the same direction. The image of a buccal object will move in the opposite direction. The movement of the lingual or buccal object is compared to objects whose locations are known; this will usually be an erupted tooth.

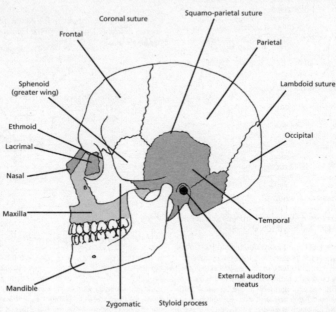

The bones of the skull

SEE WEB LINKS
- This website provides a graphic illustration of how the rule operates.

slough *n.* Dead tissue shed from the body such as is seen in *necrotizing gingivitis.

smear layer A thin layer of organic and inorganic debris compacted onto the dentinal or enamel surface of a cavity which has undergone instrumentation. It can be removed with a *conditioner or by means of the *acid-etch technique. Its presence can influence the adhesion of a bonded restoration. In endodontic therapy it may be removed with citric acid and sodium hypochlorite or ethylene diamine tetraacetic acid (EDTA), a chelating agent, along with sodium hypochlorite to dissolve the organic portion.

smoking *n.* The act of burning *tobacco and other substances and drawing the hot vapour containing fine particles of carbon and other products of combustion into the mouth and lungs. **Cigarette smoking** is a risk factor for tooth loss and one of the most important risk factors for periodontitis, which is thought to be due to a reduction in gingival blood circulation, impaired white cell mobility and function, impaired wound healing, and an increased production of inflammatory substances (**cytokines**), particularly due to nicotine. Quitting smoking reduces the risk of tooth loss. Smoking also results in a black surface (extrinsic) pigmentation of the tooth enamel and *halitosis.

smooth muscle *See* MUSCLE.

smooth surface caries *See* CARIES.

snuff *n.* A form of smokeless tobacco usually placed in the oral cavity or inhaled into the nasal cavity. Nicotine is absorbed into the body through the mucous membranes. Early signs of mucosal change include superficial wrinkling, a colour change to white or pale grey, and a thickening with the formation of deep furrows. The use of snuff can result in a number of *malignant or potentially malignant oral lesions such as squamous cell *carcinoma, verrucous carcinoma, *leukoplakia, and *erythroplakia.

Snyder's test [M. L. Snyder (1907–69), American bacteriologist] A colorimetric test for evaluating caries activity or susceptibility. It is based on the rate of acid production by *acidogenic micro-organisms e.g. *Lactobacillus* in a glucose medium using bromocresol green as an indicator. The glucose medium is inoculated with a saliva sample; any lactobacilli present will ferment the glucose, forming lactic acid and thereby lowering the pH. A rapid colour change from blue-green to yellow due to the pH change is claimed to indicate a susceptibility to the formation of dental caries.

social determinants of health Specific features of and pathways by which societal conditions affect health and which potentially can be altered by informed action. Examples are income, education, occupation, family structure, service availability, sanitation, exposure to hazards, social support, racial discrimination, and access to resources linked to health.

SEE WEB LINKS
- 'Social determinants of health' overview document on the Department of Health website.

socket *n.* Any concavity into which a corresponding part fits such as the eye socket or the socket in the alveolar bone of the jaw into which a tooth root fits. **Dry socket** *See* ALVEOLITIS.

sodium fluoride *n.* An ionic compound (NaF) which was formerly used for water *fluoridation (hexafluorosilicic acid and disodium hexafluorosilicate are now the only two compounds of fluoride permitted for artificial fluoridation in the UK; disodium hexafluorosilicate is most commonly used in the USA). Sodium fluoride is added to toothpaste to reduce caries and may also be mixed with kaolin and glycerine to provide a topically applied *desensitizing paste for the treatment of dentine *hypersensitivity. Sodium fluoride poisoning is characterized by mottled tooth enamel (*fluorosis) and *osteosclerosis.

sodium hypochlorite *n.* A chemical compound (NaClO) used as a bleaching agent. In dentistry it is used in a dilute aqueous solution for the *disinfection of dentures and impressions and as a disinfectant (0.5–6.0% aqueous solution) for irrigating root canals. Although antimicrobial efficiency is improved with higher concentrations it can result in enhanced cytotoxicity and may have a detrimental effect on dentine.

Further Reading: Clarkson R. M., Moule A. J. Sodium hypochlorite and its use as an endodontic irrigant. *Aust Dent J* 1998;43(4):250–56.

sodium monofluorophosphate *n.* A chemical compound (Na_2FPO_3) frequently added to toothpaste in concentrations of 500–1500 parts per million to inhibit caries. *See also* FLUORIDE.

sodium perborate *n.* A water-soluble chemical compound ($NaBO_3$) manufactured by the reaction between sodium tetraborate, *hydrogen peroxide, and sodium hydroxide.

S

It releases hydrogen peroxide when in contact with water and has antiseptic and bleaching properties. Because it is oxygen liberating it has been used in the treatment of *necrotizing ulcerative gingivitis and the internal *bleaching of pulpless teeth. In the latter case, sodium perborate is either mixed with water or 30% hydrogen peroxide to form a paste and then sealed in the pulp cavity for an extended period of time. Prolonged use of sodium perborate can lead to mucosal irritation and *hyperplasia of the filiform papillae of the tongue (black *hairy tongue) Trade name: **Bocasan®**.

sodium phosphate *n.* A chemical added to alginate impression material to delay the reaction time between calcium sulphate and the soluble alginate salt, thereby prolonging the setting time (*retarder) and increasing the working time.

sodium pump *n.* The mechanism of active transport, using energy derived from the oxidative metabolism of **adenosine triphosphate**, by which sodium (Na^+) is extruded from a cell and potassium (K^+) is brought in, so as to maintain the gradients of these ions across the cell membrane; the conduction of a stimulus down a nerve fibre is dependent upon these changes. The action of a local *analgesic solution inhibits the passage of sodium ions into the nerve cell, thus preventing the transmission of the stimulus.

sodium thiosulphate *n.* A colourless crystalline compound ($Na_2S_2O_3$), also known as **hypo (hyposulphite)**, used as a photographic fixing solution in the processing of dental radiographs. It dissolves undeveloped silver halide crystals.

soft lining *n.* A resilient semipermanent denture base lining material which allows more even distribution of loading. Examples of soft lining materials are silicone rubber (poly dimethyl siloxane polymer with added filler) and acrylic soft liners containing either leachable or polymerizable *plasticizers. Soft linings are indicated for older patients with thin atrophic mucosa, following prosthetic surgery, or to utilize soft tissue undercuts for retention. Soft liners are contraindicated in patients with low salivary flow because of the tendency to cause uncomfortable friction on the mucosal surface.

soft palate *n. See* PALATE.

solder *n.* A fusible alloy used to unite two metal surfaces such as the units of a gold alloy *bridge. It is used in conjunction with a *flux.

solid solution *n.* A mixture of elements at the atomic level. Metals used in dentistry which readily form solid solutions with gold are copper, platinum, palladium, and silver. Steel is an example of a solid solution of a small amount of carbon in iron.

solubility *n.* A measure of how much of a given substance will dissolve in a liquid.

solute *n.* The dissolved substance in a solution. In a liquid–liquid solution, it is the name given to the minor component.

solution *n.* A homogeneous mixture of two or more substances; frequently (but not necessarily) a liquid solution. A **saline solution** is a mixture of sodium chloride (common salt) dissolved in water used for the irrigation of extraction sockets and root canals; **physiological saline solution** contains 0.9% sodium chloride in distilled water and has the same molecular concentration as blood (isotonic); it is used as a solvent for local *analgesic solutions. A **disclosing solution** contains a *disclosing agent capable of rendering *plaque deposits visible.

solvent *n.* A substance, normally a liquid, which is capable of absorbing another liquid, gas, or solid to form a homogeneous mixture.

sorbitol *n.* An alcohol derivative of sugar used as a sweetening agent in such products as chewing gum and sugar-free confectionery; it is only half as sweet by weight as *sucrose. Studies have shown sorbitol to be less cariogenic than sucrose.

Further Reading: Burt B. A. The use of sorbitol- and xylitol-sweetened chewing gum in caries control. *J Am Dent Assoc* 2006;137(2):190–96.

sordes *n.* Debris, especially the hard coating of food, epithelial matter, and micro-organisms that collect on the oral mucosa, lips, and teeth in a dehydrated individual or during a prolonged fever. The material may appear as a dark brown or blackish crust-like deposit on the lips.

sore, cold *n. See* HERPES.

sore denture *n. See* DENTURE STOMATITIS.

space analysis A process that estimates the amount of space required in a dental arch to align teeth orthodontically.

space closure The process of reducing any residual interproximal spacing during orthodontic therapy. It may be achieved by using a variety of auxiliary attachments such as active *tiebacks, nickel titanium coil *springs, and *elastics.

space maintainer A passive removable or fixed appliance used to prevent closure of a space into which a tooth is expected to erupt, usually following the extraction or premature loss of a tooth. There are a number of designs of fixed space maintainers. *See* NANCE APPLIANCE. The unilateral **band and loop** or **crown and loop** space maintainer has a band or crown cemented onto the tooth adjacent to the space; a stainless steel wire loop attached to the band or crown extends into the space and touches the tooth on the other side of the space to hold both teeth in place. The bilateral **lingual** or **palatal arch** space maintainer usually consists of metal bands cemented on to the molar teeth on both sides of the arch distal to the spaces connected by a stainless steel wire behind the incisors.

space of Donders [F. C. Donders (1818–89), Dutch physician and ophthalmologist] The space between the dorsum of the tongue and the hard palate when the mandible is in the rest position.

spasm *n.* A sudden involuntary muscular contraction.

spasticity *n.* An involuntary increased resistance to passive muscle stretching. It is a symptom of damage to the *central nervous system.

spatula *n.* (*v.* **spatulate**) A flexible, flat-bladed hand instrument without sharp edges used for mixing dental materials such as impression paste and *plaster of Paris.

spatulator, automatic *n.* A mechanical device for mixing ingredients to form a homogeneous mass.

special care dentistry That branch of dentistry that aims to secure the oral health of, and enhance the quality of life for, people who by virtue of illness, disease, disability, lifestyle, or cultural practices are considered to be at greater risk of poor oral health, who experience barriers to the access and receipt of oral care, or for whom the management of dental care presents other health risks. It usually requires an interprofessional approach supported by appropriate behaviour management techniques.

specialist list A list held by the *General Dental Council (GDC) in the UK of registered dentists who have undergone an approved period of postgraduate training that has led to the attainment of a relevant specialist qualification and have been given the right by the GDC to call themselves a 'specialist'. There are currently 13 specialist lists.

(⊕) SEE WEB LINKS
• The General Dental Council website, which provides lists of all specialists entered on the specialist lists.

special waste *n. See* CLINICAL WASTE.

specificity *n.* A measure of the ability of a diagnostic or screening test to exclude the presence of a disease (or condition) when it is truly not present. *See also* SENSITIVITY.

speech therapy The corrective or rehabilitative treatment of patients who have physical or cognitive disorders which result in a difficulty in verbal communication. Speech and language therapists must complete a recognized three- or four-year degree programme and register with the **Health Professions Council** before being able to practise in the UK.

(⊕) SEE WEB LINKS
• The Royal College of Speech and Language therapists website.

Spee, curve of *n. See* CURVE OF SPEE.

sphenoid bone *n.* A bone situated at the base of the skull located between the temporal and frontal bones and roughly resembling the shape of a butterfly. It is divided into a body, two great and two small wings extending outward from the sides of the body, and two pterygoid processes which project from it below.

sphincter *n.* A specialized circular band of muscle that surrounds an orifice e.g. the laryngeal sphincter. Muscle contraction causes partial or complete closure of the orifice.

sphygmomanometer *n.* An instrument for measuring arterial *blood pressure. It consists of an inflatable cuff (which is usually applied to the arm) connected via a rubber tube to a graduated column of mercury or aneroid pressure gauge. The cuff is inflated until the pressure is sufficient to stop the arterial blood flow. As the cuff pressure is slowly released a characteristic noise (**Korotkoff sounds**) is heard as the blood flow first starts again; this is recorded as the systolic blood pressure; the cuff pressure is further released until no sound is heard; this is recorded as the diastolic blood pressure. The technique involves the use of a *stethoscope to listen to the sounds.

spill *n. See* AMALGAM CAPSULE.

spillway *n.* A pathway through which food debris can escape during *mastication. An **interdental spillway** is formed by the interproximal contours of adjacent teeth and gingival tissues. An **occlusal spillway** is a groove that crosses a cusp or marginal ridge of a tooth. *See also* EMBRASURE.

S

spine *n.* 1. The vertebral column. 2. A small bony projection. The **anterior nasal spine** is a forward projection from the anterior surface of the maxillae clearly visible on *cephalometric radiographs. *See also* CEPHALOMETRIC ANALYSIS. The **posterior nasal spine** is a sharp bony projection from the posterior border of the horizontal plate of the *palatine bones and forms the attachment for the muscles of the *uvula. *See also* CEPHALOMETRIC ANALYSIS. **Spix's spine** [J. B. Spix (1781–1826), German anatomist] is a bony spine on the border of the inferior alveolar (dental) foramen of the mandible to which is attached the sphenomandibular ligament.

spiral filler *n.* A flexible rotary instrument with consistently spaced spirals used to distribute root canal sealer and cement evenly throughout the root canal system. Spiral fillers are marketed in different sizes. Trade name: **Lentulo® spiral filler**.

spirochaete *n.* A phylum of spiral-shaped *Gram-negative bacteria which move by a twisting motion aided by the presence of flagella on the cell walls. Most spirochaetes are *anaerobic, some of which may be associated with oral conditions, such as *Treponema denticola* associated with chronic *periodontal disease, and *Borrelia vincenti* associated with *necrotizing gingivitis and *cancrum oris.

Spix's spine *n. See* SPINE.

spleen *n.* (*adj.* **splenic**) A large dark-red oval organ on the left side of the body between the stomach and the diaphragm. It is part of the *lymphatic system. The spleen produces lymphocytes, filters the blood, stores blood cells, and produces *phagocytes which destroy old blood cells.

splint *n.* A rigid appliance used to immobilize displaced or moveable parts. An **abutment splint** rigidly bonds together adjacent tooth restorations at their interproximal contact areas; they may utilize *Maryland or *Rochette type retainers. A **bite-guard splint** is usually made of acrylic resin covering the occlusal and incisal surfaces; it immobilizes the teeth and protects them from trauma and excessive occlusal or *parafunctional forces; *see also* BITE GUARD. A **buccal splint** is usually made of plaster of Paris and is used to accurately locate the components of a fixed partial denture. A **cap splint** is usually made of metal and covers the crowns of the teeth; when cemented in position, it immobilizes the teeth and jaw fractures. A **continuous clasp splint** consists of cast clasps that follow the labial and lingual surfaces of the teeth; it is usually cemented onto the teeth to provide temporary immobilization. An **occlusal splint** is a removable appliance usually made of hard resin covering the biting surfaces of the teeth used to protect the teeth from excessive wear by preventing tooth to tooth contact. A **resin splint** is a temporary appliance made of resin composite bonded onto the enamel surfaces of two or more teeth to provide immobilization following root fracture or *subluxation. A **stabilization splint** is made of hard acrylic and is used to protect the tooth tissues as a result of muscular clenching (*bruxism).

Further Reading: Brown C. L., Mackie I. C. Splinting of traumatized teeth in children. *Dent Update* 2003;30:78–82.

split cast *n. See* CAST.

split ring *n.* A casting ring made in three parts to allow for the expansion of investment material during casting in the *lost wax process. A more commonly used technique is to line the casting ring with either an aluminosilicate or a cellulose liner.

sponge *n. See* GELATIN SPONGE.

spoon denture *n. See* DENTURE.

spoon excavator *n. See* EXCAVATOR.

sporotrichosis *n.* A disease caused by the fungus *Sporothrix schenckii* that is present naturally in soil, hay, and plant material. The disease usually affects the skin and gardeners and farmers are the most commonly infected. Very rarely it causes ulceration of the oral mucosa, larynx, and paranasal sinuses. Treatment is with potassium iodide or itraconozole.

spot grinding *See* GRINDING.

spot welding The local application of heat under pressure to components to be joined together, by means of a high electric current at low voltage. It is used in the repair and construction of appliances.

spreader *n.* A tapered fine pointed metal hand instrument used to laterally compress *gutta-percha endodontic points in a root canal during the *obturation phase of root canal therapy.

spring *n.* A coil of fine wire capable of returning to its original shape when bent. An **apron spring** is a component of a removable orthodontic appliance used to reduce an *overjet. It is a flexible spring (0.35–0.4mm diameter) attached to a high labial bow which is constructed from a stiffer archwire (0.9mm). A **Coffin spring** [C. R. Coffin (1826–91), American dentist] is an omega-shaped (Ω) spring made of heavy-gauge wire, crossing the palate as part of a removable

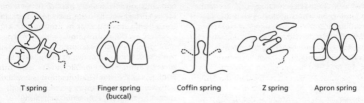

T spring | Finger spring (buccal) | Coffin spring | Z spring | Apron spring

Types of orthodontic springs

orthodontic appliance (e.g. the *Bimler or the *Crozat appliance); it provides the possibility of expansion or constriction of the maxillary dental arch. A **finger spring** consists of a short piece of wire, usually about 0.5 millimetres in diameter, forming part of an orthodontic appliance which acts as a lever to apply force to a tooth and achieve a tooth tipping movement; it may be placed buccally or palatally. Finger springs can contain helices to increase the effective wire length for added flexibility. A **flapper spring** is wire bent in the form of a 'box' incorporated into a removable appliance to tip an individual tooth or groups of teeth buccally or labially; it has the same action as a Z spring. A **rotation spring** is used in the treatment of class II and class III *jaw malocclusions and may be geometrically shaped as a 'U' or an 'S', that terminates at one end in a tube for the passage and retention of a *tie wire, and at the other end with a curved surface. The entire spring is designed to provide compression between an *archwire attached to an orthodontic bracket and a tooth band. A force is created which acts to rotate the tooth about its axis. A **T spring** is used for the buccal movement of a single molar or premolar tooth; it is activated by pulling the spring away from the acrylic base plate at an angle of 45°. A **Z spring (recurved spring)** is wire bent in the form of a 'Z', incorporated into a removable appliance used to tip an individual tooth or groups of teeth either buccally or labially.

sprue *n.* 1. Wax or metal used to form the hole or holes through which molten metal is poured into a heated mould. 2. The waste piece of metal that occupies the hole in the investment material when casting is completed. A **sprue former (sprue base, *crucible former)** is a cone-shaped base usually made of metal or resin to which the sprue is attached; it forms a crucible in the investment material which aids the passage of the molten metal during casting. A **sprue pin** is a solid or hollow length of metal used to attach the wax pattern to the sprue former.

sputum *n.* Material coughed up from the respiratory tract. It contains mucous and other substances, such as bacteria, the examination of which can provide important information for the diagnosis and treatment of respiratory disease.

squamous *adj.* Describing a flat, scaly, or plate-like cell.

squamous cell carcinoma *n. See* CARCINOMA.

squamous epithelium *n. See* EPITHELIUM.

squash bite *n.* A record taken usually in wax to register the relationship of the cusps of the upper and lower teeth. It is more appropriately termed an *occlusal record.

stability *n.* The quality or attribute of being firm and steadfast. **Denture stability** is the property of a removable denture that resists forces causing displacement of the denture from its supporting structures. **Dimensional stability** is the ability of a material to retain its size and form over a period of time.

stabilization *n.* 1. The seating or positioning of a fixed (bridge) or removable denture so that it is not displaced under pressure. 2. The control of forces on teeth or prostheses so as to minimize movement. *See also* RETENTION.

stack *n.* A set of metallic strips inserted into an *ultrasonic or sonic instrument to convert a magnetic field into high-frequency vibrations that produce movement of the instrument working tip.

Stafne's cavity (Stafne's defect) [E. C. Stafne (1894–1981), American oral pathologist] A developmental depression on the lingual surface of the mandible near the lower border which may appear radiographically as a radiolucency. It frequently contains salivary gland tissue such as the submandibular salivary gland. It is asymptomatic and no intervention is required.

staging *n.* A means of describing or measuring the progress of a tumour. A widely used system is the TNM classification that indicates the progress of the tumour by the size and spread of the primary tumour (T), the absence or presence of *metastases in *lymph nodes (N), and the absence or presence of distant metastases (M); a number after each of the letters increases with the size of the tumour and the degree of metastasis. The assessment is undertaken at initial diagnosis and before any treatment has been undertaken.

( ) SEE WEB LINKS
- A factsheet on staging from the National Cancer Institute (US).

stagnation area *n.* The location on the surface of a tissue where there is a tendency for food debris to accumulate.

stain *n.* The discoloration of a material by foreign matter. *See also* EXTRINSIC TOOTH STAINING; INTRINSIC TOOTH STAINING.

stainless steel *n.* A ferrous alloy with a minimum 12% chromium content when used for intra-oral appliances. Because of its strength and corrosion resistance, the material is used in the manufacture of hand instruments and may be used in the construction of prosthetic base plates and clasps.

stamp cusp *n. See* CUSP.

standard deviation (in statistics) A measure of the range of variation from an average of a group of measurements. 68% of all measurements fall within one standard deviation of the *mean. 95% of all measurements fall within two standard deviations of the mean.

standard error of the mean (in statistics) A measure of variability. It is the *standard deviation divided by the square root of the sample size.

standardization *n.* (in statistics) The process of converting a *variable into a standard unit of measurement (e.g. standard deviation units). This enables data to be compared when different units of measurement have been used.

standardized rate (in epidemiology) A method of predicting the number of people with a specific condition. The standardized rate is obtained by dividing the observed number of cases by the expected number of cases. **Age standardized rates** enable comparisons to be made between populations which have different age structures.

standard operating procedure A method of undertaking a procedure that outlines the preferred and safest method of undertaking it, based on a risk assessment, current clinical evidence, and established clinical practice.

standard precautions A standard of care designed to protect healthcare personnel and patients from infection by pathogenic micro-organisms, including viruses, that can be spread by blood or any other body fluid, excretion, or secretion (except sweat), whether or not they contain blood. Standard precautions also apply to contact with non-intact skin and mucous membranes. Other measures (e.g. expanded or transmission-based precautions) may be necessary in addition to standard precautions to prevent potential spread of certain diseases (e.g. tuberculosis, influenza, and varicella) that are transmitted through airborne, droplet, or contact transmission (e.g. sneezing, coughing, and contact with skin).

( ) SEE WEB LINKS
- Guidelines for infection control in dental healthcare settings from the Centers for Disease Control and Prevention (US).

Standards for Dental Professionals
Guidance published by the UK *General Dental Council (GDC) in 2005 which replaced Maintaining Standards. The new guidance applies to all members of the dental team on the *dental register. The GDC defines six general principles for dental professionals to abide by during their work. They relate to universally accepted professional standards, such as putting patients' interests first and protecting confidentiality.

stannous fluoride *n.* A *fluoride salt of tin (SnF_2) used in toothpastes, gels, and mouthrinses to inhibit *caries.

staphylion *n.* The midline point on the posterior border of the hard palate; a *craniometric landmark.

Staphylococcus *n.* A genus of *Gram-positive non-motile, spherical (cocci) bacteria occurring in grapelike clusters. *Staphylococcus epidermidis* is found on the skin and mucous membranes of the mouth and is usually of low pathogenicity but can cause oral infection if allowed to proliferate; it is often resistant to a wide variety of antibiotics, including *penicillin and methicillin. Oral strains have been shown to be the source of *septicaemia in immunocompromised patients. *Staphylococcus aureus* is a significant *pathogen and is capable of producing suppurative lesions; it has been isolated from the gingival crevice and the oral cavity. Recent studies have shown that the presence of *S. aureus* in the oral cavity is far more prevalent than previously considered. Another recent study has shown that at one week post-surgery 15% of oral titanium implants and 39.1% of teeth harboured *S. aureus*. *See also* MRSA.

Further Reading: Ohara-Nemoto Y., Haraga H., Kimura S., Nemoto T. K. Occurrence of staphylococci in the oral cavities of healthy adults and nasal oral trafficking of the bacteria. *J Med Microbiol* 2008;57:95–9.
Fürst M. M., Salvi G. E., Lang N. P., Persson G. R. Bacterial colonization immediately after installation on oral titanium implants. *Clin Oral Implants Res* 2007;18:501–8.

starch *n.* The form in which carbohydrates are stored in many plants and an important dietary constituent. Starch consists of multiple *glucose units as either α-**amylose** or **amylopectin**; it is digested by the *enzyme amylase.

statistical significance The probability that an event or difference occurred by chance alone. The significant level is the probability of making a decision to reject the *null hypothesis when the null hypothesis is actually true (*type I error). This is generally referred to in terms of the *p-value. If the p-value is found to be less than the significance level (e.g. p = 0.05), then the null hypothesis is rejected.

statistics *n.* A mathematical science concerned with the collection, analysis, interpretation, explanation, or presentation of *data.

status asthmaticus Severe, prolonged, immobilizing attack of asthma that is unresponsive to normal bronchodilator treatment. Sedatives are absolutely contraindicated and patients require immediate hospital care.

status epilepticus The repeated occurrence of *epileptic seizures without any intervening period of consciousness. It is a medical emergency and patients with a history of this condition are potentially unsuitable for dental treatment in a primary care setting.

staurion *n.* The intersection of the median and transverse palatine sutures; a *craniometric landmark.

stellate reticulum *n.* A tissue layer lying between the *stratum intermedium and the outer *enamel epithelium. It consists of star-shaped cells which protect the underlying dental tissues and maintain the shape of the tooth.

stenion *n.* The termination in either temporal fossa of the shortest transverse diameter of the skull measured from one of two *craniometric points on the sphenosquamous suture located nearest to the midline on each side.

stenosis *n.* The abnormal constriction or narrowing of a duct or canal.

stenostomia *n.* Narrowness of the oral cavity.

Stensen's duct (parotid duct) [N. Stensen (1638–86), Danish physician] The duct of the parotid *salivary gland opening into the mouth opposite the neck of the upper second molar tooth. It allows saliva to drain from the parotid duct to the mouth.

stent [C. R. Stent (1845–1901), English dentist] *n.* **1.** A tube placed inside a duct to keep it open. **2.** An acrylic resin appliance used as a positioning guide or support to maintain tissue such as bones or skin grafts in position.

Stephan's curve The curve on a graph, first described by Robert Stephan in 1943, showing the fall in pH below the critical level of pH 5.5, at which demineralization of enamel occurs following the intake of fermentable carbohydrates, acidic liquids, or sugar in the presence of acidogenic bacteria. After consumption, there is an elimination of the acid and a return to normal saliva or plaque pH, at which point repair of any destruction of the enamel structure takes place (remineralization). Repeated intakes of fermentable carbohydrates cause the low pH to be maintained for longer periods, thereby not allowing remineralization to take place.

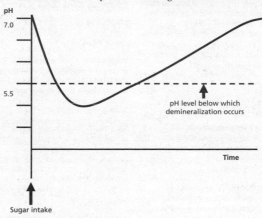

Stephan's curve

Further Reading: Stephan R. M., Miller B. F. A quantitative method for evaluating physical and chemical agents which modify production of acids in bacterial plaques on human teeth. *J Dent Res* 1943;22:45–51.

stereograph *n.* An instrument used to record mandibular movements as a series of three-dimensional arch tracings.

stereoscope *n.* An optical instrument which produces binocular vision, giving the appearance of depth for the viewing of radiographs or photographs.

sterile *adj.* Completely free from bacteria, viruses, fungi, and other organisms.

sterilization *n.* The process by which all types of micro-organisms are destroyed. **Autoclave sterilization**, utilizing both steam and pressure, is the most effective method for routine clinical dental practice. *See* AUTOCLAVE. **Dry heat sterilization** is achieved using a hot air oven on a standard setting of 160°C (320°F) for 2 hours and is useful for sterilizing powders but inappropriate for dental instruments. **Chemical sterilization** can be achieved by the immersion of materials or instruments in liquids such as *gluteraldehyde and formaldehyde solutions. This process can take 12 hours or more to kill all spores and the liquids are volatile and toxic to tissues, and is therefore inappropriate for dental instruments. **Ethylene oxide** is a gaseous form of chemical sterilization used commercially in the manufacture of many disposable medical devices. **Sterilization by flaming** an instrument until it glows red provides effective sterilization but will detrimentally alter the properties of the working tip of a metal instrument. *Glass bead sterilization and **hot salt sterilization** have been used for root canal instruments but are only effective for that part of the instrument which is in contact with the glass beads or salt, and therefore sterilization is incomplete. **Radiation sterilization**, such as x-rays or gamma rays, may be used in the commercial manufacture of some materials and equipment. **Ultraviolet (UV) sterilization** is only effective on surfaces and some transparent materials. **Boiling in water** for 15 minutes will kill most bacteria and viruses but is ineffective against *prions and many bacterial spores and is therefore unsuitable for achieving sterilization in clinical dental practice. *See also* DECONTAMINATION.

sterilizer *n. See* AUTOCLAVE.

steroid *n.* A member of a large family of structurally similar lipid substances having the same basic structure of four interconnected carbon rings. They may occur naturally such as the sex hormones and *cholesterol or produced artificially for therapeutic purposes.

stertor *n.* A snoring noise produced by a deeply unconscious person.

stethoscope *n.* An acoustic device for listening to sounds within the body (auscultation). It is most often used to listen to heart sounds and breathing, although it may also be used to listen to intestines and blood flow in arteries and veins.

Stevens–Johnson syndrome (dermatostomatitis) [A. M. Stevens (1884–1945), American paediatrician; F. C. Johnson (1894–1934), American paediatrician] *n.* A severe form of *erythema multiforme usually induced by drug *hypersensitivity. It is characterized by typically non-itchy lesions on the skin and mucous membranes, fever, and cough with a thick purulent sputum. Treatment is primarily supportive and symptomatic.

Stickler's syndrome [G. B. Stickler (1925–), German–American paediatrician] A progressive *hereditary disease of *connective tissue with onset at birth affecting ears, eyes, and joints. It is characterized by degenerative changes in the joints, *cleft palate, bifid *uvula, and progressive loss of sight.

Further Reading: Kronwith S. D., Quinn G., McDonald D. M., Cardonick E., Onyx P., LaRossa D., Borns P., Stambolian D. E., Zackai E. H. Stickler's syndrome in the Cleft Palate Clinic. *J Pediatr Ophthalmol Strabismus* 1990;27:265–7.

Stillman's cleft *n. See* CLEFT.

Stillman's method *n. See* TOOTHBRUSHING.

stimulus *n.* (*pl.* **stimuli**) Any agent that produces a response or form of activity in a cell, tissue, or other structure.

stippling *n.* An orange peel appearance of the attached gingivae caused by the attachment of the collagen bundles. It may be simulated artificially on the external surface of a denture.

stitch *n. See* SUTURE.

stomach *n.* A saclike organ forming part of the alimentary canal between the oesophagus and duodenum. Its primary function is to continue the process of digestion by the secretion of the *enzyme **pepsin** and *hydrochloric acid. The refluxing of hydrochloric acid in such conditions as *bulimia and *anorexia can result in severe tooth *erosion.

stomatalgia *n. See* STOMATODYNIA.

stomatitis

n. Inflammation of the soft tissues of the mouth. The primary cause may be bacterial, chemical, electrical, mechanical, thermal, or due to radiation therapy or reaction to an *allergen. It may also occur as a secondary manifestation of systemic disease. **Acute herpetic stomatitis** is caused by the *herpes simplex virus and is characterized by localized itchy vesicles on the hard palate and gingivae which burst to form ulcers, sore throat, enlarged lymph glands, and fever; it lasts 10–14 days. **Angular stomatitis** *See* ANGULAR CHEILITIS. **Aphthous stomatitis** is characterized by recurrent apthous ulcers. **Stomatitis areata migrans (erythema migrans)** is characterized by continuously changing red patchy lesions on the buccal and oral mucosa, similar to those seen in *geographic tongue. **Bismuth stomatitis** is characterized by a bluish-black pigmentation of the gingival tissue (bismuth line) and is caused by prolonged systemic intake of bismuth compounds. **Gangrenous stomatitis** *See* CANCRUM ORIS. **Herpetic stomatitis** *See* HERPES. **Lead stomatitis** is characterized orally by a bluish line along the free gingival margin, mucosal pigmentation, a metallic taste, excessive salivation, and swelling of the salivary glands. An excessive absorption or ingestion of mercury can result in **mercurial stomatitis** characterized orally by mucosal reddening, increased salivation, ulceration, and necrosis of the gingivae spreading to the buccal mucosa and palate, a burning sensation in the tongue (*glossodynia), and periodontal inflammation with increased mobility of the teeth; there may also be the deposition of mercurial sulphide in the inflamed tissues resulting in pigmentation similar to lead stomatitis. **Mycotic stomatitis** is a fungal infection of the oral mucosa most commonly due to *Candida albicans (*candidiasis). **Nicotinic stomatitis (smoker's keratosis)** can be caused by smoking cigars, cigarettes, and pipes, and is characterized by small raised lesions on the palate, with red centres and white borders, caused by inflammation of the minor salivary glands; the palatal mucosa also shows signs of *keratosis. **Recurrent aphthous stomatitis** *See* APHTHOUS ULCER. **Uraemic stomatitis** is a rarely reported oral mucosal disorder possibly associated with longstanding uraemia in chronic renal failure patients. It is characterized by adherent white plaques on the floor of the mouth, buccal mucosa, lateral borders of the tongue and gingivae, pain, *dysgeusia, and an ammoniacal odour. *See also* GINGIVITIS, NEPHRITIC. **Stomatitis scarlatina** is a rare oral complication of scarlet fever. **Stomatitis venenata** is the result of contact allergy, most commonly dentifrices, mouthwashes, or acrylic denture base material; symptoms may include generalized redness of the mucosa, a burning sensation, ulceration, and *vesicles. **Vesicular stomatitis** is a symptom of *hand, foot, and mouth disease.

Further Reading: Hoexter D. L. Erythema migrans. *NY State Dent J* 1980;46:350–52.

stomatodynia (stomatalgia) *n.* Sore mouth; burning mouth sensation.

stomatodysodia *n.* Malodorous breath (*halitosis).

stomatoglossitis *n.* Inflammation of the oral mucosa and tongue most commonly caused by infections, chronic malnutrition, and nutritional disorders such as vitamin B deficiency (pellagra, beriberi).

stomatology *n.* The study of the mouth and its diseases; synonymous with *dentistry.

stomatomalacia *n.* The pathological softening of any mouth structure.

stomatomenia *n.* Bleeding from the mouth at the time of menstruation.

stomatoplasty *n.* Reconstructive surgery of the mouth.

stomatorrhagia *n.* Bleeding from the gingivae or any other part of the oral cavity.

stomatoschisis *n.* Congenital *cleft or defect in the upper lip (harelip).

stomatoscope *n.* A diagnostic instrument used for illuminating and examining the interior of the mouth.

stomion *n.* A soft tissue *cephalometric landmark defining the contact point of the upper and lower lips in the mid-sagittal line when the mouth is closed.

stomodeum *n.* An invagination of the embryonic ectoderm which develops into the mouth and upper part of the pharynx. It is the embryonic precursor of the oral cavity.

stone *n.* An abrasive instrument or tool. **Carborundum stone** is an abrasive made of silicon carbide used in rotary grinding and smoothing instruments. **Diamond abrasive stone**

consists of diamond particles of varying sizes embedded in a binding material; it is used for tooth reduction, bone recontouring and grinding, or smoothing artificial dental materials. *See also* ARKANSAS STONE.

stone, dental *n.* A specially calcined gypsum derivative similar to plaster of Paris manufactured to provide improved properties of strength and hardness. It is frequently coloured yellow. Dental stone is produced by heating gypsum under steam pressure in an autoclave at 120–150°C (248–302°F). Because of its small particle size and low porosity it requires less water to form a mix than *plaster of Paris. Dental stones are classified by the American Dental Association (ADA specification no. 25) according to their properties.

The American Dental Association classification of dental stone

Type	Description	Principal uses
I	Impression plaster (plaster of Paris)	Impressions, occlusal registration
II	Model plaster (β-calcium sulphate hemihydrate)	Study models, denture flask investment
III	Dental stone (Hydrocal) (α-calcium sulphate hemihydrate)	Denture casts
IV	Dental stone, high strength (Densite) (α-calcium sulphate hemihydrate)	Wax pattern dies
V	Dental stone, high strength, high-setting expansion	Wax pattern dies for high-shrinkage alloys

High-expansion dental stone compensates for the very high shrinkage of some metal alloys.

Further Reading: *Contemporary dental materials*, ed. V. B. Dhuru, 199–200. Oxford University Press, 2004.

stone, pulp *n. See* DENTICLE.

stop *n.* 1. An orthodontic device to prevent movement of a tooth in an unwanted direction. 2. A moveable device attached to an endodontic file or reamer to indicate its depth in a root canal.

stopping *n.* 1. A colloquial term used to describe a temporary restorative material. 2. A thermoplastic temporary restorative material consisting of *gutta-percha, *zinc oxide, and white wax.

Strategic Health Authority (SHA) The *National Health Service (NHS) statutory body providing the bridge between the *Department of Health and local NHS Trust and *Primary Care Trusts. It provides strategic leadership and ensures the delivery of improvements in health, wellbeing, and health services locally.

stratification *n.* The division of a population sample in a study into specifically defined groups such as by age or sex.

stratum basale (basal cell layer, stratum germinativum) *n.* A single layer of tall, columnar, epithelial cells at the base of the *epidermis. The cells are responsible for continually renewing epidermal cells. About 25% of the cells are melanocytes that produce melanin, which provides pigmentation for the hair and skin.

stratum corneum *n. See* EPIDERMIS.

stratum granulosum (granular layer) *n.* A layer of squamous cells in the *epidermis lying between the *stratum spinosum and the stratum corneum.

stratum intermedium *n.* A thin layer of cells forming part of the *enamel organ lying over the outer *enamel epithelium; it transports nutrients to and from the *ameloblasts.

stratum spinosum (prickle cell layer) *n.* A multi-layered arrangement of cuboidal cells lying beneath the *stratum granulosum. The name comes from the spiny appearance when the adjacent *desmosomes shrink during the process of staining.

strawberry tongue *n. See* SCARLET FEVER.

strength *n.* A measure of the ability of a material to support a load. **Ultimate strength** is the greatest stress that may be induced in a material before rupture or fracture occurs; it may be compressive, tensile, or shear. **Compressive strength** is the extent of the resistance of a material to fracture when subjected to compression. **Tensile strength** is the amount of stress a material is able to withstand before permanent deformation occurs when subjected to a pulling force. **Shear strength** is the amount of stress a material is able to withstand when subjected to a tangential force or a twisting motion. *See also* STRESS.

Streptococcus *n.* (*adj.* **streptococcal**) A genus of *Gram-positive, non-motile spherical bacteria occurring in chains, some of which are pathogenic. *Streptococcus mitis* is a bacterium found in dental plaque that may play a significant role in the caries process. *Streptococcus mutans* is a facultatively anaerobic bacterial species commonly found in saliva. It has been closely associated with the development of dental caries because of its ready ability to metabolize sucrose to lactic acid and a number of distinct polymers which help its adherence to tooth enamel. It also produces a highly branched water-insoluble polysaccharide called mutan that may facilitate its establishment in dental *plaque. Recent evidence has emerged, however, that *S. mutans* is not alone in having *acidogenic and *aciduric properties and being able to produce extracellular polymers capable of promoting plaque formation. Together with *Lactobacillus*, *S. mutans* is one of the index organisms used to assess caries susceptibility. *Streptococcus pyogenes* is a pathogenic bacterium that is the cause of many significant human diseases ranging from superficial skin infections (impetigo) to life-threatening systemic disease. It frequently causes inflammation of the throat (*pharyngitis); throat infections with strains of *S. pyogenes* that produce pyogenic exotoxins can result in scarlet fever or streptococcal toxic shock syndrome. Multiplication and spread of *S. pyogenes* in deep layers of the skin during *cellulitis can result in necrotizing fasciitis, a potentially life-threatening condition. Post-streptococcal complications such as *rheumatic fever can occur in a small percentage of infections. *Streptococcus salivarius* is considered to be an opportunistic pathogen found in the upper respiratory tract, mouth, and more specifically in dental plaque, and accounts for about half the streptococci in saliva. *Streptococcus gordonii*, *Streptococcus oralis*, *Streptococcus mitis*, *Streptococcus sanguis*, and *Streptococcus anginosus* are all found in dental plaque and may have a role to play in the caries process.

streptokinase *n.* An enzyme produced by some bacteria of the genus *Streptococcus. It is capable of liquefying blood clots by enhancing the conversion of plasminogen to plasmin, and its derivatives may be used in *thrombolysis in patients presenting with acute coronary syndromes or after resuscitation from cardiac arrest.

stress *n.* 1. Any factor which has an adverse effect on the functioning of the body and capable of affecting physical or mental health. 2. The forcibly exerted pressure on a structure such as the mandibular teeth on the maxillary teeth during mastication. **Compressive stress** causes an elastic body to deform (shorten) in the direction of the applied load. **Shear stress** results from the application of forces parallel to each other, but in opposite directions. **Tensile stress** is that force which causes two parts of an elastic body, on either side of a typical stress plane, to pull apart and is the opposite to compressive stress.

stressbreaker *n.* A device incorporated into a removable partial *denture designed to reduce the *occlusal loading on an *abutment tooth (or teeth) and keep it within physiological limits.

stria *n.* (*pl.* **striae:** *adj.* **striate**) (in anatomy) A streak, longitudinal line, or thin band e.g. lateral and medial longitudinal stria.

striae of Retzius *n. See* ENAMEL STRIAE OF RETZIUS.

striated duct A glandular duct that modifies the secretory product; it derives its name from the characteristic striations in the extensive infolding of the basal membrane. They are found in the submandibular and parotid glands.

striated muscle *See* MUSCLE.

stridor *n.* A high-pitched harsh noise produced during breathing due to a partial obstruction of the upper airway (trachea or larynx).

strip crown *n. See* CROWN.

stroke *n.* A cerebrovascular accident in which the blood supply to a part of the brain is suddenly interrupted by occlusion of a blood vessel (*ischaemia), haemorrhage, or other causes. It can result in impaired vision, hearing, and speech because of the unilateral weakness or paralysis. There may also be difficulty in swallowing and clearing oral secretions, making the use of high-vacuum aspiration during operative dental procedures essential. Poor oral hygiene and reduced muscular activity can lead to an increased risk of caries and periodontal disease. Tolerance of new and existing prosthetic appliances can be poor.

S

strophulus *n.* A papular eruption or rash (*urticaria) sometimes seen on the gingivae of children during teething.

stud attachment *n. See* PRECISION ATTACHMENT.

student's alloy An alloy of mainly copper and zinc used as a substitute for gold in the teaching of gold inlay casting.

Student's t-test A statistical significance measure to test whether the differences between two means are significantly different from zero. The test is appropriate for small sample sizes (smaller than 30). It was first described in 1908 by William Sealy Gosset.

study model *n. See* CAST.

Sturge–Weber anomalad [W. A. Sturge (1850–1919), English physician; F. P. Weber (1863–1962), English physician] A rare genetic disorder characterized by excessive blood vessel growth affecting the upper part of the face which may extend intracranially. There may be associated convulsions, hemiplegia, or intellectual impairment. The condition presents risks for surgery. Treatment is symptomatic.

stylohyoid ligament A fibrous band of strong flexible connective tissue attached to the *styloid process of the temporal bone and the lesser cornu of the *hyoid bone.

styloid process A slender downward and forward pointing piece of bone which projects from the lower surface of the temporal bone below the ear. It provides attachment for muscles and ligaments of the tongue and *hyoid bone.

stylomandibular ligament A specialized band of the cervical *fascia which extends from near the apex of the *styloid process of the temporal bone to the angle and posterior border of the ramus of the mandible, between the masseter and the internal pterygoid muscle.

styptic *n.* An *astringent agent that stops or reduces external bleeding (*haemostatic).

sub-acute *adj.* Describing a condition that progresses more rapidly than a *chronic condition but does not become *acute.

sub-acute bacterial endocarditis (SBE) *n. See* ENDOCARDITIS.

sub-clinical *adj.* Describing a disease or condition in which there are no discernable *signs or *symptoms.

subcutaneous *adj.* Beneath the skin.

subgingival *adj.* Describing a location at a level *apical to the gingival margin.

sublingual *adj.* Relating to the region below the tongue. The **sublingual fossa** is a shallow depression on the inner surface of the mandible above the mylohyoid line in which lies the sublingual salivary gland. The **sublingual space** consists of loose connective tissue containing the sublingual *salivary gland, and the duct of the submandibular salivary gland together with the lingual and hypoglossal nerves.

sublingual gland *n. See* SALIVARY GLAND.

sublining *n.* A thin layer of material placed beneath a *lining in a prepared cavity. *Calcium hydroxide may be placed as a sublining on partly demineralized dentine for its therapeutic effect but will require an additional lining if further thermal insulation is required. A sublining lacks the compressive *strength of a lining material.

subluxation *n.* 1. The loosening of a tooth without displacement. It causes significant injury to the *periodontal ligament with tenderness to percussion; it is usually accompanied by gingival bleeding. Primary incisors may change colour when subluxated due to pulpal damage; treatment for a primary tooth usually involves a soft diet. A permanent tooth may require splinting to prevent excessive mobility. 2. Partial dislocation of a joint. Subluxation of the *temporomandibular joint can occur when the mandibular condyle is dislocated anterior to the articular eminence and cannot return to its normal position.

submandibular *adj.* Relating to the region below the mandible.

submandibular duct *See* WHARTON'S DUCT.

submandibular fossa A shallow depression on the inner surface of the mandible below the mylohyoid line in which lies the submandibular salivary gland.

submandibular gland *See* SALIVARY GLAND.

submandibular space An area of loose connective tissue limited above by the mucous membrane and the tongue and below by the superficial layer of the cervical fascia as it extends from the hyoid bone to the mandible. It is divided into the *sublingual and *submaxillary spaces by the mylohyoid muscle. Inflammation and cellulitis of this area is described as *Ludwig's angina and infections of the second and third mandibular molars may perforate the mandible and spread into the submandibular or *submental spaces.

submandibular triangle A region of the neck immediately below the body of the mandible which contains the submandibular gland; it is bounded above by the lower border of the body of the mandible and a line drawn from its angle to the mastoid process, anteriorly by the anterior belly of the digastric muscle, and posteriorly by the posterior belly of the digastric muscle.

submaxillary *adj*. Situated beneath the maxilla. The **submaxillary space**, which contains the submandibular salivary gland and the submental lymph nodes, is divided by the anterior belly of the digastric muscle into the central *submental space and the lateral submaxillary space.

submental *adj*. Describing the area beneath the chin. The **submental space** forms part of the *submaxillary space. *Abscesses of the second and third mandibular molars may perforate the mandible and spread into the *submandibular and submental spaces.

submental triangle Part of the *anterior triangle of the neck, also known as the **suprahyoid triangle**. It is bounded posteriorly by the anterior belly of the digastric muscle, anteriorly by the midline of the neck between the mandible and the hyoid bone, and inferiorly by the body of the hyoid bone. The triangle contains the submental lymph nodes.

submerged tooth *See* INFRAOCCLUSION.

submucosa *n*. (*adj*. **submucosal**) The layer of loose connective tissue containing vessels, nerves, and accessory *salivary glands lying beneath the *mucosa.

subnasale *n*. The point at which the nasal septum forms an angle with the *philtrum. It is used as a soft-tissue *cephalometric landmark.

subnasion *n*. The point of the angle between the septum of the nose and the surface of the upper lip in the mid-sagittal plane.

subperiosteal implant *n*. *See* IMPLANT.

subspinale *n*. A cephalometric landmark marking the posterior midline point on the premaxilla between the anterior nasal spine and the *prosthion.

substantivity *n*. A characteristic of a mouthwash whereby it remains active in the oral cavity for a prolonged period; for example, *chlorhexidine gluconate is absorbed onto the oral mucous membrane and is active in the oral cavity for up to 8 hours following rinsing.

substructure *n*. That part of an *implant which is covered by the soft tissues and in contact with the bone. It supports a *superstructure such as an implant-supported denture.

succedaneous tooth *n*. Any of the permanent teeth with primary predecessors (premolars, canines, and incisors).

succussion *n*. The process of vigorous shaking with impact in the making of a *homeopathic remedy. *See also* POTENTIZATION.

sucrose *n*. A *disaccharide ($C_{12}H_{22}O_{11}$) consisting of *glucose and *fructose. Overconsumption has been linked to obesity, diabetes, and coronary heart disease. Because it is metabolized by some bacteria to form *lactic acid, frequent consumption is associated with dental *caries.

sugar *n*. One of a number of water-soluble carbohydrates subdivided into disaccharides (e.g. *sucrose, *maltose) and monosaccharides (e.g. *glucose, *fructose). The Committee on the Medical Aspects of Food Policy classified sugars in relation to dental caries as either **intrinsic sugars** (sugar molecules inside the cell such as fresh fruit and vegetables) or **extrinsic sugars** (sugar molecules outside the cell). Extrinsic sugars were further sub-divided into non-milk extrinsic sugars (NMES) and **milk sugars** such as lactose, present in dairy products. Non-milk extrinsic sugars are sugar molecules which exist outside the plant cell and are most responsible for dental *caries. They include table sugar, confectionary, jam, and sugars which are added to foods and drinks during processing or preparation, together with sugars naturally present in fresh fruit juices, honey, and syrups. NMES have the potential to cause caries, and a safe ingestion level is dependent on the consistency and frequency of intake. Daily intake may be monitored with a *diet diary or by using a **sugar clock** which graphically illustrates the number of sugar intakes in a 24-hour period and therefore the potential number of harmful acid attacks on the teeth. The clock is divided into 24 segments corresponding to each hour of the day. The child enters the times of food or drink ingestion and when the teeth were brushed.

S

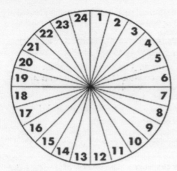

A sugar clock

Further Reading: Levine R. S., Stillman-Lowe C. R. *The scientific basis of oral health education.* British Dental Journal Books, 2004.

Fuller S. S., Harding M. The use of the sugar clock in dental health education *Br Dent J* 1991;170:414–16.

SEE WEB LINKS

• Mary Immaculate College Curriculum Development Unit. A diet teaching aid for children.

sulcular fluid *n. See* CREVICULAR FLUID.

sulcus *n.* 1. A groove or depression on the surface of a tooth. 2. A soft-tissue groove in the oral cavity. The **alveololingual sulcus** is the space between the alveolar ridge and the tongue. The **gingival implant sulcus (crevice)** is the small groove between the implant abutment post and the free gingival tissue which resembles a natural gingival sulcus. The **gingival sulcus** (also known as the gingival crevice) is the shallow groove between the free gingiva and the surface of the tooth extending around its circumference and from the crest of the free gingiva to the junctional epithelial attachment.

sulcus bleeding index (SBI) An index of gingival inflammation in which bleeding is measured from four gingival units (mesial and distal papillary units and labial and lingual marginal units), using a periodontal probe with a 0.5mm diameter tip. The scoring range around eight anterior teeth (four maxillary and four mandibular) is from 0 (healthy appearance and no bleeding on probing) to 5 (spontaneous bleeding with a marked swelling, and a change in colour).

sulcus terminalis *n.* A V-shaped groove which separates the anterior and posterior parts of the dorsum of the *tongue at the apex of which is a small pit (*foramen caecum).

sulphur, flowers of *n.* Light yellow crystalline powder made by distilling sulphur. It is mixed with calcium oxide and water to form a paste which is painted on and around a mercury spillage so that the mercury can be removed for safe disposal.

sum of squared errors (sum of squares) (in statistics) An estimate of total variability or spread of a set of data.

supernumerary tooth Any tooth additional to the normal 32 teeth in the permanent dentition or the 20 teeth in the primary dentition. They are rare in the primary dentition but common in the permanent dentition, particularly in the anterior and premolar regions of the maxilla; they tend to occur more frequently in females than males. They may be described according to their location e.g. *distomolar, *mesiodens, *paramolar, *parapremolar. The aetiology of supernumerary teeth is not completely understood. Multiple supernumerary teeth may be associated with other conditions such as *cleft lip and palate, cleidocranial *dysostosis, and *Gardner's syndrome. It has been reported that 75% of supernumerary teeth fail to erupt. *See also* SUPPLEMENTAL TOOTH.

Further Reading: Gill S. D., Tredwin C., Naini F. B. Diagnosis and management of supernumerary teeth. *Dent Update* 2008;35:510–20.

supersaturated *adj.* Describing a metastable solution in which the dissolved material exceeds the amount the solvent can hold in normal equilibrium at the temperature and other conditions that prevail. Saliva is a supersaturated solution of calcium phosphate which encourages enamel *remineralization. *See also* SATURATED.

superstructure *n.* That part of a prosthetic appliance which fits on to *implant abutments. It may consist of artificial teeth, denture resin, metal framework, connectors, precision attachments, or conventional clasps.

supine *adj.* Describing a position lying horizontally on the back, with the face upward.

supplemental tooth A type of *supernumerary tooth which is identical in morphology to a fully formed tooth. It frequently leads to localized crowding.

support *n.* The resistance of a denture to occlusally transmitted forces, gained either from the mucosa and underlying bone of the denture-bearing area, or from selected natural abutment teeth.

suppuration n. (adj. **suppurative**) The formation of *pus. It occurs in response to established bacterial infection.

supragingival adj. Situated above or coronal to the gingival margin. **Supragingival calculus** see CALCULUS.

supramentale n. A cephalometric point (point B) situated at the most posterior midline point in the concavity between the *infradentale and *pogonion. See also CEPHALOMETRIC ANALYSIS.

supraversion n. A condition in which the maxillary teeth are situated above or below their normal vertical relationships e.g. a deep *overbite.

surface n. The outside of a material or body. The **fitting surface** is that part of a restoration, prosthetic, or orthodontic appliance in contact with the supporting tissues. A **smooth surface** is a surface of a tooth on which pits and fissures are normally absent. A **surface marker** is a form of patient identification applied to the external surface of a denture; it may be either permanent or temporary (for identification during construction). *Tooth surfaces are defined by their relationship to other anatomical structures.

surfactant n. A wetting agent. Any substance that when dissolved in an aqueous solution reduces its surface tension between it and another liquid.

surgery n. 1. A room in which surgical procedures are undertaken. 2. The branch of medicine that treats diseases or conditions by manual or operative intervention. **Access flap surgery** involves the reflection of a full thickness *flap created to gain access to the *alveolar bone for the purpose of bone remodelling or the removal of apical bone prior to an *apicectomy. **Apically repositioned flap surgery** is undertaken to reposition a flap of gingival tissue apically so as to maintain or create a functionally adequate zone of attached *gingiva. **Mucogingival surgery** is undertaken to obtain or maintain a functionally adequate zone of attached gingiva, to deepen the vestibule, or to alter the position or remove a fraenal attachment. **Osseous surgery** is the removal (*ostectomy) or recontouring (*osteoplasty) of bone to treat an osseous defect, to extract a tooth, or to gain access for the removal of a tooth root or root apex (apicectomy). **Pedicle flap surgery (laterally repositioned flap)** is undertaken to repair a gingival cleft by repositioning

and suturing a tissue flap mesial or distal to the defect.

Surgically Assisted Rapid Maxillary Expansion (SARME) See RAPID MAXILLARY EXPANSION.

surgical orthodontics Correction of occlusal irregularities by the surgical repositioning of parts or all of the mandible or maxilla to improve function and aesthetics.

surgical spirit Methylated spirit to which is normally added small quantities of oil of wintergreen and castor oil. It is used to clean the skin prior to an injection.

survey line A line drawn on a dental *cast using a *surveyor which marks the greatest height of contour in relation to the orientation of the cast to the vertical marker. It assists in defining the planned path of insertion of an appliance or the positioning of retentive components.

surveyor n. An instrument used to define the relative parallelism of two or more surfaces (usually tooth surfaces) on a cast. It may have an adjustable table on which the cast is mounted that can be used to establish the path of insertion and removal of an appliance. A surveyor is used for a number of purposes, including surveying a diagnostic or master cast, contouring a wax pattern, the placement of intra-coronal attachments and internal rest seats, and the machining of cast restorations. Accessory tools used include a carbon marker to mark the height of the contour and an undercut gauge to measure the undercut depth. The increased use of *computer-aided design/computer-aided manufacture (CAD/CAM) for surveying (**virtual surveying**) may in time replace the physical surveyor.

Sutton's aphthae [R. L. Sutton (1878–1952), American dermatologist] An alternative name for recurrent *aphthous ulceration.

suture 1. n. (in anatomy) A type of immovable joint found particularly in the skull. 2. v. To sew up a wound to aid the healing process. 3. n. The material used to sew up a wound. It may be resorbable (trade names: **Dexon®**, **Vicryl®**, **Monocryl®**) or non-resorbable such as silk, nylon, or prolene (polymer polypropylene) (trade names: **Ethilon®**, **Novafil®**). Monofilament suture

S

material such as nylon causes less tissue response than braided material such as silk. A number of different types of suture technique may be used in minor oral surgery: when using a **simple interrupted suture**, each suture is tied separately; a **continuous suture** uses one continuous length of suture material; a **mattress suture** is a double stitch made parallel (horizontal mattress) or perpendicular (vertical mattress) to the wound edge.

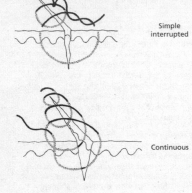

Simple interrupted

Continuous

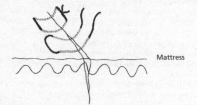

Mattress

Types of surgical suturing

suture needle *n. See* NEEDLE.

Suzanne's gland [J. G. Suzanne (1859), French physician] A mucous gland found in the floor of the mouth near the midline.

swab *n.* A pad of absorbent material which may be attached to a wooden stick or wire. It is used for cleaning or to apply medication.

swage 1. *v.* A metal forming technique in which the dimensions of an item or material are altered, using a die into which the item is forced. The technique was formerly used for the fabrication of stainless steel crowns. 2. *n.* A tool used for this purpose.

swallowing *n. See* DEGLUTITION.

sweat gland *n.* An *exocrine gland lying with a secretory duct in the *dermis of the skin. They serve a number of functions including the regulation of body temperature and excretion of waste products.

sweetener *n.* A non-nutritive *sugar substitute. Sweeteners can be beneficial in the control of dental caries and obesity. **Intense sweeteners** can be up to 3000 times sweeter than *sucrose; they include saccharin, acesulfame K, aspartame, and thaumatin. **Bulk sweeteners** are modified sugars or alcohol derivatives of sugars (polyols) such as sorbitol, isomalt, mannitol, xylitol, and hydrogenated glucose syrups. Sorbitol and mannitol are commercially used in sugar-free confectionery and chewing gum.

swelling *n.* One of the cardinal signs of inflammation caused by an increase in fluid in the tissues.

swinglock denture *See* DENTURE.

symbiosis *n.* The intimate living together of two dissimilar organisms in a mutually beneficial relationship.

sympathetic nervous system One of the two divisions of the *autonomic nervous system having nerve fibres that leave the central nervous system and supply the blood vessels, heart, lungs, intestines, sweat glands, genitalia, and salivary glands, whose functions it governs by reflex action. *See also* PARASYMPATHETIC NERVOUS SYSTEM.

symphysion *n.* The most anterior point of the alveolar process of the mandible in the midline; a *craniometric point.

symphysis *n.* 1. A fibrocartilaginous fusion between two bones creating a rigid structure. 2. The line that marks the fusion between two bones that were separate at an earlier stage of development, such as the symphysis of the *mandible.

symptom *n.* (*adj.* **symptomatic**) An indication of a disease, condition, or disorder noticed by the patient. A **presenting symptom** is one that leads the patient to obtain a professional consultation.

syn- (sym-) Prefix denoting union, fusion, or joined together.

synalgia *n.* A synonym for referred *pain.

synapse *n.* The minute gap across which a nerve impulse passes from one *neuron to another. The **chemical synapse** is the most common type of synapse in which the pre- and post-synaptic membranes are separated by a very small gap (**synaptic cleft**). During synaptic transmission a neurotransmitter is released into the synaptic cleft, having been triggered by an *action potential. The neurotransmitter is recognized by selective receptors on the post-synaptic cell, allowing further transmission of the impulse to occur.

syncheilia *n.* A congenital adhesion of the lips.

syncope (fainting) *n.* Loss of consciousness caused by a temporary insufficient supply of blood to the brain. It is characterized by pallor, sweating, blurred vision, and a feeling of nausea. The *pulse is rapid at first and then becomes slow and weak. Recovery is usually spontaneous and without any persisting ill-effects if the patient is laid flat to restore the cranial blood supply.

syndesmotome *n.* A surgical instrument used to sever the periodontal ligament fibres.

syndesmotomy *n.* The severing of the periodontal ligament fibres prior to the extraction of a tooth.

syndrome *n.* A combination of *signs and *symptoms that together form a distinct clinical picture indicative of a specific disorder.

syneresis *n.* 1. The contraction of a blood clot. 2. The process by which a fluid exudate forms on the surface of a hydrocolloid gel, such as *alginate impression material; it is accompanied by shrinkage of the gel.

syngnathia *n.* The congenital adhesion of the maxilla and mandible by fibrous bands of tissue. It may be associated with other congenital abnormalities such as *cleft lip, cleft palate, and *aglossia.

synodontia *n. See* FUSION.

synostosis *n.* The joining of two bones by the ossification of intervening *connective tissue, such as the bones of the skull.

synovial fluid A viscous, translucent fluid found within a synovial *joint that lubricates joint surfaces and supplies the joint cartilages with nutrients.

synovial joint *See* JOINT.

syntax *n.* (in statistics)   Pre-defined written commands or rules that instruct a mathematical system to carry out a task.

syphilis *n.* A sexually transmitted disease caused by the bacterium *Treponema pallidum* which may be congenital (rare) or acquired. Oral lesions include a hard ulcer (**primary chancre**), secondary mucous patches (**snail track ulcers**), and soft necrotic ulceration (**tertiary gumma**). Primary syphilis presents 9–90 days after exposure. The primary lesions may heal spontaneously despite inappropriate treatment, leading the patient to assume that they have been effectively treated. Syphilis is highly infective, particularly in the primary and secondary stages. Manifestations of secondary syphilis appear about 6 weeks after exposure while those of tertiary syphilis may develop years after the initial exposure. Treatment is by antibiotic therapy. Syphilis transmitted prenatally (**congenital syphilis**) may lead to *Hutchinson's incisors, *Moon's molars, or fissures or cracks in the skin around the mouth (*rhagades).

syringe *n.* An instrument consisting of a hollow nozzle or needle, a piston in a tight fitting tube and a plunger, used to inject solutions, aspirate material, or to irrigate tissues. A hand **air syringe** (**chip syringe**) consists of a long hollow tube, angled at the working end, with a hollow rubber bulb which is manually compressed to deliver a spurt of air. An **aspirating syringe** has a hypodermic needle used for delivering local anaesthetic solution and is modified to permit the creation of negative pressure in the cartridge, such as by a harpoon on the plunger or a narrow plunger to fit a modified bung, allowing the operator to detect in advance of delivering the anaesthetic agent, that the needle has not entered a blood vessel; it is a type of **cartridge syringe** since it accommodates a glass tube containing a sterile drug, such as local anaesthetic, for injection. A **combination syringe (triple, 3 in 1)** is usually part of the dental unit and can deliver air, water, or water spray under pressure. A **Hunt's syringe** has a sprung-loaded plunger and is used for irrigation. An **impression material syringe** has a detachable nozzle and plunger and is used for transferring impression material to the site of operation; some impression material syringes have twin barrels containing catalyst and base respectively which are mixed to a homogenous mix automatically (**automix**) within the nozzle when the plunger is depressed. An **intraligamentary syringe** is designed so that considerable force may be applied to the plunger mechanism to force the local anaesthetic into the periodontal ligament.

S

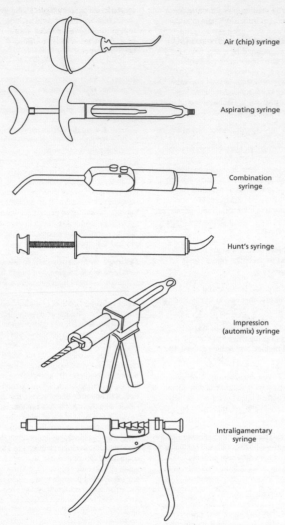

Air (chip) syringe

Aspirating syringe

Combination
syringe

Hunt's syringe

Impression
(automix) syringe

Intraligamentary
syringe

Types of syringe

systematic review A review of a clearly
described question that uses systematic methods
and a clearly defined protocol to identify and
critically appraise relevant research material, and
to collate and analyse data from the studies that
are included in the review. The results may be
combined and summarized using a systematic
approach and statistical methods (*meta-
analysis).

Further Reading: Petrie A., Bulman J. S., Osborn J. F. Further
statistics in dentistry Part 8: Systematic reviews and meta-
analyses. *Br Dent J* 2003;194(2):73–8.

⊕ SEE WEB LINKS

• The Cochrane Collaboration glossary of terms.

systemic *adj.* Relating to or affecting the whole body rather than an individual part or organ.

systemic lupus erythematosus (SLE)
n. See LUPUS ERYTHEMATOSUS.

systole *n.* (*adj.* **systolic**) The period of the cardiac cycle during which either the ventricles (**ventricular systole**) or atria (**atrial systole**) of the heart contract.

tablet *n*. A small disc containing a measured amount of drug or drugs made by compressing the powdered form. It is usually chewed or swallowed whole but may be taken by other routes e.g. as an anal suppository.

tachycardia *n*. An increase in the heart rate which may be physiological e.g. during exercise, or may be indicative of a disease or a cardiac conduction problem.

tachyphylaxis *n*. The rapidly decreasing response to a drug following continuous use or repeated administration.

tachypnoea *n*. Rapid breathing.

talc *n*. Magnesium silicate powder. It was formerly used to dust surgical latex gloves but is now no longer used because of the potential for adverse skin reactions.

talon *n*. 1. The distal cusp on an upper molar. 2. A palatal cusp projecting from the cingulum of a permanent incisor; this may be associated with other dental anomalies such as peg-shaped lateral incisors, or supplemental or congenitally missing teeth. *See also* DENS EVAGINATUS.

talonid *n*. The distal part of a lower molar crown developed from the distal part of the cingulum.

Tanner appliance [H. M. Tanner (1923–2003), American prosthodontist] *n*. A hard acrylic removable appliance worn over the mandibular teeth. It is used to provide symptomatic relief in *temporomandibular joint dysfunction or prior to comprehensive restorative procedures. *See also* SPLINT.

tannic acid *n*. A polyphenol which attaches itself to *collagen. It has been used as a cavity *conditioner prior to the placement of a restoration. It is also present in tea and coffee and can cause a brown discoloration of the salivary *pellicle.

tape, dental *n*. A ribbon of nylon, silk, or synthetic material, which may be waxed or unwaxed. It is used in the same way as *floss to remove *plaque from the *interproximal surfaces of the teeth by sliding it over the surface of the tooth in a coronal direction away from the gingival tissue.

tardive dyskinesia *n*. Involuntary movement of the facial muscles, tongue, and jaws, usually resembling a chewing action. It is associated with long-term antipsychotic medication, occurring mainly in older patients.

tarnish *n*. Surface discoloration or loss of lustre of a metal caused by the formation of hard or soft deposits e.g. sulphides and chlorides. It may involve metallic oxidation of the surface layer. Tarnish is removed by polishing. *See also* CORROSION.

tartar *n*. A colloquial term for *calculus.

tartaric acid *n*. A chemical commonly added to glass ionomer *cement to prolong the working time.

taste *n*. The sense of appreciating different flavours of substances in the mouth. The sensory organs are the *taste buds situated mainly on the *tongue. Five primary taste sensations may be described, namely sweet, sour, bitter, salt, and umami (glutamate, savoury) to which alkaline and metallic may be added. Different taste qualities are found in all areas of the tongue, although some regions are more sensitive than others.

(((⊕))) SEE WEB LINKS

- An overview of the physiology of taste on the website of Colorado State University.

taste buds The sensory receptors concerned with taste usually embedded within papillae. They are found mainly in the epithelium on the dorsum of the tongue, although they are also present in the soft palate, the epiglottis, and parts of the pharynx. Each taste bud is flask-like in shape with a broad base and a hollow neck opening at an orifice between the epithelial cells. *See also* PAPILLA.

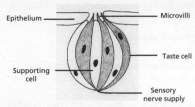

Epithelium — Microvilli

Taste cell

Supporting cell

Sensory nerve supply

Taste bud

tattoo (amalgam) *n. See* AMALGAM.

taurodontism *n.* A malformed multi-rooted tooth characterized by the crown being of normal length, the roots being abnormally short, and the *pulp chamber being abnormally large and extending deeply into the roots of the tooth; it is a condition found in Neanderthal man and ruminants.

technician *n. See* DENTAL TECHNICIAN.

teeth *pl. n. See* TOOTH.

teething (odontiasis) *n.* The process of the eruption of the *primary dentition in infants. It is often characterized by increased salivation, localized inflammation, and pain. There may also be systemic involvement with diarrhoea and a raised temperature, although these symptoms may be coincidental. Treatment is aimed at achieving symptomatic relief with an *antipyretic and *analgesic such as paediatric paracetamol (trade names: **Cupal**, **Panadol**, **Calpol**) or by the topical application of a proprietary teething gel (trade names: **Bonjela**, **Teejel**).

TEGDMA (tri-ethyleneglycol dimethacrylate) *n.* A small molecular weight monomer added to *resin composite to improve the flow characteristics.

teicoplanin *n.* A glycopeptide *antibiotic which acts by attacking the bacterial cell wall. It is not absorbed from the gut and is therefore only given by injection or infusion. It has been used *prophylactically to treat patients with a history of infective *endocarditis and who are allergic to *penicillin.

telangiectasia *n.* Multiple small enlarged blood capillary vessels (telangiectases) near the surface of the skin (**spider veins**). They occur most frequently on the face, cheeks, nose, and chin. They can present as a port-wine stain (*haemangioma), usually on the head or neck. A hereditary form (**hereditary haemorrhagic telangiectasia**, also known as **Osler–Weber–Rendu syndrome** [Sir W. Osler (1849–1919), Canadian physician; H. J. M. Rendu (1844–1902),

French physician; F. P. Weber (1863–1962), British physician]) may appear intra-orally as small raised red-blue elevations on the tongue; treatment is mainly supportive and consists of controlling and treating the bleeding.

teledentistry *n.* The use of information technology to link two or more healthcare facilities for the purpose of providing healthcare, obtaining a second opinion, seeking expert advice, or planning treatment. Information technology may include telephone, teleconference, videoconference, or the internet, without the direct personal contact with any patients involved. Teledentistry that crosses jurisdictional or national boundaries can raise complex issues of data protection, and the storage, use, processing, retrieval, access, and security of patient clinical records.

telediagnosis *n.* The process of arriving at a diagnosis by utilizing the electronic transmission of data between two geographically separated dental or medical facilities.

telemetry *n.* The electronic transmission of data between two distant points. It is used as a method of measuring the *pH of *plaque by connecting radio transmitters to electrodes placed in an intra-oral splint; it is also used in the assessment of the cariogenicity of foods.

telescope crown *n. See* CROWN.

tell–show–do technique A familiarization technique commonly used in paediatric dentistry, in which the patient is told what the operator is going to do in non-threatening terms. The operator then demonstrates what is going to be done, and then carries it out.

temazepam *n.* A *benzodiazepine used as a powerful oral sedative or strong hypnotic. It also possesses amnesic and motor-impairing properties, together with *anxiolytic, anticonvulsant, and skeletal muscle relaxant qualities. It is generally prescribed to help with insomnia. It is available in oral suspension or tablet form. Side-effects include drowsiness, dizziness, and loss of appetite. Trade name: **Restoril**.

tempering *n.* The process of hardening or toughening a metal or alloy by cold working or by controlled heating and cooling. Tempering occurs when *gold foil is cold worked by being malleted into a tooth cavity.

template *n.* A pattern or shape which forms an accurate copy of an object or structure. *Computer-aided design and manufacturing have made it possible to transfer data from *computerized tomography to the surgery using a laser-driven polymerization process that fabricates an anatomic model and **implant templates**. A **surgical template** is a thin transparent acrylic resin baseplate used as a guide to shaping the alveolar process, prior to fitting an immediate denture.

temporal bone One of a pair of bones which form part of the sides and base of the skull and consist of five parts. The **squama** forms the upper anterior part of the bone and is thin and transparent, projecting from the lower part of which is the **zygomatic process**; the **mastoid** portion forms the posterior part; the **petrous** portion is pyramidal in shape and forms part of the base of the skull and contains the organ of hearing; the **tympanic** part is a curved plate of bone lying below the squama and in front of the mastoid process. The **styloid process** is a slender pointed projection which is directed downwards and forwards, from the under-surface of the temporal bone.

(((•))) SEE WEB LINKS

• A detailed anatomical description of the temporal bone.

temporal fossa The space bounded by the *temporal lines superiorly and the infratemporal crest inferiorly; it is the origin of the temporalis muscle.

temporal lines Anatomical landmarks on the lateral side of the skull for the attachment of the temporal fascia and the temporalis muscle.

temporary anchorage device (TAD) See ONPLANT.

temporary crown See CROWN.

temporary restorative material See RESTORATION.

temporomandibular joint (TMJ) A double *synovial joint that connects the condyle of the *mandible with the squamous part of the *temporal bone. The articular surface of the temporal bone consists of a concave fossa (**glenoid** or **mandibular fossa**) and a convex **articular eminence** anterior to it. There is a saddle-shaped fibrocartilaginous disc (**articular disc**) situated between the mandibular condyle and the glenoid fossa attached anteriorly to the lateral pterygoid muscle and posteriorly fused to the temporomandibular capsule; it divides the joint into upper and lower compartments. The joint allows the mandible to rotate open and closed, translate forward and backward, and move laterally and medially. The lower compartment permits rotation of the condylar head; with further opening of the jaw, the condylar head and articular disc slide forwards in the glenoid fossa and down the articular eminence. The joint is enclosed in a fibrous capsule lined on the inner aspect with a synovial membrane which produces *synovial fluid to provide lubrication and nutrients for the joint.

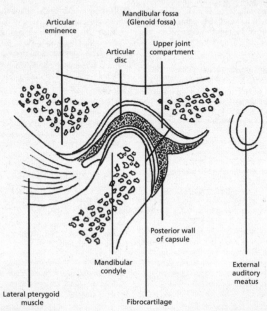

Temporomandibular joint

🌐 **SEE WEB LINKS**

- Jaw movement, on the University of Michigan Medical School website.

temporomandibular joint dysfunction syndrome (TMD) (Also known as **Costen's syndrome**, mandibular pain syndrome (**MPS**), temporomandibular joint pain dysfunction syndrome (**TMJ-PDS**), and myofascial pain dysfunction syndrome (**MPDS**)). A condition of the *temporomandibular joint (TMJ) which may be characterized by pain in the joint and masticatory muscles, limited jaw movement, or locking of the jaw. It may also be associated with pain radiating down the face, neck, and shoulders, painful clicking or grating sounds in the TMJ on opening or closing the jaw, a *malocclusion between the maxillary and mandibular teeth, and sometimes by headaches, earache, *tinnitus, or dizziness. There are many causes, which can make both diagnosis and treatment problematical; these causes include jaw malocclusion, trauma, a displaced articular disc, and stress which can induce clenching or grinding of the teeth (*parafunction). Treatment is dependent on the cause and may include counselling, non-steroidal anti-inflammatory drugs, rest, physiotherapy, *occlusal adjustment, and *splint therapy.

Further Reading: Al-Ani Z., Gray R. TMD current concepts: An update. *Dent Update* 2007;34:278–88.
Luther F. TMD and occlusion part I. Damned if we do? Occlusion: the interface of dentistry and orthodontics. *Br Dent J* 2007;202(1):E2; discussion 38–9.
Luther F. TMD and occlusion part II. Damned if we don't? Functional occlusal problems: TMD epidemiology in a wider context. *Br Dent J* 2007;202(1):E3; discussion 38–9.

tendon *n.* A tough whitish fibrous band of tissue consisting of parallel bundles of collagen fibres that serves to attach muscle to bone.

TENS *n. See* TRANSCUTANEOUS ELECTRICAL NERVE STIMULATION.

tensile stress *n. See* STRESS.

tension *n.* 1. The state of being stretched, strained, or extended. 2. The partial pressure of a gas dissolved in a liquid, such as oxygen or carbon dioxide dissolved in blood. **Surface tension** describes the attraction of molecules to each other on the surface of a liquid. **Interfacial surface tension** represents the resistance to separation possessed by the thin film of a liquid between two well-adapted surfaces such as the saliva between a denture base and the underlying mucosa.

teratoma *n.* A tumour composed of tissues not usually found at that site and which may be composed of cells capable of differentiating into

all the three primary germ layers. Teeth may therefore be found to be present, as well as hair and rarely eyes and other complex organs. They most frequently occur in the ovary and testis.

terminal hinge axis *See* HINGE AXIS.

terminal hinge position The mandibular hinge position beyond which further opening of the mandible would produce forward translatory movement rather than hinge movement.

tertiary care Medical and related care services of high complexity and usually high cost, generally only available at specialized national or international referral centres.

tertiary dentine *See* DENTINE.

tertiary prevention Those measures concerned with limiting the extent of *disability once a disease has caused some functional limitation.

Tessier classification of facial clefts An anatomical classification first described by Dr Paul Tessier in 1976, which classifies the location of facial, craniofacial, and laterofacial clefts, using the orbit as the primary structure for reference. Fifteen locations for clefts are differentiated.

🌐 **SEE WEB LINKS**

- Detailed information on Tessier clefts on the Cleft Palate Foundation website.

tetanus (lockjaw) *n.* (*adj.* **tetanic**) A condition characterized by prolonged contraction of skeletal muscle fibres caused by tetanus toxin (**tetanospasmin**). Tetanus toxin is a potent neurotoxin produced by the Gram-positive, anaerobic bacterium *Clostridium tetani*. Infection usually occurs through wound contamination with *C. tetani* spores. It is characterized by spasmodic contraction of muscles due to the effect of the bacterial *exotoxins on the nerves, leading to rigidity of the jaw (lockjaw) and neck which spreads to the rest of the body. *Immunization against tetanus is effective but temporary. *See also* CLOSTRIDIUM.

tetany *n.* Muscle spasm and cramp, particularly of the face, hands, and feet. It is caused by a reduced blood calcium level which may be due to underactive *parathyroid glands, *rickets, or *alkalosis.

tetartocone *n. See* HYPOCONE.

tetartoconid *n. See* HYPOCONID.

tetracaine (amethocaine) *n.* An ester group local anaesthetic used for topical application to mucous membranes and often used in ophthalmology. Trade name: **Ametop cream**.

tetracycline *n.* One of a group of antibiotic compounds derived from cultures of *Streptomyces* bacteria. This group are broad-spectrum antibiotics and include chlortetracycline, doxycycline, minocycline, and oxytetracycline. The use of low-dosage long-term tetracycline has been advocated for patients with aggressive *periodontitis, but there are concerns regarding the risk of the emergence of bacterial drug resistance in the oral flora. Its administration during tooth formation should be avoided because of the possibility of enamel discoloration of the permanent teeth. Trade names: Achromycin, Tetracin. 📷

Further Reading: Gilbert A. Local tetracycline is an effective adjunct in the treatment of chronic periodontitis. *Evid Based Dent* 2004;5(3):67.

thecodont *adj.* Describing a tooth embedded in a socket or *alveolus, as in mammals.

thegosis *n.* The process of sharpening teeth by grinding one anterior tooth against another to create wear facets. In some mammals it keeps the teeth sharply honed for use as weapons. It has been suggested that this is a biological process and that pathological thegosis, predominantly in response to stress, is synonymous with *bruxism.

Further Reading: Murray C. G., Sanson G. D. Thegosis—A critical review. *Australian Dental Journal* 1998;43(3):192–8.

therapeutic index *n.* The ratio of the toxic dose of a therapeutic agent to the effective dose. It indicates the relative efficacy of a treatment.

therapeutics *n.* The branch of medicine concerned with the treatment of disease particularly related to the application of drugs and other remedies for curing or healing disease.

therapist, dental *n.* A person skilled in a particular kind of therapy. A **dental therapist** is a class of *dental care professional (DCP) who in the UK must work to the written prescription of a dentist and be statutorily registered with the *General Dental Council (GDC). The clinical remit of the dental therapist varies in different countries but in the UK they can undertake the full clinical remit of a *dental hygienist, with the addition of providing simple restorative treatment on primary and secondary teeth and the extraction of primary teeth under *local analgesia. The clinical remit may be extended subject to the approval of the GDC and completion of appropriate additional training. An **orthodontic therapist** is a UK DCP legally permitted to treat orthodontic patients under the prescription from a dentist following completion of an approved

course and successfully obtaining a Diploma in Orthodontic Therapy; they must be statutorily registered with the GDC. The remit of the orthodontic therapist includes the cleaning and polishing of teeth and removal of supragingival deposits, the taking of impressions and clinical photographs, the placement, maintenance, and removal of orthodontic appliances, and the fitting of space maintainers, retainers, and orthodontic headgear.

(()) SEE WEB LINKS

• The British Association of Dental Therapists website.

thermal conductivity The ability of a solid or liquid to transfer heat.

thermocoagulation *n. See* CAUTERY.

thermogenesis *n.* The increase in energy output in response to food intake, cold exposure, and psychological influences.

thermoplastic *adj.* Describing a reversible physical phenomenon in which there is deformation with the application of heat and a return to rigidity at normal temperature. A thermoplastic process is used for making transparent celluloid *templates.

thermosetting *adj.* Having the property of becoming irreversibly hardened with the application of heat such as with *vulcanite and the curing of *acrylic resin.

thesis *n.* A written dissertation describing original research, usually submitted by a candidate as part of a university higher degree.

thiamin *n. See* VITAMIN B$_1$.

thimble *n. See* COPING.

thixotropic *adj.* Describing the property of becoming temporarily liquid when shaken or stirred and returning to a gel on standing. It is a feature of some dental restorative and impression materials.

thorax *n.* (*adj.* **thoracic**) The part of the body between the neck and the abdomen. It contains the lungs, heart, and oesophagus and is enclosed by skeletal structures consisting of the sternum, costal cartilages, ribs, and the thoracic vertebrae of the spine.

throat pack A pad of absorbent material, such as *Gamgee tissue, used to protect the patient from inhaling or swallowing liquids or foreign bodies.

thrombin *n.* A coagulation protein that acts as an *enzyme. It converts soluble *fibrinogen to insoluble fibrin in the final stage of blood coagulation. It is present in blood plasma as the precursor *prothrombin.

thrombocyte *n.* See PLATELET.

thrombolysis *n.* The process of breaking up and dissolving a blood clot (thrombus).

thrombosis *n.* The presence of a blood clot (thrombus) in a blood vessel. A thrombus in an artery supplying the brain can cause a stroke; if in an artery supplying the heart it can cause a coronary thrombosis (*myocardial infarction); and if in a vein can cause a deep vein thrombosis.

thrush *n.* See CANDIDIASIS.

thumb sucking See DIGIT SUCKING.

thymol *n.* A white crystalline phenolic substance used as an *antiseptic in some commercial mouthwashes.

thyroid collar See CERVICAL.

thyroid gland A large two-lobed endocrine gland situated at the base of the neck, each lobe being either side of the *trachea. It is concerned with the regulation of the metabolic rate by the secretion of thyroid hormone (*thyroxine), which is controlled by thyroid-stimulating hormone from the *pituitary gland. Reduced function (*hypothyroidism) may rarely be congenital (*cretinism), or may be due to autoimmune disease, surgical removal, or malfunction of the pituitary control resulting in *myxoedema. Over-activity (hyperfunction) is usually due to an exophthalmic goitre (*Graves' disease) or to an excessive production of thyroid hormones (thyrotoxicosis or Graves' disease); stress, trauma, or infection can initiate a thyrotoxic crisis if the condition is not stable.

thyrotoxicosis *n.* See GRAVES' DISEASE.

thyroxine *n.* The hormonal secretion of the thyroid gland. It may be administered orally to treat underactivity of the thyroid gland.

tic douloureux *n.* See TRIGEMINAL NEURALGIA.

tidal volume The amount of air normally inhaled or exhaled during breathing. For an adult at rest it is approximately 500ml.

tieback *n.* A ligature wire attached to a tooth either to prevent unwanted movement or to initiate active movement. It is a method whereby closed spaces in the arches are kept from re-opening during the later phases of orthodontic treatment. Tiebacks may be either active or passive.

tie wire *n.* A fine wire that is twisted around the bracket of an orthodontic appliance to hold an archwire in position.

tin *n.* A silver-white metallic element (Sn) which resists corrosion and is not easily oxidized in air. It is one of the three main constituents of *amalgam alloy. **Tin foil** is a very thin sheet of metal (usually aluminium, not tin) used as a separating medium in the construction of dentures. **Tin plating** is a process of depositing a layer of tin on a noble or precious metal alloy to provide a micromechanical retentive surface for resin bonding; this chairside procedure is primarily indicated for the intra-oral repair of fractured metal-ceramic restorations where the metal is exposed.

tincture *n.* An alcoholic solution of a drug derived from a plant.

tine *n.* The slender pointed end of a dental *explorer.

tinnitus *n.* Noises in the ears such as ringing, buzzing, or clicking in the absence of any external sound source. It is thought to be due to a misinterpretation of signals in the central auditory pathways of the brain. It may be a symptom of *temporomandibular joint dysfunction syndrome. A link between tinnitus and amalgam restorations is yet to be established.

tip-edge appliance A type of fixed orthodontic appliance similar to a *Begg appliance, but with *brackets which have pre-adjusted values.

tipping *n.* The movement which occurs when a point source is applied to a tooth. It combines rotational movement with a horizontal translation of the tooth. It is the only type of tooth movement that a removable orthodontic appliance can bring about. The force required may be as low as 30–60gm, causing rotation at a point near the junction of the middle and apical third of the root.

tissue *n.* An aggregation of similar cells performing a specialized function.

tissue adhesive A material used to unite two cut surfaces. Tissue adhesives are usually *cyanoacrylate monomers which, when they come into contact with moisture on the skin's surface, chemically change into a polymer that binds to the superficial epithelial layer. It has advantages over *sutures in that it can be applied using a topical anaesthetic without the use of needles, there is a faster repair time, it is better accepted by patients, it provides a water-resistant covering, and it does not require the removal of sutures. It is however contraindicated for use on mucosal surfaces. Trade names: **Dermabond, Indermil**.

tissue-borne *See* DENTURE.

tissue conditioner A temporary material applied to the fitting surface of the denture to allow inflammation of the tissues to resolve prior to the taking of definitive impressions; the material is resilient, allowing more even distribution of loading and thus promoting tissue recovery. It consists typically of a poly ethyl methacrylate (PEMA) mixed with a plasticizer and a solvent such as ethyl alcohol. Because the alcohol and plasticizer leach out quickly, a tissue conditioner can be regarded as a temporary *soft lining.

tissue health index A measure of oral health status defined as a weighted average of sound teeth, filled (otherwise sound) teeth, and teeth with some *caries; the weights are intended in principle to represent the relative amounts of sound tissue in the three categories of teeth, divided by 28 to create an index with a range of 0 to 1.

titanium *n.* A light lustrous metallic element (Ti). Because it is both strong and biocompatible with human tissues, commercially pure titanium or titanium alloy is widely used as an *implant material in dentistry and orthopaedic surgery; it has the inherent property of *osseointegration. Preparing titanium for implantation involves subjecting it to a high-temperature plasma arc which removes the surface atoms, exposing fresh titanium that is instantly oxidized. The surface of the titanium used for implants may be modified mechanically or chemically by adding or removing material from the metallic surface e.g. by plasma-spraying, grit blasting, acid-etching, oxidation, or coating with *hydroxyapatite material.

Further Reading: Sul Y. T., Byon E., Wennerberg A. Surface characteristics of electrochemically oxidized implants and acid-etched implants: surface chemistry, morphology, pore configurations, oxide thickness, crystal structure, and roughness. *Int J Oral Maxillofac Implants* 2008;23:631–40.

titanium nitride *n.* An extremely hard material (TiN), with the appearance of metallic gold, used to coat instruments made of titanium, steel, carbide, or aluminium, to create a non-stick surface. It may be applied as a coating to the surfaces of instruments used for placing and contouring *resin composite cements.

titratable acidity *n.* The total amount of all hydrogen ions (what makes acids 'acidic') in a solution of juice, must, or wine. Drinks with a high titratable acidity are difficult for the *saliva to neutralize and are therefore potentially particularly damaging to the teeth. Pure fruit juices have high titratable acidity, whereas carbonated water, while being acidic, has a low titratable acidity and is therefore less likely to cause tooth *erosion.

TNM staging *n. See* STAGING.

tobacco *n.* A genus of short-leafed plants of the nightshade (Solanaceae) family indigenous to North and South America, or the dried leaves of such plants. The tobacco leaves may be smoked, in the form of cigarettes, cigars, or as pipe tobacco, inhaled as *snuff, or chewed. Tobacco may be added to *betel quid and chewed; this is a common practice in India. Over 60 *carcinogens are present in tobacco smoke and 28 have been identified in tobacco for oral use; these include benzo(a)pyrine, volatile aldehydes, nitrosamines, inorganic compounds, and radionucleotides. Tobacco contains the neurotoxin **nicotine**, which is absorbed into the bloodstream and over time results in *tolerance and *dependence. Because of the absorption of nicotine, tar, and other harmful alkaloids, long-term tobacco use carries significant risks of developing various cancers, particularly oral and lung cancer, as well as strokes, and severe cardiovascular and respiratory diseases. Tobacco also causes potentially malignant disorders in the mouth including *leukoplakia, *erythroplakia, and erythroleukoplakia. Cigarette *smoking is an important risk factor for periodontal disease.

Tofflemire matrix retainer *See* MATRIX RETAINER.

tolerance *n.* A characteristic of substance *dependence that may be shown by the need for markedly increased amounts of the substance to achieve intoxication or the desired effect. It may develop after taking a particular drug over a long period of time.

tolonium chloride *n. See* TOLUIDINE BLUE.

toluidine blue (tolonium chloride) *n.* A chemical dye used as a screening method to identify potentially malignant mucosal cells. It may be applied topically to the suspected area or as a mouth rinse. It stains suspicious tissue blue. Trade names: **Orascreen, OraTest®.**

Tomes' granular layer *See* GRANULAR LAYER OF TOMES.

Tomes' process [Sir Charles Tomes (1847–1928), English dentist] The pyramidal extension at the secretory end of an *ameloblast surrounded by enamel as the ameloblast retreats from the dentine. It gives the ameloblasts a picket fence appearance under the microscope.

Tomes, Sir John (1815–95) Sir John Tomes was considered to be the father of British dentistry.

He was born in Weston-on-Avon and began medical studies at King's College, London, in 1836, later becoming a dental surgeon at Middlesex Hospital. He was active in promoting the Dental Act of 1858, which introduced obligatory training and registration for all dentists. In 1877 he was elected chairman of the Dental Reform Committee. He was the first president of the British Dental Association, formed in 1879, was elected an honorary fellow of the Royal College of Surgeons in 1883, and was knighted for his services to dentistry in 1886. He was an inventor of many dental instruments, including a new type of curved dental forceps, and he also wrote a number of papers and books including his *System of dental surgery* (1859). In 1894 he established the triennial Tomes prize for original and scientific work; it was first awarded to his son, Charles Sissmore Tomes (later Sir Charles Tomes).

tomography *n. See* COMPUTERIZED TOMOGRAPHY.

tongue *n.* A muscular organ which plays an important role in mastication, speech, swallowing, cleansing, taste, suckling, and exploring. The lower surface is covered by a thin non-keratinized layer of mucosal *epithelium, which is continuous with the floor of the mouth. The tongue is anchored anteriorly by the lingual *fraenum (frenulum linguae), either side of which lie the fimbriated (frilly) folds of tissue. The upper surface of the tongue (*dorsum) is divided into an anterior two thirds within the oral cavity and a posterior third that faces the pharynx separated by a V-shaped groove (*sulcus terminalis) at the apex of which is a small depression (*foramen caecum). The tongue is divided into two halves mesio-distally by a fibrous septum. The anterior two thirds of the tongue are covered by a specialized *keratinized mucosa containing the circumvallate, filiform, fungiform, and foliate *papillae in which (except for the filiform) are embedded *taste buds.

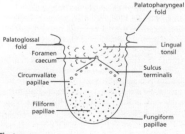

Palatopharyngeal fold

Palatoglossal fold

Foramen caecum

Lingual tonsil

Circumvallate papillae

Sulcus terminalis

Filiform papillae

Fungiform papillae

The tongue

The tongue consists of **intrinsic muscles**, which alter the shape of the tongue, and extrinsic muscles which alter its position to facilitate speech, swallowing, and eating. Because the tongue is divided into two halves by the median septum, all the intrinsic muscles are paired and consist of superior and inferior longitudinal, transverse, and vertical fibre bundles. The **extrinsic muscles** of the tongue (hyoglossus, styloglossus, palatoglossus, genioglossus) arise from structures outside the tongue and insert into it. The primary **blood supply** is from the lingual artery and venous drainage is via the lingual or facial veins. The **nerve supply** consists of motor innervation from the hypoglossal nerve (except for the palatoglossal muscle, which is supplied by the pharyngeal branch of the vagus nerve) and sensory innervation of the oral anterior two thirds of the tongue via the lingual nerve. The tongue may become enlarged in conditions such as *Down's syndrome (Down syndrome), *myxoedema, and *acromegaly.

tongue, atrophic *n. See* GLOSSITIS.

tongue, bifid *n.* A tongue divided by a midline cleft extending from the tip.

tongue, black hairy (lingua villosa nigra) A black discoloration of the dorsum of the tongue caused by elongated filiform *papillae, an accumulation of dark pigments, and an overgrowth of bacteria. It is characterized by a black or brown discoloration of the tongue, giving rise to its name. The cause is unknown but predisposing factors include poor oral hygiene, pigment-producing bacteria or fungi, certain mouthwashes, antibiotic therapy, medications such as bismuth preparations, *smoking, drinking tea or coffee, and chewing *tobacco. The discoloration can usually be mechanically removed by a *tongue scraper or tongue brushing. 📷

tongue, cobblestone Describes the appearance of the tongue due to *hyperplasia and *hyperaemia of the fungiform and filiform *papillae caused by riboflavin (*vitamin B_2) or biotin deficiency.

tongue, fissured A condition of uniformly arranged fissures radiating laterally and anteriorly from the medium raphe. It is usually asymptomatic and non-inflammatory and is more common with increased age.

tongue, geographic (benign migratory glossitis) Irregular denuded erythematous patches on the surface of the tongue, which give a map-like appearance and which can vary on a daily basis. It is caused by filiform papilla depapillation on the dorsal and lateral aspects of the tongue; the underlying connective tissue is infiltrated by mixed chronic inflammatory cells. The condition may be

t

persistent and uncomfortable, although most lesions are asymptomatic. The cause is unknown although stress, *allergies, and *vitamin B, iron, and zinc deficiency have been implicated. *See also* GLOSSITIS.

tongue, magenta A purplish-red discoloration of the tongue due to *vitamin B_2 (riboflavin) deficiency. It is also characterized by oedema and flattening of the filiform *papillae on the dorsum of the tongue.

tongue scraper A hand instrument used to remove surface deposits on the dorsum of the tongue by dragging it across the surface from back to front. There is little evidence to suggest that tongue scrapers are more effective at reducing *halitosis than toothbrushes.

Further Reading: Seemann R. Tongue scrapers may reduce halitosis in adults. *Evid Based Dent* 2006;7(3):78.

tongue, smooth *See* GLOSSITIS.

tongue, strawberry *See* SCARLET FEVER.

tongue thrust An orofacial muscular imbalance, due to a retained infantile pattern of swallowing in which the tongue is pushed forward against the anterior teeth. It may be characterized by mouth breathing, an open *bite condition of the teeth, an open mouth posture when at rest, and difficulty with speech. Treatment is by muscular therapy or the provision of a preventive appliance.

tongue-tie *n. See* ANKYLOGLOSSIA.

tonsil *n.* (*adj.* **tonsillar**) A mass of *lymphoid tissue concerned with protection against infection. The **palatine tonsils** are situated on either side of the back of the mouth between the palatoglossal and palatopharyngeal arches (the pillars of the *fauces), and the **lingual tonsils** are situated either side of the pharyngeal third of the tongue.

tonsillitis *n.* Inflammation of the *tonsils due to bacterial or viral infection characterized by sore throat, fever, and difficulty in swallowing. Streptococcal tonsillitis, if untreated, may progress to *rheumatic fever.

tooth *n.* (*pl.* **teeth**) One of the hard mineralized structures embedded in the maxillary and mandibular alveolar processes of the mouth. The exposed part of the tooth (*crown) is covered with enamel and the part within the bony socket (*root) is covered with *cementum and attached by means of the *periodontal membrane to the *alveolar bone. The bulk of the tooth is made up of *dentine, which surrounds the pulp chamber and pulp canals. In the permanent dentition there are four different morphological types of tooth: *incisors,

*canines, *premolars, and *molars. In the primary (deciduous) *dentition there are only three different types of tooth: incisors, canines, and molars.

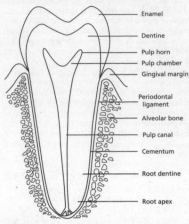

Tooth structure

tooth abutment *n. See* ABUTMENT.

toothache (odontodynia) *n.* A pain associated with a tooth or its surrounding supporting structures. Common causes of toothache include inflammation of the pulp (*pulpitis), an acute abscess associated with a tooth root, a cracked or fractured tooth, exposed root surface tissue, and acute inflammation of the bone or soft tissue surrounding the tooth.

tooth-borne *See* DENTURE.

toothbrush *n.* A device with a handle and bristles at one end designed to remove soft deposits from the oral structures and to stimulate the gingival tissues. The head size is selected to meet the needs of the individual. The bristles are normally multitufted, round-ended, and made of nylon to reduce the risk of toothbrush *abrasion. Natural bristles have a less predictable texture, and may be porous and therefore more likely to harbour bacteria. The handle of the brush may be modified to suit patients with limited dexterity. The toothbrush is normally used with a *dentifrice to improve the effectiveness of the brush. **End-tuft (single-tuft, unituft, interdental) brushes** have a small tuft of bristles set at an angle to the handle to assist in accessing difficult-to-reach areas. An **interdental brush** has a small tuft of bristles with an angled head, designed to fit into the space between two teeth. **Powered toothbrushes (automatic toothbrushes)** use a battery or electrical power source and produce a vibratory or oscillating action in the brush head. Evidence suggests that a rotation oscillation action removes plaque and reduces gingival inflammation more effectively than manual toothbrushing and that oscillating/pulsating power toothbrushes are more effective at plaque removal and improvement of the gingival condition than high-frequency power toothbrushes.

Further Reading: Davies R. M. Manual versus powered toothbrushes: what is the evidence? *Dent Update* 2006;33 (3):159–62.

toothbrushing *n.* The process of using a toothbrush to remove soft deposits and provide gingival stimulation. A faulty toothbrushing technique can result in ineffective cleansing, inadequate stimulation, gingival damage, and excessive tooth abrasion. The **scrub toothbrushing technique** involves short horizontal brush strokes with the bristles placed at right angles to the teeth. Using the **Bass technique**, first described by C. C. Bass in 1948, the brush head is placed at an angle of 45° to the posterior teeth, directed towards the gingival tissues and vibrated with firm pressure using a side-to-side motion to work the bristles into the *gingival crevice without the bristle tips losing contact with the gingival tissues; for the anterior teeth, the brush is held in a vertical position. **Charters technique** is a method of toothbrushing first documented by W. J. Charters in 1928, in which the bristles of the toothbrush are placed at a 45° angle to the tooth surface and pointed in a coronal direction with half the bristles on the gingivae and half on the teeth. Pressure is applied and the bristles are moved in a small rotational movement so that the bristles move into the interproximal spaces, remove plaque debris, and massage the gingival tissues. **Fones' method** is a toothbrushing technique in which, to brush the buccal and labial tooth surfaces, the teeth of the opposing jaws are placed in contact, the brush is placed at right angles to the tooth surfaces, and the brush is moved with a circular motion. This motion is repeated for the lingual and palatal surfaces with the jaws apart; the occlusal surfaces are brushed with an antero-posterior movement. Using the **Stillman's method**, the brush head is placed on the junction between tooth and gingivae and vibrated with short strokes. This may be terminated with a rolling action of the bristles over the tooth surface (**modified Stillman**).

tooth charting *n. See* TOOTH NOTATION.

tooth development

A process which starts at about the 6th week of intrauterine life from a thickening of the *ectodermal epithelium, which forms the *primary epithelial band (**initiation stage**); from this develops the *dental lamina, on which swellings (*enamel organs) differentiate through a series of stages (bud, cap, and bell) to form the tooth structure with the formation of both enamel (*amelogenesis) and dentine (*dentinogenesis). The **bud stage** occurs at about 8 weeks of intrauterine development. Clumps of *mesenchymal cells induce the *dental lamina to form swellings known as *enamel organs or tooth buds. These swellings are subsequently responsible for the development of each tooth. Ten buds develop per arch representing the primary (deciduous) teeth; subsequently the permanent tooth buds develop lingually to the primary tooth buds. The **cap stage** starts at about 9–11 weeks of intrauterine life, when the cells on the inner aspect of the *enamel organ change from cuboidal to columnar in shape. Unequal cell growth leads to the characteristic shape: the peripheral cells (outer *enamel epithelium) are cuboidal and the cells in the concavity are tall and columnar (inner enamel epithelium); the cells in between differentiate to form a delicate cellular network (*stellate reticulum). The **bell stage** takes place at about the 12–14th week of intrauterine life. The *enamel organ is bell-shaped and consists of an *inner enamel epithelium covered by the *stratum intermedium, and these two layers are separated by the *stellate reticulum. The internal enamel epithelium induces the adjacent cells of the dental papilla to differentiate into *odontoblasts and form *dentine; the dentine then induces the internal enamel epithelium to differentiate into *ameloblasts and form *enamel. The stellate reticulum expands by increasing the amount of intracellular fluid and then collapses before the formation of enamel. The enamel organ forms *Hertwig's sheath, which determines the shape of the root and initiates the formation of root dentine.

Bud   Cap   Bell

Stages of tooth development

During development, teeth may become *ankylosed, *dilacerated, or *geminated. The number of teeth may be greater (*hyperdontia) or fewer (*hypodontia) than normal, resulting in *supernumerary or *supplemental teeth, or they may be altered in shape (*peg-shaped, *Moon's molars, *Hutchinson's incisors). Abnormalities of tooth structure include enamel *hypomineralization, *amelogenesis imperfecta, and *dentinogenesis imperfecta. *See also* DENTITION.

Further Reading: Katchburian E., Holt S. J. Studies on the development of ameloblasts. *Journal of Cell Science* 1972;11:415–47.

(((🌐))) SEE WEB LINKS

• A video on YouTube describing the histological changes during tooth development.

tooth eruption *See* ERUPTION.

tooth extraction (exodontia) The planned removal of a tooth from its socket in the *alveolar bone. It is usually accomplished by the use of *forceps and *elevators, although historically *pelicans and *tooth keys have been used. **Serial extraction** is the planned selective and sequential extraction of primary and sometimes permanent teeth to relieve anticipated *overcrowding in the permanent dentition. It involves the extraction of selected primary teeth over a period of years. The primary canine teeth are removed when the upper and lower permanent incisors have erupted. This makes room for the permanent incisors. After 2 years, when the first premolars and permanent canines are ready to erupt, more teeth may be removed if necessary, including possibly the first premolars. **Surgical extraction** requires a mucoperiosteal flap to be raised, followed by the removal of alveolar bone. Extraction may be indicated for many reasons, including caries, pain, *sepsis, trauma, failed restorative treatment, periodontal disease, *ankylosis, overcrowding, poor patient cooperation, insufficient tooth structure for restorative therapy, pulpal involvement, and a relevant medical history. Complications arising during tooth extraction may include tooth or root fracture, primary *haemorrhage, *haematoma, nerve damage, and inhalation or swallowing of the tooth or tooth fragment. Complications which may occur following tooth extraction include reactionary or secondary haemorrhage and infection (*alveolitis) and, where the extraction has been undertaken using local analgesia, self-inflicted soft tissue trauma and prolonged analgesia due to nerve damage from the analgesic needle.

Further Reading: Luyten C. Guided tooth eruption via serial extraction. *Rev Belge Med Dent* 1995;50(2):67–78.

tooth extrusion *See* EXTRUSION.

tooth germ (tooth bud) *n.* The formative structures of the developing tooth made up of the *enamel organ (*ectodermal component) and the dental *papilla (*mesodermal component).

tooth inhalation The passage of a tooth or tooth fragment into the trachea or lungs. It is most likely to occur during tooth extraction, particularly if the patient is unconscious when protection of the airway is essential.

tooth intrusion *See* INTRUSION.

tooth jewellery *See* ORAL JEWELLERY.

tooth key *n.* An instrument which was formerly used for extracting teeth. It superseded the *pelican and was first described by Alexander Monro in 1742. It consisted of a bolster, shaft, and claw. The bolster was placed against the root of the tooth and the claw positioned over the crown. On rotation of the key, the intended tooth was dislocated. Forceps replaced the tooth key as the principal extraction instrument in the early 20th century.

tooth loss The separation of a tooth from its investing and supporting structures. It may occur due to normal *exfoliation (primary dentition only), trauma, excessive bone resorption, *periodontal disease, or planned extraction. Tooth loss is usually associated with loss of the supporting *alveolar bone. It can lead to speech, masticatory, and aesthetic problems.

tooth, milk *See* PRIMARY DENTITION.

tooth mobility The horizontal or vertical displacement of a tooth beyond its normal physiological boundaries. It may be due to trauma, *periodontal disease, *occlusal traumatism, or loss of *alveolar bone support. Tooth mobility may be assessed by applying alternate pressure on the outer and inner aspects of the crown of the tooth using two hand instruments, but this assessment is very operator-dependent. The results can be recorded using a **mobility index**.

A tooth mobility index	
Grade	Mobility
0	Detectable movement of up to 0.2mm.
I	Horizontal movement of the crown between 0.2 and 1.0mm.
II	Horizontal movement of the crown greater than 1.0mm.
III	Horizontal movement of the crown greater than 1.0mm and additional vertical movement.

Mechanical instruments for measuring mobility more accurately have been developed, such as the **Periotest** * which uses an accelerometer to measure the resistance of the tooth to a force applied 16 times over a 4 second period. Vertical *tooth movement may be detected on the occlusion of the tooth (*fremitus).

tooth movement The change of position of a tooth within the alveolar bone in response to an external force. When induced by an orthodontic appliance, it may involve **rotation**, bodily movement of a tooth in a mesial or distal direction without rotation (**translation**), vertical movement (*intrusion or *extrusion), or a combination of rotation and translation (*tipping). The tooth is capable of movement because of *osteoclastic activity, where there is an increase in pressure resulting in bone resorption, and *osteoblastic activity, where there is a decrease in pressure creating bone formation.

tooth, natal *n. See* NATAL TEETH.

tooth, neonatal *n. See* NEONATAL.

tooth notation

A means of graphically recording the presence and location of teeth and associating information with them within a dentition. More than 32 different systems have been described but only a few have achieved widespread acceptance. These include the **Palmer tooth notation system** (originally termed the **Zsigmondy system** after the Hungarian dentist Adolf Zsigmondy who developed the idea in 1861, using a **Zsigmondy cross** to record quadrants of tooth positions: also known as **chevron**, or **set square system**). The mouth is divided into four quadrants and each permanent tooth is assigned a number from 1 to 8 starting at the midline and each primary tooth assigned a letter of the alphabet from A to E also starting at the midline. The number or letter is placed inside an L-shaped symbol to indicate the quadrant. e.g ⌐D describes the upper left primary first molar and 5⌐ describes the upper right second premolar.

With the advent of electronic recording, the quadrant indicator may be replaced by UL, UR, LL, and LR to indicate the respective quadrants. The designations 'left' and 'right' on the chart correspond to the patient's left and right, respectively. The *Federation Dentaire Internationale (FDI) notation system (also known as ISO-3950 notation) was first developed in 1971 and is used more internationally than the Palmer system. The mouth is divided into quadrants and a two-digit code is used to designate each tooth, the first digit representing the quadrant and the second the tooth position. The quadrants are numbered 1 to 4 in the permanent dentition and 5 to 8 in the primary dentition, such that the upper right quadrant is 1 or 5, upper left is 2 or 6, lower left is 3 or 7, and the lower right is 4 or 8, depending on the dentition. The designations 'left' and 'right' on the chart correspond to the patient's left and right, respectively.

The **universal/national numbering system** is a dental notation system for associating information to a specific tooth, and is commonly used in the United States and has been adopted by the American Dental Association. The permanent teeth are numbered from 1 to 32 and the primary teeth are labelled A to T using upper case letters (an alternative system labels them 1d to 20d). The designations 'left' and 'right' on the chart correspond to the patient's left and right, respectively; however, the orientation of the

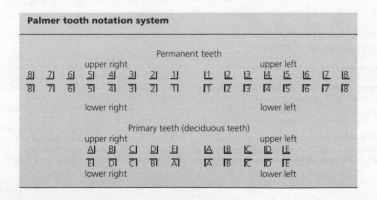

Palmer tooth notation system

Permanent teeth

upper right   upper left

8⌐ 7⌐ 6⌐ 5⌐ 4⌐ 3⌐ 2⌐ 1⌐   ⌐1 ⌐2 ⌐3 ⌐4 ⌐5 ⌐6 ⌐7 ⌐8

8⌐ 7⌐ 6⌐ 5⌐ 4⌐ 3⌐ 2⌐ 1⌐   ⌐1 ⌐2 ⌐3 ⌐4 ⌐5 ⌐6 ⌐7 ⌐8

lower right   lower left

Primary teeth (deciduous teeth)

upper right   upper left

A⌐ B⌐ C⌐ D⌐ E⌐   ⌐A ⌐B ⌐C ⌐D ⌐E

E⌐ D⌐ C⌐ B⌐ A⌐   ⌐A ⌐B ⌐C ⌐D ⌐E

lower right   lower left

FDI tooth notation system

Permanent teeth

	upper right								upper left				
18	17	16	15	14	13	12	11	21	22	23	24	25	26	27	28
48	47	46	45	44	43	42	41	31	32	33	34	35	36	37	38
			lower right								lower left		

Primary teeth (deciduous teeth)

upper right						upper left			
55	54	53	52	51	61	62	63	64	65
85	84	83	82	81	71	72	73	74	75
lower right						lower left			

The universal/national tooth numbering system

Permanent Teeth

	upper left								upper right				
16	15	14	13	12	11	10	9	8	7	6	5	4	3	2	1
17	18	19	20	21	22	23	24	25	26	27	28	29	30	31	32
		lower left								lower right				

Primary teeth (deciduous teeth)

upper left						upper right			
J	I	H	G	F	E	D	C	B	A
K	L	M	N	O	P	Q	R	S	T
lower left						lower right			

Alternative system for primary teeth

upper left						upper right			
10d	9d	8d	7d	6d	5d	4d	3d	2d	1d
11d	12d	13d	14d	15d	16d	17d	18d	19d	20d
lower left						lower right			

chart is traditionally 'patient's view', i.e. patient's right corresponds to notation-chart right.

toothpaste *n.* A paste form of *dentifrice.

toothpick *n. See* WOOD POINT.

tooth positioner *See* POSITIONER.

tooth separator *See* SEPARATOR.

tooth, submerged A tooth that has failed to erupt sufficiently to make contact with the teeth in the opposing arch. It may be caused by *ankylosis to the alveolar bone.

tooth surface Any of the outer portions of a tooth. Tooth surfaces are labelled according to their relation to the midline or to structures in the oral cavity. Abbreviations may be used when describing cavities or restorations involving these surfaces e.g. MOD for a cavity or restoration involving the mesial, occlusal, and distal surfaces.

tooth trauma *n. See* TRAUMA.

tooth wear The non-bacterial loss of tooth substance by *abrasion, *attrition, or *erosion. **Abnormal occlusal tooth wear** is that wear on the biting surfaces of the teeth that exceeds the normal physiological wear pattern due to attrition; it is usually as a result of *bruxism or an unusually abrasive diet. Occlusal wear may be seen as part of the normal physiological ageing process. **Interproximal wear** is the loss of tooth substance at the proximal contact areas due to functional wear; it creates broader and flatter

Tooth surfaces

Tooth surface	Description
Mesial (M)	Nearest to the midline of the dental arch
Distal (D)	Furthest from the midline of the dental arch
Labial	Next to the lips (incisors and canines)
Buccal (B)	Next to the cheeks (molars and premolars)
Lingual	Next to the tongue (mandibular teeth only)
Palatal	Next to the palate (maxillary teeth only)
Occlusal (O)	The biting surface of posterior teeth (molars and premolars)
Incisal (I)	The cutting edge of anterior teeth (incisors and canines)
Proximal (interproximal, aproximal)	Mesial and distal surfaces
Facial (F)	Buccal and labial surfaces
Cervical	The junction between the crown and root
Apical	At the apex of the tooth root

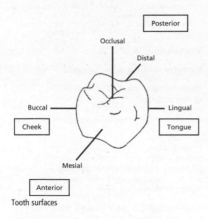

Tooth surfaces

contact areas and reduces the mesio-distal dimension of the dental arch. The **tooth wear pattern** is the distribution of areas of tooth wear resulting from *attrition, the masticatory pattern, or *parafunction.

tooth wear index A method of measuring the extent of tooth wear and expressing it as a numerical value. Many indices have been developed but none have achieved universal acceptance. The tooth wear index of Smith and Knight (1984) is an index that is commonly used.

Further Reading: Donachie M. A., Walls A. W. The tooth wear index: a flawed epidemiological tool in an ageing population group. *Community Dent Oral Epidemiol* 1996;24(2):152–8.

tooth whitening *See* BLEACHING.

topical *adj.* Pertaining to the surface of a part of the body. Used as a route for the application of a drug.

topical analgesia *See* ANALGESIA.

torquing *n.* The intentional movement of the root of a tooth in a bucco-lingual direction with either minimal or no movement of the crown in the opposite direction. It can only be achieved by the use of rectangular wires using a fixed *orthodontic appliance, and is usually undertaken towards the end of active *orthodontic therapy.

torus mandibularis *n.* A rounded bony swelling (*exostosis) occurring on the lingual aspect of the *mandible between the canines and the molars above the attachment of the mylohyoid muscle. In most cases the swelling is bilateral. 🔘

torus palatinus *n.* A rounded bony swelling (*exostosis) usually found in the midline of the hard *palate. Most are less than 2cm in diameter, but their size can change throughout life. 🔘

toxaemia *n.* Blood poisoning caused by *toxins formed from a local focus of bacterial infection passing into the bloodstream. It is characterized by fever, diarrhoea, and vomiting. *See also* SEPTICAEMIA.

toxic *adj.* Poisonous and potentially lethal.

toxin *n.* A poisonous substance produced by a living organism, such as a *bacterium, that is active at low concentrations. Bacterial toxins may be either *exotoxins or *endotoxins and are neutralized in the body by special *antibodies (antitoxins).

TPS probe *n. See* PROBE.

trabecula *n.* (*pl.* **trabeculae**) **1.** A septum extending from the outer part of an organ to its interior, dividing it into separate chambers. **2.** Any of the thin lamellae found in cancellous *bone.

trachea *n.* The cartilaginous tube forming the air passage (windpipe) between the *larynx and the left and right bronchi. The upper part of the trachea is crossed by the isthmus of the *thyroid gland.

tracheostomy (tracheotomy) *n.* A surgical procedure to create a hole through the neck into the trachea to relieve obstruction to breathing. A tube is usually inserted into the opening and taped in position to maintain the aperture.

tracing *n.* A pattern scribed by a pointed instrument on some form of tracing material. A **cephalometric tracing** is a tracing of the salient features of a cephalometric radiograph made on a piece of transparent material placed over the radiograph. An **intra-oral tracing** is a recording of mandibular movements using a device with a stylus attached to one jaw contacting a coated plate on the other jaw. The tracing shapes are referred to as **Gothic arch**, **arrow point**, or **sea gull tracings**; the apex of the tracing indicates the most retruded relation of the mandible to the maxilla in normal function (*centric relation).

tract *n.* **1.** A group of fibres passing from one part of an organ to another such as the *dead tracts found in dentine. **2.** An organ or collection of organs providing for the passage of something, e.g. the alimentary tract. **3.** A communication between a pathological area and a body cavity or the skin (*sinus tract).

traction *n.* The application of a pulling force. **Extra-oral traction (EOT)** is the process of applying a backwards (distal) pressure on the maxillary teeth during orthodontic therapy by the use of external headgear consisting of a *facebow, *headcap, or *neckstrap and some form of force mechanism, usually a *spring attached to a plastic tag. Extra-oral or external traction is also used for fracture reduction appliance therapy, with rigid connectors between points of fixation in the oral cavity and over the cranial area. **Intra-oral (intermaxillary) traction (IOT)** is the attachment of elastic bands or other devices to the upper and lower teeth in order to produce the force necessary to move teeth.

tragus *n.* The projection of cartilage that extends over the opening of the external auditory meatus.

training base *n. See* BASE.

trait *n.* A genetically inherited set of bodily characteristics e.g. *sickle-cell trait.

tranexamic acid *n.* An antifibrinolytic which inhibits the activation of plasminogen to *plasmin and therefore encourages blood clotting. It is used as a post-operative mouthwash following surgical procedures in patients with blood disorders such as *haemophilia. Trade names: **Cyklokapron**, **Transamin**.

transcutaneous electrical nerve stimulation (TENS) The passage of pulses of a low-voltage electric current into tissue for the relief of pain. It has been used in dentistry as a form of local analgesia. The treatment is believed to stimulate the body's production of *endorphins or natural pain killers.

Further Reading: Caroll D., Moore R. A., McQuay H. J., Fairman F., Tramér M., Leijon G. Transcutaneous electrical nerve stimulation (TENS) for chronic pain (Cochrane Review), *Cochrane Library* 2003; issue 4. Chichester: Wiley.

transexamic acid *n. See* TRANEXAMIC ACID.

transfer coping *n. See* COPING.

transformation *n.* (in statistics) The application of a mathematical function to all observations in a data set. For example, the correction of an abnormal distribution such as a *skew.

transfusion *n.* The injection of blood products from one individual (the donor) to a patient (the recipient) to replace blood that is lost during surgery, from injury, or because the recipient's blood is deficient in quality.

transient ischaemic attack (TIA) The result of a temporary disruption of the circulation, and therefore a temporary reduction in oxygen supply, to part of the brain due to blockage of the arteries to the brain (*thrombosis) or spasm of the vessel walls. The symptoms are similar to those of a *stroke but the patient recovers within 24 hours.

transillumination *n.* The illumination of part of the body by shining a bright light, such as a resin curing lamp, through it. **Fibre-optic transillumination (FOTI)** is a method of assisting in the diagnosis of interproximal caries in anterior teeth using a specially designed fibre-optic device; a carious lesion appears as a darkened shadow surrounded by a normal coloured zone.

translucent *adj.* Describing a material which allows some light to pass through it, absorbs some of the remainder, and reflects the rest from its surface or internal interfaces. It is an important property of aesthetic restorative materials and denture base resins.

translucent zone *n.* The area of gradual loss of mineral underneath an advancing carious lesion; the translucent zone has only slight loss of mineral, whereas the outer and narrower **dark zone** represents an area of previous mineralization.

transmissible spongiform encephalopathies (TSEs) A group of fatal degenerative brain diseases, including *Creutzfeldt-Jakob disease (CJD), that occur in humans and several other animal species caused by altered forms of naturally occurring *prion proteins normally present in brain tissue.

transmucosal *adj.* Through the mucous membrane. It may be applied to the administration of a drug or to that part of an *implant which penetrates the mucosal tissue.

transplantation *n.* The transfer of tissue from one person (donor) to another (recipient) or from one site to another in the same individual. **Autogenous transplantation** is the implantation of tissue, such as a tooth, from one site to another in the same individual. **Homogenous transplantation** is the implantation of tissue from a donor to a recipient of the same species.

transposition *n.* The migration of a tooth from its usual position such that the normal order of the teeth is changed e.g. a canine distal to a first molar or a lateral incisor mesial to a central incisor. It is often associated with a history of trauma. Management is usually by orthodontic therapy or restorative treatment to produce the best aesthetic and functional result.

transudation *n.* The passage of a liquid (**transudate**) through a membrane due to a hydrostatic or *osmotic pressure gradient e.g. blood through the walls of a capillary vessel.

trauma *n.* A physical wound or injury. Trauma to the oral tissues may involve only the hard dental tissues and pulp (enamel crack with no tooth loss, enamel fracture, crown fracture involving dentine, crown fracture involving dentine and pulp, or root fracture), or it may involve trauma to the periodontal tissues (*subluxation, partial *avulsion, lateral *luxation, intrusive luxation, or total avulsion), the supporting bone (compression of the alveolar socket, fracture of the socket wall, fracture of the alveolar process, or fracture of the mandible or maxilla), or the oral mucosa (laceration, *contusion, or *abrasion). *See also* CHILD ABUSE.

traumatic *adj.* Pertaining to or caused by injury. **Traumatic occlusion** is damage to the tooth or supporting structures caused by the application of a force, in excess of that which the tooth or supporting structures can withstand. The damage caused may be reversible or irreversible, depending upon the extent and duration of the forces applied. *See also* TRAUMATISM.

traumatism *n.* The physical or psychological condition produced by trauma. **Periodontal traumatism** describes the degenerative changes in the periodontium which occur when occlusal forces exceed physiological limits. If severe enough, it can result in *thrombosis of blood vessels, haemorrhage, *hyalinization of the periodontal fibres, and possibly *necrosis of the periodontal fibres and bone in areas of excessive pressure. In areas where there is tension, the periodontal ligament is widened, bone and cementum resorption occurs and is sometimes additionally associated with tearing of the cementum or bone. Clinically, the teeth may show increased mobility and tenderness to *percussion; there may also be pulpal hypersensitivity.

tray *n. See* IMPRESSION TRAY.

Treacher Collins syndrome [E. Treacher Collins (1862-1919), British ophthalmologist] A hereditary disorder of facial development. It is characterized by underdevelopment of the jaw and cheek (zygomatic) bones and a variety of ear and facial malformations.

treatment plan *n.* A schedule of procedures, usually listed in chronological order, detailing the advice, care, or intervention required to restore the oral health of a patient.

trench mouth *n. See* GINGIVITIS, NECROTIZING.

Trendelenburg position [F. Trendelenburg (1844-1924), German surgeon] *n.* A position in which the patient is supine with the head and chest at a lower level than the legs.

trephine bur *n. See* BUR.

Treponema *n.* A genus of parasitic *anaerobic *spirochaete bacteria, several of which may be found in the mouth. These include *T. mucosum* and *T. denticola*, found in periodontal infections, and *T. vincentii*, associated with necrotizing ulcerative *gingivitis. *T. pallidum* causes *syphilis in humans.

triage *n.* A process in which patients are sorted according to their need so that treatment priorities can be defined. It is used in the emergency dental service in the UK to determine which patients should receive urgent care.

triamcinolone acetonide *n.* A synthetic *corticosteroid used topically as a paste in the treatment of localized inflammatory lesions in the mouth such as aphthous ulceration. Trade name: **Adcortyl in Orabase***.

triclosan *n.* A chlorinated aromatic compound with antibacterial, anti-inflammatory, and antifungal properties. It targets bacteria by inhibiting fatty acid synthesis and can be effective in reducing periodontal disease. Triclosan lacks the staining effects of cationic agents such as *chlorhexidine; its oral retention can be increased by its combination with co-polymers of methoxyethylene and maleic acid. Triclosan is an ingredient of many *dentifrices.

Further Reading: Niederman R. Triclosan-containing toothpastes reduce plaque and gingivitis. *Evid Based Dent* 2005;6(2):33.

triconodont 1. *adj.* Describing a tooth having three cones or cusps. 2. *n.* A very small mammal that lived from the Triassic period until the Cretaceous period; so named because it had three-cusped teeth.

tricuspid *adj.* 1. Describing a tooth having three cusps. 2. (in anatomy) Having three prongs or points such as the tricuspid valve of the heart.

tri-ethylene glycol dimethacrylate (TEGDMA) *n.* See TEGDMA.

trifurcation *n.* The point at which a structure, such as a tooth root, divides into three branches or roots.

trigeminal neuralgia *n.* See NEURALGIA.

trigger point A hypersensitive part of the body which when stimulated produces local or *referred pain.

trigone *n.* The anterior part of the upper primitive molar tooth which usually carries three cusps (*protocone, *paracone, and *metacone).

trigonid *n.* The anterior part of the lower primitive molar tooth which usually carries three cusps (*protoconid, *paraconid, and *metaconid).

tri-helix appliance *n.* A fixed slow-expansion orthodontic appliance with only one anterior coil. It is less efficient than the *quadhelix appliance and limited to the treatment of narrow or high palatal vaults or a combination of both.

trimmer *n.* An instrument used for modifying the contour of a tooth or material. A

gingival margin trimmer is a single-bevelled, double-ended type of chisel; the blade is curved with a straight cutting edge; it forms a pair of instruments shaped to bevel the mesial or distal margins or to accentuate the mesial or distal axio-gingival angles of a cavity. A **Mitchell's trimmer** is a multi-purpose double-ended hand instrument with a spoon-shaped end and a triangular pointed blade. A **model trimmer** is a piece of equipment used to shape or trim the sides and edges of a plaster or stone cast; it may take the form of a mechanical instrument or a rigid knife (plaster knife).

triple syringe See SYRINGE.

trismus *n.* The spasm of the muscles of mastication resulting in difficulty in opening the jaw. It is a characteristic symptom of *tetanus but may also occur with some oral inflammatory lesions such as *pericoronitis. It can also be associated with *temporomandibular joint dysfunction.

Further Reading: Dhanrajani P. J., Jonaidel O. Trismus: aetiology, differential diagnosis and treatment. *Dent Update* 2002;29:88–94.

tritubercular theory A theory which described the evolution of heterodont mammalian teeth from simple peg-like (*haplodont) teeth with the development of two smaller cones, one in front (*paracone) and one behind (*metacone) the main one. This *triconodont stage underwent further adaptation with the paracone and the metacone becoming external to the original cone (*protocone) in the upper jaw and internal in the lower jaw to create a triangular-shaped tooth with a cone at each angle (**tritubercular tooth**). These tritubercular teeth are a very common occurrence in ancestral mammals.

trituration *n.* The mixing or grinding of a powder such as the mixing of silver alloy and mercury to form *amalgam. This may be achieved by hand using a *pestle and *mortar or by using a mechanical device (*amalgamator).

troche *n.* See LOZENGE.

troph- (tropho-) Prefix denoting nourishment or nutrition.

-trophy Suffix denoting development, growth, or nourishment e.g. **dystrophy** (defective growth).

-tropic Suffix denoting 1. Turning towards e.g. *thixotropic. 2. Having an affinity for; influencing e.g. **inotropic** (affecting muscle contraction).

Trotter's syndrome A clinical triad of unilateral deafness, neuralgia affecting the mandibular branches of the trigeminal nerve, and defective mobility of the soft palate, first described by Wilfred Trotter in 1911. There may also be associated trismus. The condition is caused by malignant tumours invading the lateral wall of the nasopharynx.

Trousseau's sign [A. Trousseau (1801–67), French physician] Spasmodic contraction of muscles, particularly the muscles of mastication in response to nerve stimulation such as tapping the surface. It is a characteristic sign of low blood calcium level.

try-in *n.* The preliminary placement of teeth in wax as part of the process of constructing a complete or partial denture to evaluate the appearance and the correct relationship of the individual artificial teeth and arch forms to each other and to any natural teeth present. Where a significant number or all the teeth are being replaced, the try-in stage is normally preceded by jaw *registration. **Try-in paste** is a resin composite or glycerine based material used to provisionally locate a porcelain veneer to check for fit and colour prior to cementation; the resin composite material may exclude a light sensitive *initiator to give prolonged try-in time.

t-test *See* STUDENT'S T-TEST.

tube *n.* A hollow, usually cylindrical structure. A **discharge tube** is any vacuum tube, such as an x-ray tube, in which a high voltage electric current is discharged. An **endotracheal tube** is a catheter inserted through the mouth or nose (*intubation) in order to maintain an open airway or to allow the passage of gases such as nitrous oxide or oxygen. An **orthodontic tube** allows a wire to slide through it and may be round or square in cross-section; it is usually welded onto a band cemented onto a molar tooth but may be bonded directly onto the tooth using *resin composite (**bondable tube**).

tubercle *n.* A small rounded nodule or elevation on the surface of a tissue such as bone or teeth. The **tubercle of Carabelli** [G. C. Carabelli (1787–1842), Austrian dentist] is an elevation sometimes found on the mesiopalatal surface of the crown of a maxillary primary second molar or permanent maxillary first molar. The **genial tubercles (genio-hyoid tubercles, mental spine)** are small bony projections located on either side of the midline of the internal surface of the lower border of the body of mandible that give attachment below to the geniohyoid muscle and above to the genioglossus muscle. The **labial tubercle** (procheilon) is the central prominence on the upper margin of the upper lip. The **tubercle of Zuckerkandl** [E. Zuckerkandl (1849–1910), Austrian anatomist] is a

prominence sometimes found on the mesial half of the buccal surface of the primary maxillary first molar.

Further Reading: Kannapan J. G., Swaminathan S. A study on a dental morphological variation. Tubercle of Carabelli. *Indian J Dent Res* 2001;12(3):145–9.

tuberculosis (TB) *n.* An infectious disease caused by the bacillus *Mycobacterium tuberculosis* characterized by the formation of granulomatous lesions in the tissues, particularly in the lungs. It may also affect the jaws, oral mucosa, temporomandibular joint, and the lymph nodes of the head and neck (*scrofula). There has been a recent increase in the disease because of the association with *HIV infection and bacterial resistance. Prevention is aided by x-ray screening and *vaccination and treatment is by combinations of antibiotics.

tuberoplasty *n.* The surgical reshaping or reduction of the maxillary *tuberosity, usually prior to the construction of a prosthetic appliance.

tuberosity (tuber) *n.* A rounded protuberance on a bone. The **maxillary tuberosity** is the most distal posterior extension of the maxillary alveolar bone; fracture of the tuberosity is a surgical risk during the extraction of maxillary third molars.

tubule *n.* A small tube such as those seen in *dentine.

tuft *n.* A small cluster of bristles on a *toothbrush head. Also used to describe areas of incomplete enamel formation (*enamel tufts).

tularaemia (rabbit fever) *n.* A bacterial infection caused by the bacterium *Francisella tularensis*, contracted from rodents by direct contact or from drinking contaminated water. It is characterized by flu-like symptoms lasting several weeks with *necrotic ulceration at the site of infection such as the *mucosa of the mouth. Treatment is by antibiotic therapy.

tumor *n.* Swelling; one of the classical signs of tissue *inflammation. It is due to the accumulation of fluid between the cells.

tumoral calcinosis *n.* A rare inherited *autosomal disorder characterized by the presence of a periarticular mass containing calcific deposits in the joints affected. It may occur either in a familial form or a sporadic form secondary to other systemic disorders. It most commonly affects children and adolescents. Dental manifestations may include obliteration of the pulp chambers of the teeth with calcified deposits and short or absent roots predisposing to early mobility and tooth loss; the condition has been known to affect the *temporomandibular joint.

Further Reading: Naikmasur V., Guttal K., Bhargava P., Burde K., Sattur A., Nandimath K. Tumoral calcinosis with dental manifestations—a case report. *Dent Update* 2008;35:134–8.

tumour *n.* An abnormal growth of tissue which may be either *benign or *malignant. The progressive development of tumours is assessed by *staging. *See also* CARCINOMA; CYST; SARCOMA.

tungsten carbide *n.* An alloy of the metal tungsten and carbon. It is four times harder than titanium and is therefore used as an abrasive in grinding wheels and instruments. It is combined with other metals in the manufacture of cutting instruments and *burs.

tunnel preparation A technique of preparing a cavity in a carious posterior tooth by gaining access to the carious lesion on the proximal surface from an access cavity created on the occlusal surface without removal of the marginal ridge.

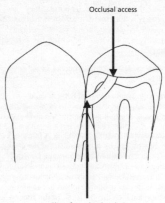

Occlusal access

Site of proximal caries

Tunnel preparation

turbinate bone *See* CONCHA.

turbine handpiece *n.* A *handpiece which incorporates a rotor driven by compressed air. It

was first patented in New Zealand in 1949 and first commercially manufactured as the Borden Airotor in 1957.

Turner's tooth (Turner's hypoplasia) [J. G. Turner (1870–1955), English dentist] *n.* An area of localized enamel *hypoplasia on a permanent tooth usually resulting in an area of white or yellow discoloration. It may be caused by trauma to an associated primary tooth or due to a primary tooth with a periapical inflammatory lesion; the result is a disturbance in the enamel formation (*amelogenesis) of the developing unerupted permanent tooth. The labial surface is the most likely surface affected.

tweezers *pl. n.* A hand instrument with two straight or curved beaks fixed at one end used for grasping small objects. They may have a locking device so that the beaks remain closed when the digital pressure is removed.

twin block appliance A removable *activator-type *functional *orthodontic appliance utilizing two blocks of acrylic resin with intervening expansion screws used to modify the lateral growth of the jaws to correct a *malocclusion by increasing the arch width. Early treatment is effective in reducing the *overjet and the severity of *malocclusion.

Further Reading: Gill D., Sharma A., Naini F., Jones S. The twin block appliance for the correction of Class II malocclusion. *Dent Update* 2005;32(3):158–60, 163–4, 167–8.

two-tailed test *See* ONE-TAILED TEST.

Type I error (in statistics) The chance of accepting the research hypothesis when the *null hypothesis is actually true (a false positive). It is represented by the Greek letter α. A **Type II error** is the chance of accepting the null hypothesis when the research question is actually true (a false negative). It is represented by the Greek letter β.

typodont *n.* An artificial, articulated model containing artificial or natural teeth set in wax or resin and used as a demonstration and teaching aid.

U

uberwulf *n.* An instrument which was formerly used for the extraction of teeth. It was a development of the *pelican with an elevator instead of a bolster. The tooth was extracted in an arc instead of using an oblique force required by the earlier pelicans, a technique which was considered to be less successful. It was superseded by the *tooth key in the early 18th century.

ugly duckling stage A stage of dental development, usually between the ages of 7 and 12 years, preceding the eruption of the permanent canines when the upper central and lateral incisors are tipped laterally due to the crowding created by the unerupted canines, to produce a midline space (median diastema). The midline space is normally transitory and the incisors usually assume normal alignment when the upper canines erupt into position. 📷

ulalgia *n.* Pain in the gingival tissues.

ulatrophy *n.* *Atrophy of the gingival tissue associated with recession and exposure of the root portion of the tooth. **Afunctional ulatrophy** is gingival atrophy occurring in a *congenital *malocclusion. **Atrophic (*ischaemic) ulatrophy** describes gingival atrophy due to a deficient blood supply to the gingival tissues. **Traumatic ulatrophy** is gingival atrophy due to trauma to the gingival tissues.

ulcer *n.* A break in the skin or *mucosa so that the underlying connective tissue is exposed. The margins are inflamed and the surface is covered by slough. *See also* ORAL ULCERATION; APHTHOUS ULCER.

ulcerative colitis *n.* A chronic inflammatory disease of the mucosa and submucosa of the colon manifested clinically by pain, diarrhoea, and rectal bleeding. Oral symptoms may include necrotic mucosal lesions indistinguishable from *aphthous ulcers. The condition is closely related to *Crohn's disease.

(⊕) SEE WEB LINKS
• MedicineNet factsheet on the symptoms, causes, and treatment of ulcerative colitis.

ulitis *n.* An alternative name for *gingivitis.

ultimate strength *n.* *See* STRENGTH.

ultrasonic *adj.* Describing sounds with frequencies above 20,000 Hz and therefore beyond the range of human hearing. An **ultrasonic cleaner** is a piece of equipment that creates high-frequency vibrations in a fluid-filled container; it is used to remove debris and particulate matter from dental instruments and appliances by a process of *cavitation. The fluid is usually an enzymatic *detergent designed to digest biological material. This method of cleaning is suitable for stainless steel instruments but is not appropriate for plastic items. **Ultrasonic scaler** *see* SCALER. **Ultrasonic tips** may be used to locate fine root canals when undertaking endodontic therapy.

ultrasound *n.* A technique using ultra-high frequency sound waves (1–20KHz) to visualize soft tissues. Sound waves are produced by mechanical vibrations using a piezoelectric transducer to convert electrical signals into sound waves, which are transmitted through the tissues as a series of pulses. It is becoming increasingly used for disagnostic purposes in the head and neck region in which shorter wave lengths (7–12MHz) are utilized; it is often the first imaging modality of choice for soft tissue lesions including lymph nodes and salivary gland masses. An important advantage of ultrasound as a diagnostic tool is that it is non-ionizing. 📷

Further Reading: Kotecha S., Bhatia P., Rout P. G. J. Diagnostic ultrasound in the head and neck. *Dent Update* 2008;35:529–34.

ultraviolet light *n.* That part of the electromagnetic spectrum having a wavelength between 200 and 400 nanometres and which is shorter than the wavelength of visible light. It was formerly used as a light source for curing resin composite materials but has been replaced by alternative light sources because of its potential health hazard.

undercut *n.* 1. That part of a tooth cavity that provides an area of resistance to withdrawal or removal of a restoration. It is a desirable feature

The classification of units of dental activity

Band	Type of treatment	UDA allowance
1	Diagnosis and preventative advice	1
2	Diagnosis, preventative advice, and one or more restorations	3
3	Diagnosis, preventative advice, and one or more restorations and one or more crowns	12
Emergency treatment		1.2

for an amalgam restoration but is undesirable for cast restorations. 2. That portion of a tooth surface that lies between the gingival margin and the height of contour of the tooth. It is an area in which a prosthetic clasp arm may engage to provide resistance to displacement. 3. The contour of a cross-section of an alveolar ridge that would prevent the vertical placement of a denture or appliance. The depth of undercut can be measured with an undercut *gauge.

underjet *n.* A malocclusion in which the maxillary incisors are measurably within the perimeter of the mandibular incisors.

unerupted *adj.* Describing a tooth or tooth root not having penetrated the oral mucosa.

unilateral *adj.* Pertaining to one side only.

unit *n.* A single undivided whole. A **dental unit** comprises all the equipment, both fixed and mobile, in a dental surgery or clinic which provides the means for delivering dental treatment. An **x-ray unit** is the equipment designed to take radiographs.

United States Department of Health and Human Services (USDHHS) A cabinet-level government organization comprising 12 agencies, including the Food and Drug Administration and the Centers for Disease Control. It is the US government's principal agency for protecting the health of all Americans and providing essential human services, especially for those who are least able to help themselves.

 SEE WEB LINKS
• The United States Department of Health and Human Services website.

United States Occupational Safety and Health Administration (OSHA) A unit of the US Department of Labor, created to develop and promulgate occupational health and safety standards.

SEE WEB LINKS
• The United States Occupational Safety and Health Administration website.

United States Pharmacopeia (USP) The official public standards-setting authority for all prescription and over-the-counter medicines, dietary supplements, and other healthcare products manufactured and sold in the United States. It is a compendium recognized by the Federal Food, Drug and Cosmetic Act as the official source of the descriptions, uses, strengths, and standards of purity for selected drugs.

SEE WEB LINKS
• The website of the US Pharmacopeia.

Unit of Dental Activity (UDA) A method of measuring dentists' activity within the *National Health Service under the new dental contract introduced in 2006. UDAs are banded broadly according to the clinical activity undertaken.

univariate *n.* (in statistics) A process or mathematical expression with only one *variable.

universal curette *n. See* CURETTE.

universal precautions A standard of care developed by the Centers for Disease Control and Prevention (CDC) based on the concept that all blood and body fluids should be treated as infectious because patients with blood-borne infections can be asymptomatic or unaware they are infected. The main role of universal precautions is to protect the healthcare worker and every individual in their care and reduce the opportunities for transmission of micro-organisms. The relevance of universal precautions to other aspects of disease transmission has been recognized and in 1996 the CDC expanded the concept and changed the term to *standard precautions.

SEE WEB LINKS
• Guidelines for infection control in dental healthcare settings from the Centers for Disease Control and Prevention.

universal tooth designation system *n.* *See* TOOTH NOTATION.

unloading reflex The reflex inhibition of the muscles of mastication which occurs when food or other material between the jaws suddenly breaks or collapses and which helps stop the jaws forcefully coming together.

unmet need *n. See* NEED.

upper face height *n. See* FACE HEIGHT.

upper removable appliance (URA) *n. See* ORTHODONTIC APPLIANCE.

urethane dimethacrylate (UDMA) *n.* A high-viscosity, high molecular weight liquid *monomer used to form the resin base of some *resin composite restorative materials.

urticaria (nettle rash, hives, weal) *n.* A skin reaction that results in slightly elevated patches that are redder or paler than the surrounding skin and often are accompanied by itching. It is caused by the release of *histamine. It may be **acute**, representing an allergic response to allergens such as strawberries or seafood, or **chronic**, where it may last for years. It can involve the lips, eyes, and tongue (**angio-oedema, angioneurotic oedema**), which can swell rapidly; this constitutes a medical emergency. Treatment is by antihistamines.

usual, customary and reasonable (UCR) **plan** *n.* A dental benefits plan in the US that determines benefits based on a community's usual, customary, and reasonable fee criteria.

usual fee *See* FEE.

uveoparotitis (uveoparotid fever) *n.* Inflammation of the uvea (iris, ciliary body, and choroid) of the eye, low-grade fever, swelling of the parotid salivary gland, and facial nerve palsy. It is a symptom of *sarcoidosis. Also known as **Heerfordt's syndrome** [C. F. Heerfordt (1871–1953), Danish ophthalmologist].

uvula *n.* A small soft tissue extension on the posterior border of the soft palate that hangs from the roof of the mouth. It consists of muscle, connective tissue, and mucous membrane. It plays an important role in speech. Dehydration, excessive smoking, infection, and allergic reactions can cause the uvula to swell (**uvulitis**). A congenital cleft can result in a split uvula (**bifid uvula**).

u

vaccination *n.* A means of producing immunity (*immunization) to a disease by the administration of a preparation of antigenic material (**vaccine**) to stimulate the formation of appropriate antibodies. Vaccination is usually given by injection and over two or three stages to reduce the potentially unpleasant side-effects.

vacuum formed appliance *n.* *See* ORTHODONTIC APPLIANCE.

vacuum mixing *n.* *See* MIXING, VACUUM.

validity *n.* 1. The degree to which data or the results of a study are correct. 2. The extent to which a clinical sign or test is a true indicator of the disease being tested.

vallate *adj.* Having a surrounding wall or rim. *See also* PAPILLA.

valve antiretraction A valve or device integrated into a variety of dental instruments connected to *dental unit waterlines (DUWLs). They are used in the patient's mouth (e.g. ultrasonic scalers, turbine and conventional handpieces) to prevent back siphonage of oral fluids into DUWLs. The requirement for antiretraction devices has been emphasized by studies that demonstrated that oral fluids can be retracted into DUWLs during instrument use. The detection of oral bacterial species and other human-derived microbial pathogens and potential pathogens in dental unit water has provided convincing evidence for probable failure of antiretraction devices. Currently, best practice recommends that dental handpieces should be operated to discharge water and air for a minimum of 20–30 seconds after each patient to flush out patient material and oral fluids that may have been retracted into the handpiece air, or waterlines.

Further Reading: Coleman D. C., O'Donnell M. J., Shore A. C., Swan J., Russell, R. J. The role of manufacturers in reducing biofilms in dental unit waterlines. *Journal of Dentistry* 2007;35:701–11.

Van Buchem's syndrome (generalized cortical hyperostosis) An inherited skeletal *dysplasia resulting in an excessive deposition of endosteal bone throughout the skeleton. It is characterized by enlargement of the lower jaw and thickening of the long bones and the top of the skull. The face may appear swollen with some facial paralysis and deafness. There may also be widening of the bridge of the nose and angles of the mandible. The symptoms are not painful and there is no bone tenderness. It was first described by Van Buchem, a Dutch physician, in 1955. *See also* HYPEROSTOSIS.

vancomycin *n.* A glycopeptide *antibiotic used in the *prophylaxis and treatment of serious life-threatening infections caused by Gram-positive bacteria. It has been given as a prophylactic measure to patients about to receive invasive dental treatment and who are considered to be at special risk or who have a history of infective *endocarditis; however, the *National Institute for Health and Clinical Excellence (NICE) clinical guideline 64 recommends that *antibiotic prophylaxis should no longer be offered routinely for defined interventional procedures. Vancomycin is delivered by slow intravenous infusion. Trade name: **Vancocin**.

Vancouver citation system A referencing system which uses a number series to indicate references. Bibliographies list these in numerical order as they appear in the text. Vancouver style is so named as it is based on the work of a group, first meeting in Vancouver in 1978, which became the International Committee of Medical Journal Editors (ICMJE). *See also* HARVARD CITATION SYSTEM.

Van der Woude syndrome *n.* *See* LIP PITS.

vapour (*US* **vapor)** *n.* The gaseous form of a solid or liquid, subsequent to its change in state due to alteration in the heat or pressure of the environment or to an alteration of both.

variable 1. *adj.* Able to vary in quantity or magnitude. 2. *n.* The properties of an object which can take on different values. A **continuous variable** can be found at any point on a continuous scale (e.g. height). A **dependent variable (response variable)** is a factor whose values in different treatment conditions are compared: that is, the researcher is interested in determining if the value of the dependent variable varies when the values of another variable (the **independent variable**) are varied, and by how much; the independent variable is said to cause an apparent change in, or simply affect, the dependent variable. A **dichotomous variable** has two categories (e.g. gender: male and female). A **discrete variable** can be found only at fixed points and is expressed in whole units or mutually exclusive categories (e.g. numbers of teeth). **Interval data** is measured on a scale of which the intervals are equal. **Nominal variables** classify *data into categories (e.g. male, female). **Ordinal variables** rank data according to degree; they indicate only that one data point is ranked higher or lower than another. A **predictor variable** tries to predict values of another variable (the **outcome variable**). A **quantitative variable** takes a numerical value e.g. DMF score; a **qualitative variable** takes a non-numerical value or defines a characteristic e.g. sex (M or F).

variance *n.* (in statistics) A measure of variability. *See also* ANALYSIS OF VARIANCE.

varicella *n. See* CHICKENPOX.

varicosities *n.* Enlarged and superficial veins or other blood vessels. They increase with age and are common underneath the tongue.

varnish, cavity *See* CAVITY VARNISH.

varnish, fluoride *See* FLUORIDE VARNISH.

vascular *adj.* Relating to or supplied with blood vessels.

vasoconstrictor *n.* An agent that causes constriction of blood vessels which reduces local blood flow to an area, and temporarily raises blood pressure. Vasoconstrictors such as *adrenaline (epinephrine) and *felypressin may be added to dental local analgesic agents to prolong their effectiveness. They also reduce local haemorrhage, which can be helpful during surgical procedures. Intravenous deposition should be avoided as *hypertension may occur. Vasoconstrictors have a rapid effect on mucous membranes and may be used to relieve nasal congestion. *Compare* VASODILATOR.

vasodentine *n.* A modified form of *dentine, with branching blood vessels but lacking dentinal tubules, such as is found in marine fishes of the cod family.

vasodilator *n.* An agent that causes widening of the blood vessels and therefore an increase in blood flow. Vasodilators are used to lower the blood pressure in cases of *hypertension. *Glyceryl trinitrate (GTN) increases the blood

flow to the heart and is used to relieve or prevent *angina. *Compare* VASOCONSTRICTOR.

vasomotor *adj.* Controlling the muscular walls of blood vessels creating either expansion or contraction and therefore modifying their diameter. A **vasomotor nerve** is any nerve, usually belonging to the *autonomic nervous system, that controls the passage of blood through blood vessels by its action on the muscular walls or its action on the heartbeat.

vasopressin (anti-diuretic hormone, ADH) *n.* A hormone secreted by the *pituitary gland that causes constriction of the blood vessels and increases the reabsorption of water by the kidneys.

vasovagal attack Excessive activity of the vagus nerve resulting in a slowing of the heart and a drop in blood pressure which leads to fainting (*syncope).

vault, palatal *n.* 1. The arched form of the maxillary palate. 2. The form of a denture adapted to the maxillary palate.

Veau's cleft classification *See* CLEFT CLASSIFICATION.

Veau's operation [V. Veau, (1871–1949), French surgeon] A surgical technique for the repair of a cleft palate which includes dissection and suturing of the nasal mucosa.

vegetation *n.* A mesh of *fibrin and *platelets that can form on the surface of heart valves in patients suffering from infective *endocarditis; it can trap micro-organisms present in the bloodstream.

vehicle *n.* Any substance, usually a liquid, that acts as the medium in which a drug is administered.

Veillonella *n.* A genus of non-motile, *Gram-negative bacterial diplococci that are part of the normal flora of the mouth and the intestinal and respiratory tracts. **Veillonella** species have been isolated from plaque and have the ability to use lactic acid produced by other bacterial species to generate energy for growth. *Veillonella alcalescens* has been isolated from the flora of periodontal pockets and may be associated with the periodontal disease process.

vein *n.* (*adj.* **venous**) A blood vessel conveying blood towards the heart. Only the pulmonary veins carry oxygenated blood. Small veins (**venules**) drain blood from the capillaries and unite to form a vein. The walls of a vein consist of three layers: an inner endothelium (**tunica**

V

interna, tunica intima), a middle smooth muscle layer (**tunica media**), and an outer fibrous tissue layer (**tunica adventitia**). The walls are thinner and less elastic than those of arteries. Unlike arteries, the larger veins contain valves which assist the flow of blood back to the heart. Veins, especially those in the legs, can become enlarged and twisted (**varicosed**). See also Appendix E for the principal veins of the head and neck.

veneer *n.* A layer of tooth-coloured material, usually porcelain (**indirect veneers**), or composite resin fabricated in the mouth (**direct veneers**), attached to the surface of a tooth frequently used to improve aesthetics by modifying the colour, shape, or position of a tooth. It may be likened to a false finger nail. The tooth normally requires some enamel reduction to accommodate the thickness of the veneer but provides a more conservative restorative technique than crowning. The veneer may have no incisal involvement, be extended to the incisal edge, or overlap the incisal edge. Palatal veneers may be used to restore tooth loss (usually due to acid erosion), reduce dentine sensitivity, restore aesthetics, or to protect the tooth pulp. 📷

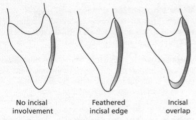

| No incisal involvement | Feathered incisal edge | Incisal overlap |

Types of veneer preparations

ventricle *n.* 1. Either of the two inferior thick-walled muscular chambers of the heart. 2. One of the four fluid-filled cavities within the brain.

vermilion border *n.* The junction between the lip (*vermilion zone) and the facial skin.

vermilion zone The red margin of the upper and lower lip that extends from the exterior edge of the intra-oral labial *mucosa to the extra-oral junction of the lips with surrounding facial skin. It is a thinly *keratinized layer of stratified squamous *epithelium deeply penetrated by well-vascularized dermal papillae which impart the typical red appearance of the lips. It is frequently the site of *herpetic lesions.

verruca vulgaris (common wart) *n.* A benign growth on the skin caused by infection with the human papillomavirus (HPV). They are characterized by small raised swellings with a roughened surface usually found on the hands, knees, or feet. Treatment is by the application of salicylic acid but cryotherapy with liquid nitrogen is probably more effective. *See also* PAPILLOMA.

verruciform *adj.* A wart-like appearance projecting above the surface of the tissue.

verrucous carcinoma *n. See* CARCINOMA.

vertebra *n.* (*pl.* **vertebrae**) One of the 33 bones which form the backbone. The seventh cervical vertebra (C7) is known as the **vertebra prominens** due to its long spinous process.

vertical bitewing radiograph *See* BITEWING RADIOGRAPH.

vertical bone loss An abnormal decrease in alveolar bone on one proximal surface of a tooth in comparison to the tooth on the adjacent side. This uneven reduction in the height of the alveolar bone is less common than horizontal bone loss and produces an infrabony *pocket. *See also* PERIODONTAL DISEASE.

vertical dimension 1. A vertical measurement of the face between two points located one above the oral cavity and one below it. 2. The vertical height of the face recorded with the teeth in occlusion. The vertical dimension may be reduced by attrition of the natural or artificial teeth, the total loss of the natural dentition, or the resorption of the alveolar bone. The vertical dimension may be increased by modification of the natural or artificial teeth. The **vertical rest dimension** is the vertical dimension with the lower jaw in the rest position with minimum muscular activity; it is a measurement used in prosthetic treatment when assessing the correct aesthetic proportion of the face; it can be measured using a Willis bite *gauge.

vertical maxillary excess (VME) *n.* A vertical *skeletal discrepancy in which there is excessive gingival tissue visible either at rest or when smiling.

vesicant *n.* A substance that causes blistering of the skin or mucous membrane.

vesicle *n.* (*adj.* **vesicular**) A small blister on the skin or mucous membrane containing a clear fluid (*serum). It is a characteristic of many lesions including *herpes simplex, recurrent herpes, *varicella, *erythema multiforme, *pemphigus vulgaris, and *pemphigoid.

vestibular band One of the two processes (the other being the *dental lamina) formed from the *primary epithelial band at about the 7th week of intrauterine life. It eventually develops into the *vestibule separating the lips and cheeks from the teeth and gingivae.

vestibule *n.* That part of the oral cavity bounded anteriorly and laterally by the lips and the cheeks, posteriorly and medially by the teeth or gingivae, and above and below by the reflections of the mucosa from the lips and cheeks to the gingivae. It extends posteriorly to the distobuccal end of the retromolar pad.

vestibuloplasty *n.* Any of a series of surgical procedures designed to restore *alveolar ridge height by repositioning muscles attaching to the buccal, labial, and lingual aspects of the jaws. It may be undertaken for many reasons, such as to deepen the vestibular trough, reposition the *frenum or muscle attachments, or to broaden the zone of attached gingiva after periodontal treatment.

vibrating line *n.* An imaginary line drawn between the soft and hard *palate, marking the division between the moveable tissue and the immovable tissues supported by bone.

vibrator *n.* A machine with a vibrating plate used to remove air bubbles from plaster and investment materials during mixing.

Vickers hardness test A method of testing the hardness of a material by using a diamond indenter that produces a square indent on almost any metallic material. It is indicative of the resistance to wear and scratching. The **Vickers hardness number (VHN)** is a function of the test force divided by the surface area of the indent. *See also* BRINELL HARDNESS TEST; KNOOP HARDNESS TEST.

villiform *adj.* Having hair-like projections.

Vincent's angina *n. See* GINGIVITIS, NECROTIZING.

Vincent's gingivitis *n. See* GINGIVITIS, NECROTIZING.

vinculum *n.* (*pl.* **vincula**) A connecting band of tissue or anatomical ligament that produces limitation of movement.

Vipeholm study A classical study undertaken between 1945 and 1953 in the Vipeholm Hospital, Sweden, to investigate the relationship between *caries and the ingestion of sugar. It concluded that the risk of sugar increasing caries activity is greatest if the sugar is consumed between meals

and is in the form in which the tendency to be retained on the surfaces of the teeth is pronounced with a transiently high concentration of sugar on those surfaces. This study would now be considered as unethical.

Further Reading: Gustafsson B. E., Quensel C. E., Lanke L. S., Lundqvist C., Grahnen H., Bonow B.E., Krasse B. The Vipeholm Dental Caries Study. The effect of different levels of carbohydrate intake on caries activity in 436 individuals observed for five years. *Acta Odont Scand* 1954;11: 232-364.

viraemia *n.* The presence of a virus in the bloodstream either as free virus or cell associated.

Virchow's angle [R. L. K. Virchow (1821–1902), German pathologist] The angle formed by a line joining the nasofrontal suture and the most prominent point on the lower border of the maxillary *alveolar process with a line joining the lower border of the orbit to the external auditory meatus.

virologist *n.* A person who specializes in the field of *virology.

virology *n.* The scientific study of viruses and virus-like agents, and the diseases caused by them.

virus *n.* (*adj.* **viral**) A non-cellular infectious biological entity that is unable to grow or multiply outside a host cell. An individual virus is called a viral particle or **virion** and consists of nucleic acid (DNA or RNA) contained within a protein coat (**capsid**). Viruses are much smaller than bacteria, cannot be seen under a light microscope, and are too small to be trapped by filters. The shape of the capsid can vary considerably between different viruses. Some viruses contain an additional outer envelope surrounding the capsid consisting of a host cell membrane (**enveloped viruses**) such as hepatitis B virus (DNA virus) and HIV virus (RNA virus), whereas other viruses lack such an envelope (**naked viruses**) e.g. poliovirus (RNA virus). Many scientists consider that viruses are non-living for a variety of reasons; one important feature that distinguishes viruses from all other living organisms is that viruses do not have cells. However, they do have genes and they evolve by natural selection like all other living organisms. Viruses cause a wide range of infectious diseases in humans including measles, mumps, herpes, chickenpox, influenza, polio, and AIDS. Protection against infection by some viruses can be afforded by *vaccines. Some currently available antiviral drugs are designed to help combat viral infections caused by HIV and herpes viruses.

viscerocranium *n.* The part of the skull which comprises the facial skeleton.

vital *adj.* Necessary to or pertaining to life. It is the description applied to a tooth pulp containing living tissue. *Compare* NON-VITAL.

vital capacity *n.* The volume of air that can be expelled from the lungs from a position of full inspiration, with no limit to the duration of expiration.

vitality *n.* The state of being alive. **Pulp vitality** may be tested by a thermal or electrical stimulus (**vitality test**), a positive response by the patient indicating possible vitality. A thermal stimulus may be either extreme cold, such as by the application of *ethyl chloride to the surface of the tooth crown, or heat from hot *gutta-percha. An electrical stimulus can be provided by one of the many commercially available electrical pulp testers which are generally considered to be more accurate than thermal testing.

Vitallium® *n.* The trade name for an alloy of 60% cobalt, 20% chromium, and 5% molybdenum. It is used in the construction of prostheses because of its light weight and resistance to corrosion. Vitallium was formerly used for dental implants but has now been largely replaced by *titanium.

vitalometer *n.* A device for applying variable intensities of an electrical current to individual teeth to measure the level of reaction, and hence the *vitality of the dental pulp.

vital signs Signs that a patient is alive based on a number of measurements, including body temperature, *blood pressure, *heart rate, and *respiration rate; it can also include an assessment of consciousness and urine output.

vitamin *n.* Any of a group of substances that are required in very small amounts for healthy growth and development; they cannot be synthesized by the body and are essential components of the diet. They are either water-soluble (e.g. vitamin B complex and vitamin C) or fat-soluble (e.g. vitamins A, D, E, and K).

vitamin A (retinol) A fat-soluble vitamin found especially in milk products, egg yolk, and liver and formed in the body from β-carotene found in some vegetables (e.g. carrots, and cabbage). Retinol is essential for growth, vision, and the maintenance of mucous tissue.

vitamin B₁ (thiamin, aneurine) A colourless water-soluble compound active in the form of thiamin pyrophosphate. It is a *coenzyme which plays an important role in helping the body convert carbohydrates and fat into energy. It is present in cereals, beans, nuts, meat, and

potatoes. A deficiency of vitamin B_1 can lead to **beriberi**.

vitamin B₂ (riboflavin) A water-soluble compound. Like its close relative *vitamin B_1, vitamin B_2 plays a crucial role in certain metabolic reactions, particularly the conversion of carbohydrates into sugar. It is required for the health of the mucous membranes and helps with the absorption of iron and vitamin B_6. It is found in milk, liver, and eggs. A deficiency of vitamin B_2 can lead to cracks at the corners of the mouth (*angular cheilitis), inflammation of the mouth and tongue, eye disorders, and skin lesions.

vitamin B₆ (pyridoxine) A water-soluble compound found in most foods.

vitamin B₁₂ (cyanocobalamin) A water-soluble compound exclusively synthesized by bacteria and found primarily in meat, eggs, and dairy products. Vitamin B_{12} is necessary for the synthesis of red blood cells, the maintenance of the nervous system, and growth and development in children; a deficiency, usually due to a failure to absorb the vitamin in the intestine, affects nearly all body tissues, especially those containing rapidly dividing cells, and can lead to *anaemia and degeneration of the nervous system.

vitamin C (ascorbic acid) A water-soluble compound with *antioxidant properties which help to counter the detrimental effects of free radicals produced by the body's normal metabolic processes. Vitamin C is essential in maintaining healthy connective tissues and the integrity of cell walls, and synthesizing collagen. A deficiency leads to *scurvy. Humans are unable to synthesize vitamin C and the main source is citrus fruits and vegetables.

vitamin D A fat-soluble compound occurring mainly in two forms, **ergocalciferol (vitamin D₂)** manufactured by plants and **cholecalciferol (vitamin D₃)** produced in the skin exposed to sunlight. Vitamin D has an important role in regulating the calcium and phosphorous levels in the blood, and in promoting bone formation and *mineralization. Good sources of vitamin D are liver and fish oils. A deficiency due to poor diet or lack of sunlight can lead to decalcified bones and the development of *rickets and *osteomalacia.

vitamin E (tocopherol) A fat-soluble vitamin in eight forms with *antioxidant properties thought to stabilize cell membranes by preventing oxidation of their unsaturated fatty acid components. It is found in vegetable oils, eggs, butter, and wholemeal cereals.

vitamin K A fat-soluble compound essential for the synthesis of a number of blood clotting factors including *prothrombin. Vitamin K is synthesized by bacteria in the large intestine, and therefore a dietary deficiency is rare. It is also widely available in green leaf vegetables and meat.

vitremer *n. See* CEMENT.

vocal folds (vocal cords) Two folds of tissue covered with mucous membrane stretched across the larynx to form a narrow slit. They vibrate, modulating the flow of air being expelled from the lungs during phonation.

vocational dental practitioner (VDP) A recently qualified dentist, formerly called a **vocational trainee**, who continues to train and work during the first year of practice under the guidance of an experienced general dental practitioner (vocational dental practitioner trainer) as part of the **vocational training scheme**. It is a requirement for dentists qualifying at a UK dental school to complete one year's vocational training at an approved practice in order to have their name entered on a National Health Service dental list.

(⊕) SEE WEB LINKS

• NHS web pages giving an overview of career opportunities for dental students within the NHS.

vocational dental technician (VDT) A recently qualified dental technician undergoing a training scheme to enhance existing vocational skills and broaden experience within the profession of dental technology. It is a Scottish provision for newly qualified dental technicians within the European Economic Area (EEA).

(⊕) SEE WEB LINKS

• The website for the National Health Service (NHS) Education for Scotland.

vocational related qualification (VRQ) A type of award developed independently by individual awarding bodies rather than a specific national award, and having a vocational focus. The level 3 VRQ in dental nursing accredited by the **Qualifications and Curriculum Authority**

(QCA) allows learners to develop the knowledge required for employment and career progression within the dental sector. *See also* NATIONAL VOCATIONAL QUALIFICATION.

vomer *n.* A somewhat quadrilateral-shaped bone forming the posterior and lower portion of the nasal septum. It is one of the unpaired bones of the facial skeleton located in the mid-sagittal plane. It is bounded anteriorly by the ethmoid bone and the septal cartilage, inferiorly by the maxillae and the palatine bones, and superiorly by the sphenoid bone; the posterior border is free, concave, and separates the *choanae.

von Ebner's glands *See* EBNER'S GLANDS.

von Ebner's lines *See* EBNER'S LINES.

von Korff's fibres *See* KORFF'S FIBRES.

von Willebrand's disease [A. von Willebrand (1870–1949), Swedish physician] A hereditary *blood coagulation abnormality arising from a qualitative or quantitative deficiency of **von Willebrand factor**, a glycoprotein that is required for normal platelet adhesion. It binds with *factor VIII and prevents its rapid breakdown within the blood. It is characterized by bleeding from mucous membranes, nose bleeds, gingival haemorrhage, and gastrointestinal blood loss. Excessive haemorrhage may occur after dental treatment and surgery.

vulcanite *n.* A thermo-hardening material made from an irreversible chemical reaction where the physical properties of an *elastomer are changed by causing it to react with sulphur or other cross-linking agents (**vulcanization**). Vulcanization typically decreases plasticity and improves resistance to swelling by organic liquids. Vulcanite was originally used as a baseplate material for complete and partial dentures prior to the use of *acrylic resin; it was patented by the Goodyear Company in 1864. Although it had good dimensional stability it had poor aesthetics and colour stability, deteriorating with time to a dark red or brown colour.

v

Waldeyer's ring [H. W. G. Waldeyer (1836–1921), German anatomist] A band of *lymphoid tissue that encircles the *nasopharynx and *oropharynx. It consists of the lymphatic tissue of the pharynx, the palatine *tonsil, and the lingual tonsil, as well as other smaller collections of lymphoid tissue in the region.

wall *n.* One of the enclosing surfaces of a tooth cavity. It is named after the tooth surface towards which it faces (e.g. mesial, distal, buccal, lingual, gingival, incisal). The **enamel wall** is that part of the prepared cavity wall that consists of enamel; it meets the external unprepared surface of the tooth (cavosurface) at the *cavosurface angle.

Wand® A computer-controlled dental local anaesthetic injection device. The computer-controlled system maintains constant pressure and volume ratios of the anaesthetic solution regardless of variation in tissue resistance. The system is designed to reduce the incidence of pain during injection.

Ward's wax carver *n. See* CARVER.

warfarin *n.* An anticoagulant used to reduce the risk of thrombosis; it may be prescribed for patients with prosthetic heart valves. Although there is the potential for excessive haemorrhage following dental surgery, patients who require dental surgical procedures in primary care and who have an INR (*international normalized ratio) below 4.0 should continue warfarin therapy without dose adjustment. Trade names: **Marevan, Panwarfin, Coumadin, Sofarin**.

Further Reading: Randall C. Surgical management of the primary care dental patient on warfarin. *Dent Update* 2005;32 (7):414–16, 419–20,
Perry D., Noakes T., Helliwell P. Guidelines for the management of patients on oral anticoagulants requiring dental surgery. *Br Dent J* 2007;203:389–93.

wart *n. See* VERRUCA VULGARIS.

Warthin's tumour *See* ADENOLYMPHOMA.

Warwick James elevator *n. See* ELEVATOR.

washer-disinfector An automated machine designed to clean, decontaminate, and thermally disinfect **reusable invasive medical devices** (RIMD) used in dentistry such as dental instruments. There are a number of automated stages including pre-rinsing, cleaning, interim rinsing, thermal disinfection, final rinsing, and drying. Disinfection is achieved by flushing with water at 90°C (194°F) for 1–10 minutes. The machine is unsuitable for heat-sensitive items. The specification of the washer-disinfector should comply with requirements of EN ISO 15883, parts 1 & 2. Each washer-disinfector should be fitted with an independent process monitoring system in accordance with EN ISO 15883 part 1. When lumened devices, such as dental handpieces, are being reprocessed, the washer-disinfector should be provided with load carriers that permit the irrigation of the lumened device. Washer-disinfectors and accessories should be specified, installed, validated, commissioned, tested, and operated in accordance with EN ISO 15883, parts 1,2 & 5 or UK standard HTM 01–05. Washer-disinfectors should be subject to planned preventative maintenance.

waste *n. See* CLINICAL WASTE.

water fluoridation *See* FLUORIDATION.

water irrigator *See* ORAL IRRIGATOR.

water–powder ratio *See* RATIO.

wax *n.* An ester of ethylene glycol and two fatty acids or a combination of other fatty alcohols with fatty acids. Dental waxes are compounds of different waxes combined to provide the appropriate physical characteristics. **Baseplate wax** is a hard pink wax used for making occlusal rims and for holding artificial teeth to baseplates during the fabrication of dentures; it is composed mainly of beeswax, paraffin, and a colouring agent. **Beeswax** is a natural wax with a high melting point (62–64°C, 144–147°F) which historically was formerly used in the *lost wax process; it is a constituent of other dental waxes and may be utilized in the manufacture of waxed dental *floss. **Bite registration wax** is a metal-impregnated (usually aluminium) wax in sheet form; it is used to record the occlusal relationships between a patient's opposing arches (*occlusal record) and to later transfer this relationship to the cast for articulation; it is hard at mouth temperature. **Carding wax** is used mainly to form a box around impressions of the mouth prior to pouring a *plaster of Paris or *gypsum stone cast; it is red in colour and soft and pliable at room temperature. **Carnauba wax** is a hard, high melting point wax used to control the melting temperature of many dental waxes. **Disclosing (pressure indicator) wax** is painted onto the mucosal surface of a denture to identify areas of unequal pressure; the wax flows away from the area needing relief. **Inlay (casting, burnout) wax** is used to fabricate wax patterns for cast alloy inlays and removable partial dentures; it is soft when heated but hardens at room or mouth temperature when it can be carved with great accuracy. It is capable of close adaptation to the prepared surfaces and minimal distortion after carving. It is available in blue, green, ivory, and deep purple sticks. **Low fusing impression wax** flows under controlled pressure and may be used in relining or rebasing complete or partial dentures. **Occlusal indicator wax** is used to indicate occlusal contact areas; it is manufactured in thin strips, about 0.5mm thick, of soft, brightly coloured wax with an adhesive on one surface so that it can be moulded around the previously dried teeth; occlusal contact areas show as perforations in the wax which can then be identified with a marking pencil. **Sticky wax** is composed of beeswax, paraffin, and resins and has many uses particularly in the dental laboratory; it is brittle at room temperature and becomes a sticky thick liquid when heated. **Boxing** or **utility wax** is tacky and pliable at room temperature without the addition of heat and is used for adapting impression trays, building up the post-dam area on impressions, or forming a border on preliminary or final impressions. It is usually coloured red or white and available in stick form; it may also be supplied in rope form (**rope wax**).

wax carver (Ward's) *n. See* CARVER.

waxing up The contouring of a wax pattern or a wax denture base to produce the desired shape.

wax pattern A *wax model of an *inlay or metal denture casting. It is invested in casting *investment and, when heated, the wax is eliminated and the resulting space is replaced with metal alloy (*lost wax process).

weaning *n.* The act of substituting other food for the mother's milk in the diet of a child. If sugar is added to bottle milk, or reservoir feeders are supplemented with fruit syrup, there is a strong relationship between their use and the incidence of dental *caries.

wear *n. See* TOOTH WEAR.

wear facet *n.* A flat polished area on the biting (occlusal or incisal) surface of a tooth produced by physiological or *parafunctional contact of an opposing tooth or teeth.

Weber's glands [M. I. Weber (1795–1875), German anatomist] *n.* Any of the various *mucous secreting (**muciparous**) glands on either side of the posterior border of the tongue.

Wedelstaedt chisel *n. See* CHISEL.

wedge *n.* A small triangular-shaped piece of wood or plastic used to temporarily separate two teeth or to apply pressure to a *matrix band and prevent a gingival overhang of restorative material when restoring a tooth that has a cavity involving the proximal surface. Plastic wedges have been used because of their ability to transmit light when using a light-cured restorative material.

Weil's basal layer *n. See* BASAL LAYER OF WEIL.

Weisbach's angle [A. W. Weisbach (1837–1914), Austrian anthropologist] *n.* The angle formed at the alveolar point between lines passing from the basion and from the middle of the frontonasal suture. It is a *craniometric measurement.

wet bonding *n.* A term applied to bonding of resin composite to dentine in which the dentine is damp dried and not completely dried or *desiccated, since desiccating has been linked to post-operative sensitivity and low bond strengths.

wetting agent *n.* A substance that reduces the surface tension of water e.g. a substance applied to the surface of a wax pattern prior to investment to produce a smooth and bubble free surface. **Wettability** is the relative degree to which a fluid will spread into or coat a solid surface.

Wharton's duct (submandibular duct, submaxillary duct) [T. Wharton (1614–73), English anatomist] *n.* A tube about 5cm long which drains the saliva from the submandibular (submaxillary) salivary gland and opens into the oral cavity via a narrow orifice at the side of the lingual frenum.

Whitehead's varnish [W. Whitehead (1840–1913), English surgeon] *n.* A liquid containing iodoform, benzoin, storax, balsam of tolu, and solvent ether. It may be applied to ribbon gauze and used as a dressing in the treatment of inflammatory conditions such as *alveolitis (dry socket) and as a post-operative dressing after maxillectomy. Iodoform has

w

marked anaesthetic properties when applied to mucous membranes.

white spot lesion *n.* A visibly lighter area on the enamel surface which may be diagnostic of *fluorosis or early *caries.

whitlow (paronychia) *n.* A localized infection of the nail folds. It is associated with secondary infection with *Candida albicans* and occurs mainly in those who habitually engage in wet work. It is characterized by pain in the affected fingers, often accompanied by infection of the lymph vessels and nodes (**lymphangitis**) lasting up to several weeks. It can also be caused by *Herpes simplex* (**herpetic whitlow**) and is therefore a potential hazard in clinical dentistry if protective gloves are not worn when treating a patient who is infected.

Widman flap *See* FLAP.

Wilcoxon's rank sum test [F. Wilcoxon (1892–1965), American statistician] *See* MANN–WHITNEY TEST.

Williams probe *See* PROBE.

Williams syndrome *n.* A hereditary condition caused by a chromosomal defect, first described by J. C. P. Williams, a New Zealand cardiologist, in 1961. It is characterized by large eyes, a wide mouth, a small chin, high blood calcium level, short stature, and learning difficulties.

(((∰))) SEE WEB LINKS
• The website of the Williams Syndrome Foundation.

Willis bite gauge *See* GAUGE.

Winter's elevator *See* ELEVATOR.

Winter's lines A method of assessing the angulation and extent of impaction of mandibular third molars, first described by G. B. Winter in 1926. A line drawn along the occlusal surfaces of the erupted mandibular molars demonstrates the axial inclination of the wisdom tooth; this also gives some indication of the depth of the tooth in the mandible. A second line, extending from the surface of the bone distal to the third molar to the crest of the interdental septum between the first and second molars, indicates the amount of alveolar bone enclosing the impacted tooth. A third perpendicular line is drawn from the second line to the amelo-cemental junction on the mesial surface of the impacted tooth (elevator application point) and is used to determine the depth of impaction of the tooth within the bone.

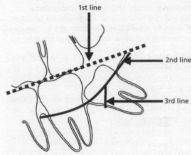

Winter's lines

wire, wrought *n.* A wire formed by drawing a cast structure through a die into a desired shape and size; used in dentistry for partial denture clasps and orthodontic appliances.

wiring *n.* An arrangement of a wire or wires. **Circumferential wiring** is used as a method of immobilization of a jaw fracture; a splint is held in place by wires passing around the bone and through the soft tissues with the ends exiting in the oral cavity. **Continuous loop (multiple loop) wiring** is a means of jaw fracture fixation and reduction by wiring the teeth.

wisdom tooth A lay term for a third molar tooth. They are generally thought to be called wisdom teeth because they appear so late after the other teeth erupt, at an age where one is supposedly wiser than as a child. Their eruption period is normally between the ages of 17 and 25, although they may erupt considerably later or not at all. *See* MOLAR, PERMANENT MAXILLARY THIRD.

witness *n. See* EXPERT WITNESS.

wood point (wooden interdental cleaner) An *oral hygiene aid made from wood such as birch, bass, or linden wood shaped with a flat surface tapering to a point. It is used to remove *plaque and food debris from proximal tooth surfaces, wide interdental spaces, exposed root surfaces, and *furcation areas in periodontally involved teeth. Wood points may be impregnated with *chemotherapeutic agents. 🔲

working length The length of a root canal measured from a fixed point at the apical region to a fixed point on the crown or root face of a tooth used to define the depth of instrumentation during *root canal therapy.

working side The side towards which the mandible is moving during *mastication i.e. opposite to the *balancing side.

working time The period of time that a material can be manipulated without a negative effect on its properties; the working time includes the *mixing time and the *manipulation time.

Workplace (Health, Safety and Welfare) Regulations 1992 Legislation introduced by the UK parliament in 1992 to cover a wide range of basic health, safety, and welfare issues. The regulations apply to most workplaces, including dental clinics, practices, and laboratories.

(⊕) SEE WEB LINKS

• The Workplace (Health, Safety and Welfare) Regulations 1992 (Office of Public Sector Information).

World Health Organization The directing and coordinating authority for health within the United Nations system. It is responsible for providing leadership on global health matters, shaping the health research agenda, setting norms and standards, articulating evidence-based policy options, providing technical support to countries, and monitoring and assessing health trends.

wound *n.* An injury to a tissue or organ caused by an external agent. **Wound healing** is the body's natural process of regenerating dermal or epidermal tissue. There is an initial phase of inflammation with the removal of bacteria and debris and blood coagulation, followed by a proliferative phase with the deposition of *collagen and formation of *granulation tissue, and completed by a final phase of *epithelialization. Healing is described as by **primary intention** when there is a healing together of clean closely opposed wound edges, usually held by sutures, and by **secondary intention** when there is substantial loss of tissue or where the edges of the tissue cannot always be joined during healing. In the latter case a larger clot develops and more *granulation tissue is formed. Healing by secondary intention may occur due to a wound being left open, the presence of infection, excessive trauma, or excessive skin loss. Alveolar socket wound healing following tooth extraction is a complex example of healing by secondary intention.

w

xanthoma *n.* A condition of the skin characterized by irregular yellow nodules particularly on the eyelids, neck, and back. It has been attributed to disturbances of *cholesterol metabolism. A **verruciform xanthoma** is an uncommon solitary xanthoma of the oral tissues usually occurring later in life. It is a painless *benign lesion resembling a *papilloma; it is usually covered with a rough yellowish-white *keratinized layer and is most commonly found on the gingivae or alveolar mucosa. It may occur in response to local trauma but may also be associated with more serious diseases, even immune suppression. It is treated by conservative surgical excision.

X-bite *n. See* BITE.

xenograft (heterograft) *n.* A piece of tissue transplanted or grafted from one species to another species, for example pig to human. Xenograft material may be used in periodontal surgery or bone augmentation for intraosseous *implants. The material is obtained from animals certified disease-free from accredited herds and treated to render it safe and non-*antigenic. *See also* GRAFT.

xerostomia *n.* Abnormal dryness of the mouth resulting from decreased secretion of *saliva. It is characterized by a smooth, red *mucosa, difficulty with speech and eating, reduced taste sensation, a greater incidence of *periodontal disease, an increased potential for cervical and smooth surface *caries, and a tendency towards fungal infections. It also has a detrimental effect on the retention of complete dentures. Xerostomia may be a sign of underlying disease such as *Sjögren's syndrome, *diabetes, and connective tissue diseases, or it may result as a side-effect from medication such as *chemotherapy and some antidepressants, alcohol, radiation therapy, or the taking of drugs such as *cannabis and *methamphetamine. Tumours or trauma to the salivary glands may also reduce salivary secretion. Treatment is usually directed at the underlying condition but where this is impossible it is focused on relieving the symptoms by the use of mouthwashes, saliva substitutes, reservoir *bite guards, sugar-free chewing gum, and extensive oral hygiene instruction and monitoring.

x-rays *n.* High-energy electromagnetic radiation of shorter wavelength than ultraviolet radiation which passes through matter in varying degrees depending on its density. It is used in high doses to treat cancer (*radiotherapy) or in low doses to diagnose disease (diagnostic *radiology) by the production of a visible film which distinguishes between hard and soft tissues (*radiograph).

xylitol *n.* A sugar alcohol (polyol) derived from xylose by reduction of the carbonyl group; it is as sweet as sucrose and is used as a non-cariogenic sweetener in chewing gum and other food products and also as a sugar substitute in diabetic diets.

Xylocaine *n. See* LIGNOCAINE.

yaws (pian, framboesia) *n.* A tropical infectious disease affecting the skin and its underlying tissues. It is characterized by fever, pains, and itching followed by small tumours on the hands, face, legs, and feet. In the final stages there is destructive and deforming lesions of the skin, bone, and *periosteum. Growths on the nasal maxillae can lead to severe damage to the nose and palate. It is caused by the spirochaete *Treponema pertenue* and commonly affects children. Treatment is with antibiotics.

yield point The point at which a material permanently deforms with no increase in load. It is an important physical property of many dental materials.

York Review *See* FLUORIDATION.

zinc *n.* A metallic element which used to be added to *amalgam alloy during manufacture to act as a scavenger for oxygen; however, its presence can cause the amalgam to expand in the presence of moisture, which can lead to tooth fracture. The addition of zinc is now avoided by manufacturing the alloy powder in an oxygen-free inert atmosphere.

zinc chloride *n.* A compound used as an *astringent to control localized bleeding. Absorbent cord may be impregnated with zinc chloride for gingival retraction. It is added to toothpaste as a *desensitizing agent and for its bacteriostatic properties.

zinc oxide cement *See* CEMENT.

zinc oxide eugenol (ZOE) impression paste *n.* A non-elastic irreversible impression material used for relining partial or complete dentures. It is supplied as a **base paste** containing zinc oxide, olive oil, linseed oil, zinc acetate, and a trace of water and a **catalyst paste** containing eugenol, filler, accelerator, gum rosin, and oils. When the two pastes are mixed together, **zinc eugenolate** is formed. The trace of water initiates the reaction and the zinc acetate speeds up the setting process. Eugenol may be substituted with other compounds such as lauric acid to eliminate the odour and taste of eugenol, or for patients allergic to eugenol. The mixed material adheres well to denture bases, has adequate rigidity to prevent distortion of the impression borders, can be added to, has good accuracy of surface detail, and has good dimensional stability. It is, however, difficult to remove from instruments, and because of its adherence to dry skin the lips benefit from protection with petroleum jelly.

zinc phosphate cement *See* CEMENT.

zirconia *n.* A white crystalline oxide of zirconium (zirconium dioxide, ZrO_2) which exists in monoclinic, tetragonal, and cubic forms. **Yttrium tetragonal zirconia polycrystals (Y-TZP)** is the tetragonal form, with the addition of 3% yttrium oxide to act as a stabilizing agent, used as a core material for ceramic crowns and bridges (trade names: **Lava, Cerec, Procera**). The material has high resistance to fracture and degradation by water present in the saliva; it is fabricated using *CAD/CAM technology. Zirconia may also be infiltrated with aluminium (70% aluminium, 30% zirconia) to produce a strong core material. Trade name: **In-Ceram**.

Further Reading: Burke F. J., Ali A., Palin W. M. Zirconia-based all-ceramic crowns and bridges: three case reports. *Dent Update* 2006;33(7):401–2, 405–6, 409–10.

zoning *n.* A method of delineating areas of contamination within an operating environment to simplify, speed up, and make more effective the *decontamination process. Areas that are likely to become contaminated by direct contact or splatter during treatment procedures can be clearly distinguished from those areas unlikely to be directly contaminated.

(((●))) SEE WEB LINKS

• Description of the zoning of areas and the use of barrier protection on the Infection Control Services Ltd website.

Z-plasty *n.* A surgical technique that is used to improve the functional and cosmetic appearance of healing tissue as in the repair of a *cleft lip or in *ankyloglossia. The middle line of the Z-shaped incision is made along the line of greatest tension or contraction, and triangular flaps are raised on opposite sides of the two ends and then transposed.

z-score A statistical measure that quantifies the distance a data point is from the *mean of a data set measured in *standard deviations.

Zsigmondy–Palmer system *n. See* TOOTH NOTATION.

zygomatic arch The arch on the lateral aspect of the skull formed by the union of the zygomatic process of the *temporal bone and temporal process of the *zygomatic bone.

zygomatic bone (malar bone) A paired bone of the skull. It articulates with the *maxilla, the *temporal bone, the *sphenoid bone, and the *frontal bone, and forms part of the orbit. It is situated at the upper and lateral part of the face; it forms the prominence of the cheek, part of the lateral wall and floor of the orbit, and parts of the temporal and infratemporal fossae. It has lateral, temporal, and orbital surfaces and frontal and temporal processes.

Appendix A: Symbols and abbreviations

An asterisk against a word used in a definition indicates that it has its own entry in the main body of text.

∇	*diagnosis	AAMP	American Academy of Maxillofacial Prosthetics
–ve	negative		
+ve	positive	AAO	American Association of Orthodontists
↑	increased		
↓	decreased	AAOGP	American Academy of Orthodontics for the General Practitioner
<	less than		
>	greater than	AAOM	American Academy of Oral Medicine
≤	less than or equal to	AAOMS	American Association of Oral and Maxillofacial Surgeons
≥	greater than or equal to		
≠	not equal to	AAOP	American Academy of Oral Pathology
#	*fracture		
~	approximately	AAP	American Academy of Periodontology; American Academy of Pedodontics
μ	micro (e.g. μg microgram		
1^0	primary		
2^0	secondary	AAPD	American Academy of Pediatric Dentistry
3^0	tertiary		
©	copyright	AAPHD	American Association of Public Health Dentistry
®	registered trade mark		
™	trade mark	ABDSA	Association of British Dental Surgery Assistants
AACD	American Academy of Cosmetic Dentistry	ABG	arterial blood gases
		ABO	American Board of Orthodontists
AACOMS	Academic Advisory Committee in Oral and Maxillofacial Surgery	ABP	American Board of Pedodontics; American Board of Periodontics; American Board of Prosthodontics
AAD	Association of Associate Deans		
AADGP	American Academy of Dental Group Practice	ABSTD	Association of Basic Science Teachers in Dentistry
		ACD	American College of Dentists
AADP	American Academy of Dental Prosthetics	ACDT	Advisory Committee on Dental Training
AADPA	American Academy of Dental Practice Administration	ACLS	advanced cardiac life support
		ACP	American College of Prosthodontists
AADR	American Academy of Dental Radiology	ACPA	American Cleft Palate Association
		ACTH	*adrenocorticotrophic hormone
AADS	American Association of Dental Schools	ADA	American Dental Association; Australian Dental Association
AAE	American Association of Endodontists	ADAA	American Dental Assistants Association
AAGO	American Academy of Gnathologic Orthopedics	ADEE	Association of Dental Education in Europe
AAHD	American Academy of the History of Dentistry; American Academy of Hospital Dentists; American Association of Health and Disabilities	ADH	Association of Dental Hospitals
		ADH	anti-diuretic hormone
		ADHA	American Dental Hygienists Association
AAID	American Association of Implant Dentistry	ADHD	attention deficit hyperactivity disorder

ADI	Association of Dental Implantology (UK)	BADT	British Association of Dental Therapists
ADJ	*amelo-dentinal junction	BAFO	British Association for Forensic Odontology
ADM	Academy of Dental Materials		
ADP	Academy of Denture Prosthetics	BAO	British Association of Orthodontists
ADS	American Denture Society	BAOMS	British Association of Oral and Maxillofacial Surgeons
ADSA	American Dental Students Association		
		BAOS	British Association of Oral Surgeons (formerly British Association of Surgical Dentists)
ADTA	American Dental Trade Association		
AED	*automated external defibrillator		
Ag	*antigen	BASCD	British Association for the Study of Community Dentistry
AHF	antihaemophilic factor		
AIDS	Association of Industrial Dental Surgeons; *acquired human immunodeficiency syndrome	BCC	*basal cell carcinoma
		BChD	Baccalaureus Chirugiae Dentalis (a primary degree from the University of Leeds, equivalent to BDS)
ALS	*advanced life support		
ANUG	acute necrotizing ulcerative *gingivitis	BCLS	basic cardiac life support
		bd	(Latin) *bis die*, twice daily
AOB	anterior open *bite	BDA	*British Dental Association
AOD	Academy of Operative Dentistry	BDEF	British Dental Editors Forum
APL	accredited prior learning	BDentSci	Bachelor in Dental Science
APS	American Prosthodontic Society	BDHA	British Dental Hygienists' Association; now known as the British Society of Dental Hygiene and Therapy (BSDHT)
ARF	annual retention fee (of the General Dental Council, UK)		
ARR	absolute *risk reduction		
ASA	American Society of Anesthesiologists	BDHF	*British Dental Health Foundation
		BDJ	British Dental Journal
ASAAD	American Society for the Advancement of Anesthesia in Dentistry	BDPMA	British Dental Practice Managers Association
		BDRA	British Dental Receptionists Association
ASAASD	American Society for the Advancement of Anesthesia and Sedation in Dentistry		
		BDS	Bachelor of Dental Surgery
		BDSA	British Dental Students' Association
asap	as soon as possible	BDTA	British Dental Trade Association
ASD	atrial septal defect	BES	British Endodontic Society
ASDA	American Society for Dental Aesthetics	BFS	British Fluoridation Society
		bid (b.i.d.)	(Latin) *bis in die*, twice a day
ASDC	American Society of Dentistry for Children	BIDST	British Institute of Dental and Surgical Technologists
ASDHHS	*United States Department of Health and Human Services	BIPP	*bismuth iodoform paraffin paste
		BLS	*basic life support
ASDR	American Society of Dental Radiographers	BMA	*British Medical Association
		BMI	*body mass index
ASGD	American Society of Geriatric Dentistry	BMJ	British Medical Journal
		BMP	*bone morphogenic protein
ASO	American Society of Orthodontists	BMR	*basal metabolic rate
ASOS	American Society of Oral Surgeons	BNF	*British National Formulary
ATDT	Association of Teachers of Dental Technology	BOS	British Orthodontic Society; British Orthoptic Society
ATLS	advanced trauma life support	BP	British Pharmacopoeia; blood pressure; boiling point
AUT	Association of University Teachers		
AV(N)	*atrioventricular (node)	BPS	British Paedodontic Society; British Pharmacological Society
BADN	British Association of Dental Nurses		

BSCD	British Society for Computer assisted learning in Dentistry	CC	chief complaint
BSDH	British Society of Dentistry for the Handicapped	cc	cubic centimetre
		CCCDS	Central Committee for Community Dental Services (British Dental Association)
BSDHT	British Society of Dental Hygiene and Therapy (formerly known as the British Dental Hygienists' Association)	CCCPHD	Central Committee for Community and Public Health Dentistry (British Dental Association)
		CCD	charged couple device
BSDMR	British Society of Dental and Maxillofacial Radiology	CCHADT	Central Council for Health Authority Dental Technology
BSDR	British Society for Dental Research	CCHDS	Central Council for Hospital Dental Services (British Dental Association)
BSE	bovine spongiform encephalopathy		
BSI	British Standards Institute	CCST	Certificate of Completion of Specialist Training
BSMDH	British Society of Medical and Dental Hypnosis	CCU	coronary care unit; critical care unit
BSOM	British Society for Oral Medicine	CCUDT&RW	Central Committee for University Dental Teachers and Research Workers (British Dental Association)
BSP	British Society of Periodontology		
BSPD	British Society of Paediatric Dentistry		
BSRD	British Society for Restorative Dentistry	CDA	certified dental assistant (US)
		CDC	Centers for Disease Control (US)
BSS	black silk suture	CDDS	Council of Deans of Dental Schools
BSSO	British Society for the Study of Orthodontics	CDE	continuing dental education
		CDLE	chronic discoid *lupus erythematosus
BSSPD	British Society for the Study of Prosthetic Dentistry	CDO	Chief Dental Officer; community dental officer
BST	basic specialist training		
BT	bleeding time	CDS	Community Dental Service
BTEC	Business and Technical Educational Council	CDT	clinical dental technicians
		CDTA	Clinical Dental Teachers Association
BUOLD	Bristol University Open Learning for Dentists	CEJ	*cemento-enamel junction
		Cf.	(Latin) *confer*, compare or bring together
b/w	*bitewing* *radiograph		
Bx	*biopsy	CHD	congenital heart defects
CABG	coronary artery bypass graft	CJD	*Creutzfeldt–Jakob disease
CAD	*coronary artery disease	CL/P	*cleft lip/palate
CAD/CAM	*computer aided design/computer aided manufacture	cm	centimetre
		CME	continuing medical education
CADO	chief administrative dental officer	CMI	cell mediated *immunity
CAL	*computer aided (computer assisted) learning	CMO	Chief Medical Officer
		CMOS	complementary metal oxide semiconductor
Cal	large *calorie		
cal	small *calorie	CNS	*central nervous system
CAM	*complementary and alternative medicine	c/o	complaining of
		CO$_2$	*carbon dioxide
CAP	Central Audit Panel; chronic adult periodontitis	CODE	Confederation Of Dental Employers
		COPDEND	Conference of Postgraduate Dental Deans and Directors (UK)
CAPD	continuous ambulatory peritoneal dialysis	CoSHH	*Control of Substances Hazardous to Health
CAPRAP	Central Audit and Peer Review Advisory Panel		
		CP	*cerebral palsy
CAT	*computerized (axial) tomography	CPD	*continuing professional development
CATS	Credit Accumulation and Transfer Scheme		
		CPE	continuing professional education

CPR	*cardiopulmonary resuscitation	DPF	Dental Practitioner's Formulary
CRDG	Consultants in Restorative Dentistry Group	DPH	doctor of public health; doctor of public hygiene
CRHP	Council for the Regulation of Health Professionals	DPMA	*Dental Practice Managers Association
CSAG	Clinical Standards Advisory Group	DPT	*dental panoramic tomogram
CSF	*cerebrospinal fluid	DRD	Diploma in Restorative Dentistry
CSI	*calculus surface index	DRO	*dental reference officer
CSSD	central sterile supply department	DRS	*Dental Reference Service
CT	computed tomography	DRSG	Dental Rates Study Group
CV	*cardiovascular	DSA	dental surgery assistant
CVA	*cerebrovascular accident	DSASTAB	Dental Surgery Assistants Standards
CVS	*cardiovascular system		and Training Advisory Board (now
CVT	Committee on Vocational Training		*DNSTAB)
	for England and Wales	DSSA	Dental System Suppliers Association
DAC	*Dental Access Centre; *Dental	DSTG	Dental Sedation Teachers Group
	Auxiliaries Committee	DTA	Dental Technicians Association
DCI	Dental Council of Ireland	DTAI	Dental Technicians Association
DCP	*dental care professional		Ireland
DCS	*Dental Complaints Service (General	DTETAB	Dental Technicians Education and
	Dental Council)		Training Advisory Board
DCU	*dental chair unit	DUWL	*dental unit water lines
DDA	Dental Defence Agency; *Disability	DVT	deep vein *thrombosis
	Discrimination Act	DVTA	Dental Vocational Training Authority
DDH	Diploma in Dental Health		England and Wales
DDO	district dental officer	DwSIs	*dentists with special interests
DDOrth	Diploma in Dental Orthopaedics	Dx	*diagnosis
DDPH	Diploma in Dental Public Health	EADPH	European Association of Dental
DDS	doctor of dental surgery; *Defence		Public Health
	Dental Service	EBD	*evidence-based dentistry
DDSc	doctor of dental science	EBM	*evidence-based medicine
DEAC	Dental Education Advisory Council	EBV	*Epstein–Barr virus
DEF (def)	*decayed, extracted, filled (index)	ECF	extracellular fluid; extended care
DGDP(UK)	Diploma in General Dental Practice		facility
	(UK)	ECG	*electrocardiogram
DH or DoH	Department of Health (England);	ECT	electroconvulsive therapy
	*dental hygienist	EDH	enrolled dental hygienist
DHA	District Health Authority	EDS	European Dental Society
DLA	Dental Laboratories Association	EDTA	*ethylene diamine tetraacetic acid
DMD	doctor of dental medicine	EEC	European Economic Commission
DMF (dmf)	*decayed, missing, filled	EEG	electroencephalogram
DN	*dental nurse	EFP	European Federation of
DNA	did not attend		Periodontology
DNR	do not resuscitate	EMD	*enamel matrix derivative
DNSTAB	*Dental Nurses Standards and	EMLA	*eutectic mix of lignocaine and
	Training Advisory Board		prilocaine
DO	dental officer	ENAP	*excisional new attachment
DOB	date of birth		procedure
DoH or DH	Department of Health (England)	ENT	ear, nose, and throat
DOrth	Diploma in Orthodontics	EO	extra-oral
DOS	Dental and Optical Services	EOA	extra-oral *anchorage
	(National Health Service Executive)	EOS	European Orthodontic Society
DPA	dental practice adviser	EOT	extra-oral *traction
DPB	*Dental Practice Board	EPA	European Prosthodontic Association

ERASMUS	European Scheme for the Mobility of University Students
ERV	*expiratory reserve volume
ESI	*extent and severity index
ESR	*erythrocyte sedimentation rate
EUA	examination under anaesthesia
F	female
F/-	full (complete) upper denture (and -/F for lower)
FA	fixed appliance
FACD	Fellow of the American College of Dentists
FB	*foreign body
FBC	full *blood count
FDA	Food and Drug Administration (US)
FDI	*Fédération Dentaire Internationale (World Dental Federation)
FDS	fellowship in dental surgery; Faculty of Dental Surgery
Fe	*iron
FGDP(UK)	Faculty of General Dental Practice (UK), the Royal College of Surgeons of England
FHSA	Family Health Services Authority
FMPA	Frankfort mandibular plane angle
FOA	Federation of Orthodontic Associations
FOTI	fibre-optic transillumination
FPC	Family Practitioner Committee
FPD	fixed partial *denture
FS	Fluoridation Society
f/s	fissure sealant
ft	foot
fx	*fracture
g; Gm; gm	gram
GA	general *anaesthesia
GANA	gamma-amino-butyric acid
GDC	*General Dental Council
GDP	*general dental practitioner
GDPA	General Dental Practitioners Association
GDS	*General Dental Services
GERD	gastro-esophogeal reflux disease (US spelling)
GI	*gastrointestinal; *glycaemic index
GIC	glass ionomer *cement
GMC	*General Medical Council
GMP	*general medical practitioner
GORD	*gastro-oesophageal reflux disease
GP	*gutta-percha; general practitioner
GPT	general professional training
gt.	(Latin) *gutta,* a drop
GTN	*glyceryl trinitrate
GTR	*guided tissue regeneration
Gy	*gray (unit of absorbed dose of ionizing radiation)
H & E	haematoxylin and eosoin
h/o	history of
HA	Health Authority (disbanded March 2002)
Hb, Hbg	*haemoglobin
HBsAg	*hepatitis B surface antigen
HBV	*hepatitis B virus
HC	Health Committee (General Dental Council)
HDL	high-density *lipoprotein
HDS	Hospital Dental Services
HEFCE	Higher Education Funding Council for England
HEFCW	Higher Education Funding Council for Wales
Hep B/C	*hepatitis B/C
Hg	*mercury
HIV	*human immunodeficiency virus
HIW	Health Inspectorate Wales
HO	house officer
HPI	history of present illness
HRT	hormone replacement therapy
HSE	Health and Safety Executive
HSV	*herpes simplex virus
Hx, hx	history
IADC	International Association of Dentistry for Children
IADH	International Association of Dentistry for the Handicapped
IADR	International Association of Dental Research
IADS	International Association of Dental Students
IAG	International Academy of Gnathology
IAOMS	International Association of Oral and Maxillofacial Surgeons
IAOP	International Association of Oral Pathologists
IAOS	International Association of Oral Surgeons
IAPD	International Association of Paediatric Dentistry
IBS	irritable bowel syndrome
ICON	*index of complexity outcome and need
ICP	inter-cuspal position
ICRP	International Commission on Radiological Protection
ICU	intensive care unit
ID	inferior dental; infective dose
IDB	inferior dental block

IDEA	Index of Dental Educational Activity	MDAS	modified dental anxiety scale
IE	infective *endocarditis	MEDLARS	Medical Literature Analysis and Retrieval System
i.e.	(Latin) *id est*, that is		
Ig	*immunoglobulin	MEDLINE	*MEDLARS online
IM	*intramuscular	MG	*myasthenia gravis
IMF	*intermaxillary fixation	mg	milligram
IMPT	Institute of Maxillofacial Prosthetists and Technologists	MHz	megahertz
		MI	*myocardial infarction
INR	*international normalized ratio	MIH	molar incisor *hypomineralization
IO	intra-oral	MIMS	Monthly Index of Medical Specialties
IOM	*infant oral mutilation		
IOT	intra-oral *traction	min	minute
IOTN	*index of orthodontic treatment need	ml	millilitre
		mm	millimetre
IQE	*International Qualifying Examination (General Dental Council)	MMPA	maxillary mandibular planes angle
		MMR	measles–mumps–rubella (vaccine)
		MOA	medium opening activator
IRV	inspiratory reserve volume	MOrth	Membership in Orthodontics
IS	inhalation *sedation	MPD	*maximum permissible dose
ISO	*International Standards Organization	MPDS	*myofascial pain dysfunction syndrome
IU	international units	MPS	mandibular pain syndrome
IUL	intra-uterine life	MRD	Membership in Restorative Dentistry
IV	*intravenous		
JACADS	Joint Advisory Committee for Additional Dental Specialties	MRI	*magnetic resonance imaging
		MRSA	meticillin resistant *Staphylococcus aureus*
JCSTD	Joint Committee for Specialist Training in Dentistry		
		MS	*multiple sclerosis
k	constant	MTA	*mineral trioxide aggregate
Kg	kilogram	MVP	mitral valve prolapse
LA	local *anaesthesia	N/A	not applicable
LAPRAP	Local Audit and Peer Review Advisory Panel	NACPDE	National Advice Centre for Postgraduate Dental Education
LD	*lethal dose	NAD	no appreciable disease; nothing abnormal detected
LDC	*Local Dental Committee		
LDL	low-density *lipoprotein	NAEDH	National Alliance for Equity in Dental Health
LDS	Licentiate in Dental Surgery		
LE	*lupus erythematosus	NAI	*non-accidental injury
LFH	lower *face height	NCAS	*National Clinical Assessment Service
LSD	*lysergic acid diethylamide		
M	male; *molar	NCCPED	National Centre for the Continuing Professional Education of Dentists
m	metre		
mμ	millimicron	NDA	National Dental Association
MAA	mandibular advancement appliance	NDAC	National Dental Advisory Committee (Scotland)
MAC	minimum alveolar concentration		
MAD	mandibuloacral *dysplasia	NDACCPE	National Dental Advisory Centre for Continuing Professional Education
MADEL	Medical and Dental Education Levy		
MADEN	Medical and Dental Education Network	NDHEG	National Dental Health Education Group
MALT	mucosal associated lymphoid tissue	NDTA	National Dental Technicians' Association
MAOI	*monoamine oxidase inhibitor		
MCCD	Membership in Clinical Community Dentistry	NEBDN	*National Examining Board for Dental Nurses
MCV	mean corpuscular volume	NHS	*National Health Service

NHSTA	National Health Service Training Authority
NICE	*National Institute for Health and Clinical Excellence
NIH	*National Institutes of Health
NiTi	nickel titanium
NK	natural killer (cell)
NLM	National Library of Medicine
NLP	neuro-linguistic programming
nm	nanometre
NME	non-milk extrinsic (sugars)
NMET	Non-Medical Education and Training
NMR	nuclear magnetic resonance
NNT	number needed to treat
nocte	(Latin) at night
NPSA	*National Patient Safety Agency
NRPB	National Radiological Protection Board
NSAID	non-steroidal anti-inflammatory drugs
NTN	*National Training Number
NUG	necrotizing ulcerative *gingivitis
NVQ	*National Vocational Qualification
o.d.	once daily
o/b	*overbite
O/E	on examination
o/j	*overjet
O_2	*oxygen
OFD	orodigitalfacial dysostosis
OFG	orofacial granulomatosis
OH	oral hygiene
OHAG	Oral Health Advisory Group
OHE	*oral health education
OHI	oral hygiene instruction; *oral health index
OHP	*oral health promotion
ONJ	*osteonecrosis of the jaw
OPCS	Office of Population Census and Surveys
OPG/OPT	orthopantomograph
OR	*odds ratio
ORN	*osteoradionecrosis
OSCE	objective structured clinical examination
OSHA	Occupational Safety and Health Administration (*United States)
OSVE	objective structured video examination
OT	occupational therapy
OTA	Orthodontic Technicians Association
OTC	over the counter
OVD	*occlusal vertical dimension
oz	ounce

P/-	partial upper *denture (and -/P for lower denture)
PALS	paediatric advanced life support
PAMs	professions allied to medicine
PAR	*peer assessment rating
PBL	problem-based learning
PCC	Professional Conduct Committee (General Dental Council)
PCD	professional complementary to dentistry (now known as DCP: dental care professional)
PCO_2	partial pressure of carbon dioxide
PCP	*parachlorophenol
PCT	*Primary Care Trust (England)
PD	Parkinson's disease
PDA	patent ductus arteriosus
PDGF	platelet-derived growth factor
PDH	past dental history
PDI	*periodontal disease index
PDL	*periodontal ligament
PDP	personal development plan
PDS	Personal Dental Service
PDU	Preventive Dentistry Unit
PEG	percutaneous endoscopic gastrostomy
PET	*positron emission tomography
PFM	porcelain fused to metal
PGMDE	postgraduate medical and dental education
PH	past history
PhD	philosophiae doctor: doctor of philosophy
PI	*periodontal index
PIL	*practice information leaflet
PJC	porcelain jacket *crown
PLS	*Papillon Lefèvre syndrome
PM	post mortem; *premolar; *papillary marginal index
PMGI	*papillary marginal gingival index
PMH	past medical history
PMMA	*polymethylmethacrylate
PND	paroxysmal nocturnal *dyspnoea
po	(Latin) *per orum*, by mouth
PO_2	partial pressure of oxygen
ppm	parts per million
PR	per rectum
PRN, prn	(Latin) *pro re nata*, as required
PrPC	Professional Performance Committee (General Dental Council)
PRR	*preventive resin restoration
psi	pounds per square inch
PSP	photostimulable phosphor
PSR	*periodontal screening and recording

PTFE	*polytetrafluoroethylene
PTH	*parathyroid hormone
PWS	*Prader–Willi syndrome
q.i.d.	(Latin) *quater in die*, four times a day
q.o.d.	([Latin) *quaque altere die*, every other day (recommended should no longer be used by the Joint Commission on Accreditation of Healthcare Organizations because of potential confusion with q.i.d.)
QCA	Qualifications and Curriculum Authority
qds	(Latin) *quater die sumendus*, four times a day
R&D	research and development
R/T	related to
RA	*relative analgesia
rad	radiation absorbed dose
RAE	research assessment exercise
rbc	red blood cell; red blood cell count
RCCT	randomized controlled clinical trial
RCP	*retruded contact position
RCPS	Royal College of Physicians and Surgeons
RCSEd.	Royal College of Surgeons of Edinburgh
RCSEng.	Royal College of Surgeons of England
RCSI	Royal College of Surgeons of Ireland
RCT	*randomized controlled trial; *root canal therapy
RDH	registered *dental hygienist
REM	rapid eye movement
RIDDOR	*Reporting of Injuries, Diseases and Dangerous Occurrences Regulations
RME	*rapid maxillary expansion
RMGIC	resin modified glass ionomer *cement
RNI	*reference nutrient intake
RPA	*radiation protection adviser
RPD	removable partial *denture
RPS	*radiation protection supervisor
RR	*risk ratio; *respiratory rate
RSA	root surface area
RV	*residual volume
Rx	take; treatment
s/s	signs and symptoms
SA	*sinoatrial (node)
SAAD	Society for the Advancement of Anaesthesia in Dentistry
SAD	seasonal affective disorder
SaO$_2$	arterial oxygen saturation
SARME	surgically assisted *rapid maxillary expansion
SARS	severe acute respiratory syndrome
SBE	*subacute bacterial endocarditis

SBI	*sulcus bleeding index
SC	*subcutaneous
SCC	squamous cell *carcinoma
SD	*standard deviation
SDAC	Standing Dental Advisory Committee
SDAG	Scottish Dental Audit Group
SDB	sleep-disordered breathing
SDO	senior dental officer
SDR	Statement of Dental Remuneration
SDVTC	Scottish Dental Vocational Training Committee
SDVTECC	Scottish Dental Vocational Training Equivalence and Certification Committee
SF	sugar-free
SGDS	Society of General Dental Surgery
SGDSC	Scottish General Dental Services Committee
SGUMDER	Steering Group on Undergraduate Medical and Dental Education and Research
SHA	*Strategic Health Authority
SHO	senior house officer
SI	(French) *Système International d'Unitès*; International System of Units
SIFT(R)	Service Increment for Teaching (and Research)
sig.	(Latin) *signa*, affix a label, inscribe
SIGN	Scottish Intercollegiate Guidelines Network
SLE	systemic lupus erythematosus
SMO	standard midline occlusal
sol. (soln)	solution
SRRDG	Senior Registrars in Restorative Dentistry Group
SS	stainless steel
STAC	Specialist Training Advisory Committee (of the General Dental Council)
stat.	immediately (*statim*)
STD	sexually transmitted disease
STI	sexually transmitted infection
Sx	*symptoms
tab	tablet
TAD	temporary *anchorage device
TB	*tuberculosis
TBV	total blood volume
TC	tungsten carbide
TCA	tricyclic antidepressant
tds	three times daily
TENS	*transcutaneous electrical nerve stimulation
TIA	*transient ischaemic attack

t.i.d.	(Latin) *ter in die*, three times a day	VLDL	very low-density *lipoprotein
TMD	*temporomandibular joint disorders	VME	*vertical maxillary excess
TMJ	*temporomandibular joint	Vol	volume
TMPDS	*temporomandibular pain dysfunction syndrome	VRQ	*vocational related qualification
		VSD	ventriculo-septal defect
TTP	tender to percussion	VT	vocational training; vocational
TV	*tidal volume		trainee; ventricular *tachycardia
Tx	treatment	VTS	vocational training scheme
UCR	usual, customary, and reasonable	WBC; wbc	white blood cell; white blood count
UDA	*unit of dental activity	WCPMDE	Welsh Council for Postgraduate
UDMA	*urethane dimethacrylate		Medical and Dental Education
URA	upper removable *appliance	WGDSC	Welsh General Dental Services
USP	*United States Pharmacopeia		Committee
UTI	urinary tract infection	WHO	*World Health Organization
VC	*vital capacity	WID	Women in Dentistry
VDP	*vocational dental practitioner	wt	weight
VDT	*vocational dental technician	Xbite	*crossbite
VF	ventricular fibrillation	YAG	yttrium-aluminium-garnet (*laser)
VHDL	very high-density *lipoprotein	ZOE	*zinc oxide eugenol

Appendix B: Foramina and canals of the bones of the skull

Name	Bone	Contents
Alveolar foramina	Maxilla	Posterior superior alveolar vessels and nerves
Anterior ethmoidal foramen	Ethmoid	Anterior ethmoidal nerve and artery
Anterior nasal aperture	Margins are maxilla and nasal bones	Anterior opening to the nasal cavity in the skull
Carotid canal	Temporal	Internal carotid artery carotid plexus of nerves
Choanae	Margins are sphenoid, palatine, and vomer	Posterior opening of the nasal cavity to nasopharynx
Condylar canal	Occipital	Emissary veins
Cribriform foramina	Ethmoid	Cranial nerve I
External acoustic meatus (external auditory meatus)	Temporal	Closed by tympanic membrane
Facial canal	Temporal	Cranial nerve VII
Foramen caecum	Frontal	Emissary vein
Foramen lacerum	Between sphenoid and occipital	Deep petrosal nerve
Foramen magnum	Occipital	Vertebra arteries, spinal cord – brainstem, spinal roots of cranial nerve XI
Foramen ovale	Sphenoid	Mandibular nerve (V3) and accessory meningeal nerve
Foramen petrosum	Sphenoid	Lesser petrosal nerve
Foramen rotundum	Sphenoid	Maxillary nerve (V2)
Foramen spinosum	Sphenoid	Middle meningeal artery meningeal branch of V3
Greater palatine foramen	Between maxillary and palatine	Greater palatine nerve and artery
Hiatus for the greater petrosal nerve	Temporal	Greater petrosal nerve
Hiatus for the lesser petrosal nerve	Temporal	Lesser petrosal nerve
Hypoglossal canal	Occipital	Hypoglossal nerve
Incisive canal	Maxilla	*See* Incisive foramina
Incisive foramina	Maxilla	Nasopalatine nerve sphenopalatine artery
Inferior orbital fissure	Between sphenoid and maxilla	Maxillary division of trigeminal and infraorbital artery and inferior ophthalmic vein
Infraorbital foramen	Maxilla	Infraorbital nerve branch of V2 and vessels

Name	Bone	Contents
Internal acoustic meatus	Temporal	Cranial nerve VII & VIII and labrynthine artery (internal auditory artery)
Jugular foramen	Between temporal and occipital	Internal jugular vein, cranial nerve IX, X, XI, posterior meningeal artery
Lesser palatine foramina	Palatine	Lesser palatine nerve and artery
Mandibular canal	Mandible	*See* Mandibular foramen
Mandibular foramen	Mandible	Inferior alveolar (inferior dental) nerve and vessels
Mastoid foramen	Temporal	Auricular branch of cranial nerve X, branches of occipital artery
Mental foramen	Mandible	Mental nerve and vessels
Nasal foramina	Nasal	emissary vessels
Nasolacrimal canal	Formed by maxillary and lacrimal	Drains into nasal cavity (inferior meatus)
Optic canal	Sphenoid	Ophthalmic artery and cranial nerve II
Palatovaginal canal	Between sphenoid and palatine	Pharyngeal branch of maxillary artery and pharyngeal nerve
Parietal foramen	Parietal	Emissary veins
Petrotympanic fissure	Temporal	Chorda tympani nerve
Piriform aperture *See* Anterior nasal aperture		
Posterior ethmoidal foramen	Ethmoid	Posterior ethmoidal nerve and artery
Pterygoid canal	Sphenoid	Vidian nerve or nerve of the pterygoid canal
Pterygopalatine canal	Between maxilla and perpendicular plate of palatine	Greater palatine nerve and vessels
Sphenopalatine foramen	Between sphenoid and palatine	Nasopalatine nerve sphenopalatine artery
Stylomastoid foramen	Temporal	Cranial nerve VII and stylomastoid artery
Superior orbital fissure	Between greater and lesser wings of the sphenoid	Ophthalmic division of V1, cranial nerve III, IV, VI, ophthalmic vein
Supraorbital notch (foramen)	Frontal	Supraorbital nerve and vessels
Tympanomastoid fissure	Temporal	Auricular branch of cranial nerve X
Zygomaticofacial foramen	Zygomatic	Zygomaticofacial nerve and vessels
Zygomatico-orbital foramen	Zygomatic	Zygomatico-orbital nerve Zygomaticotemporal nerve
Zygomaticotemporal foramen	Zygomatic	Zygomaticotemporal nerve

Appendix C: Arteries of the head and neck

Name	Origin	Distribution / Branches
Alveolar, anterior superior (anterior superior dental)	Infraorbital via maxillary	Maxillary canines and incisors.
Alveolar, inferior (inferior dental)	Maxillary	Mandibular teeth, buccal mucous membrane, floor of mouth.
Alveolar, posterior superior (posterior superior dental)	Maxillary	Mucous membrane of antrum, maxillary molars and premolars.
Angular	Facial	Lacrimal sac, lower eyelid, nose.
Anterior inferior cerebellar	basilar	Superior cerebellum.
Ascending pharyngeal	External carotid	Posterior meningeal, pharyngeal, inferior tympanic aa.
Auricular, posterior	External carotid	Stylomastoid, posterior tympanic, auricular, occipital and parotid branches.
Basilar	Vertebral	Anterior inferior cerebellar, pontine, mesencephalic, superior cerebellar and posterior cerebral a.
Buccal	Maxillary	Buccinator muscle, buccal mucous membrane, skin of cheek.
Carotid, common	Aortic arch (left) and brachiocephalic trunk (right)	Internal and external carotid arteries. Features include carotid sinus, and carotid body.
Carotid, external	Common carotid	Ascending pharyngeal, superior thyroid, lingual, facial, occipital, posterior auricular, maxillary, and superficial temporal branches.
Carotid, internal	Common carotid	Ophthalmic, anterior cerebral, middle cerebral, anterior choroidal, and posterior communicating branches. It has no external branches.
Cerebral, anterior	Internal carotid	Central and cortical branches, motor and somatosensory area for lower limb.
Cerebral, middle	Internal carotid	Lateral cortex including most of the motor and somatosensory areas.
Cerebral, posterior	Vertebral	Posterior cortical branches.
Choroidal, anterior	Internal carotid	Interior of brain, including choroid plexus of lateral ventricle and adjacent parts.
Communicating, anterior	Internal carotid	Suprachiasmatic, median commissural, anteromedial central aa.
Communicating, posterior	Internal carotid	Posteromedial central, chiasmatic, premammillary, hypothalamic, mammillary, and branches to oculomotor n.

Name	*Origin*	*Distribution / Branches*
Deep lingual	Lingual	Lower surface and tip of tongue.
Dental branches	Inferior alveolar	
Dental, inferior *see* Alveolar, inferior		
Dental, posterior superior *see* Alveolar, posterior superior		
Dorsal lingual	Lingual	Mucous membrane of the posterior third of the tongue, the glossopalatine arch, the tonsil, soft palate, and epiglottis.
Facial	External carotid	Ascending palatine, tonsillar, submental, glandular, inferior labial, superior labial, lateral nasal, and angular branches.
Glandular	Facial	
Infraorbital	Maxillary	Maxilla, maxillary sinus, upper teeth, lower eyelid, cheek, nose.
Internal thoracic	Subclavian	Thymic, mediastinal, tracheal, sternal, perforating, anterior intercostal, musculophrenic and superior epigastric.
Labial, inferior	Facial	Lower lip.
Labial, superior	Facial	Upper lip.
Lingual, deep	External carotid	Suprahyoid, sublingual, dorsal lingual, deep lingual.
Linguofacial trunk	External carotid	The facial and lingual may arise together as a trunk or separately.
Masseteric	Maxillary	Masseter muscle.
Maxillary	External carotid	Deep auricular, anterior tympanic, superior tympanic, inferior alveolar, middle meningeal, masseteric, deep temporal, pterygomeningeal, buccal, posterior superior alveolar, infraorbital, artery of pterygoid canal, descending palatine, sphenopalatine.
Maxillary, external *see* Facial		
Meningeal, middle	Maxillary	Named branches over meninges and superior tympanic.
Mental	Inferior alveolar	Chin.
Nasal, lateral	Facial	Ala and dorsum of nose.
Nasopalatine *see* Sphenopalatine		
Occipital	External carotid	Mastoid, auricular, sternocleidomastoid, occipital, meningeal and descending.
Ophthalmic	Internal carotid	Eye, orbit, adjacent facial structures.
Palatine, ascending	Facial	Soft palate, wall of pharynx, tonsil, auditory tube.
Palatine, descending	Maxillary	Greater and lesser palatine a.

Name	Origin	Distribution / Branches
Palatine, greater	Descending palatine	Hard palate.
Palatine, lesser	Descending palatine	Soft palate, tonsil.
Posterior inferior cerebellar	Vertebral	Inferior cerebellum and medulla.
Pterygoid, lateral	Posterior deep temporal	Pterygoid muscles.
Pterygoid, medial	Posterior deep temporal	Pterygoid muscles.
Sphenopalatine	Maxillary	Structures adjoining nasal cavity, nasopharynx.
Spinal, anterior	Vertebral	Ventral spinal cord.
Spinal, posterior	Posterior inferior cerebellar or vertebral	Dorsal spinal cord.
Subclavian	Aortic arch (left) and brachiocephalic trunk (right)	Vertebral, basilar, internal thoracic, thyrocervical trunk, costocervical trunk.
Sublingual	Lingual	Sublingual gland.
Submental	Facial	Tissues under chin.
Superior cerebellar	Basilar	Superior cerebellum.
Suprahyoid	Lingual	Muscles attached to the hyoid bone.
Supraorbital	Ophthalmic	Forehead, upper muscles of orbit, upper eyelid, frontal sinus.
Supratrochlear	Ophthalmic	Forehead medial to supraorbital.
Temporal, anterior deep	Maxillary	Zygomatic bone, greater wing of sphenoid, temporal muscles.
Temporal, posterior deep	Maxillary	Temporal muscles, pterygoid muscles.
Temporal, superficial	External carotid	Parotid, transverse facial, anterior auricular, zygomatico-orbital, middle temporal, frontal, and parietal branches.
Thyrocervical trunk	Subclavian	Inferior thyroid, ascending cervical, suprascapular, and transverse cervical.
Thyroid ima	Brachiocephalic trunk	Thyroid gland (occasionally present).
Thyroid, inferior	Trifurcation of the thyrocervical trunk, first part of the subclavian a	Inferior laryngeal, glandular, pharyngeal, oesophageal, and tracheal branches.
Thyroid, superior	External carotid	Infrahyoid, sternocleidomastoid, superior laryngeal, cricothyroid, anterior, posterior and lateral glandular.
Tonsillar	Facial	Base of tongue, fauces, and tonsil.
Vertebral	Subclavian	Prevertebral, cervical, atlantic and intercranial parts.
Willis, cerebral arterial circle of	Internal carotid	Anterior cerebral, anterior communicating, middle cerebral, posterior communicating.
	Basilar	Posterior cerebral.

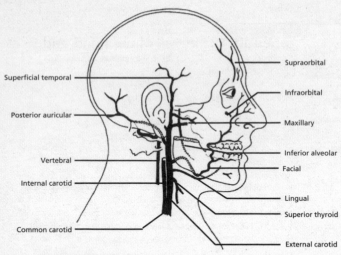

Main arteries of the head and neck.

Appendix D: Nerves of the head and neck

Cranial Nerves Summary Table

Number	Name	Principal Function
I	Olfactory	Smell
II	Optic	Vision
III	Oculomotor	Eye movement of extrinsic muscles of the eye superior rectus, medial rectus, inferior rectus and levator palpebra superioris, parasympathetic innervation
IV	Trochlear	Eye movement superior oblique muscle
V	Trigeminal	Facial sensation and mastication
VI	Abducent (abducens)	Eye movement
VII	Facial	Facial expression, taste (anterior ⅔ tongue), parasympathetic innervations salivation (incl. submandibular and sublingual), and lacrimation
VIII	Vestibulocochlear	Balance, and hearing
IX	Glossopharyngeal	Taste (posterior ⅓ tongue), parasympathetic salivation (parotid gland), and sensory innervation of the pharynx, stylopharyngeus m.
X	Vagus	Swallowing, speech, respiration, and taste, parasympathetic innervation
XI	Accessory – cranial	Pharyngeal and laryngeal muscles
	Accessory – spinal	Head and shoulder movement
XII	Hypoglossal	Tongue movement

Nerves of the head and neck

Nerve	Origin	Sensory supply	Motor supply
Abducent (Cranial n.VI) or abducens	Brain stem at the junction of the pons and medulla		Lateral rectus muscle of the eyeball
Accessory (Cranial n. XI)	Cranial part: Medulla Spinal part: upper cervical spinal cord C1-C4/5		Cranial part: contributes to recurrent laryngeal n. Spinal part: Sternocleidomastoid and trapezius muscles
Alveolar (dental) – anterior superior	*Infraorbital n.	Mucosa of nasal floor, maxillary incisors and canines and their associated structures	
Alveolar (dental) – inferior	*Mandibular n.	Teeth and gingivae of mandible	
Alveolar (dental) – middle superior	*Infraorbital n.	Maxillary premolars and associated structures	

Nerve	Origin	Sensory supply	Motor supply
Alveolar (dental) posterior superior	*Maxillary n.	Maxillary molars, gingivae and buccal mucosa; mucosa of maxillary sinus	
Ansa cervicalis	Cervical plexus (C1-C4)		Omohyoid, sternohyoid, sternothyroid, thyrohyoid and geniohyoid muscles
Auricularis – anterior	Auriculotemporal n.	Skin of auricle and external auditory meatus	
Auricularis – great	Cervical plexus (C2-C3)	External ear and region below the ear	
Auricularis – posterior	*Facial n.		Occipital part of occipitofrontalis muscle and intrinsic muscles of the auricle
Auriculotemporal	*Mandibular n.	Skin over angle of mandible and adjacent part of auricle	Secretomotor to the parotid gland via lesser petrosal n. and otic ganglion
Brachial plexus	C5-T1	Upper limb	Upper limb
Buccal	*Facial n.		zygomaticus major & minor, buccinator, orbicularis oris, and muscles of facial expression
Buccal (long)	*Trigeminal n.	Skin and mucosa of cheek	
Caroticotympanic	Tympanic plexus of glossopharyngeal n.	Tympanic region	
Carotid – external	Superior cervical ganglion		Glands and smooth muscle of head via external carotid plexus
Carotid – internal	Superior cervical ganglion		vascular smooth muscle of the brain, orbit, forehead, upper nasal cavity, sweat glands of the forehead and dilator pupillae muscles
Cervical ganglion	Sympathetic trunk Superior cervical Middle cervical Inferior cervical/ Stellate		Sympathetic innervations to the head arises from the superior cervical ganglion.

Nerve	Origin	Sensory supply	Motor supply
Cervical plexus	Ventral rami of C1-C4	Lesser occipital n. Great auricular n. Transverse cervical n. Supraclavicular n.	Form ansa cervicalis (*see* Ansa cervicalis). Part of the phrenic n. to the diaphragm. Spinal part of the accessory to vagus n. Muscular branches to deep muscles of the neck
Chorda tympani	Nervus intermedius		Taste buds on anterior two-thirds of tongue via lingual n. Submandibular and sublingual glands via lingual n. and submandibular ganglion
Cranial	Brainstem and upper cervical spinal cord. 12 pairs of nerves. *See* Cranial nerves summary table		
Dental – inferior *see* Alveolar			
Dental – superior (anterior, middle, posterior) *see* Alveolar			
Ethmoidal – anterior	Nasociliary	Mucosa of nasal cavity and anterior ethmoidal sinus, and skin of lower part of nose	
Ethmoidal - posterior	Nasociliary	Mucosa of posterior ethmoidal and sphenoidal sinuses	
Facial (Cranial n. VII)	Brain stem at lower border of pons	Surface of external auditory meatus and ear drum; taste buds on the palate and anterior two-thirds of the tongue	Muscles of facial expression, posterior belly of digastric, stapedius and stylohyoid muscles Parsympathetic innervation to lacrimal and submandibular and sublingual salivary glands
Frontal	*Ophthalmic n.	Skin of scalp, forehead, and upper eyelids, mucous membrane of frontal sinus	

Nerve	Origin	Sensory supply	Motor supply
Ganglion – ciliary	Inferior division of occulomotor n.		Parasympathetic ganglion to ciliary muscles of the eye and constrictor muscle of iris
Ganglion – geniculate	*Facial n.	Cell bodies of general somatic afferent n. from external auditory meatus and skin of ear	
Ganglion – otic	Lesser petrosal n. formed from tympanic n. plexus of glossopharyngeal n.		Parasympathetic secretomotor to the parotid gland distributed via auriculotemporal n
Ganglion – pterygopalatine	Greater petrosal n. (parasympathetic) and deep petrosal n. (sympathetic) join to form vidian n. (nerve of the pterygoid canal)		Parasympathetic fibres are secretomotor to mucous glands of the palate, nasal cavity, lacrimal gland
Ganglion- trigeminal (semilunar/ Gasserian)	Lies in a depression in the middle cranial fossa	Cell bodies for general somatic afferent fibres (except proprioception) of trigeminal nerve	
Ganglion – submandibular	Chorda tympani facial nervus intermedius		Secretomotor to the submandibular and sublingual glands and the small glands of the lingual mucosa
Glossopharyngeal (Cranial n. IX)	Medulla oblongata	Mucosa of posterior third of tongue and special visceral afferent (SVA) fibres of taste buds of circumvallate papillae	Stylopharyngeal muscle and parasympathetic secretomotor to parotid gland
Great auricular	*Cervical plexus (C2-C3)	Lateral aspect of the head, posterior aspect of the ear, part of the parotid region	
Hypoglossal (Cranial n. XII)	Medulla oblongata		All intrinsic and extrinsic muscles of tongue except the palatoglossus muscle
Incisive	*inferior alveolar n.	Lower incisors and adjacent labial gingival	
Infraorbital	*Maxillary n.	Lower eyelid, skin and mucosa of maxillary sinus, nose, and upper lip	

Nerve	Origin	Sensory supply	Motor supply
Infratrochlear	Nasociliary n.	Skin and conjunctiva of the medial upper and lower eyelids; skin of the lateral surface of the nose	
Labial – inferior	*Mental n.	Skin of lower lip	
Labial – superior	Infraorbital n.	Skin of cheek and upper lip	
Lacrimal	*Ophthalmic n.	Skin of the lateral portion of the upper eye lid and its associated conjunctiva	Secretomotor to the lacrimal gland
Laryngeal – inferior	Recurrent laryngeal n.	Mucous membrane of the larynx below the vocal fold	All intrinsic muscles of the larynx except the cricothyroid m. Secretomotor to the mucous membrane of the larynx below the vocal fold
Laryngeal – recurrent	Vagus n.	Upper oesophagus, lower pharynx, and larynx below the vocal folds	Upper oesophagus, lower pharynx, and laryngeal muscles smooth muscle of the trachea; secretomotor to mucosal glands in the upper oesophagus, lower pharynx, larynx below the vocal fold
Laryngeal – superior	Vagus n.	Mucous membrane of the larynx above the vocal folds	Cricothyroid m. and inferior pharyngeal constrictor muscles via external branch; secretomotor to mucosal glands of the larynx above the vocal folds via internal branch
Lesser occipital	*Cervical plexus (C2)	Lateral aspect of head, posterior aspect of ear	
Lingual	*Mandibular n. posterior division. Joined by chorda tympani in the infratemporal fossa	Mucosa of anterior two-thirds of tongue and floor of mouth, lingual aspect of lower gingiva	
Mandibular branch of facial n.	Facial n.		Depressor labii inferioris, mentalis muscles

Nerve	Origin	Sensory supply	Motor supply
Mandibular	Trigeminal n.	Mucosa of cheek, floor of mouth, anterior two-thirds of tongue, skin of lower part of face, and mandibular teeth	Mylohyoid m, anterior belly of digastric, tensor tympani, tensor veli palatini, masseter m, medial and lateral pterygoid muscles and temporalis m.
Masseteric	*Mandibular	Temporomandibular joint	Masseter m.
Maxillary	Trigeminal n.	Meninges, skin of upper part of face, mucosa of nose, maxillary sinus, cheeks and palate, and maxillary teeth	
Mental	*Mandibular	Skin of lower lip, chin, and gingiva	
Mylohyoid	*Alveolar – inferior		Mylohyoid and anterior belly of digastric muscles
Nasal – external	Nasociliary	Skin of nose	
Nasal – internal	Nasociliary	Nasal mucosa	
Nasal – lateral	Nasociliary	Nasal mucosa	
Nasal medial	Nasociliary	Mucosa of nasal septum	
Nasociliary	*Ophthalmic division of trigeminal n.	Eyeball, skin and mucosa of eyelid, ethmoidal and sphenoidal air sinuses	
Nasopalatine	Pteryopalatine ganglion	Mucosa of hard palate and parts of nasal cavity	
Nervus intermedius	Pons and medulla Associated with the facial nerve.	Taste from the anterior two-thirds of the tongue via chorda tympani	Secretomotor to the lacrimal gland and mucous glands of the lower nasal cavity; secretomotor to the mucosa of the maxillary sinus and palate secretomotor to submandibular and sublingual glands
Olfactory (Cranial n. I)	Olfactory bulb	Olfactory mucosa Smell	
Ophthalmic	*Trigeminal	Skin of anterior part of scalp and forehead, orbit and eyeball, meninges, and mucosa of nose, frontal, ethmoidal, and sphenoidal air sinuses	

Nerve	Origin	Sensory supply	Motor supply
Optic (Cranial n. II)	Optic tracts	Retina	
Palatine – anterior/ greater palatine	*Maxillary n. via Pterygopalatine ganglion	Mucosa of palate	
Palatine – posterior/ lesser palatine	*Maxillary n. via Pterygopalatine ganglion	Mucosa of palate, soft palate and uvula	
Palpebral	Infratrochlear n.	Upper eyelid	
Palpebral – inferior	Infraorbital n.	Lower eyelid	
Petrosal – deep	Internal carotid plexus via cervical sympathetic ganglion		Sympathetic innervations to glands, mucous membranes and smooth muscle
Pharyngeal plexus	Vagus n.		Pharyngeal muscles
	Glossopharyngeal n.	Pharyngeal mucosa	Stylopharyngeus m.
Phrenic	C3,C4,C5		diaphragm
Pterygoid, lateral	*Mandibular n.		Lateral pterygoid m.
Pterygoid, medial	*Mandibular n.		Medial pterygoid m., branches of this nerve pass to tensor tympani and tensor veli palatini
Sphenopalatine see Ganglion - pterygopalatine			
Sublingual	*Lingual n.	Area of sublingual gland	
Supraclavicular	*Cervical plexus (C3-C4)	Inferior aspect of the posterior triangle and divides into medial and lateral branches over the clavicle	
Supraorbital	*Frontal n.	Mucosa of frontal sinus, skin of forehead, and upper eyelid	
Supratrochlear	*Frontal n.	Skin of forehead, bridge of nose, and upper eyelid	
Temporalis	*Mandibular		Temporalis m.
Transverse cervical	Cervical plexus (C2-C3)	Skin on anterolateral neck up to the lower border of the mandible	
Trigeminal (Cranial n. V)	Brain stem at lower border of pons. Divides into *ophthalmic, *maxillary, and mandibular divisions (nerves)	Face, mouth, nasal cavity, sinuses, orbit, anterior scalp to vertex, and dura mater.	Muscles of mastication, mylohyoid, anterior belly of digastric, tensor veli palatini and tensor tympani.
Trochlear (Cranial n. IV)	Midbrain (only cranial nerve to exit on the posterior surface of the midbrain)		Superior oblique muscles of eyeball

Nerve	Origin	Sensory supply	Motor supply
Tympanic	Inferior ganglion of glosspharyngeal n.	Mucosa of middle ear and pharyngotympanic tube	
Vagus (Cranial n. X)	Medulla oblongata	Skin of external auditory meatus, meninges, laryngeal and pharyngeal mucosa	Striate muscles of larynx and pharynx, thoracic and abdominal viscera
Zygomatic	*Maxillary n.	Skin in temporal region and related to zygomatic bone	
Zygomaticofacial	*Zygomatic n.	Skin over zygomatic bone	
Zygomaticotemporal	*Zygomatic n.	Skin over anterior area of temporal region	

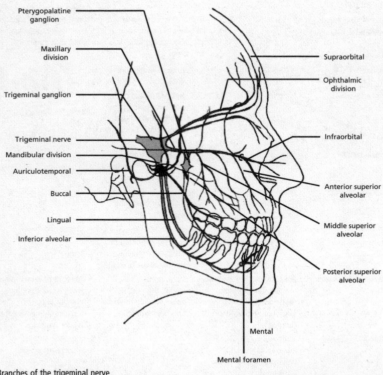

Branches of the trigeminal nerve

Functional groups of cranial and cervical spinal nerves

General afferent fibres		Sensory fibres from periphery via spinal and cranial nerves
General somatic afferent (GSA)	V, VII, X cutaneous branches of cervical plexus	Sensory fibres carrying pain temperature and touch and proprioception for sensory nerve endings
General visceral afferent (GVA)	IX, X	Sensory fibres carrying from visceral nerve endings, carotid sinus and body
Special somatic afferent (SSA)	II, VIII	Sensory fibres from special sense organs of vision, hearing and balance
Special visceral afferent (SVA)	I, VII, IX, X	Sensory fibres from smell and taste receptors
General efferent		Motor neurons arising from the brain stem, spinal cord and autonomic ganglia. Innervating all musculature except branchiomeric muscles
General somatic efferent (GSE)	III, IV, VI, XII, ansa cervicalis.	Motor fibres to muscles via ventral roots of the spinal cord or brainstem (extraocular muscles and tongue)
General Visceral efferent (GVE)	III, VII, IX, X	Autonomic fibres to smooth muscle, salivary and lacrimal glands
Special visceral efferent (SVE)	V, VII, IX, X, XI	Motor fibres to branchiomeric derived muscles e.g. muscles of mastication, muscles of facial expression, pharynx larynx, sternocleidomastoid and trapezius muscles

Appendix E: Veins of the head and neck

Name	Origin	Distribution
Angular	Formed by supraorbital and supratrochlear veins and continues on the side of root of nose and inferior margin of orbit to form the facial vein.	Empties into the facial vein at its union with the superior labial vein.
Anterior branch of retromandibular vein	Formed when the retromandibular vein splits.	Joins the common facial vein to drain into the internal jugular vein.
Anterior jugular	Formed in submandibular triangle from veins; it runs close to the midline in the anterior triangle.	Empties into the external jugular vein or subclavian vein.
Buccal		Empties into pterygoid plexus.
Common facial	Below angle of the mandible formed by the union of the facial vein and the anterior branch of the retromandibular vein.	Empties into the internal jugular vein at the level of the greater horn of the hyoid.
Deep temporal		Empties into pterygoid plexus.
Dental		Empties into pterygoid plexus.
External jugular	Formed by the union of the posterior retromandibular and occipital veins at the level of the angle of the mandible; it drains most of the face and scalp. Further on its course it receives tributaries in the neck.	Runs superficial to the sternocleidomastoid muscle and empties into the subclavian vein.
Facial	Formed by the union of the supraorbital and supratrochlear veins and runs obliquely following the facial artery ending at the angle of the mandible; its upper part is called the angular vein.	Joins the anterior retromandibular vein and empties into the common facial vein.
Greater palatine		Empties into pterygoid plexus.
Infraorbital	Lateral nose, lower eyelid and upper lip.	Enters the infraorbital foramen to empty into pterygoid plexus.
Internal jugular	Brain, superficial face and neck. It starts in the cranial cavity at the sigmoid sinus. Lying in the carotid sheath its tributaries include anterior retromandibular and common facial veins and many veins in the deep neck.	Joins with the subclavian vein to form the brachiocephalic vein in the upper thorax.
Masseteric		Empties to pterygoid plexus.

Name	Origin	Distribution
Maxillary	Found between the sphenomandibular ligament and the neck of the mandible; it receives deep veins from the pterygoid plexus. It is much shorter than the maxillary artery.	At the level of the neck of the mandible it joins the superficial temporal vein to empty into the retromandibular vein.
Nasal, external	Nasal arch; drains the dorsum of the nose.	Joins supratrochlear vein to form facial (angular) vein.
Occipital	Formed by venous plexus at posterior of scalp.	Empties by joining deep cervical and vertebral veins.
Posterior auricular	Formed from the plexus of veins on the scalp posterior to the ear.	Joins the posterior branch of the retromandibular vein to form the external jugular vein.
Posterior branch of retromandibular	Formed when the retromandibular vein splits.	Joins posterior auricular vein to drain into the external jugular vein.
Posterior external jugular	Formed in the occipital region from venous plexus.	Drains the upper and posterior neck.
Pterygoid		Empties into pterygoid plexus.
Pterygoid plexus	Forms the maxillary vein and also empties into the cavernous sinus and facial vein.	Empties regions of distribution of the maxillary artery. Found on the lateral surface of the medial pterygoid muscle.
Pterygoid plexus	Found between temporalis and lateral pterygoid muscles; it drains many structures of the infratemporal fossa and beyond.	Anastomoses with the cavernous sinus and the facial vein.
Retromandibular	Found in the parotid gland; it is formed by the union of the superficial temporal and maxillary veins.	Empties by dividing into anterior and posterior branches.
Superficial temporal	Formed from a venous plexus over the scalp in front of the ear; its tributaries drain the lateral part of the frontal and anterior parietal regions of the scalp.	Ends in the parotid gland by joining with the maxillary vein to form the retromandibular vein.
Supraorbital	Forehead from the plexus with the middle superficial temporal veins.	Empties the forehead uniting at the medial angle of the orbit with the supratrochlear vein to form the angular vein. It communicates with the superior ophthalmic vein via the supraorbital notch.
Supratrochlear	Forehead from plexus with superficial temporal veins; it follows the margin of the orbit.	Empties the forehead uniting at the medial angle of the orbit with the nasal branches and the supraorbital vein to form the angular vein.
Thyroid, (superior, middle and inferior)		Drains thyroid, larynx, and trachea.

Name	Origin	Distribution
Transverse facial		Passes posteriorly to meet the superficial temporal vein at the level of the parotid gland.
Vertebral	Follows the vertebral artery through the transverse foramen to C6.	Empties into the brachiocephalic vein.

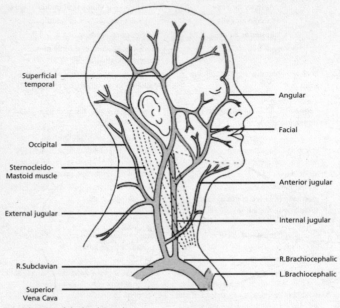

Superficial temporal

Angular

Facial

Occipital

Sternocleido-Mastoid muscle

Anterior jugular

External jugular

Internal jugular

R.Subclavian

R.Brachiocephalic

L.Brachiocephalic

Superior Vena Cava

Principle veins of the head & neck

Appendix F: Paranasal sinuses

Sinus or duct	*Subdivision of sinus*	*Enters the nasal cavity via:*
	Anterior air cells	Hiatus semilunaris of middle meatus
Ethmoidal	Middle air cells	Bulla ethmoidalis of middle meatus
	Posterior air cells	Superior meatus
Frontal		Infundibulum of middle meatus
Maxillary		Middle meatus
Nasolacrimal duct		Inferior meatus
Sphenoidal		Sphenoethmoid recess

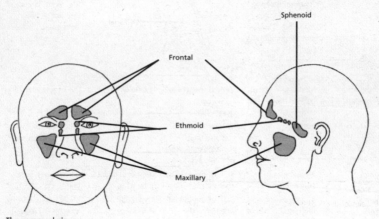

The paranasal sinuses

Appendix G: Muscles of the head and neck

Muscle	Origin	Insertion	Nerve supply	Function
Auricularis – anterior	Lateral part of galea aponeurotica.	Anterior part of helix of auricle.	Facial n.	Pulls auricle upwards and anteriorly.
Auricularis – posterior	Lateral part of mastoid process.	Cranial surface of the auricle.	Facial n.	Pulls auricle posteriorly.
Auricularis – superior	Lateral part of galea aponeurotica.	Cranial surface of the auricle.	Facial n.	Pulls the auricle upwards and backwards.
Buccinator	Posterior alveolar process of maxilla. Posterior alveolar process of mandible. The pterygomandibular raphe.	Fibres of the orbicularis oris.	Buccal branch of facial n.	Compresses the cheek(s) against the teeth and closes the lips. It is a secondary muscle of mastication.
Caninus see Levator anguli oris				
Chondroglossus (Ceratoglossus)	Medial side and base of lesser horn of hyoid.	Tongue between hyoglossus and genioglossus.	Hypoglossal n.	As hyoglossus.
Compressor naris	Maxilla	Passes upwards and medially towards the bridge of the nose.	Facial n.	Compresses vestibule of nasal cavity.
Corrugator supercilii	Medial part of superciliary arch.	Skin of medial eyebrow.	Temporal branch of facial n.	Draws eyebrows medially.
Corrugator supercilii	The superciliary arch on the frontal bone just above the nose.	Skin of the medial portion of the eyebrows above the middle of the orbital arch.	Zygomatic branch of facial n.	Pulls the eyebrows downward and medially producing vertical wrinkles on the forehead (frowning).
Depressor anguli oris	Oblique line of the mandible.	Skin at the angle of the mouth.	Facial n.	Pulls down the angle of the mouth. A muscle of facial expression associated with frowning.
Depressor labii inferioris	Oblique line of the mandible, between symphysis and mental foramen.	Skin of lower lip blending with the orbicularis oris.	Mandibular branch of facial n.	Pulls the lower lip downward and laterally. A muscle of facial expression.
Depressor septi nasi	Maxilla above the central incisor.	Nasal septum.	Facial n.	Widens the nasal aperture.

Muscle	Origin	Insertion	Nerve supply	Function
Digastric	Anterior belly: digastric fossa on the internal surface of the mandible. Posterior belly: mastoid process of temporal bone.	Lateral aspect of the body of hyoid bone by a pulley tendon.	Posterior belly: facial n. (CN VII). Anterior belly: mylohyoid n. (CN V).	When the hyoid is held in place (by the infrahyoid muscles), it will tend to depress the mandible (open the mouth).
Dilator naris	Maxilla	Cartilaginous alar of nose.	Facial nerve.	Widens the nasal apertures.
Epicranius	Muscle of the scalp made of frontal and occipital bellies joined by the membranous galea aponeurotica. See frontalis and occipitalis.			
Frontalis (frontal belly of occipitofrontalis)	Galea aponeurosis covering the upper part of the cranium, anterior to the coronal suture.	Skin above the eyes and nose.	Temporal branch of facial nerve.	Draws back the scalp to raise the eyebrows and wrinkle the brow.
Genioglossus	Inner surface of the mandible near the symphysis (superior part of mental spine).	Hyoid bone and underside of the tongue.	Hypoglossal n.	Raises the hyoid bone, depresses and protrudes the tongue.
Geniohyoid	Inner surface of the mandible from the inferior mental spine on the back of the symphysis menti.	Anterior surface of the body of the hyoid bone.	Branch from C1 (via the hypoglossal nerve).	Elevates the tongue, depresses the mandible and works in conjunction with the mylohyoid and digastric muscles.
Hyoglossus	The side of the body and the greater cornu of the hyoid bone.	Base and sides of the tongue.	Hypoglossal n.	Depresses the sides of the tongue. It is important in singing.
Inferior constrictor	Oblique line and inferior horn of thyroid cartilage to cricoid cartilage.	Posterior pharyngeal raphe.	Pharyngeal plexus.	Functions in swallowing.
Inferior oblique	Orbital surface of maxilla lateral to the lacrimal groove.	Lower lateral quadrant of the posterior half of the sclera of the eye.	Occulomotor n.	Elevates, laterally rotates, and abducts the eye.

Muscle	Origin	Insertion	Nerve supply	Function
Intrinsic muscles of the tongue	Within the tongue.	Within the tongue.	Hyoglossal n.	Superior longitudinal, inferior longitudinal, transverse and vertical muscles change the shape of the tongue.
Levator anguli oris	Anterior surface of maxilla below the infraorbital foramen.	Angle of the mouth.	Buccal branch of facial n.	Lifts the angle(s) of the mouth (as in smiling).
Levator labii superioris	Medial half of infraorbital margin.	Skin and muscles of upper lip.	Buccal branch of facial n.	Elevates and everts the upper lip.
Levator labii superioris alaeque nasi	Frontal process of maxilla.	Upper lip muscles and skin of nasal cartilage.	Buccal branch of facial n.	Elevates the upper lip and dilates the nostrils.
Levator palpebrae superioris	Inferior aspect of the lesser wing of sphenoid just above the optic foramen.	The skin of the upper eyelid and the superior tarsal plate.	Occulomotor n. and sympathetic innervation.	Elevates and retracts the upper eyelid.
Levator veli palatini	Apex of the petrous part of the temporal bone and the medial rim of the cartilage of the pharyngotympanic tube.	Aponeurosis of soft palate.	Pharyngeal branch of vagus n. with its motor fibres from the accessory n.	Raises, retracts and laterally deviates the soft palate. It may open the pharyngotympanic tube on swallowing.
Longus capitis	Anterior tubercles of third to sixth vertebrae.	Basilar part of the occipital bone.	Ventral rami of C1–C3.	Flexes the head.
Longus colli	Anterior surface of first cervical to third thoracic vertebrae.	Bodies and transverse process of cervical vertebrae.	Ventral rami C2–C6.	Flexes neck and rotates head to opposite side
Masseter	Superficial part: zygomatic process of the maxilla and the inferior border of the zygomatic arch. Intermediate part: inner surface of the zygomatic arch. Deep part: Posterior aspect of inferior border of zygomatic arch.	Superficial: angle of mandible and lateral surface of mandibular ramus. Intermediate: ramus of mandible. Deep: superior ramus of mandible and coronoid process of mandible.	Masseteric n. V3.	Elevates the mandible (clenching the teeth). It may deviate the mandible to the opposite side of contraction.

Muscle	Origin	Insertion	Nerve supply	Function
Mentalis	Incisive fossa on the anterior aspect of the mandible.	Skin of the chin.	Mandibular branch of the facial n.	Protrudes lower lip and elevates and wrinkles the skin of the chin.
Middle constrictor	Lesser horn of the hyoid, stylohyoid ligament, greater horn of hyoid.	Posterior pharyngeal raphe.	Pharyngeal plexus.	Functions in swallowing.
Musculus uvulae	Posterior nasal spine of palatine bones, palatine aponeurosis.	Mucous membrane.	Vagus nerve (pharyngeal plexus).	Contracts and elevates uvula.
Mylohyoid	The inner surface of mandible along the mylohyoid line.	Anterior three quarters: midline raphe. Posterior quarter: upper border of body of hyoid bone.	Mylohyoid n. V3.	Elevates hyoid bone, supports and raises the floor of the mouth. It aids in mastication and swallowing.
Nasalis	Alar (dilator naris) and transverse (compressor naris) parts. *See* dilator naris and compressor naris.			
Oblique capitis inferior	Spine and lamina of axis.	Transverse process of atlas.	Suboccipital nerve (C1).	Rotates head to same side on the axis.
Oblique capitis superior	Transverse process of atlas.	Between superior and inferior nuchal lines.	Suboccipital nerve (C1).	Extends and rotates head on the axis.
Occipitofrontalis *see* Epicranius				
Occipitalis: Occipital belly of occipitofrontalis	Lateral two thirds of superior nuchal line of the occipital bone and from the mastoid part of the temporal bone.	Galea aponeurosis, over the occipital bone.	Posterior auricular branch of facial n.	Draws back the scalp to raise the eyebrows and wrinkle the brow.
Omohyoid	Superior scapular border medial to the suprascapular notch and the suprascapular ligament.	Inferior border of hyoid bone (via a fascial sling attached to the medial end of the clavicle).	The upper part from the superior root of the ansa cervicalis and the lower part from the inferior root of the ansa cervicalis.	Depresses, retracts, and stabilizes the hyoid bone and larynx.

Muscle	Origin	Insertion	Nerve supply	Function
Orbicularis oculi	Oval sheet of muscle. Lacrimal portion: lacrimal crest of lacrimal bone. Orbital portion: medial orbital margin between supraorbital notch and infraorbital foramen. Palpebral portion: medial palpebral ligament.	Circumferentially around orbit meeting at the lateral palpebral raphe.	Temporal and zygomatic branches of facial n.	Sphincter of the eyelids. Closes the eyelids and aids the passage and drainage of tears dilating the lacrimal sac and spreads lacrimal secretions.
Orbicularis oris	Near the midline on the anterior surface of the maxilla and mandible and modiolus at the angle of the mouth. Receives deep fibres from buccinator m. It has a marginal and labial part.	Circumferentially around mouth. It merges with other muscles.	Buccal branches of facial n.	Sphincter of the mouth. Closes and protrudes the lips. It narrows the orifice of the mouth.
Palatoglossus	Soft palate and pharyngotympanic tube.	Posterolateral part of the tongue.	Pharyngeal branch of vagus n. with its motor fibres from the accessory n.	Raises tongue, constricts the anterior fauces and aids the initiation of swallowing.
Palatopharyngeus	Soft palate and pharyngotympanic tube.	Aponeurosis of pharynx and the posterior border of the thyroid cartilage.	Accessory n. via pharyngeal plexus.	Depresses the soft palate, narrows the fauces, elevates the pharynx and larynx and aids the process of swallowing.
Platysma	Subcutaneous skin over the neck and the upper lateral part of the chest.	Inferior border of mandible and the skin over the lower face and the angle of the mouth.	Cervical branch of facial n.	Depresses mandible and lower lip and tenses and wrinkles the skin over the neck.
Procerus	Lower part of nasal bone and lateral nasal cartilages.	Skin of lower forehead between eyebrows and mixes with frontalis.	Superior buccal branch of facial n.	Draws down medial angle of eyebrows.

Muscle	Origin	Insertion	Nerve supply	Function
Pterygoid – lateral	Superior (upper) head: lateral surface of the greater wing of the sphenoid bone. Inferior (lower) head: lateral surface of the lateral pterygoid plate.	Neck of the mandibular condyle and the articular disk of the TMJ.	Lateral pterygoid n. V3.	Moves the mandible to the opposite side of contraction during chewing. The inferior head opens the mouth by protruding the mandible. The superior head closes the mouth by elevating the mandible.
Pterygoid – medial	Deep head: the medial side of the lateral pterygoid plate and the fossa between the medial and lateral plates. Superficial head: tuberosity of maxilla and the pyramidal process of the palatine bone.	Inner surface of mandibular ramus and the angle of the mandible.	Medial pterygoid n. V3.	Elevates the mandible (clenches the teeth) and can protrude move the mandible from side to side in combination with the lateral pterygoid muscle.
Rectus – inferior	Common annular tendon from the body and lesser wing of the sphenoid bone and the margins of the optic canal.	Posterior to the sclerocorneal junction (each muscle inserting along its own directional axis).	Inferior division of occulomotor n.	Depresses, laterally rotates and adducts the eye.
Rectus – lateral	Common annular tendon which comes of the body and lesser wing of the sphenoid bone and the margins of the optic canal.	Medial sclera anterior to the equator of the eyeball (each muscle inserting along its own directional axis).	Abducens n.	Abducts the eye.
Rectus – medial	Common annular tendon (tendinous ring) from the body and lesser wing of the sphenoid bone and the margins of the optic canal.	Medial sclera anterior to the equator of the eyeball (each muscle inserting along its own directional axis).	Inferior division of the occulomotor n.	Adducts the eye.
Rectus – superior	Common annular tendon (tendinous ring) from the body and lesser wing of	Superior sclera anterior to the equator of the eyeball (each	Superior division of occulomotor n.	Elevates, medially rotates and adducts the eye.

Muscle	Origin	Insertion	Nerve supply	Function
	the sphenoid bone and the margins of the optic canal.	muscle inserting along its own directional axis).		
Rectus capitis anterior	Lateral mass and root of transverse process of atlas.	Basilar process of occipital bone anterior to foramen magnum.	Ventral rami of C1 and C2.	Flexes head.
Rectus capitis lateralis	Transverse process of atlas.	Jugular process of occipital bone.	Ventral rami of C1 and C2.	Flexes head to side.
Rectus capitis posterior major	Spinous process of axis.	Inferior nuchal line.	Suboccipital nerve (C1).	Extends and rotates head to same side.
Rectus capitis posterior minor	Posterior arch of the atlas.	Inferior nuchal line.	Suboccipital nerve (C1).	Extends head.
Risorius	Deep fascia of the face and parotid gland.	Skin and modiolus at the angle of the mouth.	Buccal branch of facial n.	Retracts the mouth laterally (as in smiling).
Salpingopharyngeus	Inferior surface of auditory tube.	Blends with palatopharyngeus.	Pharyngeal plexus.	Elevator of the pharynx.
Scalene (scalenus)	Anterior scalene: anterior tubercle of transverse processes third to sixth cervical vertebrae. Middle scalene: posterior tubercle of transverse processes second to seventh cervical vertebrae. Posterior scalene: posterior tubercle of transverse processes fourth to sixth cervical vertebrae.	Anterior scalene: scalene tubercle of first rib. Middle scalene: upper surface of first rib. Posterior scalene: second rib.	Anterior scalene: Ventral rami C4–C6. Middle scalene: Ventral rami C3–C8. Posterior scalene: Ventral rami C5–C8.	Flexion, lateral rotation and functions as accessory respiratory muscles.
Stapedius	Pyramidal eminence.	Posterior surface of neck of stapes.	Facial nerve.	Protective dampening of sound vibrations.
Sternocleidomastoid	Anterior and superior part of the manubrium of sternum and medial third of the clavicle.	Lateral aspect of mastoid process of temporal bone and anterior half of superior nuchal spine.	Motor supply is from the spinal accessory n. and sensory supply is from the ventral rami of C2.	Rotates the head to the side opposite to the muscle contracting. It laterally flexes to the contracted side. Bilaterally it flexes the neck and protracts the head.

Muscle	Origin	Insertion	Nerve supply	Function
Sternohyoid	Posterior aspect of the manubrium and the sternal end of the clavicle.	Inferior border of the body of the hyoid bone.	The upper part from the superior root of the ansa cervicalis and the lower part from the inferior root of the ansa cervicalis.	Depresses hyoid bone and larynx.
Sternothyroid	Posterior aspect of manubrium.	Oblique line of thyroid cartilage.	The upper part from the superior root of the ansa cervicalis and the lower part from the inferior root of the ansa cervicalis.	Depresses hyoid bone and larynx.
Styloglossus	Anterior surface and apex of the styloid process of the temporal bone and the upper quarter of the stylohyoid.	Sides of the tongue.	Hypoglossal n.	Raises and retracts the tongue. It aids the initiation of swallowing.
Stylohyoid	Base of styloid process of the temporal bone.	Lateral margin of hyoid bone.	Mandibular branch of the facial n.	Raises and retracts the hyoid bone. It aids swallowing and elevates the larynx.
Stylopharyngeus	Medial side of the styloid process.	Passing between the superior and middle constrictor muscles it blends with the muscles of pharynx.	Glossopharyngeal n.	Elevator of the pharynx.
Superior constrictor	Pterygoid hamulus, pterygomandibular raphe and end of the mylohyoid line, tongue.	Posterior pharyngeal raphe and pharyngeal tubercle.	Pharyngeal plexus.	Functions in swallowing.
Superior oblique	Body of sphenoid.	Upper lateral quadrant of the posterior half of the sclera (via the trochlea, as a pulley).	Trochlear n.	Depresses, medially rotates, and adducts the eye.
Temporalis	Temporal fossa between the inferior temporal line and the infratemporal crest.	Medial surface, apex and anterior border of the coronoid process, and anterior border of the	Deep temporal branches of the anterior division of the mandibular n. division of the trigeminal.	Retracts the protruded mandible and elevates it (closes the mouth).

Muscle	Origin	Insertion	Nerve supply	Function
		ramus of the mandible.		
Temporoparietalis	Aponeurosis above the auricularis.	Galea aponeurotica.	Facial nerve.	Tenses the galea.
Tensor tympani	Greater wing of sphenoid and length of the auditory tube in its own canal.	Handle of the malleus.	Trigeminal nerve.	Protective dampening of sound vibrations.
Tensor veli palatini	Scaphoid fossa of sphenoid bone and cartilage of pharyngotympanic tube.	Aponeurosis of soft palate (via a pulley of the pterygoid hamulus).	Mandibular division of the trigeminal n.	Contracts and tenses the soft palate and opens the pharyngotympanic tube.
Thyrohyoid	Oblique line of thyroid cartilage.	Lower border of great horn of hyoid bone.	Cervical plexus via Hypoglossal n.	Depresses hyoid bone or raises larynx.
Zygomaticus major	Anterior surface of the zygomatic bone anterior to the zygomatic-temporal suture.	Modiolus at the angle of the mouth.	Buccal branch of facial n.	Lifts and draws back the angle(s) of the mouth (as in smiling).
Zygomaticus minor	Zygomatic bone, posterior to maxillary-zygomatic suture.	Skin and muscle of the upper lip.	Buccal branch of facial n.	Elevates and everts the upper lip.

Summary of muscles of the tongue
Genioglossus, hyoglossus, chondroglossus, styloglossus, superior and inferior longitudinal muscles, transverse muscle, vertical muscle, palatoglossus. For details see table.

Summary of muscles of the soft palate and fauces
Palatine aponeurosis, levator veli palatine, tensor veli palatini, musculus uvulae, palatoglossus, palatopharyngeus. For details see table.

Summary of extraocular muscles
Superior rectus, inferior rectus, medial rectus, lateral rectus, superior oblique, inferior oblique, levator palpebrae superioris, common tendinous ring. For details see table.